Health Promotion in the Workplace

3rd edition

*This book is dedicated to my
mother Ellen who has been an inspiring model
of balance and my father Kevin who has been
an excellent model of lifestyle enhancement*

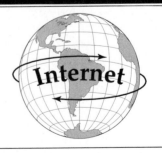

Health Promotion in the Workplace

THIRD EDITION

Michael P. O'Donnell, Ph.D., M.B.A., M.P.H.
Editor in Chief and President, American Journal of Health Promotion

and Associates

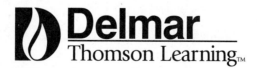

Delmar
Thomson Learning™

Africa • Australia • Canada • Denmark • Japan • Mexico • New Zealand • Philippines
Puerto Rico • Singapore • Spain • United Kingdom • United States

NOTICE TO THE READER

Delmar Staff:

Business Unit Director: William Brottmiller

Product Development Manager: Marion S. Waldman

Project Development Editor: Jill Rembetski

Editorial Assistant: Robin Irons

Executive Marketing Manager: Dawn F. Gerrain

Project Editor: Mary Ellen Cox

Production Coordinator: Nina Lontrato

Art/Design Coordinator: Timothy J. Conners

COPYRIGHT © 2002

Delmar, a division of Thomson Learning, Inc. Thomson Learning™ is a trademark used herein under license.

Printed in the United States of America
2 3 4 5 6 7 8 9 10 XXX 05 04 03 02

For more information, contact Delmar, 3 Columbia Circle, PO Box 15015, Albany, NY 12212-0515; or find us on the World Wide Web at http://www.delmar.com

Library of Congress Cataloging-in-Publication Data

Health promotion in the workplace / edited by Michael P. O'Donnell—3rd ed.
    p. cm.
  Includes bibliographical references and index.
  ISBN 0-7668-2866-2
  1. Employee health promotion. 2. Industrial hygiene. I. O'Donnell, Michael P.
(Michael Patterson), 1952–

RC969.H43 H454 2001
658.3'82--dc21

00-060290
CIP

INTERNATIONAL DIVISION LIST

ASIA (including India):
Thomson Learning
60 Albert Street, #15-01
Albert Complex
Singapore 189969
Tel 65 336-6411
Fax 65 336-7411

AUSTRALIA/NEW ZEALAND:
Nelson
102 Dodds Street
South Melbourne
Victoria 3205
Australia
Tel 61 (0)3 9685-4111
Fax 61 (0)3 9685-4199

LATIN AMERICA:
Thomson Learning
Seneca 53
Colonia Polanco
11560 Mexico, D. F. Mexico
Tel (525) 281-2906
Fax (525) 281-2656

CANADA:
Nelson
1120 Birchmount Road
Toronto, Ontario
Canada M1K 5G4
Tel (416) 752-9100
Fax (416) 752-8102

UK/EUROPE/MIDDLE EAST/AFRICA:
Thomson Learning
Berkshire House
168-173 High Holborn
London WC1V7AA
United Kingdom
Tel 44 (0)20 497-1422
Fax 44 (0)20 497-1426

Business Press:
Berkshire House
168-173 High Holborn
London WC1V7AA
United Kingdom
Tel 44 (0)20 497-1422
Fax 44 (0)20 497-1426

SPAIN (Includes Portugal):
Paraninfo
Calle Magallanes 25
28015 Madrid
España
Tel 34 (0)91 446-3350
Fax 34 (0)91 445-6218

DISTRIBUTION SERVICES:
ITPS Cheriton House
North Way
Andover,
Hampshire SP10 5BE
United Kingdom
Tel 44(0)1264 34-2960
Fax 44 (0)1264 34-2759

INTERNATIONAL HEADQUARTERS:
Thomson Learning
International Division
290 Harbor Drive, 2nd Floor
Stamford, CT 06902-7477
Tel (203) 969-8700
Fax (203) 969-8751

FOREIGN RIGHTS DEPARTMENT (Headquarters):
Thomson Learning
Berkshire House
168-173 High Holborn
London WC1V7AA
United Kingdom
Tel 44 (0)20 497-1422
Fax 44 (0)20 497-1426

FOREIGN RIGHTS-ASIA:
Thomson Learning
60 Albert Street, #15-01
Albert Complex
Singapore 189969
Tel 65 336-6411
Fax 65 334-1617

FOREIGN RIGHTS-SPAIN:
Paraninfo
Calle Magallanes 25
28015 Madrid
España
Tel 34 (0)91 446-3350
Fax 34 (0)91 445-6218

FOREIGN RIGHTS-LATIN AMERICA:
Thomson Learning
Seneca 53
Colonia Polanco
11560 Mexico, D. F. Mexico
Tel (525) 281-2906
Fax (525) 281-2656

CONTRIBUTORS

Jeffrey S. Harris, MD, MPH, MPA,
Chief Executive Officer,
Med-Fx,
Mill Valley, California

Jim Fries, MD,
Professor of Medicine,
Stanford University School of Medicine,
Palo Alto, California

Michael P. O'Donnell, PhD, MBA, MPH,
Editor-in Chief-and President,
American Journal of Health Promotion,
Keego Harbor, Michigan

John Harris,
President,
Harris Health Trends,
Toledo, Ohio

Tim McDonald, MHSA, PA,
Manager,
Corporate Health Promotion,
General Motors Health Care Initiative,
Detroit, Michigan

William B. Baun, EPD, FAWHP,
Manager,
Human Resource Programs & Wellness,
The University of Texas,
M.D. Anderson Cancer Center,
Houston, Texas

Ron Z. Goetzel, PhD,
Vice President and Director of Consulting Services,
The Medstat Group,
Washington, DC

Ronald J. Ozminkowski, PhD,
Senior Economist and Research Manager,
The Medstat Group,
Ann Arbor, Michigan

Larry S. Chapman, MPH,
Chairman,
Summex Corporation,
Seattle, Washington

Kenneth A. Wallston, PhD,
Professor of Psychology in Nursing,
Vanderbilt University School of Nursing,
Nashville, Tennessee

Colin Armstrong, PhD,
Director of Corporate Health Psychology Services,
The Kim Dayani Health Promotion Center,
Vanderbilt University Medical Center,
Nashville, Tennessee

Judd Robert Allen, PhD,
President,
Human Resources Institute, Inc.,
Burlington, Vermont

David Anderson, PhD,
Vice President of Programs and Services,
The StayWell Company,
St. Paul, Minnesota

Seth Serxner, PhD, MPH,
Vice President, Research,
StayWell,
San Bruno, California

Paul E. Terry, PhD,
Vice President of Education,
Park Nicollett, Institute for Research and Education,
St. Louis Park, Minnesota

Mark G. Wilson, HSD,
Associate Professor,
University of Georgia,
Department of Health Promotion and Behavior,
Athens, Georgia

C. Shannon Griffin-Blake, MA,
Doctoral Candidate,
University of Georgia,
Department of Health Promotion and Behavior,
Athens, Georgia

David DeJoy, PhD,
Professor,
University of Georgia,
Department of Health Promotion and Behavior,
Athens, Georgia

Karen Glanz, PhD, MPH,
Professor and Researcher,
University of Hawaii,
Honolulu, Hawaii

Alan R. Kristal, PhD
Associate Member,
Fred Hutchinson Cancer Research Center,
Seattle, Washington

Gordon D. Kaplan, PhD,
Chief Science Officer,
McLaughlin Young Institute for Corporate Health,
Denton, Texas

Valerie Brinkman-Kaplan, MS, RD,
Director Operations and Development,
McLaughlin Young Institute for Corporate Health,
Denton, Texas

Edward M. Framer, PhD,
Chief Operating Officer,
McLaughlin Young Institute for Corporate Health,
Denton, Texas

Nell H. Gottlieb, PhD,
Professor,
Department of Kinesiology and Health Education,
University of Texas at Austin,
Austin, Texas

Paul E. Terry, PhD,
Vice President of Education,
Park Nicollett, Institute for Research and Education,
St. Louis Park, Minnesota

Lawrence R. Murphy, PhD,
Research Psychologist,
National Institute for Occupational Safety and Health,
Cincinnati, Ohio

R. Paul Maiden, PhD,
Associate Professor of Social Work,
College of Health and Public Affairs,
University of Central Florida,
Orlando, Florida

Donald B. Levitt, PhD,
President,
The New World of Work Network,
Ann Arbor, Michigan

Kenneth R. McLeroy, PhD,
Associate Dean,
Texas A & M University,
School of Public Health,
College Station, Texas

Catherine A. Heaney, PhD,
Associate Professor,
School of Public Health,
Ohio State University

Daniel Stokols, PhD,
Professor and Dean,
University of California at Irvine,
School of Social Ecology,
Irvine, California

Shari G. McMahan, PhD,
Associate Professor,
Department of Kinesiology and Health Promotion,
California State University,
Fullerton, California

Kimari Phillips, MA,
Health Psychology Project Coordinator,
University of California,
Irvine, Health Promotion Center,
Irvine, California

David C. Gobble, PhD,
Associate Director and Professor,
Fisher Institute for Wellness and Geronotology,
Ball State University,
Muncie, Indiana

Wolf Kirsten, M. Sc,
K2 Consulting Corporation,
Washington, DC

Michelle Nunn,
Executive Director,
Hands On Atlanta, and City Cares of America,
Atlanta, Georgia

Don R. Powell, PhD,
President,
American Institute for Preventive Medicine,
Farmington Hills, Michigan

Elaine Frank, MEd, RD,
Vice President,
American Institute for Preventive Medicine,
Farmington Hills, Michigan

CONTENTS

PREFACE

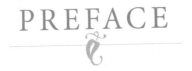

Evolution of Workplace Health Promotion

The first edition of this book was published in 1984. The art and science of health promotion was just emerging as an organized field of study and practice in the United States. Fewer than 10% of employers offered programs. Most program managers had training in exercise physiology and little training or experience in managing a program or working within a business setting. The concept of comprehensive health promotion had been articulated, but most programs were dominated by a fitness center with a focus on exercise and followed a superficial educational model for reaching employees. Very little formal documentation existed on programming methodology. In fact the first edition of this text was the first reference text for the field. Most of the academic programs offering bachelor's and master's degrees to support the field were in departments of physical fitness. The field was full of excitement and promise but very little science.

By 1994, when the second edition of this book was published, over 80% of employers with 50 or more employees had programs in place. The Association for Worksite Health Promotion (the dominant association in the field) reached its peak in membership and conference attendance, and a number of other health-related professional associations added special interest groups for workplace health promotion or health education. Major research universities offered degree programs in related areas, and hundreds of studies had been published on the health and financial impact of programs. A number of scientific and trade journals emerged to document the field. Over half of the hospitals, hundreds of entrepreneurs, and many insurance companies were selling a wide range of health promotion products and services. The business of health promotion had indeed established itself. Exercise was still a dominant element, but most programs addressed nutrition, weight control, stress management, smoking control, and medical self-care. Programs were often managed by nurses, health educators, psychologists, and nutritionists in addition to exercise physiologists. These new disciplines brought rich knowledge and perspective to the field but contributed to its fragmentation. Communication between the many academic disciplines and between the researchers and practitioners was limited. Most programs still had strong educational components, but most also recognized the importance of concentrating on changes in actual behavior instead of merely changing knowledge and attitudes; many programs made concerted efforts to create environments that encouraged healthy lifestyle practice.

The field has continued to evolve as we have entered the twenty-first century. Growth in the proportion of employers offering programs has been only moderate, increasing from 81% in 1992 to 90% in 1999 (Association for Worksite Health Promotion, U.S. Department of Health and Human Services, & William M. Mercer, Inc., 2000). However, most of the growth has been in organizations that have not historically had programs. For example, employers in large industrial settings have greatly expanded their programs. General Motors is in the process of implementing the largest workplace health promotion program in the world, and Chrysler (now DaimlerChrysler) continues to expand a maturing program.

There has been substantial growth in the science supporting health promotion. A systematic review of the literature on the health impact of workplace health promotion programs (Wilson, Holman, & Hammock, 1996) identified 378 published studies, and half of these studies were randomized controlled designs or quasi-experimental designs. A review on the financial impact of programs (Aldana, 1998) identified 40 studies on the impact of programs on medical care costs and absenteeism, and 52% of these were randomized controlled designs or quasi-experimental designs. From the perspective of methodological rigor, this body of literature is comparable in quality to the literature supporting most nonpharmacological medical treatments.

For the first time, we have sufficient evidence to make a number of strong statements about health promotion. First, there is no doubt that modifiable lifestyle risk factors such as smoking, sedentary lifestyle, poor nutrition, obesity, excess stress, and quality of social interactions are related to health outcomes, including morbidity and mortality. Second, there is also no doubt these risk factors are related to medical care costs and productivity. Third, we can persuasively conclude that workplace health promotion programs can improve health-related knowledge, attitudes, behaviors, and objective health conditions such as muscle strength and endurance, body fat, blood pressure, heart rate, respiratory function, blood lipid levels, back pain, and emotional and physical symptoms of stress—at least on a short-term basis. Fourth, a small number of intensive clinical programs (Gould, 1995) have been able to reduce underlying health conditions including heart disease and coronary artery stenosis, something medical interventions had not been able to do. Fifth, many programs have demonstrated the ability to reduce medical care costs and absenteeism rates, sometimes producing returns well in excess of program costs.

Having the data to answer these five questions marks an important milestone for this field, but at least two very important questions remain unanswered by the research literature. First, we have little evidence to show that programs are able to produce lifelong or even multiyear changes. Many of the programs reported in the literature are discontinued after the one- or two-year period of the study. In other cases, the programs continue, but the evaluation effort ceases after a year or two. At this point it is probably safe to speculate that few short-term programs are able to produce lifelong changes. If we want to create lifelong changes, we probably have to maintain programs on a long-term basis, and we probably have to create environments that encourage healthy lifestyle practices. Second, the research literature says very little about what strategies or protocols are most effective in producing change. Our knowledge is especially weak concerning the best strategies to reach older adults, racial minority groups, young adults, and people with low education levels. This is not to say that many experienced health promotion practitioners do not have a good sense of the most effective strategies; it just means we have not been able to test their ideas with empirical research or even to document them in less rigorous formats.

Despite the growth in the science base supporting health promotion, it remains an orphan among most scientific groups. For example, the Director of Prevention at the

National Institutes of Health estimated that 25% of NIH's research budget is devoted to prevention (Harlan, 1998). However, this includes research on early intervention surgeries and other medical treatments, medical screening, reduction of iatrogenic diseases, and many other procedures that have little relation to health promotion. The percent of NIH funds spent on health promotion is certainly less than 5% and probably less than 1%. Most research in workplace health promotion is funded by employers who are evaluating the effectiveness and impact of their own programs. Rigorous research of this nature often costs as much as the programs. It is unlikely that employers will continue to fund this type of research for their programs.

Other factors that have influenced health promotion in the past decade have included outsourcing of programs, the explosive growth of computer technology, increasing medical care costs, the influx of managed care and pharmaceutical companies, and an increasingly global economy.

When the second edition of this book was published, programs managed internally by the employer were the predominant program model. Today, externally managed or "outsourced" programs are the norm. This has opened up new career paths for health promotion professionals, facilitated the development of standardized operating protocols, and created operating efficiencies. It has also caused some organizations to be less involved in their programs and some to view what used to be a very special "warm and fuzzy" endeavor as a commodity, much like a company cafeteria or parking lot, which can be disposed of during tight financial times. It has also stimulated the growth of a small number of large program management organizations that now dominate the field.

Technology has also had a significant impact on programs. General business operating systems, including word processing, spreadsheets, presentation software, database programs, and program management software, are a standard element in all programs. This has allowed a dramatic improvement in internal communication, recordkeeping, and program evaluation. The advent of the Internet as an education and communication tool has expanded the range of program offerings and the ability to reach remote sites beyond most people's expectations. However, it has also caused a dangerous shift in program focus. Programs that used to pride themselves on establishing warm rapport with their members have sometimes become programs dominated by impersonal e-mail and Internet interactions. Program managers who are skilled communicators, who thrive on human interaction, have often become technocrats. To avoid this peril, technology must be harnessed to improve efficiencies and thus free up program staff from routine administrative details and allow them to spend *more* time with people.

The growth of managed care organizations in the 1990s seemed to hold up the promise of substantial growth for workplace health promotion and the potential to pull health promotion into the medical mainstream. One of the basic philosophical tenets of managed care was to keep members healthy, thereby preventing the need for medical care and reducing medical costs. Indeed, a number of managed care organizations developed substantial health promotion units and encouraged their employer clients to implement and expand health promotion programs. They sometimes provided free health promotion services to their employer clients. Employers quickly accepted their managed care organization as a natural provider of health promotion services, and some eliminated their internally managed programs. Unfortunately, most managed care organizations did not develop sufficient internal skills to implement high-quality programs or sufficiently large staff to serve more than a small portion of their employer clients. Many of these programs were seen as marketing vehicles and never established linkages within the medical leadership of the organization. When profit margins in the managed care industry dropped, many managed care organizations cut or severely reduced their health promotion programs. Ironically, many employers still see their managed care organization as having primary responsibility for their health promotion programs (Goldman, 2000) and have reduced internal program funding. Involvement of managed care has done little, if anything, to improve the quality of programs and has caused the closure of some programs. At this point, this foray into health promotion by the managed care industry has probably been a detriment to the field.

A number of the large pharmaceutical companies have had long-standing excellent health promotion programs for their own employees. In the mid-to-late 1990s, a number of pharmaceutical companies entered the business side of the health promotion field when they launched their disease management programs. Disease management programs consisted of a combination of behavioral, pharmaceutical, and medical treatment protocols to provide optimal care for a number of diseases. Some of these protocols required people to stop smoking, eat better foods, exercise, and manage excess stress. Of course all of these protocols required people to take more drugs, so behavioral protocols to increase compliance needed to be implemented as well. Disease management programs were quickly followed by new drugs for weight loss, quitting smoking, sleep enhancement, and mood management. Traditional health promotion programs were usually companions to these programs as well. In an effort to reach a broader market, many of these companies offered free health promotion programming and materials to employer groups. They have also supported health promotion research efforts and been generous contributors to professional activities. The long-term impact of the pharmaceutical industry on workplace programs is yet to be seen. If their medicinal products are so successful that they allow people to have positive health outcomes without developing healthy lifestyles, they will undermine the basic principles of the field. Giving programs to employers tends to decrease employers' willingness to take responsibility for supporting their own programs. If the pharmaceutical companies can continue to add sophistication to the science of health promotion and provide financial support for professional activities, they will make a positive contribution. However, if they lose interest in behavioral interventions and pull their financial support from the field, it will be worse than it was before they entered.

With the exception of a number of programs in Australia, Japan, Europe, and South America, workplace health promotion has been primarily a North American phenomenon, and the United States certainly leads the world in terms of the number and sophistication of the programs. That position of dominance will likely continue for decades, but increasing numbers of programs are emerging all over the world. One of the reasons for this growth is the increasing number of U.S. companies that are expanding their overseas operations. Another reason is that there are no geographical boundaries to the clear business advantages that health promotion presents.

Watching the evolution of health promotion has been much like watching the growth of a child. You see a small child grow in small ways every day. Progress is continual but slow. Then you turn around and that child has become an adult.

The field of health promotion has not yet reached adulthood, but it is clear that the field has grown and become more sophisticated. Like a child, it has probably lost some of its innocence and perhaps some of its soul. Despite its growth, it is still floundering. It lacks stature. It is not part of mainstream business. It is not part of mainstream medicine. It is a minor player in national policy. Its science base is limited. It has no natural champion to carry it forward. It also lacks national leadership. The Association for Worksite Health Promotion, the dominant professional association in the field, has had declining membership for a number of years and now has fewer members than it did 20 years ago.

A number of factors may have a huge impact on workplace health promotion in the next few years. The first is the relationship between health and productivity. Health promotion advocates have long argued that there is a relationship between health behaviors and productivity, and few people have argued with this. The basic concept is that people who exercise, have a balanced emotional state, don't smoke, eat a healthy diet, and practice other health enhancing behaviors, are absent less often and are more productive when they are at work (O'Donnell, 2000). As Chapter 2 discusses, if a program is to pay for itself through medical care cost reductions, savings of approximately 5% are required; if the same program is paid for through productivity enhancements, savings of only 0.33% are required. However, the research supporting these linkages has been quite limited. Few tools have existed to measure productivity, and longitudinal studies have not been funded to study these relationships. Fortunately, the Health Enhancement Research Organization (HERO) is launching a major initiative to correct this situation (O'Donnell, 2000). These initiatives could significantly increase the demand and budget allocations for worksite health promotion programs.

The second factor is increased funding for behavioral research. Research exploring how to change health behaviors most effectively has been very limited, primarily because of lack of funding for this research. A significant increase in federal and foundation funding for behavioral research could have a significant impact on the success of workplace health promotion programs. Research on the most effective ways to produce lasting change and how to create environments that support long-term healthy lifestyle are two areas that are especially important. As a profession, we need to lobby Congress and private foundations to allocate funding for behavior research.

The third area of opportunity is government policy. The federal government has traditionally given only lip service support for health promotion, but that may change in the next decade. The concept of health promotion is an integral part of the federal government's health goals, which are described in the Healthy People 2010 Objectives (U.S. Department of Health and Human Services, 1999). In fact, specific goals have been set for the prevalence and intensity of workplace health promotion programs. Unfortunately, very little funding has been allocated to achieve these goals. As a profession, we need to make sure Congress allocates sufficient funding to implement programs that can achieve these goals. Furthermore, selected officials at the Health Care Finance Administration are open to the concept of health promotion because they are searching for ways avoid bankrupting Medicare in light of the aging U.S. population.

Here again, as a profession, we need to advocate Medicare and Medicaid support for health promotion procedures. This would stimulate the refinement of the science of health promotion and thus raise the quality of programs.

AUDIENCE

The focus of this book is the nuts and bolts of designing and managing workplace health promotion programs, not the policy level issues discussed above, but it is written within the context of these larger issues.

This book will be most valuable to three groups of people: students at the graduate and undergraduate level courses on health promotion; professionals working within employer settings who are responsible for developing, managing, or supervising health promotion programs; and consultants responsible for designing health management programs.

WHAT'S NEW IN THIS EDITION?

Ninety percent of this book is brand new.

The conceptual framework that guided the development of this book is the same that guided the second edition. Therefore, the basic list of chapter titles is very similar to the second edition, and many of the authors are the same. Furthermore, the basic structure of the chapters on program design, program evaluation, employee assistance, and social health are the same, but they have been updated to incorporate new concepts and recent studies. The rest of the chapters have been completely rewritten.

The first section, the Health Promotion Concept, explains why health promotion makes sense from the perspective of individual and organizational health and as an investment for employers.

The second section, Program Management, describes the process of designing, managing, and evaluating a program.

The third section, Strategies, discusses three levels of change which programs can impact: awareness, behavior change, and supportive environments.

The fourth section, Interventions, describes the kinds of programs that are used to operationalize a health promotion program. The physical dimension includes chapters on fitness, nutrition, weight control, tobacco control and cessation, and medical self-care. The emotional dimension includes chapters on stress management and employee assistance programs. The social dimension is discussed in only one chapter. The concept of social health is just emerging within workplace health promotion, but it is expected to have a major impact on program strategies and outcomes in the next decade.

We have not included a chapter on the intellectual dimension because we have not seen many workplace health promotion programs implemented on this topic.

One chapter is devoted to health assessment, which is not a specific intervention area but is the entry point for many programs.

The fifth section, on Perspectives, discusses major issues impacting our field. It has chapters on programs for small business and programs for retirees and older adults. It also includes chapters on the emerging global perspective, the concept of corporate and community partnerships, and a peek at one future that might materialize.

Conceptual Framework

The conceptual framework for this edition is based on the definitions of health promotion and optimal health presented in the *American Journal of Health Promotion:*

> "Health promotion is the science and art of helping people change their lifestyle to move toward a state of optimal health. Optimal health is defined as a balance of physical, emotional, social, spiritual and intellectual health. Lifestyle change can be facilitated through a combination of efforts to enhance awareness, change behavior and create environments that support good health practices. Of the three, supportive environments will probably have the greatest impact in producing lasting changes" (O'Donnell 1989).

These five dimensions of optimal health and three levels of health promotion programs are discussed next.

Dimensions of Optimal Health

Many of the early health promotion programs focused primarily on physical fitness. Current programs have expanded beyond fitness to address smoking cessation, nutrition, weight control, and stress management. With the exception of stress management, all of these areas address the physical dimension of optimal health. Given the medical genesis of health promotion and the overwhelming research supporting the relationship between physical health, morbidity, and mortality, this focus on the physical dimension is not unexpected. Nevertheless programs limited to physical health will not address all of the modifiable influences on an employee's health. As we gain experience in health promotion, we are beginning to realize that employees' health is affected by many dimensions of their home and work life. For example, an employee who does not smoke, works out every day, and eats a perfect diet can also be a workaholic, have insufficient social support, be depressed, and be highly susceptible to debilitating emotional or physical breakdown. Another employee who exercises regularly, eats well, avoids abusive substances, and manages stress well can suffer from physical exhaustion due to the demands of caring for children or an invalid parent. Still another employee who seems to be a high-energy, well-liked, and productive worker can also be a cocaine addict.

Recognizing the need to look beyond physical health and building on the work of others, such as Bill Hettler (1977), led us to develop the five dimensions of optimal health. This remains a conceptual model, but the evidence supporting each of the dimensions is growing and much of it is reviewed in this text. Each of the five dimensions is briefly described here (O'Donnell 1991).

Physical health refers to the physiological condition of one's body. The impacts on health of smoking, physical activity, alcohol, and nutrition have all been very well documented, and most health promotion programs address all these areas.

Emotional health refers to one's mental state of being. It encompasses the stresses in a person's life, how one reacts to those stresses, and the ability to relax and devote time to leisure. There is growing evidence linking emotional health to health care utilization, susceptibility to disease, and unhealthy lifestyle practices. Worksite health promotion programs designed to address this area include stress management, employee assistance programs, and recreation and leisure programs.

Social health is the ability to get along with others, including family members, friends, professional colleagues, and neighbors. Social support has been shown to be very important in facilitating recovery and rehabilitation from disease, reducing the impact of stress on physical and emotional health, and even lowering disease and mortality rates. Additionally, social norms have a tremendous impact on lifestyle behaviors. Social health programs might include child and frail-parent care programs; support groups; peer leadership development opportunities; culture change efforts; group recreation and sports teams; and skill development programs in communication, parenting, and assertiveness. Incorporating social health programs into workplace health promotion may represent the greatest opportunity available to us for improving the impact of our efforts.

Spiritual health is the condition of one's spirit, including having a sense of purpose in life, the ability to give and receive love, and feeling charity and goodwill toward others. For some people, religion will be a central component of spiritual health programs; for others it will not. Programs might include life-planning workshops, service to voluntary and charitable organizations, and cooperative programs with religious groups. Research in this area is limited but growing.

Intellectual health is related to achievements in life, which can occur through work, school, community service, hobbies, or cultural pursuits. Intellectual health manifests its impact on overall health through relationships between education and healthy lifestyle practices; unemployment and disease; socioeconomic status and medical care utilization; and self-esteem, self-efficacy, and health practices. Psychoneuroimmunology and neuropsychology are beginning to help us understand these relationships. Intellectual health programs are unusual in workplace health promotion, but in the future might include programs to enhance self-esteem and career planning and development efforts. Some of these might be best coordinated by training departments.

The Importance of Balance

Striving to achieve excellence in all five dimensions of optimal health is an overwhelming goal that would discourage most people from even attempting it. Therefore the key message to convey to employees is the importance of achieving a **balance** in all these areas and not sacrificing one area to achieve excellence in another. This message is probably best conveyed to employees by sharing examples of people who have focused on one area at the expense of other areas and then have faced a setback. An example—very tangible in the workplace—is the business executive determined to make whatever sacrifices are necessary to be successful in his career, including neglecting his family, not developing friendships outside work, working long hours at the expense of regular exercise and adequate sleep, and developing a hard driving personality not able to relax. This approach might produce short and even midterm success, but what will happen to this person if he loses his job through retirement, layoff, or even poor performance? The adjustment will be very difficult because he has little to fall back on. He will not receive much social support because he is not close to his family and he has few nonwork friends. The emotional stress of this situation could lead to health problems because his body is already weak from the strains of poor diet and sedentary lifestyle. His self-esteem will be very low because his life is wrapped up in his work. Some men in these circumstances will never recover.

Another example tangible to most people is the wife who drops out of college to finance her husband's education, further delays her own career to raise children, and supports his career by creating a comfortable home and entertaining his clients and coworkers. What happens to this woman when she is middle-aged, the children are off to college, and her husband divorces her? In most cases she will be unable to support herself because she has not developed work skills. She will be socially isolated because most of her friends are tied to her husband's work or are at least part of a couple also close to her husband. This is a very difficult adjustment that thousands of women face each year.

One final example less common to the personal experience of most employees but still highly visible due to media coverage is the skilled athlete who devotes his or her life to success in sports. He or she might neglect school work in deference to practice or physical conditioning. Friends might be limited to those involved in sports. A balanced physical fitness program might even by neglected in favor of playing despite injuries and taking growth enhancing drugs such as steroids. What happens to these athletes when their athletic career ends? This might happen if they are not good enough to make the jump from junior varsity to varsity, high school to college, college to professional sports or the Olympics. It also might happen through a career-ending injury or after they reach their prime and are no longer able to compete at age 25, 35, or 40. Athletes who develop all aspects of their lives can do very well when they finish sports. Those who do not develop all aspects of their lives often find themselves with no means of financial support, a broken body, and a distorted view of what is required for success.

It is not difficult for employees to realize that these traps are easy to fall into given the norms in our society. What ideal is held higher in our society than striving for career success? What is more commendable than devoting your life to your spouse and children? What, on the surface, is more consistent with health promotion than developing your body to the fullest extent and succeeding in sports? Until recently we have done very little in health promotion to focus on a broad view of health or to stress the importance of balance.

Three Levels of Health Promotion Programs

Another limitation of early programs was the failure to clarify or even understand the different levels of program impact. Workplace health promotion programs can have three levels of effect. They can enhance awareness, help employees make lifestyle changes, and create environments that support healthy lifestyles. Of course, programs that create supportive environments will have the greatest chance of success in helping employees develop and maintain long-term healthy lifestyle practices. The impact of each level of program and the basic components are described next (O'Donnell 1992).

Level I: Awareness

An awareness program increases an employee's level of awareness or interest in the program topic. In very few cases does the employee actually change health behavior or improve health as a result of these programs. Examples of awareness programs include newsletters, posters, flyers, health fairs, educational classes, weekend retreats, and health screening without feedback, goal setting, and interactive counseling.

The intended impact of many of these programs is often health behavior change or improved health, but the outcome usually falls short. Many health education classes have this shortcoming. Their design is based on an antiquated model of health education that suggests that changes in the individual's beliefs, attitudes, and knowledge can result in changes in behavior. This may occur in some cases, but not in most.

If the goal of the health promotion program is to improve the employee's health, awareness programs by themselves are of almost no value. However if the awareness programs are offered in conjunction with other programs, they can be very useful; in fact, they can be used as a direct feeder to the lifestyle change programs.

Additionally, awareness programs can be of value to the employer apart from their impact on health goals. Such programs can be made very visible to employees and the outside community and thus provide a public relations function or act as a morale booster. Awareness programs can also be an inexpensive way to get started in health promotion and can stimulate management to develop more extensive programs.

Level II: Lifestyle Change Programs

Lifestyle change programs go a step beyond awareness programs by setting lifestyle-related behavior change as the desired outcome. Changes might include quitting smoking, exercising on a regular basis, successfully managing stress, eating more nutritious foods, or combining exercise and nutritious eating to lose weight.

The most successful lifestyle change programs use a combination of health education, behavior modification, experiential practice, and feedback opportunities. Successful programs also allow sufficient time to elapse for behavior changes to occur and take root. This process probably takes at least twelve weeks to start.

In addition to beginning to improve employees' health, lifestyle change programs are also of greater value to the employer than awareness programs. First, behavior changes can result in improved health status, which in turn can lead to reduced medical problems and thus reduced medical costs. Second, lifestyle change programs have a greater chance of improving an employee's outlook and physical and emotional capacity to be more productive at work. Third, these programs can provide a bigger morale boost and publicity angle, simply because they are more extensive. Finally, the extended nature of the programs provides employees additional opportunities to get to know one another, which can in turn help them learn to work together more effectively.

The problem with lifestyle change programs is their failure to sustain long-term behavior change. Unfortunately most smokers who quit smoking resume the habit. Most people who lose weight gain it back within a year. Very few people are able to maintain regular ongoing physical fitness programs. The best way to reduce these lapses is through supportive environment programs.

Level III: Supportive Environment

The goal of a supportive environment program is to create an environment within the work setting that encourages a healthy lifestyle. A supportive environment is critical to helping people maintain newly acquired healthy lifestyle habits. For example, after employees leave the supportive group setting of a quit smoking program, they must return to work, home, and favorite social spots. Much of their lives have been built around smoking. Their offices and homes are filled with ashtrays, lighters, and matches, and they know just where they can buy cigarettes all over town. Many of their closest friends are smokers, and many of them will not be ready to quit. If indeed they continue to not smoke, they will usually have to spend less time with their friends who still smoke. During the last decade we have seen a switch in many social and workplace environments from a setting that makes it very easy to smoke to settings that make it more difficult. Smoking rates have dropped dramatically as this has occurred.

We have also seen changes that make physical fitness and nutritious eating more palatable. For example, regular exercise used to be popular primarily among young athletes, most of whom were male. Today regular exercise provides a recreational and social outlet for people regardless of age or gender. We have seen an explosion of fitness fashions and health clubs to support this change. Finally, we have seen similar changes in food. It is far easier to buy foods low in fat, salt, and sugar in grocery stores and restaurants than in the past.

Many of those changes have occurred independent of any intentional health promotion efforts, but we can make intentional changes in the workplace to make it more health inducing. We can create environments that support healthy lifestyles by

- changing the physical setting, corporate policies, and corporate culture
- implementing ongoing programs
- and enhancing employee ownership of programs

Improvements in the physical environment that can encourage healthy lifestyles include construction of lockers, showers, and workout areas; stocking vending machines and cafeterias with healthful foods; and removing cigarette machines and ashtrays from common areas.

Corporate policies that foster healthy lifestyles include instructing managers to encourage employees to participate in programs, allowing flexible work scheduling to permit employees to exercise during the day, instituting nonsmoking policies, funding medical care coverage programs so they reward good health practices instead of poor health, and restructuring absenteeism policies to reward coming to work instead of taking days off.

The corporate culture can be adjusted to support positive health by applauding employees' involvement and successes in the program, featuring top management and other key employees as role models of healthy lifestyles, and providing regular information reports on the health status and practices of each department.

Ongoing structures such as a permanent formal health promotion program with a program manager, program materials, and an office, as well as ongoing activities such as classes, health screenings, activity groups, special events, and regular promotion, can help make the program a stable part of the organization.

Employee ownership of the program means that employees know that the program serves their best interests and that they can use it actively. This feeling of ownership can be fostered by maintaining confidentiality of all health-related employee data, by actively involving employees in managing and delivering the program, and by requiring employees to pay for a portion of the cost of the program.

This supportive environment will provide the employer with the best opportunity to achieve related organizational goals of reducing health care costs, enhancing image, and stimulating improvements in productivity.

MICHAEL P. O'DONNELL

About the Editor

Michael P. O'Donnell, PhD, MBA, MPH, is founder, editor-in-chief, and president of the *American Journal of Health Promotion, Inc.,* the first scientific journal to address the health promotion field. As editor-in-chief, Dr. O'Donnell has completed composite editorial reviews of over 1,400 manuscripts. As president, he has organized 10 national conferences. Dr. O'Donnell is also founder and president of the Health Promotion Research Foundation and research director of the Health Enhancement Research Organization (HERO). Prior to starting the *Journal,* Dr. O'Donnell worked in hospital management for seven years and in management consulting for four years. He has served on the faculties of five universities and is currently an adjunct professor in the School of Public Health at the University of Michigan.

During the 1998–1999 academic year, Dr. O'Donnell moved to Seoul, Korea, with his family to serve as a Senior Fulbright Scholar and visiting professor in the department of preventive medicine at Catholic University and the Graduate School of Health Sciences at Yonsei University. While in Korea, he also helped to create the first systematic employee health promotion program in Korea and helped to conceive and fund the first nationwide smoke-free workplace campaign in Korea.

Dr. O'Donnell's publications include over 100 articles, book chapters, columns, books, and workbooks. His awards include Alumni of the Year from Seoul Foreign School (1999), Distinguished Leadership and Service Lifetime Achievement Award from the Association for Worksite Health Promotion (1997), Young Professional Award from the Society for Public Health Education, Great Lakes Chapter (1990), selection as a Fellow by the Association for Fitness in Business (1985), and the Bausch Lomb Award in Science from the University of Rochester (1970).

Dr. O'Donnell earned a PhD in Health Behavior and Health Education from the School of Public Health at the University of Michigan, an MBA in Entrepreneurship and General Management, and an MPH in Hospital Administration from the University of California, Berkeley. He completed his undergraduate work in Psychobiology at Oberlin College.

References

Aldana, S. (1998). Financial impact of worksite health promotion and methodological quality of the evidence. *The Art of Health Promotion,* 4, 1, 1–8.

Association for Worksite Health Promotion, U.S. Department of Health and Human Services, & William M. Mercer, Inc. (2000). *1999 national worksite health promotion survey.* Northbrook, IL: Association for Worksite Health Promotion and William M. Mercer, Inc.

Goldman, P. (2000, March 9). *Market potential of worksite health promotion.* Paper presented at Art and Science of Health Promotion Conference, Colorado Springs, CO.

Gould, L., Ornish, D., Scher, W., Brown, S., Edens, R., Hess, M., Muller, N. et al. (1995). Changes in myocardial perfusion abnormalities by positron emission tomography after long-term, intense risk factor modification. *Journal of the American Medical Association,* 274, (11), 894–901.

Harlan, W. R. (1998). Prevention research at the National Institutes of Health. *American Journal of Preventive Medicine, 14*(4), 302–307.

Hettler, B. (1977). Patient handout.

O'Donnell, M. (1989). Definition of health promotion: Part III: Expanding the definition. *American Journal of Health Promotion* 3(3):5.

_____ . 1991. The third and fourth steps in the evoltion of worksite health promotion. Preface in *Worksite Health Promotion: Needs, Approaches, and Effectiveness*, edited by J. Mayer and K. David. Michigan Department of Public Health.

O'Donnell, M. P. (2000). Health and productivity management: The concept, impact and opportunity. *American Journal of Health Promotion, 14*(4), 211–214.

U.S. Department of Health and Human Services. (1999). Healthy people 2010 objectives, Washington, DC: U.S. Government Printing Office.

Wilson, M., Holman, P., & Hammock, A. (1996). A comprehensive review of the effects of worksite health promotion on health related outcomes. *American Journal of Health Promotion, 10*(6), 429–435.

CHAPTER

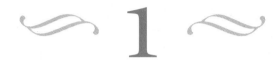

The Health Effects of Health Promotion

Jeffrey S. Harris and James F. Fries

INTRODUCTION

The Ottawa Charter for Health Promotion, sponsored by the World Health Organization, defined health promotion as "the process of enabling people to increase control over, and to improve their health" (World Health Organization, 1986). The Charter defined health as "a resource for everyday life . . . a positive concept emphasizing social and personal resources as well as physical capabilities." Health is therefore considered an instrumentality for successful living. "Health" clearly goes beyond physical health to include coping and problem solving skills, a rational balance between self-care and health service use, accomplishment at home and at work, successful social interactions, and a positive attitude and outlook. Research has related these characteristics, interestingly enough, to reduced symptomatology and lower health service use. Disability associated with age is substantially postponed in those with positive health habits, particularly exercise. Self-management of minor illness is both a result and a cause of increased personal autonomy. Self-management of

chronic illness can improve outcomes as well. Autonomy may also be exercised by executing Living Wills and Durable Power of Attorney for Health Care documents. Effective health promotion programs are health improvement programs; they go beyond providing information to effect behavioral change.

The emphasis of most health promotion programs and evaluative research in the past two decades has been on physical risk factors, physical health status, and health insurance costs (see Chapter 2). Often studies of insurance costs infer that the health promotion program could reduce morbidity from disease. However, there are several areas for health promotion, broadly defined, beyond disease prevention. In the short run (less than 10–15 years), the social, production, and monetary costs of disability may well be greater than the costs of medical care. Disability is very strongly related to present and future health service use.

Breslow (1999) has noted that true health extends beyond the prevention of disease and activity limitation to the development of more effective coping skills and enhanced abilities to accomplish various tasks. Research in this area, particularly that associated with increased personal self-efficacy, provides the missing link between provision of health information and reduction in disabilities, cost, and absence from work that may not be directly connected to the risks or diseases affected. Further, more effective problem-solving skills and abilities should translate to more effective work and home life.

In this chapter, we will summarize currently available data. First, we will briefly review the leading causes of morbidity, mortality, and disability in the United States. We will then summarize the evidence linking health behaviors to illness, disability, and positive health and productivity. Finally, we will discuss the evidence that health promotion efforts in general, and those at the worksite in particular, can reduce health risks, prevent disease, decrease medical care costs, and increase all aspects of health. The conceptual paradigm is the Compression of Morbidity. The theoretical basis for interventions is improvement in personal self-efficacy.

THE BURDEN OF ILLNESS

Leading Causes of Mortality

Mortality statistics are often the starting place for analysis of the drivers of negative health in a population because they are universally available, at least in industrialized nations, relatively accurate, and the endpoint, death, is clear. Their chief drawback is that they do not directly relate to morbidity, health, and quality of life.

Health promoters should review the leading causes of death in their populations as reflected in life insurance statistics in order to target disease prevention efforts, with the caveat that changes in the demographics of the work force may affect the mortality burden and antecedent morbidity and disability. In the absence of specific data, United States population figures are often close to the mark if applied by age group.

The leading causes of death in the U.S. in 1997, in order of the number of deaths, are shown in Table 1-1. There were 2,314,245 deaths in the U.S. in 1997.

By age group, the leading causes of death for the U.S. population as a whole are accidents (primarily motor vehicle) for ages 1–44, cancer for ages 45–64, and heart disease for those ages 65 and over. For the black population, however, the leading cause for ages 15–24 was homicide and for ages 25–34, HIV infection. Tables 1-5–1-14 display the relationships between the leading causes of death and specific behaviors; we discuss specifics in the following pages.

Leading Causes of Morbidity and Disability

Health practices have an influence on illness, disability, and the use of health care services, as well as on mortality. Many of the leading causes of morbidity and disability are related to lifestyle, including failure to seek preventive services. To obtain specific rates of morbidity or disability, one can survey the target pop-

Table 1-1 Leading Causes of Death in the United States, 1997

Cause of Death	Proportion Attributable to Lifestyle	Number of Deaths
Heart disease	57%	726,974
Cancer	37%	539,577
Cerebrovascular disease	50%	159,791
Chronic obstructive pulmonary disease		109,029
Accidents	60%	95,644
Pneumonia	23%	86,449
Diabetes	34%	62,636
Suicide	60%	30,535
Chronic liver disease and cirrhosis	70%	25,125
HIV		16,516

Source: National Center for Health Statistics, *Advance report of final mortality statistics, 1997,* 1999.

ulation or analyze health insurance claims data. (Keep in mind, however, that claims data omit the 40% of total health care expenses not covered by insurance, and therefore underestimate the total cost of ill health.) Good quality-of-life data are not frequently available but may be obtained by survey.

In 1995, the leading causes of acute morbidity among the U.S. population were respiratory conditions, with influenza outranking the common cold. The reported chronic conditions with the highest prevalence were sinusitis, arthritis, orthopedic impairments, and hypertension, each affecting more than 10% of the population (National Center for Health Statistics [NCHS], 1998). Among those under 45 years of age, sinusitis was by far the most common condition, followed by other upper respiratory disorders. For those between 45 and 64, high blood pressure topped the list, followed by heart disease and sinusitis. Heart disease and arthritis become most prevalent over age 65. Tables 1-7–1-14 display the relationships of the leading causes of morbidity and disability to specific behaviors; we discuss specifics below.

Leading Causes of Health Service Use

Use of health services follows a similar pattern. On average, individuals in the United States had almost six physician contacts in 1995 – a total of more than 1.5 billion contacts. The main reasons for the visits, in rank order, are shown in Table 1-2, from three points of view: patient surveys, physician coding in a national survey, and codes submitted on medical claims.

The leading causes of physicians' office visits, according to patient survey, were cough, sore throat, stomach symptoms, earache, and back pain for females, and cough, sore throat, earache, fever, and back pain for males (NCHS, 1992). The leading causes of physicians' office visits, described by diagnostic code assigned by the examining physician, were hypertension, otitis media, acute URI, diabetes, pharyngitis, allergic rhinitis, bronchitis, neurotic disorders, and sinusitis for females, and hypertension, otitis media, acute URI, diabetes, allergic rhinitis, bronchitis, pharyngitis, back pain, and ischemic heart disease for males. The most common reasons for visits (based on physician billing codes) were general medical examinations, cough, routine prenatal visits, throat symptoms, postoperative visits and well-baby visits. At least three of these types of visits could be considered preventive.

The reasons for visits varied by age. Those younger than 15 were the only group with earache and fever listed among the top 10 most frequent reasons. Routine pregnancy examination was the most frequently listed reason for a visit among females 15–44 a years of age. Depression was a leading reason for a visit only among those in the 25–44-year-old age group. Hypertension and visual dysfunction were among the top 10 for those 45 years of age and older.

Table 1-2 Leading Reasons for Use of Health Services, 1995

Patient Survey		Physician Diagnostic Code		
Male	Female	Male	Female	Billing Data
cough	cough	hypertension	hypertension	general medical exam
sore throat	sore throat	otitis media	otitis media	cough
earache	stomach symptoms	acute URI	acute URI	routine prenatal exam
fever	earache	diabetes	diabetes	throat symptoms
back pain	back pain	allergic rhinitis	pharyngitis	well-baby visits
		bronchitis	allergic rhinitis	

Table 1-3 Leading Causes of Hospital Admission in the United States, 1992

Cause of Admission	Rank
Heart disease	1
Mental disorders	2
Cancer	3
Pneumonia	4
Fractures	5

Source: National Center for Health Statistics, *National hospital discharge survey, 1992,* 1996.

Six percent of individuals in the United States have at least one hospital stay in a given year, with one percent having two or more (NCHS, 1996). The most common reasons for admission are shown in Table 1-3. Many hospitalizations are for childbirth, although that reason is usually excluded from federal statistics. Respiratory disorders are by far the most common cause of admission among those under 15 years of age, followed by trauma and digestive disorders. Mental disorders and trauma are the most common reasons for admission for those 15–44 years old. Circulatory disorders, digestive diseases, and cancer topped the list for those 45 and older.

The most costly disorders for commercial health plans are typically neoplasms, injuries, non-specific complaints, and cardiovascular disorders. For Medicare, with an older population, the most expensive entities are cardiovascular disease, neoplasms, and respiratory disorders.

LEADING CAUSES OF DISABILITY

Disability is often mediated by a disease state that causes functional impairment. In the 1992 National Health Interview Survey (NHIS), 38 million Americans reported 61 million disabling conditions. (Disability, as used here, is generally longer term than activity limitation.) In one recent study, 73% of disabilities reported in the NHIS in 1992 were linked to a disease or injury. The other 27% were related to physical impairments, which are defined as deficits of body structure or function (LaPlante, 1996). Yet there

Table 1-4 Activity Limiting Conditions and Disability in the United States, 1992

Condition	Activity Limitation	Disability
Musculoskeletal/orthopedic deformities and disorders	27.5%	31.3%
back and spine	12.6%	
arthritis and related disorders	8.3%	
lower extremities	4.6%	
shoulder and/or upper extremities	2.0%	
Heart disease/circulatory disorders	13.0%	16.7%
Asthma/respiratory disorders	4.2%	7.8%
Diabetes	4.2%	
Diseases of the nervous system		7.2%

Source: M. LaPlante, 1996.

are people with disabilities but without obvious physical impairment, and people with severe handicaps who are quite functional. About 5% of the disabilities in the NHIS were ascribed to signs, symptoms, and ill-defined conditions. Among impairments, many were orthopedic, hearing, and visual impairments for which there are accommodations or accommodative devices. One important challenge is finding other actionable variables that link impairment and disability, so that disability can be managed and reduced.

The most common disorders associated with disability in the NHIS were musculoskeletal and connective tissue disorders (17.2%); a further 14.1% were classified as orthopedic impairments (see Table 1-4). Injury codes were attached to 12 disorders and 72 impairments, accounting for 13.4% of all disabling conditions.

LEADING CAUSES OF ACTIVITY LIMITATION

Musculoskeletal problems account for the largest overall proportion (27.5%) of temporary activity limitation (see Table 1-4). Injuries (off-the-job as well as work-related) were the leading acute cause of work loss (123 days/100 workers), followed by respiratory conditions (110/100). The rates were highest in both instances among workers 25–44 years old.

Acute and chronic conditions caused individuals in the United States to spend an average of 6 days in bed, workers to lose more than 5.3 days of work, and students to miss an average of 4.5 days of school. The leading acute causes of "bed disability" were respiratory conditions and injuries. Interestingly, the total number of hospital bed-days per 1,000 population was almost twice as great in the South as in the Northeast.

BEHAVIORAL RISK FACTORS

A number of health behaviors have been strongly linked to morbidity, disability, and mortality. Diseases, injuries, or disabilities may have several risks associated with them. Thus, attributable risk must be divided among a number of factors.

The most detailed analysis has been applied to causes of death. McGinnis and Foege (1993) synthesized the evidence about factors associated with the leading causes of death in the United States in 1990. Analysis of attributable risk factors yielded associations of lifestyle factors with about half of all deaths in the U.S. (see Table 1-5). The effects vary among different age, gender, and racial groups.

An important analysis by Amler and Dull in 1988 calculated the burden of illness as both deaths and premature years of life lost (PYLL) before age 65. This is a useful technique, although obviously there are also many PYLL lost after age 65. Their analysis indicated that 27% of premature deaths were associated with tobacco use, 24% with high blood pressure, and 23% with over-nutrition. In terms of PYLL, the frequencies are different (see Table 1-6). The proportions are probably somewhat different today, as the number of overweight individuals has increased, but hypertension is better controlled. The study also attributed 21% of hospital days and 16% of direct medical costs to lifestyle factors.

Breslow and colleagues (Breslow & Breslow, 1993) analyzed longitudinal data from the Alameda County Human Population Laboratory and demonstrated that people with poor health habits have twice the relative risk of death of those with good health habits. The habits in question were smoking, excessive alcohol consumption, being obese, very little physical activity, getting more or less than 7-8 hours of sleep each night, eating between meals, and not eating breakfast. They further demonstrated that social support has an independent and cumulative effect on mortality and disability.

Cumulative risk, often seen as multiple risks in certain high-risk individuals, markedly increases the

Table 1-5 Lifestyle-related Causes of Death in the United States, 1990

Lifestyle Risk	Estimated Number of Deaths per Year
Tobacco use	400,000
Diet and activity patterns	300,000
Alcohol misuse	100,000
Microbial agents	90,000
Toxic agents	60,000
Motor vehicles	47,000
Firearms	36,000
Sexual behavior	30,000
Illicit use of drugs	20,000

Source: J. M. McGinnis and W. Foege, *Journal of the American Medical Association*, 1993.

Table 1-6 Lifestyle Factors Contributing to Premature Years of Life Lost before Age 65 (PYLL) in the United States, 1988

Lifestyle Factor	PYLL
Injury without alcohol use	21%
Injury with alcohol use	19%
Tobacco use	18%
Gaps in primary prevention	15%
Unintended pregnancy	6%
Other alcohol-related problems	4%
Handguns	4%
High blood pressure	4%

Source: R. Amler and H. B. Dull, *Closing the gap: The burden of unnecessary illness*, 1988.

risk of disability. In follow-up studies of the Alameda County cohort, the survivors who had poor health habits in the original cohort had twice the odds of disability as those who had good health habits. As with mortality, the social network index had an independent effect on disability. More recently, Vita, Terry, Hubert, and Fries (1998) showed reductions in cumulative lifetime disability by one-half for those who exercised, did not smoke, and maintained a good body weight.

THE EFFECTS OF SPECIFIC RISK FACTORS

Individual risk factors, as well as pooled risk factors, affect morbidity, disability, and mortality (Wallace, Doebbeling, & Last, 1998). Health promoters must be familiar with these links in order to design programs and to conduct rigorous evaluative re-

search. More complete tables (see Tables 1-7–1-16) indicating these linkages are provided at the end of this chapter.

Substance Use and Abuse

The use or abuse of legal and illegal substances has major negative effects on health. Smoking, the leading cause of mortality in the U.S. and many other countries, has been linked with a wide range of problems. These range from acute respiratory illnesses, ear infections, and sudden infant deaths to gingivitis, as well as over 20 types of cancer, emphysema, and circulatory disease (see Table 1-7). [Odds ratios and attributable percentages, as well as other specifics, can be found in Fries, Singh, et al., 1994.] Second hand smoke poses risks for respiratory and ear infections, heart disease, and other illnesses as well as ex-

Table 1-7 Some Adverse Health Effects of Tobacco Use

Mortality	Morbidity	Disability	Productivity
• Arteriosclerosis	• Atherosclerosis	• Respiratory compromise	• Cigarette breaks
• Coronary artery disease	• Angina pectoris	• Paralysis	• Accidents
• Aortic aneurysm	• Stroke sequellae	• Activity limitation	• Slow output
• Sudden cardiac death	• Peripheral vascular disease	• Attention deficit disorder	• Fires
• Cancer:	• Burns	• Cognitive delays	• Work time lost
Respiratory	• Pneumonia	• Amputations	
GI	• Bronchitis	• Claudication	
GU	• Asthma	• Halitosis	
• Stroke	• Emphysema	• Congestive heart failure	
• COPD	• Otitis media		
• Pneumonia and influenza	• Tracheitis		
• SIDS	• Low birth weight		
• Neonatal mortality	• Prematurity		
• Fetal mortality	• RDS		
• Burns	• Ulcer disease		
• Injuries	• Periodontal disease		
• Ulcer disease	• Gastroesophageal reflux disease		
	• Low back and neck pain		
	• Epilepsy		
	• Cerebral palsy		
	• Facial wrinkles		
	• Thrombophlebitis		
	• Congestive heart failure		

acerbations of asthma, sinusitis, heart disease, and other health problems (see Chapter 13).

Other substance abuse has a variety of effects ranging from markedly elevated use of health services to significant morbidity and increased risk of death (see Chapter 16). The effect depends on the substance. Tobacco, of course, is the most commonly abused substance, followed by alcohol, cocaine, and intravenous narcotic use. Tobacco is also the most addictive, followed by heroin. These effects are listed in Table 1-8. Note that moderate alcohol intake (1–2 drinks per day) is associated with decreased overall morbidity and morbidity as compared with abstainers, particularly with regard to heart disease, but higher rates of cancer and liver disease.

Table 1-8 Health Effects of Other Substance Use

Risk factor	Mortality	Morbidity	Disability	Productivity
Alcohol use	• Cirrhosis • Accidents • Homicide • Suicide • Cancer: 　GI 　Respiratory • Stroke • Heart disease • AIDS	• Trauma • Pneumonia and influenza • COPD • Tuberculosis • Pancreatitis • Cirrhosis • Alcoholic hepatitis • Peptic ulcer disease • Gastritis • Hypertension • Angina • Cardiomyopathy • Dementia • Psychosis • Migraine • Neuropathy • Epilepsy • Unintended pregnancy • Fetal alcohol syndrome • Withdrawal	• Mental abilities: 　Acute 　Chronic • Developmental 　delay • Developmental 　disability • Domestic violence	• Mental abilities: 　Acute 　Chronic • Accidents
Other drugs (cocaine, heroin, stimulants, depressants, other "recreational" drugs)	• Overdose • Trauma • AIDS • Stroke • Heart attack • Renal failure	• Unintended pregnancy • Pregnancy complications • Low birth weight • Crack baby syndrome • Injury • Nasal perforation • Systemic infections • Withdrawal • Child abuse and neglect • AIDS • Renal disease	• Developmental 　delay • Developmental 　disability	• Absenteeism • Drug seeking 　behavior • Theft • Poor performance

Fitness

Exercise has a strong protective effect against mortality, morbidity, and disability. Having a sedentary lifestyle has a profound effect on the prevalence of disability, supporting the theory of the compression of morbidity (see Table 1-9). The teams at Stanford University conducting several longitudinal studies have demonstrated an inverse relationship between mortality and exercise intensity for Harvard alumni (Lee, Hsieh, & Paffenbarger, 1995), members of a runners club (Fries, Singh et al., 1994), and alumni at the University of Pennsylvania (Vita et al., 1998). Exercise may be acting through intermediary effects, such as reduction in serum low-density lipoproteins and glucose, and body mass, as well as reduction of stress effects and improvement in muscle mass, metabolic rate, and respiratory efficiency. The University of Pennsylvania study also showed increased mortality with increased body-mass index and smoking independent of exercise effects.

Simonsick and colleagues (1993) found a protective effect of recreational physical activity on the risk of mortality, while high level activity protected against functional decline. Fries and associates (Fries, Singh et al., 1994) demonstrated slower development of disability among members of a runners club and alumni at the University of Pennsylvania who engaged in vigorous exercise and, in the latter case, among those who were nonsmokers and had lower body-mass indices. In the University of Pennsylvania study, the onset of disability was postponed approxi-mately 7.75 years in the low risk group as compared to the high risk group (see also Chapter 10).

Nutrition

Nutrition is an issue for several reasons (see Chapter 11). The best-known nutritional risk is consumption of excessive saturated fat. Saturated fat intake leads to increased low-density lipoprotein (LDL) levels, a risk for heart and cerebrovascular disease. In addition, since fat has a caloric density over twice that of carbohydrates or protein, fat consumption can easily lead to excess body mass, an independent risk factor for vascular disease and type II diabetes. (See Tables 1-10 and 1-11). Moderate to vigorous exercise reduces both LDL levels and body mass. There are a number of theories about glucose intake, anti-oxidants, and carbohydrates that are less well-established.

Social Role, Social Support, and Stress

Social role and social support clearly have independent effects on mortality and disability, as demonstrated in classic and continuing studies by Breslow, Berkman and Syme, and Kasl, among others (see Chapter 17).

Stress reactions, both acute and chronic, affect health and well-being in a variety of ways (see Table 1-12). Responses to stressors often lead to physical symptoms, causing people to seek medical care that should be no more than symptomatic or a reinforcement of coping skills. On a more global level, job stress, particularly

Table 1-9 Adverse Health Effects of Sedentary Lifestyle

Mortality	Morbidity	Disability	Productivity
• Heart disease • Diabetes	• Heart disease • Diabetes • Falls • Low back pain • Other musculoskeletal pain • Herniated disks • Fractures	• All-cause • Muscle atrophy • Aerobic deconditioning • Balance and coordination • Osteoporosis • Arthritis • Musculoskeletal pain • Atelectasis • GI dysmotility	• Reduced creativity • Reduced endurance

Table 1-10 Adverse Health Effects Related to Poor Nutrition Risks

Risk Factor	Mortality	Morbidity	Disability
Dietary fat intake	• Heart disease • Stroke • Atherosclerosis • Diabetes • Cancer	• Overweight • Angina pectoris • Stroke sequellae • Digestive diseases	• Mobility • Endurance
Dietary fiber intake	• Heart disease • Colorectal cancer • Breast cancer • Prostate cancer	• Angina pectoris • Stroke sequellae • Digestive diseases • Diabetes	• Constipation • Irritable bowel syndrome

Table 1-11 Adverse Health Effects Related to Both Nutrition Risks and Lack of Exercise

Risk Factor	Mortality	Morbidity	Disability
Overweight	• Heart disease • Diabetes	• Angina pectoris • Arthritis • Gallbladder disease • Breast and endometrial cancer • Osteoarthritis • Slipped capital femoral epiphysis	• Arthritis • Activity limitation
Elevated serum cholesterol	• Heart disease • Stroke	• Angina pectoris • Stroke	
Elevated blood pressure	• Heart disease • Stroke • Nephrosclerosis • Renal failure	• Angina pectoris • Stroke sequellae • Renal failure	

Table 1-12 Health Effects of Stressors and Reactions to Them

Risk Factor	Mortality	Morbidity	Disability	Productivity
Stress	• Heart disease	• Prematurity		
Hostility	• Heart disease • Violence	• Angina • Conflict		
Social support	• All-cause		• All-cause	
Social class	• All cause	• Depression • Personality disorders		

Table 1-13 Reproductive Risks

Risk Factor	Mortality	Morbidity	Disability
Sexual behavior	• AIDS	• STDs • Urinary tract infections	• Sterility
Oral contraceptives	• Heart disease in smokers • Stroke in smokers	• Migraine	
Pregnancy history	• Breast, ovarian, endometrial cancer		
Unintended pregnancy	• Maternal deaths • Infant deaths	• Prematurity	• Birth defects
Low birth weight	• Decreased survival	• Respiratory distress	• Developmental delays

Table 1-14 Other Risk Factors for Preventable Health Effects

Risk Factor	Mortality	Morbidity	Disability
Lack of immunization	• Infectious diseases	• Hepatitis • Measles • Rubella	• Birth defects • Encephalitis
Driving	• Trauma	• Low back and neck pain • Herniated disk	• Musculoskeletal pain
Firearms	• Homicide • Suicide	• Injury	• Residual damage from gunshot wounds
Sunlight	• Melanoma	• Basal cell cancer • Squamous cancer	

Chemical exposure	• Cancer:
	  Respiratory
	  GU
	  Hematopoietic
		• Asthma
		• Allergy
		• Dermatitis	

high demand—low control situations, has been correlated with excess mortality as well as morbidity and lost productivity (Karasek & Theorell, 1990). In individuals with pre-existing cardiac disease, stress-induced vasoconstriction can increase symptoms (see Chapter 17). Social networks and social status, on the other hand, buffer the effects of stressors.

Various behaviors related to reproduction are major risks for children and younger adults. These may be the areas of highest impact for employers with younger work forces (see Table 1-13). There are a number of other behavioral risks that contribute to mortality, morbidity, and disability. These are listed in Table 1-14.

Some risk factors are synergistic, as noted in Table 1-15. Some disease states also interact to multiply the risk of other diseases (Table 1-16).

TRENDS IN ILLNESS, DISABILITY, AND RISK FACTORS

Since 1979, the federal government has published a series of documents assessing preventable health risks and the burden of illness and setting targets for improvement (U.S. Department of Health and Human Services [DHHS], 1991; U.S. Surgeon General, 1979). *Healthy People 2000* (Office of Health Promotion & Disease Prevention, 1991), *Healthy People 2010* (Of-

Table 1-15 Risk Factor Interactions

Risk Factor	Reduces	Increases
Sedentary lifestyle		• Blood pressure • Blood sugar • Serum cholesterol • Weight
Tobacco use	• Fitness	• Heart disease in diabetics • Drug use • High risk sexual behavior • Combativeness
Fat intake		• Serum cholesterol • Weight
Sodium intake		• Blood pressure
Social class		• Substance abuse
Overweight	• Physical fitness	• Blood pressure • Serum cholesterol
Other drug use		• High risk sexual behavior
Alcohol use	• Serum LDL cholesterol	• Triglyceride levels • Drug use • High risk sexual behavior

Table 1-16 Disease State Interactions

Disease State	Increases
Diabetes	• Heart disease • Stroke • Renal failure • Retinopathy • Peripheral vascular disease • Neuropathy • Birth defects
HIV	• Renal disease • Cancers • Infections • Dementia
Migraine	• Stroke
Cardiac disease	• Stroke
Depression	• Suicide • Arthritis symptoms • Other somatic symptoms • Sleep disturbance

fice of Health Promotion & Disease Prevention, 2000), and related updates and studies provide examples of performance measures and targets that may be useful at a given health promotion site, depending on the site-specific rates of illness and disability.

There has been significant progress in a number of areas. In 1990, the leading causes were in almost the same rank order as in 1997 (NCHS, 1993). However, chronic obstructive pulmonary disease (COPD) has now replaced accidents as the 4th leading cause, presumably due to population aging and the delayed effects of smoking. HIV became the 8th leading cause in 1996, up from 10th in 1990, but then plummeted to 14th in 1997, most likely due to the introduction of more effective multi-drug therapy (NCHS, 1999b). The number of accidental deaths rose 21.7%, and diabetes deaths increased from 48,000 to 62,636, a 30.5% rise. The number of heart disease deaths increased by only 1%, cancer by 6.8%, and stroke by 11%. Influenza and pneumonia deaths increased by almost 6%. The factors responsible for the differential changes in various lifestyle-related health problems are not immediately clear, especially since these chronic illnesses develop slowly. More certainly, one could conclude that secular changes in risk factors, whatever their cause, have affected their primary targets, heart disease and accidents. Laws about seatbelts, child restraints, and drunk drivers, and changes in motor vehicles and highways affected the latter as well.

When age-adjusted death rates, rather than absolute numbers, are used to adjust for population increases and aging, we see a continuation of the decline in chronic disease mortality that began in the 1970's. The adjusted death rates for coronary heart disease and stroke have dropped significantly, more so for whites than blacks (DHHS, 1999). Previously, there had been a sharp drop from 1930 to 1955 and a plateau from 1955 to 1970. The crude death rate in 1997 was 864.7 per 100,000 population, but the adjusted rate was a record low of 479.1. The age-adjusted rate declined for each of the four major race-sex groups. The largest decreases were for ages 25–34 (9.2%), 33–44 (8.2%), and ages 1–4 (6.5%). The largest reduction was in HIV infection-related deaths, affecting ages 1–14 and 25–54. Significant declines in rates of death from accidents, homicide, and suicide were seen for those ages 15–24. Reductions in heart disease had the greatest effect on the decline for those 55 and over. On the negative side of the ledger, adjusted death rates increased for drug-induced causes and kidney disease.

There is still a disparity among racial groups. Blacks have significantly higher age-adjusted death rates for all causes and the highest rates of any racial group for infant mortality (twice the total population rate), homicide (four times the total population rate), HIV, cardiovascular disease, lung cancer, and breast cancer (Plepys & Klein, 1995).

As discussed in the progress report, *Healthy People 2000 Review, 1998-1999*, part of an annual series published by the U.S. Centers for Disease Control, there have been advances since the publication of *Healthy People 2000* in some areas and not in others (DHHS, 1999). Smoking prevalence among adults has decreased from 29% in 1987 to 25% in 1995. There has been progress among all ethnic, gender, and occupational groups measured, with the most dramatic decrease noted among military personnel. Cholesterol and hypertension awareness have increased substan-

tially from 1990 to 1997. The prevalence of high cholesterol has dropped during the same period. The prevalence of being overweight has increased markedly and has not changed for physical activity. Diabetes incidence has increased, as have diabetic end stage renal disease and other reported complications.

The rates of infant and fetal deaths are down significantly. However, the U.S. still ranks 25th in these areas. The death rate for sudden infant death syndrome (SIDS) is down by 66%. Prenatal care has improved substantially among all ethnic and racial groups. Breast feeding and abstinence from tobacco and alcohol during pregnancy have increased as well, although not to the same extent. However, the prevalence of teenage mothers who smoke is increasing.

Basic immunization rates have improved by 15–75%, depending on type of immunization and geographical region. However, increases in preventive screening for cholesterol, cervical cancer, and mammography have been minimal.

Rates of activity limitation due to chronic conditions have apparently increased somewhat, from 9.4–10% of the population. Reported back pain disability has increased by almost one third. Average number of years of healthy life have not changed from 1990 to 1996.

THE COMPRESSION OF MORBIDITY

Health promotion has had a great need for an underlying theoretical paradigm. Lacking such a paradigm, the health promotion community has been subject to criticisms of mistaking association for causality on the one hand or of promoting a world of long-lived, disabled, and demented individuals on the other.

The Compression of Morbidity paradigm envisions a potential reduction of overall morbidity and of health care costs, now heavily concentrated in the senior years, by compression of the period of morbidity between an increasing average age of onset of disability and the age of death, which is increasing perhaps more slowly (Fries, 1980). The healthy life is seen potentially as a life vigorous and vital until shortly before its natural close.

Intuitively, the concept of delaying the onset of disability through prevention of diseases and reduction in health risks seems natural enough. However, in the seventies and eighties, many observers believed that there was movement away from this ideal, with a steady increase in the proportion of a typical life spent ill or infirm (Gruenberg, 1977; Verbrugge, 1984). The previously prevalent acute illnesses had given way to chronic diseases with longer periods of disability and morbidity. As people took better care of themselves and lived longer, the contrarians suggested, they would live into those later years in which disability is greatest and would experience an increase in overall lifetime disability. Such critics feared that good behavioral health habits would lead to an epidemic of Alzheimer's disease and a huge population of enfeebled, demented elders who would pose an immense strain upon medical care resources (Myers & Manton, 1984). Thus, the direct test of compression (or extension) of morbidity depends upon the effects, studied prospectively and longitudinally, of reduced health risks upon cumulative lifetime disability.

New and emerging data document that the early fears were unfounded. First, life expectancy from advanced ages has plateaued rather than having increased markedly as predicted. In the U.S. the life expectancy of women from age 65 has increased only 0.6 years over a 17-year period. From age 85, female life expectancy in the U.S. has been constant at 6.4 years since 1980 (Kranczer, 1998). Second, recent longitudinal data document the ability to greatly postpone the onset of disability with age. For the past 14 years, a research group at Stanford has studied the effects of long distance running on patient outcomes in 537 members of a runners club, with participants at least 50 years old, compared with 423 age-matched community controls (Fries, Singh et al., 1994). The study was designed as a test of the Compression of Morbidity hypothesis. Appropriate controls for self-selection bias were included, and disability levels were assessed yearly, allowing the area under the disability curve to be assessed. Runners, exercising vigorously for an average of 280 minutes per week, delayed the onset of disability *by about 10 years* compared with controls. Both male and female runners increased disability at a rate only one-third that of the controls, after adjusting for age, initial disability, educational level, smoking behavior, body mass index, history of arthritis, and the presence of comorbid disease. As

these subjects moved from age 58 toward age 70, the differences in physical function between the exercising and the control population increased rather than decreased. Lifetime disability (the aggregate time spent disabled over a lifetime) in exercisers is only one-third to one-half that of sedentary individuals (Kranczer, 1998; Stewart, King, & Haskell, 1993).

Recently, in the University of Pennsylvania study, we studied 1,741 university attendees, surveyed in 1962 at an average age of 43 and then annually since 1986. This unique data set contains over 50 years of longitudinal follow up since the participant's days at University. Health risk strata were developed for persons at high, moderate, and low risk, based on the three risk factors of smoking, body mass index, and lack of exercise (Fries, Singh et al., 1994). Cumulative disability from 1986 (at an average age of 67) to 1994 (at an average age of 75) or until death served as a surrogate for lifetime disability. Persons with high health risks in 1962 or in 1986 have approximately twice the cumulative disability of those with low health risks. Results were consistent across survivors and deceased members of the study cohort, males compared to females, and over the last one and two years of observation. Deceased low-risk subjects had only one-half the disability of high-risk subjects in their last one and two years of life. High-risk subjects, in addition to having increased mortality, had greatly increased lifetime disability. Onset of disability was postponed by approximately 7.75 years in the low-risk stratum as compared with the high-risk stratum. The 100% reduction in disability rates was balanced against only a 50% reduction in mortality rates, documenting compression of morbidity.

Recent major studies by other groups confirm these findings. Daviglus and colleagues (1998) showed substantial decreases in Medicare costs for those with few risk factors in midlife. Freedman and Martin (1998) showed significant age-specific functional improvement in seniors over a seven year period. Reed and colleagues (1998) related healthy aging to prospectively-determined health risks, with results closely similar to ours.

Compression of Morbidity is readily demonstrable in those who exercise vigorously compared with those who do not, those with low behavioral health risks versus those with high such risks, and those with high educational attainment as compared with low attainment (Fries, Singh et al., 1994; House, Kessler, Herzog et al., 1990; Leigh & Fries, 1994; Stewart et al., 1993; Vita et al., 1998). Health risk behaviors, as determined in midlife and late adulthood, strongly predict subsequent lifetime disability (Fries, Singh et al., 1994; Reed, Foley, White et al., 1998; Vita et al., 1998). Both cumulative morbidity and morbidity at the end of life are decreased in those with good health habits (Vita et al., 1998). Morbidity is postponed and compressed into fewer years in those with fewer health risks. The paradigm of a long healthy life with a relatively rapid terminal decline represents an attainable ideal (Nusselder & Mackenbach, 1996). Health policies must be directed at modifying those health risks that precede and cause morbidity if this ideal is to be approached for a population (Fries, Koop, Sokolov, Beadle et al., 1998).

EFFECTS OF HEALTH PROMOTION

Perhaps the key question in the chain linking lifestyle risks to health is whether health promotion interventions can change health risks or health behaviors such as medical service use. The next question is whether the reduced risks or behaviors lead to decreases in mortality, morbidity, costs, and disability (sometimes referred to as the "total burden of illness"). There is good evidence that healthier lifestyles are associated with lower mortality, morbidity, costs, and disability. However, one should not assume that the presence of a health promotion program, or even reduction in weighted health risks, automatically confers better outcomes. Health promotion efforts are targeted at reducing health risks or changing behaviors, particularly health risk or health service use behaviors. As a necessary condition, they must be successful at changing risks over an extended time in order to be effective in improving health. Whether risk change by itself is sufficient is another question; in healthy populations, the events to be prevented may be decades in the future and impossible to measure directly. In contrast, as noted above, many other health promotion goals, such as self-management and improved self-efficacy, can yield first-year positive results.

Both individual risk factor reduction interventions and comprehensive programs have been shown to reduce risk levels. Exercise programs have been effective in reducing cardiac risk and the prevalence of disability (Hunt, Donato, & Crespo, 1996). For example, Stewart, King, and Haskell (1993) demonstrated that previously sedentary adults who participated in a structured exercise program had better physical health a year later than did controls, although there was no change in general psychological well-being.

Multifaceted programs with community reinforcement should have greater long-term success than individual counseling-based interventions because they include a series of reinforcers. In a sense, they are broader based and less controllable versions of multifaceted worksite health promotion programs (Green, 1998). Examples include the North Karelia Project in Finland, the Stanford Three-Community and Five-Community Projects, the Pawtucket Heart Health Project, the Minnesota Health Program, and the Community Intervention Trial for Smoking Cessation (COMMIT). The results seem to be good for some segments of the population and not others. Also, in contrasting the effects of a community-directed program (such as in North Karelia) and an externally developed program (such as COMMIT), it appears that developing the process of community involvement and allowing local prioritization of efforts increases the effectiveness of the intervention (Ferguson, 1998). The issue of self-determination is relevant to worksite health promotion as well.

HEALTH PROMOTION AT THE WORKSITE

The worksite should be an ideal location for health promotion efforts because it is a defined community with access to populations and social support and has economic reasons for improving health and productivity. The proportion of employers offering health promotion programs has increased significantly in the last two decades. However, the scope and design of these programs vary widely, and it is likely that many poorly constructed and poorly performed interventions are not effective.

Yet, there are many caveats to a singular focus on the worksite. The government should have the major role to play with senior citizens, who have the largest illness burden and the greatest need for effective interventions. The health insurer has a large stake involved with insured populations. About half of Americans are employed by small businesses and half by large companies; small businesses lack resources to mount their own programs and are better served by distributed programs, delivered, for example, by mail. Thus, traditional worksite-based programs may miss many of the persons most in need of health promotion services.

A key evaluation issue is a clear definition of the intervention so that it can be reproduced. Another is comparison to reasonable control groups in order to isolate the effects of secular trends. Strongest of all, and essential for rigorous evaluation, is the need for randomized controlled trials.

Reviews of Program Effectiveness

The Centers for Disease Control and the *American Journal of Health Promotion* (Wilson, Holman, Hammock, 1996) presented a series of analyses of the health impact of health promotion programs at the worksite. Almost 400 studies were reviewed. These are summarized below. The evidence varied by intervention and problem addressed. One methodologic issue was the comparability of the interventions, both in specific type (the technology) and in intensity (the dose).

Health Risk Appraisal

Many have assumed that simply assessing risk and giving feedback would lead to behavior change. In fact, health risk appraisals are aimed at allowing specific interventions to change awareness and prepare people to change behaviors (Anderson & Staufacker, 1996). Not surprisingly, then, the available data suggest that health risk appraisals (HRAs) have their only impact as part of a comprehensive program. There is some research on direct effects of HRAs, but the logic connecting the HRA with a health outcome is sometimes tenuous. According to a review by Anderson and Staufacker (1996), there are so many methodologic threats to the validity of existing studies on HRAs alone that the evidence must be regarded as weak at this time.

We should note that conventional HRAs are standardized, or "one size fits all." They are not customized for individual risks. Offering targeted assessment of progress at follow-up increases the individual impact of the instrument by initiating a dialog with the participant. Further, while all the HRAs look at mortality risk, only a few assess the risk of morbidity or health service use. The latter are of much more concern to employers and employees in the near term. The term "HRA" is itself gradually being less utilized because it connotes a goal of quantitative overall health risk computation rather than triaging personalized interventions, assessing quality, measuring change, and meeting other goals. Newer terms include "Health Assessment Questionnaire" and "Health Improvement Questionnaire". As such, the newer questionnaire instruments are an essential part of the most effective comprehensive health promotion programs.

Fitness and Exercise

Shephard (1996) has thoughtfully reviewed the evidence for the effectiveness of worksite fitness programs. Among program participants, regular participants reduced body mass by 1–2% with a reduction of body fat of 10–15%. Muscle strength and aerobic capacity can be increased by up to 20%. The impact on high-risk persons can be substantial when fitness programs are combined with cholesterol and blood pressure reduction, weight control, and other applicable heart disease prevention interventions. However, when the effects are averaged across the entire employee population, the impact is reduced. Shephard suggests that a better return on investment might be obtained by providing access to off-site fitness facilities.

Evidence about the positive effects of exercise on cardiac risk, satisfaction, well-being, and claims cost is still preliminary. Long term gains also need better documentation.

Weight Control

Hennrikus and Jeffery (1996) concluded that worksite weight control programs can produce weight loss of 1–2 pounds per week among participants. Some studies reported improvement in eating habits and employee satisfaction. Weight loss was less than that reported for clinic-based programs, but the participants were generally less obese initially and limits on loss rates were usually set. Most interventions were individual counseling. Other than contests and incentives, social interventions have not been explored. The research supports better access to overweight employees at the worksite, but methodologic problems cause the evidence to be rated "indicative" rather than conclusive.

Nutrition and Cholesterol Control

The main strategies used for both nutrition and cholesterol management programs were individual counseling, group education, mediated programs, and cafeteria-based programs. Most were nonrandomized. Targeted behaviors were increases in dietary fiber intake, reduction in fat consumption, and increases in fruit and vegetable intake. Cholesterol reductions in the 5–9% range were achieved, and dietary habits changed to some extent. It appears that the more intensive strategies have greater effect on short-term results. Longer-term results were not yet clear (Glanz, Sorenson, & Farmer, 1996).

Smoking Cessation

Smoking cessation research has changed focus, probably along with the focus of cessation programs themselves. Before 1985, smoking cessation was offered in clinics. In the late 1980s, contests and incentives became a primary emphasis. In the 1990s, worksite-wide efforts have become the norm. Group programs have reported success rates of 20–60% at 6 to 18 months. Minimal interventions, which attract more participants, report success rates ranging from 1 to 20%. Twenty-five percent quit rates are viewed as realistic in the long run, but few studies include long-term follow-up. Incentives and contests increase participation but may not increase quit rates (Eriksen & Gottlieb, 1998).

Smoking Policy

Studies of worksite policies that restrict or ban smoking are suggestive for reduction of smoking at work and reduction of environmental tobacco smoke exposure as measured by nicotine and cotinine levels. The evidence was reported as weak for effects on smoking cessation or overall consumption of cigarettes. Consumption at work dropped by an average of three cigarettes (Eriksen & Gottlieb, 1998).

Hypertension Control

As described in a review by Foote (as cited in O'Donnell, 1997), participation rates are high for hypertension control programs, with 79% of employees involved on average. Between 60 and 85% of those with high blood pressure report pressure control to normal limits while programs are in place. However, education without medical treatment is ineffective.

Stress Management

The growing number of stress management programs at work suggests that job stress is a recognized and probably growing issue. Lawrence Murphy Ph.D. of the National Institute for Occupational Health and Safety (NIOSH) critically reviewed the literature evaluating the effects of worksite stress management programs. He found it difficult to compare programs since programs used a variety of interventions ranging from muscle relaxation to cognitive techniques and combinations of interventions. Outcomes examined ranged from somatic complaints and physiologic measures to absenteeism and job satisfaction. None apparently assessed turnover, productivity, disease prevalence, health service use , or health care costs. Methodology varied greatly. The results were mostly positive but somewhat variable. None of the interventions produced consistent effects on job satisfaction or absenteeism.

As Murphy (1996) noted, we may be looking for calm, joy, and productivity in all the wrong places. For more than twenty years, the emphasis in this text's various editions, as well as the epidemiology, social science, and management literature as a whole, has been on changing organizational stressors and assessing organizational outcomes. Yet health promotion programs still generally focus on training individuals to cope with stressors. While that is a worthy first step, it does not address the source of the problem or the most direct mechanism to improve organizational effectiveness.

Substance Abuse

Roman and Blum (1996), in a review of worksite alcohol control programs, concluded that programs are effective in changing supervisors' attitudes but that there is little evidence to conclude there was substantial change in alcohol use. The change in attitudes may have increased detection and referral. The primary preventive component of the programs, if present, was not evaluated.

Employee assistance programs have also been used to treat or triage other types of substance abuse, with varying success. They can also deal with workplace conflict and other issues. They have been used as the base for primary programs to prevent substance abuse. Stress management programs should also be used to reduce the drive to use drugs as a means of coping with stress.

Seatbelts

There are only 14 studies on worksite seatbelt interventions. While the evidence is inadequate to derive a clear view of the impact of these programs, it is suggestive of effectiveness (Eddy, Fitzhugh, Wojowicz, & Wang, 1996). We should note that there is other evidence of increased seatbelt use as the result of interventions that were part of comprehensive programs. Programs that provided significant incentives and immediate reinforcement appeared to be the most effective. Although several programs included incentives for the use of child safety restraints, these were not included in the review. The literature exists mostly for the general population rather than the worksite.

Multicomponent Programs

Multicomponent programs are directed at multiple risk factors. They vary tremendously in scope, intensity, and duration (Pelletier, 1991, 1993, 1996, 1999). All programs examined in a recent review (Heaney & Goetzel, 1996) provided some form of health education to employees. In most cases, the programs provided an opportunity to learn and practice new skills as well. Some, but by no means all, included changes in organizational policy or the work environment. Interestingly, according to one meta-analysis (Heaney & Goetzel, 1996), awareness programs alone were more effective (e.g., had a higher success rate) than awareness programs plus skill building interventions. Success rates for awareness programs were measured as knowledge change, while success rates for skill building were measured as behavior change. These two rates may not be combinable because they measure different outcomes; measuring behavior change itself is complex since different behaviors are not necessarily linearly combinable. The ideal measure would be health outcome. Offering individual counseling for high-risk employees appears to be the critical component of these programs. Programs must also be of sufficient duration (typically a year) to achieve results. In addition, anecdotally and from the point of view of organizational and social theory, organizational leadership and support should be necessary reinforcers to sustain more healthy behaviors in the long run.

There are several advantages of multicomponent programs. First, components may reinforce each other. For example, fitness, stress management and nutrition/weight control programs are important to mitigate the weight gain and anxiety that often follow smoking, alcohol, or other drug cessation. Second, the highest risk employees often have more than one health risk that they should address. Third, the presence of a comprehensive program reinforces management's commitment to a healthy work force.

DEMAND MANAGEMENT

"Demand management" is a relatively recent term introduced to differentiate supply-side approaches to medical care cost reduction (rationing access, changing financial responsibility to providers) from demand-side approaches (preventing health problems, shifting financial responsibility to patients to align costs and demand decisions, information and skill-building for more appropriate decision-making). In the context of this chapter, a heart attack that does not occur or a cold that is treated at home both represent reduction in demand for medical services. Health promotion is a demand-side intervention. As such, it includes not just preventive activities but also provision (and reception and discussion) of information to make cost-effective and efficient decisions about self- and professional care, development of medically related decision-making skills, and development of self-management skills. These latter aspects of health promotion can be provided as free-standing activities or can be quite effectively integrated into primary care and case management activities to improve their long-term benefit.

Americans have developed a strong appetite for health services, far above that of the citizens of other nations. This occurred for several reasons: the out-of-pocket cost of medical care is reduced by health insurance; our fascination with technology, medicines, and now alternative therapies; and our interest in perfect health and eternal youth. And to a significant extent, providers paid on a fee-for-service basis have induced demand for their services.

Many health services produce minimal benefit for their cost. Others pose risks in excess of their benefits, particularly if they are not clearly needed. And consumers, as a group, are less than well-informed about what works, what does not, and what is necessary to improve health. Self-management coping skills may be more important than more pills or procedures.

A number of programs now have proven effective in improving the appropriateness of health service use for acute as well as chronic conditions, presumably by improving self-efficacy (Fries, Carey, & McShane, 1997; Vickery et al., 1988). An increase in self-efficacy related to health is associated with increased productivity and other aspects of positive health.

A Role for Self-Management

Self-management is a central component of the broad definition of health promotion with which we began this chapter. Good health is, in part, a function of the assumption of responsibility for personal health by each person. Educating employees, spouses, and dependents to make more informed choices decreases the use of health services. The autonomous individual who is enabled to make better decisions in his or her own interest can improve health and moderate costs. Greater individual responsibility for health is a necessary, but not sufficient, requirement for optimal health. Many studies have demonstrated that providing consumers with information and guidelines for

self-management can lower health service use by 7–17% (Fries, Carey, & McShane, 1997; Moore, LoGerfo, & Inui, 1980; Vickery et al., 1983, 1988). These approaches appear to work through two mechanisms: more reliable consumer information and increased confidence (personal self-efficacy) that many illnesses can be safely treated at home (Fries, Koop, Sokolov, Beadle et al., 1998).

Self-efficacy theory helps explain effective self-management. It states that 1) the strength of belief in one's capability is a good predictor of behavior; 2) one's self-efficacy beliefs can be enhanced through performance mastery, modeling, and reinterpretation of physiological symptoms and social persuasion; and 3) enhanced self-efficacy leads to improved behavior, thinking patterns, and emotional well-being.

Changing an individual's personal self-efficacy is one mechanism by which effective health promotion programs work. In the absence of personal self-efficacy ("I believe that there are things that I can do which will improve my health now and in the future") there is unlikely to be personal behavior change. Self-efficacy assessments are the gold standard against which stages-of-change and other models are tested and validated (Bandura, 1997). Experienced program evaluators can judge the degree to which self-efficacy contracts are included in a program. Successful self-efficacy programs are optimistic, provide specific reasons for behavior change, increase personal autonomy and the participant's belief in personal autonomy, and decrease reliance on outside authority figures.

End-of-Life Care

Again, health promotion as a broad-based approach to increased personal autonomy for health decisions includes critical decisions about life and death. A proportion of the high costs of medical care in the last year of life represent overly intensive approaches to the treatment of terminal illness. This is another form of unnecessary demand, often provider-induced. Some 18% of lifetime costs for medical care are estimated to be incurred in the last year of life; nearly 28% of Medicare and Medicaid payments are for persons in their last year of life (Scitovsky, 1994). Seventy percent of people do not desire aggressive, invasive technical treatments when they are dying, and 85% express a desire for living wills and other advanced directives (Hanson, Tulsky, & Danis, 1997). Yet fewer than 9% of the population have executed such directives, and fewer yet have distributed them so they will be available when needed. Clearly, we need to better understand the link between personal desires and actual actions.

Rigorously Evaluated Programs: The Health Project Consortium

The Health Project Consortium, a public/private volunteer group that has met unofficially at the White House for the past 7 years, has recognized 42 programs to date that improve health and reduce costs. These C. Everett Koop Award-winning programs, provided by employers or insurers, average savings of 20% of medical claims costs through various health promotion interventions. (See www.healthproject. stanford.edu for further details.)

Through analysis of the Koop Award-winning programs, the Consortium has observed an evolution from single-purpose programs to multiple-intervention programs, and now to programs that address both need and demand. Available data suggest that while programs aimed at the need for health services may take a minimum of two to three years to show an effect on health and costs, need/demand programs have achieved cost reductions in their first year.

POLICY ISSUES

The question of funding and support for health promotion remains a critical one both for the population as a whole and for employers and employees for at least two reasons. At the worksite, there may be a perceived conflict between encouraging health and the bottom line. Some of the benefit of health promotion accrues to the community rather than to a specific employer because of turnover, the long delay in effects of the reduction of some risk factors, and the diffusion of health practices into the family and community. Further, while disability and associated health service use later in the life cycle have a direct impact on pub-

lic programs such as Medicare, employers and employees pay the premiums for those programs now.

If the cost-saving effects of health promotion are emphasized, then there is a strong business case to be made to a corporation, a private insurer, or a federal or state government (whoever is at risk for the costs of poor health) that the funding for health promotion should come out of the savings. Decreased medical costs, decreased absenteeism, decreased workers compensation claims, decreased employee turnover, increased productivity, and increased employee morale represent large benefits to the business executive, even as improved health is a large benefit to the employee.

CONCLUSION

Health promotion programs, broadly defined, can produce a variety of effects, including disease prevention, increases in health awareness, risk reduction, and reduction in demand for marginal health services. The most immediate impact should be seen on morbidity and disability from common problems such as respiratory and musculoskeletal conditions, and reduction in demand for medically marginal or unnecessary services.

Because they address interrelated risks as well as health service use, integrated programs should have the greatest cost-benefit impact. They may include treatment and counseling at teachable moments. They may address risks in the population, not just those individuals seeking care. They also demonstrate and generate organizational support for healthier practices. The most effective programs include organizational commitments, such as policy changes, on-site facilities, benefits changes, and support from senior management. Follow-up and reinforcement are critical for sustained improvement.

Programs that target higher risk individuals appear to increase their cost-effectiveness, as they logically should. The "dose" of intervention should be graded as risk increases, again a logical approach to changing entrenched behaviors. In studying the results of such programs, one would want to stratify the risk-benefit calculations by risk level to more clearly define the relationship between inputs and outputs.

Another area deserving attention is clarification of the relationship between intervention and results. Cost effects that have not been directly related to the disease state targeted by the intervention are often seen. For example, total costs of health services tend to drop or increase more slowly than one would expect with interventions targeted at a specific problem or issue (Ozminkowski, Dunn, Goetzel, Murnane, & Harrison, 1999). More specific research is needed to follow effects from intervention through the steps of awareness, specific immediate changes in morbidity and disability, and ultimately to costs and longer range effects.

Finally, programs should build self-management skills. They must go beyond the development of awareness and readiness to development of the skills to make changes and sustain them. A related issue is to look at effects on all the dimensions of health, not just the absence of disease. This view will be needed to clarify the chain of causation from messages to awareness to changes in health and productivity in both the short and long term.

References

Amler, R. & Dull, H. B. (1988). *Closing the gap: The burden of unnecessary illness.* Hyattsville, MD: U.S. Department of Health and Human Services.

Anderson, D. R. & Staufacker, M. J. (1996). The impact of worksite-based health risk appraisal on health-related outcomes: A review of the literature. *American Journal of Health Promotion, 10,* 499–508.

Bandura, A. (1997). *Self-efficacy.* New York: W. H. Freeman and Company.

Breslow, L. (1999). From disease prevention to health promotion. *Journal of the American Medical Association, 281,* 1030–1033.

Breslow, L. & Breslow, N. (1993). Health practices and disability: Some evidence from Alameda County. *Preventative Medicine, 86–95.*

Daviglus, M. L., Kiang, L., Greenland, P. et al. (1998). Benefit of a favorable cardiovascular risk-factor profile in middle age with respect to Medicare costs. *New England Journal of Medicine, 339(16),* 1122–1129.

Eddy, J. M., Fitzhugh, E. C., Wojowicz, G. G., & Wang, M. Q. (1996). The impact of worksite-based safety belt programs: A review of the literature. *American Journal of Health Promotion, 11,* 281–289.

Erikson, M. P. & Gottlieb, N. H. (1998). A review of the health impact of smoking control at the workplace. *American Journal of Health Promotion, 13,* 83–104.

Ferguson, J. E. (1998). Community intervention programs. In R. B. Wallace & B. N. Doebelling (eds.), *Maxcy-Rosenau-Last public health and preventive medicine* (14th ed., pp. 881–887). Stamford, CT: Appleton & Lange.

Freedman, V. A. & Martin, L. G. (1998). Understanding trends in functional limitations among older Americans. *American Journal of Public Health, 88 (10),* 1457–1462.

Fries, J. F. (1980). Aging, natural death, and the compression of morbidity. *New England Journal of Medicine, 303,* 130–136.

Fries, J. F., Carey, C., & McShane, D. J. (1997). Patient education in arthritis: Randomized controlled trial of a mail-delivered program. *Journal of Rheumatology, 24,* 1378–1383.

Fries, J. F., Koop, C. E., Sokolov, J., Beadle, C. E. et al. (1998). Beyond health promotion: Reducing health care costs by reducing need and demand for medical care. *Health Affairs, 17,* 70–84.

Fries, J. F., Singh, G., Morfeld, D., Hubert, H. B., Lane, N. E., & Brown, B. W., Jr. (1994). Running and the development of disability with age. *Annals of Internal Medicine, 121,* 502–509.

Glanz, K., Sorenson, G., & Farmer, A. (1996). The health impact of worksite nutrition and cholesterol intervention programs. *American Journal of Health Promotion, 10,* 453–470.

Green, L. W. (1998). Prevention and health education in clinical, school and community settings. In R. B. Wallace & B. N. Doebelling (eds.), *Maxcy-Rosenau-Last public health and preventive medicine* (14th ed., pp. 889–904). Stamford, CT: Appleton & Lange.

Gruenberg, E. M. (1977). The failure of success. *Milbank Memorial Fund Quarterly, 55,* 3–34.

Hanson, L. C., Tulsky, J. A., & Danis, M. (1997). Can clinical interventions change care at the end of life? *Annals of Internal Medicine, 126,* 381–388.

Heaney, C. A. & Goetzel, R. Z. (1996). A review of health-related outcomes of multi-component worksite health promotion programs. *American Journal of Health Promotion, 11,* 290–307.

Hennrikus, D. J. & Jeffery, R. W. (1996). Worksite interventions for weight control: A review of the literature. *American Journal of Health Promotion, 10,* 471–498.

House, J. S., Kessler, R. C., Herzog, A. R. et al. (1990). Age, socioeconomic status, and health. *Milbank Memorial Fund Quarterly, 68,* 383–411.

Hunt, J. P., Donato, K. A., & Crespo, C. J. (1996). *Physical activity and cardiovascular health* (CBM 95-7). Bethesda, MD: National Library of Medicine.

Karasek, R. & Theorell, T. (1990). *Healthy work: Stress, productivity, and the reconstruction of working life.* New York: Basic Books.

Kranczer, S. (1998, October/December). U.S. life expectancy. *Statistical Bulletin,* 8–15.

LaPlante, M. (1996). Health conditions and impairments causing disability. *Disability Statistical Abstract* (No. 16).

Lee, I., Hsieh, C., & Paffenbarger, R. S. (1995). Exercise intensity and longevity in men. *Journal of the American Medical Association, 273,* 1179–1184.

Leigh, J. P. & Fries, J. F. (1994). Education, gender and the compression of morbidity. *International Journal of Aging and Human Development, 39,* 233–246.

McGinnis, J. M. & Foege, W. (1993). Actual causes of death in the United States. *Journal of the American Medical Association, 270,* 2207–2212.

Moore, S., LoGerfo, J., & Inui, T. (1980). Effect of a self-care book on physician visits. *Journal of the American Medical Association, 243,* 2317–2320.

Murphy, L. R. (1996). Stress management in work settings: A critical review of the health effects. *American Journal of Health Promotion, 11,* 112–135.

Myers, G. C. & Manton, K. G. (1984). Compression of mortality: Myth or reality? *The Gerontologist, 24,* 346–353.

National Center for Health Statistics (1992). *National ambulatory medical care survey, 1989* (PHS Publication No. 92-1771). Hyattsville, MD: National Center for Health Statistics.

National Center for Health Statistics (1993). *Advance report of final mortality statistics, 1990.* Hyattsville, MD: U.S. Department of Health and Human Services.

National Center for Health Statistics (1996). *National hospital discharge survey, 1992* (PHS Publication No. 96). Hyattsville, MD: National Center for Health Statistics.

National Center for Health Statistics (1998). *Current estimates from the National Health Interview Survey, 1995 (Series 10, No. 199)* (PHS Publication No. 98-1527). Hyattsville, MD: National Center for Health Statistics.

National Center for Health Statistics (1999a). *Advance report of final mortality statistics, 1997.* Hyattsville, MD: U.S. Department of Health and Human Services.

National Center for Health Statistics (1999b). *National vital statistics report. Deaths: Final data for 1997* (Vol. 47, No. 19). Hyattsville, MD: National Center for Health Statistics.

Nusselder, W. J. & Mackenbach, J. P. (1996). Rectangularization of the survival curve in the Netherlands. *The Gerontologist, 36,* 773–782.

O'Donnell, M. P. (1997). Health impact of workplace health promotion programs and methodological quality of the research literature. *Art of Health Promotion, 1 (3).*

Office of Health Promotion and Disease Prevention, U.S. Centers for Disease Control (1991). *Healthy people 2000: National health promotion and disease prevention objectives for the nation,* (PHS Publication No. 017-001-00474-0). Pittsburgh, PA: U.S. Government Printing Office.

Office of Health Promotion and Disease Prevention, U.S. Centers for Disease Control. (2010). *Healthy people 2010: Understanding and improving health.* (Pub. No. 017-001-00543-6). Pittsburgh, PA: U.S. Government Printing Office.

Ozminkowski, R. J., Dunn, R. L., Goetzel, R. Z., Murnane, J., & Harrison, M. (in press). A return on investment evaluation of the Citibank, N.A. health promotion program. *American Journal of Health Promotion.*

Pelletier, K. (1991). A review and analysis of the health and cost-effective outcome studies of comprehensive health promotion and disease prevention programs. *American Journal of Health Promotion, 5,* 311–315.

Pelletier, K. (1993). A review and analysis of the health and cost-effective outcome studies of comprehensive health promotion and disease prevention programs at the work site: 1991-1993. *American Journal of Health Promotion, 8,* 50–62.

Pelletier, K. (1996). A review and analysis of the health and cost-effective outcome studies of comprehensive health promotion and disease prevention programs at the work site: 1993-1995 update. *American Journal of Health Promotion, 10,* 380–388.

Pelletier, K. (1999). A review and analysis of the clinical and cost-effectiveness studies of comprehensive health promotion and disease prevention programs at the work site: 1995-1998. *American Journal of Health Promotion, 14.*

Plepys, C. & Klein, R. (1995). *Healthy people/statistical notes, 10.* Hyattsville, MD: National Center for Health Statistics.

Reed, D. M., Foley, D. J., White, L. R. et al. (1998). Predictors of healthy aging in men with high life expectancies. *American Journal of Public Health, 88 (10),* 1463–1468.

Roman, P. M. & Blum, T. C. (1996). Alcohol: A review of the impact of worksite interventions on health and behavioral outcomes. *American Journal of Health Promotion, 11,* 136–149.

Scitovsky, A. A. (1994). The high cost of dying revisited. *Milbank Quarterly, 72,* 561–591.

Shephard, R. J. (1996). Worksite fitness and exercise programs: A review of methodology and health impact. *American Journal of Health Promotion, 10,* 436–452.

Simonsick, E. M., Lafferty, M. E., Phillips, C. L., Mendes de Leon, C. F., Kasl, S. V., Seeman, T. E. et al. (1993). Risk due to physical inactivity in physically capable older adults. *American Journal of Public Health, 83,* 1443–1450.

Stewart, A. L., King, A. C., & Haskell, W. L. (1993). Endurance exercise and health-related quality of life in 50–65 year-old adults. *The Gerontologist, 33,* 782–789.

U.S. Department of Health and Human Services (1991). *Healthy people 2000: National health promotion and disease prevention objectives.* Washington, DC: U.S. Government Printing Office.

U.S. Department of Health and Human Services (1999). *Healthy people 2000 review, 1998-99.* Washington, DC: U.S. Government Printing Office.

U.S. Surgeon General (1979). *Healthy people: The surgeon general's report on health promotion and disease prevention.* Washington, DC: U.S. Government Printing Office.

Verbrugge, L. M. (1984). Longer life but worsening health? Trends in health and mortality of middle-aged and older persons. *Milbank Memorial Fund Quarterly, 62,* 475–519.

Vickery, D. M. et al. (1983). Effects of self-care education program on medical visits. *Journal of the American Medical Association, 250,* 2952–2956.

Vickery, D. M. et al. (1988). The effect of self-care interventions on the use of medical care services in a Medicare population. *Medical Care, 26,* 580–588.

Vita, A. J., Terry, R. B., Hubert, H. B., & Fries, J. F. (1998). Aging, health risks, and cumulative disability. *New England Journal of Medicine, 338,* 1035–1041.

Wallace, R. B., Doebbeling, B. N., & Last, J. N. (1998). *Maxcy-Rosenau-Last public health and preventive medicine* (14th ed.). Stamford, CT: Appleton & Lange.

Wilson, M., Holman, P., Hammock, A. (1996). A comprehensive review of the effects of worksite health promotion on health related outcomes, *American Journal of Health Promotion, 196,* 429–435.

World Health Organization (1986). *Ottawa charter for health promotion.* Copenhagen, Denmark: World Health Organization, European Regional Office.

CHAPTER

2

Employer's Financial Perspective on Workplace Health Promotion

Michael P. O'Donnell

INTRODUCTION: WHY DO EMPLOYERS INVEST IN HEALTH PROMOTION PROGRAMS?

Approximately 90% of all workplaces with 50 or more employees and virtually all employers with over 750 employees offer some form of health promotion program at their workplace (Association for Worksite Health Promotion et al., 2000). Comparisons to previous years (USDHHS, 1993) show continual growth in the total number of programs (see Table 2-1) and in specific types of programs (see Table 2-2). (Direct comparisons between 1999 and earlier years on the prevalence of some of the specific types of programs is not possible because the 1999 survey measured presence of "programs," while the earlier surveys measured presence of "activities or information.")

It is apparent from these data that most workplaces have some form of health promotion program. This begs the question: "Why do employers invest in health promotion programs?" That is the focus of this chapter.

Table 2-1 Percent of Employers Offering Health Promotion Programs at the Worksite

Employer Size	1999	1992	1985
50–99	86%	75%	NA*
100–249	92%	86%	NA*
250–749	96%	90%	NA*
750+	98%	99%	NA*
All employers	90%	80%	66%

Source: Association for Worksite Health Promotion et al., *National Worksite Health Promotion Survey,* 2000.
*The 1985 survey did not measure program prevalence by employer size.

Historically, we have argued that employers invest in health promotion programs to reduce medical care costs, enhance productivity and enhance image (O'Donnell and Harris, 1994); and, since most of our published research focuses on those areas, discussions of those studies will be the focus of this chapter. Savings in these areas can justify a health promotion program, just as savings in electricity can justify using

Table 2-2 Percent of Employers Offering Specific Types of Health Promotion Programs at the Worksite

Type of Program	1999	1992	1985
Blood pressure screenings	29%	32%	NA*
Cholesterol screenings	22%	20%	NA*
Cancer screening	9%	12%	NA*
Health risk assessment	18%	14%	NA*
Fitness programs	25%	NA*	NA*
Nutrition or cholesterol education	23%	NA*	NA*
Weight control classes or counseling	14%	NA*	NA*
Quit smoking classes or counseling	13%	NA*	NA*
Stress management classes or counseling	26%	NA*	NA*
Alcohol or drug abuse programs	28%	NA*	NA*
Back injury prevention	53%	NA*	NA*
Maternal or prenatal programs	12%	NA*	NA*
Balancing work/family education	18%	NA*	NA*
HIV/AIDS education	25%	NA*	NA*
Workplace violence prevention programs	36%	NA*	NA*
Smoking policy	79%	59%	27%

Information or Activities		1992	1985
Job hazard/injury prevention		64%	22%
Exercise/physical fitness		41%	36%
Smoking control		40%	27%
Alcohol/other drugs		36%	29%
Back care		32%	17%
Nutrition		31%	16%
High blood pressure		29%	NA*
AIDS education		28%	NA*
Cholesterol		27%	NA*
Mental health		25%	15%
Weight control		24%	NA*
Cancer		23%	NA*
Medical self care		18%	22%
Off-the-job accidents		18%	NA*
Sexually transmitted diseases		19%	NA*
Prenatal education		9%	NA*

Source: Association for Worksite Health Promotion et al., *National Worksite Health Promotion Survey*, 2000; DHHS, National Survey of Worksite Health Promotion Activities, Summary, 1993.
*The 1992 and 1985 surveys did not collect information in as much detail as the 1999 survey.

a new energy efficient light bulb. But a health promotion program that contributes only cost savings will suffer the same fate as a light bulb. When it burns out, it will be discarded.

A subtle but important shift in the way we perceive and investigate the financial, or broader organiza-tional, return of a health promotion program may help to prevent such a fate. To survive and be suc-cessful, a health promotion program must contribute to the mission, long-term goals, and short-term prior-ities of the organization it serves and to the special in-terests of those who approve its budgets.

This concept was crystallized by the results of a benchmark study on the best health promotion programs in the United States (O'Donnell et al., 1997). This study illustrated that the best programs really did take a different approach to the direction and evaluation of their programs. Most of them have well-structured studies on health improvements, medical care cost savings, and absenteeism savings, but they also had something else. They had qualitative impressions of how their program contributed to the organization mission, long-term goals, short-term goals, and the personal priorities of those who approved their funding. Studies that show medical care cost savings or absenteeism reduction are important only to the extent that controlling costs in these areas is an important priority for the organization. They might also be important if external visibility or external validation of their programs is one of the short- or long-term goals of the organization, or the priorities of the person approving the program.

A recent worksite survey (Association for Worksite Health Promotion et al., 2000) lends further support for this conclusion. Only 4% of senior managers listed employee health as their top priority, and only 35% listed it as near the top of their priority list (see Table 2-3). Health promotion programs must be tied to the items that are number one on the priority list or near the top of the list.

Much of our future research and evaluation efforts must address this new area of concentration . . . the impact of our programs on the organization mission, long-term goals, short-term goals, and the personal priorities of those who approved their funding.

Table 2-3 Where Does Employee Health and Well-Being Fall on Senior Management's Priority List? (Percentage of Companies)

The number one priority	4%
Near the top of the priority list	35%
At the middle of the priority list	33%
Low on the priority list	16%
Not on the priority list	12%

Source: Association for Worksite Health Promotion et al. *National Worksite Health Promotion Survey,* 2000.

The purpose of this chapter is to help readers understand why employers invest in health promotion programs. The conceptual argument and the evidence to date linking health promotion programs to medical care cost containment, productivity enhancement, and image enhancement are described. This is followed by a brief review of the methodological quality of the evidence. Side bar discussions recognize that the decision to start, continue, or discontinue a health promotion program are not always rational. Even so, employers can use this conceptual framework to project the financial impact of their program and to help them determine if a program will be a prudent investment for their organization.

RATIONAL REASONS FOR INVESTING IN HEALTH PROMOTION PROGRAMS

There are a number of rational reasons employees invest in health promotion programs. The most widely cited among these are medical care cost containment, productivity enhancement, and image enhancement.

Medical Care Cost Containment

Medical care costs have risen substantially during the past four decades in many developed nations around the world. Increases have been most dramatic in the United States. As a percent of gross domestic product (GDP), medical care costs in the United States have been increasing for 40 years, growing from 5.1% in 1960 to 7.1% in 1970, 12.2% in 1990, and 13.9% in 1998 (G. Anderson, 1998). In dollars, medical care costs in the United States increased from $26.9 billion in 1960 to $1.149 trillion in 1998 (Health Care Finance Administration [HCFA], 2000). The value in 1998 was greater than the gross national product of all but eight countries in the world. In 1997, the United States spent twice as much as the average of the 24 developed nations participating in the Organization for Economic Cooperation and Development at that time and 75% more than Germany, the nation spending the second most. In 1997, medical care costs accounted for 13.6% of the GDP in the United States and 10.4% in Germany; the median cost was 7.6% of GDP in the 24 participating countries.

These cost increases have been of special concern to employers because employers have assumed a disproportionate share of the increases. In 1965, employers paid 17% of the total cost, and employees paid 61% (Levit & Cohen, 1990). By 1989, employers paid 30%, and employees paid only 37%. By 1994, employers were paying 35.3%. As this trend has continued, employers have become much more aggressive about managing their costs and passing more costs on to employees; by 1999, employers were paying only 29.2% of total costs (Koretz, 2000).

During the late 1980s and 1990s, employers implemented a wide range of medical care cost strategies, including sharing some costs with employees, training employees to be better consumers of medical care, forming coalitions of employers to negotiate bulk purchase discounts directly with medical care providers rather than insurers, and offering managed care as a preferred option–and sometimes the only option–to their employees. By 2000, an estimated 92,000,000 people were covered by health maintenance organizations (HMOs), compared to 54,000,000 in 1995 and 34,000,000 in 1990 (The Interstudy Competitive Edge, 1999). An estimated 92,000,000 additional people were members of preferred provider organizations (PPOs) by 1998. (Hoechst, Marion, & Russell, 2000). Medical care providers also became very aggressive in their pricing. Development of health promotion programs was very compatible with these schemes and was often a part of cost-containment strategies. The Balanced Budget Act also decelerated spending for Medicare. This combination of strategies was apparently successful in beginning to control costs. Quite to the surprise of many forecasters, projections that medical care costs would continue to increase dramatically, and reach 16% of GDP by 1998 (Sonnefeld, 1991), did not prove accurate. Although total medical care expenditures for the United States continued to increase in absolute dollars as a percent of GDP, medical care costs peaked in 1993 at 13.7%, dropped to 13.6% in 1994, increased to 13.7% in 1995, then dropped to 13.6% in 1996, and 13.4% in 1997 (HCFA, 2000). Average medical care costs paid by employers seemed to be under control in the mid 1990s, dropping 1.1% in 1994, increasing only 0.2%

in 1995, 1.4% in 1996, and dropping 2.9% in 1997 (14th Annual National Survey, 2000).

Unfortunately, the success in medical care cost containment of the 1990s may be over, and most experts agree that medical care costs are now increasing and will continue to increase. It may be that administrative efforts have squeezed out all the slack that can be eliminated. Some are concerned that managed care organizations have actually cut costs too low, to the point that they are jeopardizing patients' safety, and creating organizations that are financially unstable. Others suggest that costs have stopped increasing primarily because general inflation has been at almost record lows during this period. Whatever the cause, medical care costs are again increasing. As a percent of GDP, total national medical care cost spending increased from 13.4% in 1997 to 13.5% in 1998 (HCFA, 2000). Average costs per employee increased 6.2% in 1998 and 7.3% in 1999 (14th Annual National Survey, 2000) and are projected to surge to 12% in 2000 (Towers Perrin, 2000). (The estimates of medical care costs as a percent of GDP just cited are slightly different between the G. Anderson source (1998) and the Health Care Finance Administration source (2000) because a slightly different method was used to estimate GDP by Anderson in order to allow direct comparisons with other nations. Both estimates are correct within the context in which they are used.)

Even without dramatic increases, 1,149 trillion dollars is an incredible sum of money, and it is prudent business practice to take aggressive efforts to control it. A modest investment in a health promotion that has a good chance of keeping employees healthy and out of the hospital is conceptually appealing, even without a lot of data to support the connection between health status and medical care costs, and most executives relied on their gut instincts to make decisions to invest in programs. However, in the past decade, an impressive body of research has emerged to support this connection.

The first significant study was conducted by Control Data Corporation (Brink, 1987). After following 10,000 employees for four years, Control Data found that medical care claims were lowest for employees who exercised regularly, ate nutritious foods, fastened their seat belts, did not smoke cigarettes, and were not hypertensive. Consistent results were found at Steelcase (Yen, 1991, 1992). Between 1985 and 1990, employees with zero risk factors had average annual medical care costs of only $250, while employees with six risk factors had costs of $1600.

One of the most impressive studies to date (Goetzel, 1998) on the link between medical care costs and risk factors, was produced through a collaboration of six employers (Chevron, Health Trust, Hoffman-La Roche, Marriott, State of Michigan, State of Tennessee) that was organized by the Health Enhancement Research Organization (HERO). StayWell (a health promotion vender) had health risk data and MEDSTAT (a medical care cost data management organization) had medical care cost data on these six employers. With the assistance of HERO and the permission of the employers, these two data bases were merged to determine the relationship between ten modifiable risk factors and medical care costs. The strengths of this study include the large sample size, measurement of a wide range of risk factors, and the multivariate nature of the analysis. As Table 2-4 shows, eight of the risk factors (depression, stress, blood glucose, body weight, current or previous tobacco use, hypertension, and sedentary lifestyle) are associated with higher costs even after controlling for the other risk factors. Depression and stress were the most expensive risk factors; employees with those risk factors had costs 70% and 46% higher than individuals without those risk factors (see Table 2-4).

Costs were higher for those with elevated cholesterol but not after adjusting for the other nine risk factors. The finding that higher levels of alcohol consumption are not related to higher costs is initially surprising but has been found in other studies; people who drink excessively often neglect their health and do not seek medical care when they need it. The finding related to nutrition was surprising. This study showed the medical costs for those with good nutrition habits were actually higher both before and after adjustment. Our suspicion is that the tool used to measure nutrition habits within the HRA was too short to capture the full scope of nutrition habits that would impact health and medical care utilization.

This study also showed that employees who had a cluster of risk factors had strikingly higher costs. Employees with a cluster of seven heart disease risk factors had an average annual cost of $3,804, those with a cluster of risk factors for stroke had average annual

Table 2-4 Medical Care Costs Associated with Risk Factors

Risk Factor	Mean Cost With Risk Factor	Mean Cost Without Risk Factor	% Difference (unadjusted)	% Difference[a] (adjusted)
Depression	$3,189	$1,679	90%	70%
Stress	$2,287	$1,579	45%	46%
Blood glucose	$2,598	$1,691	54%	35%
Body weight	$2,318	$1,571	48%	21%
Tobacco (former)	$1,950	$1,503	25%	20%
Tobacco (current)	$1,873	$1,503	30%	14%
Blood pressure	$2,123	$1,716	24%	12%
Exercise	$2,011	$1,567	28%	10%
Cholesterol	$1,962	$1,678	17%	−1%
Alcohol use	$1,431	$1,726	−17%	−3%
Nutrition	$1,498	$1,772	−15%	−9%

[a]The adjusted differences are the differences between those with and without each risk factor which persisted after adjusting for all of the other risk factors in a multivariate analysis.
Source: R. Goetzel, *Journal of Occupational and Environmental Medicine*, 1998.

Table 2-5 Medical Care Costs Associated with Clusters of Risk Factors, United States

Risk Factor Cluster	With Risk Factors	Without Risk Factors	% Difference
Heart disease risks	$3,804	$1,158	228%
Stroke risks	$2,349	$1,272	85%
Psychosocial risks	$3,368	$1,368	147%
No risk factors		$1,166	

Source: Goetzel, et al., *Journal of Occupational and Environmental Medicine,* 1998.

cost of $2,349, and those with a cluster of psychological risk factors had average annual cost of $3,368. Employees with no risk factors had average costs of $1,166 (see Table 2-5).

A follow-up study coordinated by HERO (Anderson, Whitmer, Goetzel, Ozminkowski, Wasserman, & Serxner, 2000), used the data in the earlier study to estimate the percent of total costs attributable to these risk factors. The first study identified the most expensive risk factors among those who had these risk factors. The second study identified the total cost of the risk factors, factoring in the number of employees who had each of those risk factors. This changed the order of the most costly risk factors. For example, in the first study, depression was the most costly risk factor per person, but because less than 3% of employees suffered from depression, it did not have as significant an impact on total costs. Stress was the most costly risk factor because almost 20% of employees experience high levels of stress. Almost 8% of total medical care costs were attributable to stress. Furthermore, this study showed that 24.9% of total costs were attributable to these 11 risk factors, all of which we feel are manageable through health promotion programs. This study is very important because it indicates that 25% of annual medical care costs, or about $1,000 per employee, are attributable to risk factors that health promotion programs have been shown capable of managing. This information will better help an employer make a decision to invest the $50, $100, or $200 needed to pay for a program or at least will give the employer the objective data required to justify an emotional or gut level decision to invest in a program (see Table 2-6).

Table 2-6 Cost of Risk Factors as a Percent of Total Medical Care Costs

Risk Category	Cost/ High Risk	# At High Risk	Total Cost Due to Risk	% of Total Costs	Cost/ Capita
Stress	$732	8,518	$6,236,880	7.9%	$136
Former tobacco smoker	$311	14,329	$4,455,029	5.6%	$97
Body weight	$352	9,197	$3,239,919	4.1%	$70
Exercise habits	$173	14,908	$2,574,760	3.3%	$56
Current tobacco user	$228	8,797	$2,004,045	2.5%	$44
Blood glucose	$587	2,271	$1,332,646	1.7%	$29
Depression	$1,187	997	$1,183,439	1.5%	$26
Blood pressure	$199	1,827	$363,317	0.5%	$8
Excess alcohol use	−$52	1,723	−$89,027	−1.1%	$2
High cholesterol	−$14	8,641	−$117,431	−1.5%	−$3
Nutrition habits	−$162	9,278	−$1,500,623	−1.9%	−$33
Total expenditures attributable to high risk per capita			$19,682,953	24.9%	$428
Total medical care expenditures			$78,959,286		

Source: D. Anderson, et al., *Relationship between modifiable health risks and health care expenditures: A group level analysis of the HERO Research Data Base, American Journal of Health Promotion,* 2000.

Table 2-7 Medical Care Costs Associated with Clusters of Risk Factors, Korea

Risk Factor Cluster	With Risk Factors	Without Risk Factors	% Difference
Heart disease risks	190,568 won	99,457 won	149%
Stroke risks	157,922 won	98,707 won	52%
No risk factors		41,515 won	

Source: S. Jee, M. O'Donnell, I. Suh, and I. Kim, *Impact of Modifiable Health Risks on Future Medical Care Cost Expenditures: The Korea Medical Insurance Corporation (KMIC) Study*, in press.

A similar study was recently completed in South Korea and had similar findings (Jee, O'Donnell, Suh, & Kim, in press). Data on a randomly selected sample of over 180,000 employees were analyzed using a protocol similar to the HERO studies. This study found that employees with six heart disease risk factors had medical care costs 149% higher than those with none of these risk factors, and employees with three stroke risk factors had costs 52% higher than those with none of these risk factors (see Table 2-7). It is remarkable that similar trends persisted, even in a country where annual medical care costs are only one, eighth, or about $587 per year (1997 data), of those in the United States (Anderson, G., 1998).

The work of The Health Management Research Center (formerly the Fitness Research Center) at the University of Michigan provides additional support for the connection between health risks and medical care costs. This Center has collected health care utilization and lifestyle behavior data during the past 20 years on almost 2,000,000 individuals working in over 1,000 worksites. They have established long-term data management relationships with nine large employers. These data have allowed them to formulate and test a wide range of relationships between health risks and medical care costs, which are summarized in Table 2-8. A number of these "learnings" are discussed in more detail.

Wellness scores are highly correlated with medical costs. As Table 2-9 shows, individual "wellness

Table 2-8 Key Research Learning and Date Discovered, Health Management Research Center at the University of Michigan

Learnings	Year Discovered
1. High-risk persons are high cost (prospective data)	1990
a. individual risks	
b. cumulative risks	
2. Absenteeism shows the same relationship as medical costs	1993
3. Excess costs are related to excess risks	1993
4. Changes in costs follow changes in risks	1994
5. Risk combinations are the most dangerous	1995
6. Low-risk maintenance is an important program strategy	1996
7. Changes in risk drive changes in cost when targeted to specific risk combinations	1996
8. Wellness scores are highly correlated with medical costs	1997
9. Program participation is related to risk and cost moderation	1998
10. Wellness program opportunities are in preventive services, low- and high-risk interventions, and disease management	1998

Source: D. Edington, *Worksite Wellness; 20 Year Cost Benefit Analysis and Report: 1979 to 1998*, 1998.

Table 2-9 Relationship Between Wellness Scores and Medical Care Costs

Wellness Score	Annual Medical Costs
95	$1,415
90	$1,643
85	$1,800
80	$2,087
75	$2,369
70	$2,508
65	$2,817
60	$2,638
55	$2,818
50	$2,970

Source: D. Edington, *Worksite Wellness; 20 Year Cost Benefit Analysis and Report: 1979 to 1998*, 1998.

scores" derived from the Health Management Research Center's health risk appraisal are highly correlated with annual medical care costs for the same group of individuals. This relationship is important because it allows a proxy measure of medical care costs that can be measured through a simple questionnaire.

The relationship between medical care costs and health risks is further illustrated in Table 2-10, which shows the relative cost of high-risk versus low-risk conditions for actual illness, perceived health problems, physiological measures, and lifestyle habits. Not surprisingly, the difference in medical care costs is greatest for people who actually have a disease compared to those who do not have a disease, averaging 267% higher. Those who have risk factors measured by biometric tests have differences averaging 53% higher, which is very close to the differences for people who perceive problems related to health, satisfaction, and stress. Costs for people with lifestyle risk factors are lowest among these four major categories but still average 16% higher than those without these risk factors. The methodology of this study is different

Table 2-10 Medical Care Costs and Health Factors

Health Measure	Low Health Risk	High Health Risk	Difference
No Illness	$1,773	$4,168	140%
Disease			
Heart disease	$1,875	$8,299	340%
Diabetes	$1,975	$4,669	140%
Cancer	$1,981	$3,456	70%
Other diseases	$1,871	$4,162	120%
raw average difference			267%
Biometric			
Blood pressure	$1,810	$3,732	110%
Relative body weight	$1,881	$2,633	40%
Cholesterol	$2,033	$2,276	10%
raw average difference			53%
Psychological Perceptions			
Physical health	$1,751	$3,756	110%
Life satisfaction	$2,023	$2,769	40%
Stress	$1,857	$2,572	30%
Job satisfaction	$2,056	$2,298	10%
raw average difference			48%
Lifestyle Habits			
Medication/drug usage	$1,874	$3,034	60%
Physical activity	$1,865	$2,462	30%
Smoking	$2,023	$2,290	10%
Seat belt usage	$2,059	$2,007	−3%
Alcohol usage	$2,072	$1,695	−18%
raw average difference			16%

Source: D. Edington, *Worksite Wellness; 20 Year Cost Benefit Analysis and Report: 1979 to 1998*, 1998.

from the Goetzel study (1998) of using the HERO database, so it is difficult to directly compare these results. However, the findings are consistent with each other in general terms.

The Center has collected much of this data to advise its employer clients but to date has published very little of its work in peer reviewed journals. Therefore, the methodology used to draw these conclusions has not been scrutinized by external reviewers and should be interpreted with caution. This work has also not been widely publicized. However, much of their work is summarized in a large monograph titled "Worksite Wellness; 20 Year Cost Benefit Analysis and Report: 1979 to 1998" (Edington, 1998). This monograph also includes almost 600 abstracts of articles published from a wide range of journals and magazines. As the Center's work is published in peer reviewed journals, it will receive wider distribution and provide a recognized valuable contribution to our knowledge base.

One of the Center's most interesting findings involves the relationship between changes in cost and changes in risk. The Center has found that medical care costs decrease an average (median) of $153 with every decrease in number of risk factors and increase an average (median) of $350 with every increase in number of risk factors. The finding that reduced risk factors are associated with reduced costs provides further support for the risk reduction programs advocated throughout this book. The finding that increases in risk factors are associated with increases in costs is a breakthrough discovery if it holds up to further scrutiny, because it demonstrates how important it is to keep healthy employees healthy. This is a critical finding because health promotion programs have often been criticized for attracting the people who already practice healthy lifestyles and not attracting people who do not. Programs do need to learn how to better attract those with unhealthy lifestyle practices, but this finding underscores the importance of also helping those with healthy practices to continue those healthy practices.

The link between medical costs and risk factors that can be modified by health promotion programs is fairly clear from the studies cited above. However, a separate question is whether health promotion programs can reduce medical care costs. At least two dozen studies have addressed this question, and a number of reviews have attempted to summarize these findings (Pelletier, 1991, 1993, 1996, 1999). The most systematic of these reviews was written by Aldana, (1998). He conducted a thorough review of the literature to identify research on the impact of workplace health promotion programs on medical care costs. He then examined the methodology of each study, and determined which ones had experimental, quasi-experimental and pre-experimental designs.

Aldana found 24 studies: 21 (88%) of these studies showed that programs reduced medical care costs, and 3 (12%) showed no impact on medical care costs. Eight of the studies reported the cost of the program and the amount of savings achieved, thus allowing a calculation of the cost/benefit ratio. Savings ranged from $2.30 to $5.90 for every dollar invested and averaged $3.35 (see Table 2-11). Also, the studies having experimental designs reported the highest levels of savings. How should we interpret these findings? The total number of studies published (24) is smaller than we would prefer to have, and it is likely that studies that found negative or neutral results were not submitted for publication or were more likely to be rejected if they were submitted. Nevertheless, the trend is very persuasive. We can conservatively conclude that some health promotion programs are clearly able to reduce medical care costs. The number of studies (8) reporting cost/benefit ratios is far too small to be conclusive,

Table 2-11 Impact of Health Promotion on Medical Care Costs

Medical Care Costs	# of Studies	% of Total
Reduced Medical Care Costs	21	88%
No Change	3	12%
Increased Medical Care Costs	0	0%
Total	24	100%

Cost/benefit analysis: 8 studies
range of savings: $2.30–$5.90 per $1.00 invested
average savings: $3.35 per $1.00 invested

Source: S. Aldana, *The Art of Health Promotion,* 1998.

but again the findings are very impressive. We can also conclude that some programs are apparently able to produce medical care cost savings that far exceed their cost. We need to put these cost/benefit values in perspective. An employer never expects to **make money** on an employee benefit (like a health promotion program) and rarely expects the program to pay for itself in directly measurable savings. Almost any employer would be more than satisfied with an employee benefit that produces a cost/benefit ratio of 1.00, $1.00 in savings for every $1.00 invested; returns of $3.35 for every dollar invested are clearly outstanding.

In conclusion, the relationship between medical care costs and risk factors that can be modified by health promotion programs is quite clear. Also, research on the impact of programs on medical care costs does support the claim that programs can reduce medical care costs. The quality of the research methodology is also adequate. This body of research should be sufficient to persuade an employer that health promotion programs can reduce medical costs. We could not make this statement in 1994, when the 2nd edition of this book was published (O'Donnell & Harris). Furthermore, we can probably increase the savings potential of health promotion programs if we design programs with the explicit goal of reducing medical care costs. To do this, we need to focus more attention on the health risks that are most costly, such as injury and musculoskelatal problems, instead of the health risks with the strongest links to death and chronic disease, such as cardiovascular disease and cancer. We also need to incorporate programs on the wise use of medical services in our programs. A large percentage of services provided are medically unnecessary, and it is possible to train employees to avoid using unnecessary services. (See Chapter 14.) Finally, we need to focus on improving the health of the small number of employees who are at greatest risk for high cost **and** to focus more attention on keeping the healthy employees healthy. Many programs have already adopted the strategy of focusing on high-risk employees, but few have recognized the importance of keeping healthy employees healthy as a strategic focus (Edington, 2000).

Productivity Enhancement

We have long argued that health promotion programs enhance productivity, yet little research has attempted to measure this impact, primarily because productivity is often difficult to measure and the impact of a specific factor, such as a health promotion program, is even more difficult to measure.

In general terms, employee productivity is defined as output per unit of labor. Among blue collar workers, this might be measured in terms of automobiles, toys, tables, or any other product produced per hour. For white collar workers, it might be pages typed, insurance claims processed, or airplane reservations taken per hour. For a sales person, it might be sales closed per month, and for a film producer, it might be films produced per year. In addition to the quantity of units produced, the quality of each unit produced is an important element of productivity; the automobiles, toys, and tables must meet all production standards. To be of value to the organization, pages typed, claims processed, and reservations taken must be free of errors. The sales closed must not be canceled, and the films made must be well-made.

Within the health promotion community, most of our focus to date on productivity has been on absenteeism, primarily because absenteeism is easy to measure. Absenteeism is an important part of productivity. When a worker is absent, he or she normally continues to get paid but produces no work. In some cases, he or she is replaced by someone else. This raises the cost of producing the same level of output. In other cases, he or she is not replaced, and co-workers are required to disrupt their work to fill in for the absent employee. This reduces total output. In either case, output per unit of labor (i.e., productivity) drops. Health promotion programs are expected to reduce absenteeism by helping people stay healthy and thus reduce the need to be absent. This is reasonable as long as illness is the cause of the absence. Some times people take a "mental health" day when they need a break. Other times they call in sick when, in fact, they are staying home with a sick child. The impact of a heath promotion program on these cases is more complex and is better explained

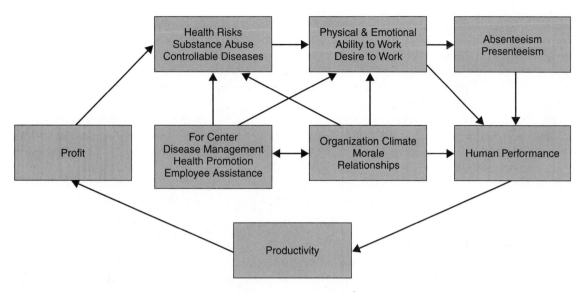

Figure 2-1 Mechanisms Linking Health, Productivity, and Profit
Source: M. O'Donnell, *American Journal of Health Promotion*, 2000.

within a broader conceptual approach, which is illustrated in Figure 2-1.

The Concept

The basic concept, as illustrated in Figure 2-1, is that human performance is higher when people are physically and emotionally able to work and have the desire to work. Higher levels of human performance lead to higher levels of productivity, which in turn can lead to higher profit levels. Health promotion programs play a central role in this model because they can improve health by reducing health risks, helping to manage controllable diseases, and reducing use of avoidable substances. These health improvements lead to improved physical and emotional ability to work. Health promotion programs also improve organization climate, which enhances people's desire to work and directly enhances human performance. This model also asserts that improved organization climate and higher profit levels directly reduce health risks. We recognize that this is a preliminary model that must be tested and refined. We fully expect that the elements within each of the boxes will change and that new mechanisms will be discovered.

Why Is This Concept of Enhancing Productivity So Important Now?

The basic reason is that increased human productivity can lead to increased profits. In operational terms, higher productivity in a manufacturing setting means more product is produced with fewer labor hours of input. Increased productivity in research and development means more and better product enhancements emerge from research labs. Increased productivity in sales and marketing means more products are sold and sales revenues are higher. Increased productivity in management means people receive more effective guidance and coordination. Productivity enhancement has always been important for these reasons, but American business is now in a new era.

The United States is experiencing an extended period of economic growth, full employment, and low inflation. The combination of economic growth and full employment usually stimulates high inflation. Economists have speculated that inflation has been held in check because productivity increases caused by use of computers has allowed growth without increasing costs. This experience has made executives very interested in discovering other new ways to increase productivity.

Their desire to improve productivity is also important because American businesses have entered an increasingly competitive global business environment. American businesses lead the world in most measures of productivity; however, labor costs in the United States are among the highest in the world, and U.S. markets have fewer limitations on imports than virtually any other major market in the world. If U.S. businesses want to continue to compete successfully, they must have higher quality products produced at lower cost through more productive processes.

The situation is further exacerbated by the current labor market in the United States. The labor shortage created by the current economic boom will become more pronounced as the work force continues to age. In the next few decades, more workers will reach 65 and leave the work force than will turn 18 and enter the work force.

Finally, existing developments in computer technology and emerging developments in measurement theory are enabling businesses to measure productivity with greater accuracy and efficiency than ever before.

Just as double digit medical care cost increases in the 1970s sparked a decades-long focus on medical care cost containment, this combination of events has sparked what we expect will be a decades-long focus on productivity enhancement.

How much more productive will employees be who are physically and emotionally able to work and motivated to work because they feel their employer is concerned about their well-being? This remains an open question, one which we expect will receive considerable attention in the next decade. The author has posed this question in formal discussions with dozens of executives and dozens of scientists during the past few years. The most common response from scientists is that employees will be 5% to 10% more productive. The most common response from executives is that employees will be 100% more productive! As we would expect and hope, scientists are more conservative in their estimates. However, executives think of themselves when they answer this question. They know how much more productive they are

when they are full of energy, not distracted by emotional problems, and really want to work. They know they are far more likely to be effective in their creative thinking, negotiating, efforts to motivate people, strategic planning, and any other challenging activity when they feel good and are motivated.

In reality, a factory worker or clerk who has little control over his or her work environment might be able to increase productivity by 5%, 10%, or even 30%. A knowledge worker, such as a lawyer, scientist, writer, salesperson, or senior manager, might be able to increase productivity by 50%, 100%, or even more.

To make this relevant to business, we need to quantify the value of productivity increases. The data supporting a financial payoff from health promotion are probably strongest in the area of medical cost savings, but the greatest potential payoff for health promotion is probably in productivity enhancement. The reason for this is simple. The maximum benefit we can achieve in medical cost savings is to eliminate the cost, or more realistically, to eliminate the costs related to lifestyle risk factors. If we eliminate the total medical care cost, this will save approximately $4,000 per year per employee. If we eliminate the 25% of costs that are related to lifestyle risk factors, we will save approximately $1,000 per year per employee. More realistically, if we eliminate one quarter of the 25% of costs that are related to lifestyle risk factors, we will save approximately $250 per year per employee. Savings at any of these levels would be significant and more than enough to pay for the healthy promotion program, but they are minor compared to the additional revenue and profit we could earn by increasing productivity.

If productivity increases by 1% in a company with a 10% profit margin and that increased productivity can be translated into increased revenues, this will increase profits by 10%. If the profit margin is 5%, profits will increase by 20%. If productivity increases by 10%, profits will increase by 100% with a 10% profit margin and by 200% with a 5% profit margin. A 1% increase in profits in the United States would be worth $80 billion per year, a 10% increase worth $800 billion, and a 20% increase worth $1.6 trillion. Potential returns of this magnitude will grab the attention of even the most skeptical executives and policy makers.

Measuring productivity is very difficult. Measuring the impact of programs on productivity is even more difficult. As we recognized above, most efforts to measure the impact of health promotion on productivity have focused on absenteeism as an outcome measure. Aldana (1998) reviewed the research on the impact of absenteeism on productivity. He found 16 studies on this topic; 14 (87%) of the studies reported reductions in absenteeism after the introduction of the health promotion programs, 1 study reported no change, and 1 study reported an increase in absenteeism as a result of the program. Five of the studies reported cost/benefit analysis values, with a range of $2.50 to $10.10 saved for every $1.00 invested and an average savings of $4.90. The studies with experimental designs had the highest level of savings values (see Table 2-12).

These results are very encouraging, and we should be comfortable in concluding that some health promotion programs can reduce absenteeism and that, in some cases, those savings may more than pay the cost of the program. However, given the small number of studies, we should view these results as preliminary.

Productivity enhancement has become an important focus for American business, and efforts are underway to measure the impact of health promotion on productivity. In the next decade, we should be able to say a lot more about the impact of health promotion on productivity.

Table 2-12 Impact of Health Promotion on Absenteeism

Absenteeism	# of Studies	% of Total
Reduced Absenteeism	14	87
No Change	1	6
Increased Absenteeism	1	6
Total	16	100

Cost/benefit analysis: 5 studies
range of savings: $2.50–$10.10 per $1.00 invested
average savings: $4.90 per $1.00 invested

Source: S. Aldana, *The Art of Health Promotion*, 1998.

Image Enhancement

We have very little data to support the impact of health promotion on image, but it remains a very important motivation for many employers who develop health promotion programs. The recent survey of workplace health promotion programs did show that attracting new employees was identified as an important reason for developing a health promotion program by 67% of employers and retaining existing employees was cited by 76% of employers (Association for Worksite Health Promotion, et al., 2000).

Some of the early health promotion programs were developed primarily for image-related reasons. For example, when the Silicon Valley was emerging in the 1970s at the southern tip of the San Francisco Bay, engineers were in great demand. Companies, such as Apple Computer, Advanced Micro Devices, and Rolm, were growing from zero to thousands of employees in just a few years. College graduates with bachelor's degrees were commanding salaries of $50,000 . . . thirty years ago. Also, many of these companies were developing competitive products with great growth potential. Knowledge of how to develop these products had great market value, so retaining existing employees was even more important than attracting new ones.

Many of these companies realized they could not survive financially by competing for employees solely through salaries; it was much less expensive, and initially more distinctive and effective, to compete based on benefits. For example, an elaborate club-type fitness center could be built for an amortized cost of $500 per employee per year and serve as a beacon to new employees and a morale-boosting perk for existing employees. If that same $500 were added to an employee's salary, it would work out to an increase of about $.24 an hour, still less after taxes. Most professional employees already earning a large salary would not even notice such an increase.

The Silicon Valley is a unique environment, but we have seen similar growth of new health promotion programs in other geographic areas that have gone through rapid industrial growth. For example, this also occurred in the New York City/Connecticut/New Jersey area populated by new corporate headquarters in the 1970s.

Some companies add health promotion programs when it is consistent with their products. For example, during the late 1970s and early 1980s, over half of the hospitals in the United States started selling health promotion programs to corporations and individuals in their communities. Prospective employer clients naturally asked these hospitals how well the health promotion program for their own hospital employees was working. Most of these hospitals did not initially have programs in place but scrambled to launch them. Unfortunately, when hospitals realized it was very difficult to run a profitable hospital-based health promotion program, many discontinued their corporate and community programs, as well as their internal employee health promotion programs.

Programs also seem to develop in industry clusters. For example, health promotion programs are common among employers in high technology, oil, insurance, consumer products, public utilities, government agencies, and, more recently, auto companies.

This industry cluster effect illustrates how benefits are typically added. A rational perspective would lead us to conclude that companies conduct organized prospective cost/benefit analyses to decide which benefits to add and retain. As discussed below, a rational analysis is not always the driving force in decisions about health promotion programs. How many companies have ever tried to measure the impact of their medical care coverage on productivity or even on the health of their employees? Very few. Instead, companies typically look at the benefits offered by their primary competitors and try to match those benefits. This does not mean that they spend their dollars frivolously. They are very aggressive in securing the best price/quality balance and in containing overall costs of their benefits . . . they just don't use the methods we might expect them to use to select benefits based on the returns they provide.

The auto industry in Detroit provides a good example of the clustering effect, the desire to have benefits comparable to competitors, and the nonscientific method by which programs are often added. In the Detroit area, large automobile companies have set the standard of high pay and excellent benefits. This started when the first large auto company was started by Henry Ford. Much like the high technol-ogy companies in California in the 1970s (and the present day), Henry Ford needed to hire a huge number of employees to keep up the exploding demand for cars created when he was able to reduce the cost of each car with the development of the assembly line. He offered hourly wages that were more than double the normal wages for a factory worker. In recent history, the labor unions have been successful in keeping those wages and benefits above market levels. Major employers in the Detroit area set their salary and benefit packages to try to keep up with the automobile companies. During the early 1980s, Ford, then Chrysler, started to add employee health promotion programs. These programs continued to grow in the late 1980s and 1990s despite the fact that in 1991 the United States auto industry had the worst financial performance in its history. Ford, Chrysler, and General Motors lost a combined $7.5 billion in 1991. (Kerwin & Treece, 1992.) A few years later, General Motors began developing plans for its employee health promotion program, a program that is now the largest employee health promotion program in the United States and probably the world. General Motors did have good rational reasons to develop a program: they were the only major U.S. auto company that did not have a program, and they had a relatively old work force and very high medical care costs. Despite these rational motivators, the impetus came from two new members of their corporate board, one of whom was a previous Secretary of Health and Human Services. These board members figured out how to divert existing health-care-related funds; within a few months, efforts to develop a program were underway. Following the lead of the auto companies, employers in southeastern Michigan have continued to develop and maintain employee health promotion programs.

This desire to match the benefits of major competitors is likely to help spread health promotion to workplaces internationally. As companies around the world start to compete globally, they will need to establish an image at least as polished as their major American competitors. They will also need to recruit employees from the same labor pools, and having comparable benefits will be part of the strategy to achieve this. This will be especially true in Asia, where establishing position and saving "face" is such an important part of the culture. (See Chapter 20.)

Combined Motives

It is important to stress that most organizations will have multiple motives for establishing their health promotion programs; some of these motives may not be entirely rational (See side bar: A Counter Perspective: The Emotional Factor). Also, as suggested by Green and Cargo (1994), health promotion programs are so common now that some employers will adopt programs because they realize health promotion makes good business sense. A process to help managers determine if a proposed health promotion program is likely to produce sufficient returns is described in the side bar (See page 42.) titled "How Can an Employer Determine if a Health Promotion Program Will Be a Good Investment?"

A COUNTER PERSPECTIVE: THE EMOTIONAL FACTOR

Why, indeed, do employers invest in health promotion programs for their employees? In the past three decades we have spent untold hours examining this question. We have felt our efforts to answer this question were well spent, because the future of our programs depended on this data. We were right in that feeling, but we may have made a basic mistake in our assumptions.

We have assumed that a decision to invest in a health promotion program is made through a fully rational process, and we have scrambled to accumulate data that show the financial returns of programs.

Ironically, now that we have good data to support the financial returns that can be realized from health promotion programs, we need to recognize that this process of deciding to start or continue a program is not fully rational.

Basically, what we need to start or continue a health promotion program is the emotional buy-in of the person who has the authority to say "YES," the emotional buy-in of the individual who has the authority to approve spending of $50 to $200 per employee per year. That's how much health promotion programs cost. To most organizations that is not very much. On the lower end, it is the equivalent of taking all the employees out for a holiday dinner. At the upper end, it is about as much as landscaping or carpeting a new facility. Spending at this level is not frivolous. Spending at this level does require close supervision to make sure the money is well-spent. However, it does not require the level of sophisticated cost/benefit analysis we have conducted to defend health promotion investments. Major investments, such as the acquisition of another company or the launch of a new product, often have less data to support their returns than we have to support investments in health promotion.

If a health promotion program has the emotional buy-in of top management, it will be approved and continued. If not, the program will never start or will be discontinued when budget problems occur. In a small- to medium-sized company, the president will have sufficient authority to approve investment in a health promotion program. In a large company, a senior vice president will have authority to make an investment of this order of magnitude.

I have come to this conclusion based primarily on my own experience in talking to the top managers who have approved, continued, and discontinued programs. However, there are a few studies that support this position. For example, a study by Wolfe, Slack, and Rose-Hearn (1993) of a small group of Canadian companies showed that senior managers did not list financial savings as the primary management motivation for establishing and continuing programs, although program managers did. Senior managers wanted to enhance morale, and they were not looking for direct quantifiable financial returns.

Also, in a national survey of employers conducted by William M. Mercer, Inc., for the Department of Health and Human Services (Association for Worksite Health Promotion et al., 2000), "keeping employees healthy" was cited by 84% of employers as an important reason for establishing a program. Reducing medical care costs was listed by 75%, and improving productivity was listed by 64% (see Table 2-13). Cost containment was important but not the most important reason.

The Dupont and Pacific Bell health promotion programs may provide further support for this concept. Both of these programs received the C. Everett Koop Award from the Health Project in

Table 2-13 Reasons Contributing to a Business Decision to Offer Health Promotion Program

Keep workers healthy	84%
Improve morale	77%
Retain good employees	76%
Reduce medical care costs	75%
Attract good employees	67%
Improve productivity	64%

Source: Association for Worksite Health Promotion et al., *National Worksite Health Promotion Survey*, 2000.

recognition of the outstanding quality of these programs. Both had published good quality studies illustrating cost savings (Bertera, 1991; Goetzel et al., 1999), yet both programs were discontinued. The reasons these programs were discontinued were never publicized, so we cannot conclude that an "emotional" factor was the cause. However, we can conclude that something other than the medical care cost containment or absenteeism reduction outcomes, which these programs demonstrated, was more important to their respective organizations.

I have always been, and continue to be, a strong advocate for excellent program evaluation and research on the health and financial benefit of health promotion programs, but I think it is important that we be more aware of why and how organizations make decisions to develop and continue or to discontinue our programs. To be successful and survive, a health promotion program must contribute to the mission, long-term goals, and short-term priorities of the organization it serves, and to the special interests of those who approve its budgets. Sometimes these specific interests are unstated emotional factors. Our research and evaluation efforts should address all of these factors.

How Good Is the Quality of the Evidence?

When the first edition of this book was published in 1984, we could only speculate about the financial impact of health promotion programs. Only a handful of studies had been published, and all of them had serious methodological flaws. By the time the second edition was published in 1994, hundreds of studies had been published on the impact of workplace health promotion programs; a large number of them addressed financial outcomes. Our general conclusion in that edition was that most of the studies did have some flaws in methodology that prevented us from making conclusive statements that programs do save money. We devoted a number of pages in that text explaining the methodological flaws of the research and

encouraging researchers to conduct higher quality studies. It is still important for practitioners to be aware of these problems, so we are reprinting a list (see Table 2-14) in this edition on the most common potential threats to internal validity (Conrad, Conrad, & Walcott-McQuigg, 1991). Despite these flaws, we made it very clear that the amount and quality of research supporting the financial returns from health promotion programs was, even then, far superior to the research supporting business investments for decisions with costs similar to those of a health promotion program. After all, these programs cost only from $50 (or less) per employee for a basic program to $250 for the best comprehensive programs in the country. As mentioned earlier, this cost is about as much as a year-end party, carpeting, landscaping, etc. The qual-

Table 2-14 Potential Threats to Internal Validity

Validity Threat	Definition/Description
1. Selection	A threat when effect may be due to pre-existing differences between the kinds of people in the study groups.
2. Attrition	Refers to the dropping out of subjects over time such that the characteristics of remaining subjects at posttest are different from the characteristics of the full group at pretest.
	In multiple group studies, differential mortality occurs when the characteristics of subjects leaving the study are different between the experimental and comparison groups.
3. Maturation	Processes occurring within the respondents as a function of the passage of time; growing older, more experienced, more motivated. In multiple group studies, selection may interact with maturation such that respondents in one group "mature" faster than respondents in another group, regardless of the treatment.
4. History	Refers to the specific unintended events occurring between the pretest and posttest measurements in addition to the treatment variable. In multiple group studies, local history is a threat when events other than the treatment affect one group but not another.
5. Instrumentation	Operates due to improper precalibration of measuring instrument: changes in the calibration of the instrument between the pretest and posttest; or because scale intervals are not equal and change is easier to detect at some points on the measurement scale than on others.
6. Statistical Regression	Tendency for an unusually high or low score to regress or return to a more usual or mean level on subsequent measures.
7. Treatment Fidelity	Refers to the ability to infer that the treatment, or worksite health promotion program, exists in sufficient strength to cause the intended outcome.
8. Diffusion of Treatments	Occurs when experimental and comparison groups have contact, and the comparison group may receive the treatment or part of the treatment from the experimental group.
9. Testing	The effects of taking a test upon the scores of a future testing. Also referred to as *reactiveness of measures*.
10. Compensatory Rivalry among Respondents Receiving the Less Desirable/No Treatment	May operate in multiple group studies when rivalry is engendered among the subject receiving the less desirable treatment or no treatment. Also referred to as the *John Henry effect*.
11. Resentful Demoralization of Respondents Receiving the Less Desirable/No Treatment	May operate in multiple group studies when the comparison group gets discouraged because they were not given the favorable treatment and, as a result, their behavior is negatively affected.
12. Compensatory Equalization of Treatments by Administrators	May operate in multiple group studies when there is administrative reluctance to tolerate inequality of treatments among groups.
13. Ambiguity about the Direction of Causal Influence	Not clear if A caused B or B caused A.

Source: Conrad, Conrad, and Walcot-McQuigg. Threats to internal validity in worksite health promotion program research: Common problems and possible solutions. *American Journal of Health Promotion* 6(2):120. Reprinted with permission.

ity of the evidence we had in 1994 was more than sufficient for an employer to make a decision to invest in a health promotion program. Indeed, by 1990, 81% of employers surveyed had decided to develop some form of health promotion program (Association for Worksite Health Promotion et al., 2000).

Since 1994, numerous additional studies have been published, and the quality of studies continues to improve. The Aldana review cited previously (Aldana, 1998) is probably the best review of the literature on the financial impact of workplace health promotion programs from the perspective of having a systematic search process and summarizing results of the literature as a whole. In addition to summarizing the impact of the studies, this review also critiqued the methodology of each study using the criteria in Table 2-15. The numbers of studies with each level of research rating are in Table 2-16.

Table 2-15 Research Rating Criteria for Individual Studies

*****properly conducted study with randomized control group
**** properly conducted study with comparison group but not with randomized control group
***   evaluation without comparison or control group
**   no intervention but might include long-term or dramatic results from dissemination of information or introduction of a medical agent into a population
*   descriptive, anecdotal, or authoritative

Source: M. Wilson, P. Holman, & A. Hammock, *American Journal of Health Promotion*, 1996.

Table 2-16 Research Ratings of Studies on Medical Care Cost and Absenteeism Reduction

	5 Star	4 Star	3 Star	Total
Absenteeism Reduction	2	9	5	16
Medical Care Cost Reduction	4	6	14	24
total	6	15	19	40

Source: S. Aldana, *The Art of Health Promotion*, 1998

If this body of literature is scored using the criteria developed by David Anderson (Wilson, Holman, & Hammock, 1996), this body of research would receive a rating of indicative to acceptable, which is comparable to the rating I would give (see Table 2-17).

The most important methodological problems in the research on the financial impact of workplace health promotion programs are the lack of sufficient randomized controlled designs, small sample sizes, short duration of the studies, inadequate measurement tools, and inappropriate analysis (Aldana, 1998). Despite these limitations, it is difficult to find many higher quality bodies of research in health care, business, or any of the social sciences for investments of similar order of magnitude. From a practical perspective, the quality of evidence is certainly good enough for a business executive trying to determine if health promotion is a good investment.

Does this mean we rest on our laurels? Should we stop conducting research on the organizational or financial impact of workplace health promotion programs? Definitely not, but we should refocus our efforts in terms of methodology, the scope of our research outcomes, and where the research is conducted. The most important problems with health promotion research are listed in Table 2-18, and suggestions on how to address these problems are discussed below.

Individual employers should continue to conduct high quality evaluations of their programs, examining both the health and organizational outcomes of their programs. However, the primary focus of these evaluation efforts should shift to focus on how well the program supports the organization's mission, long-term goals, and current priorities. To the extent that these goals and priorities include containing medical care costs and enhancing productivity, those outcomes should be studied. Indeed, we suspect there will be a big focus on productivity enhancement in the next decade. These individual program evaluation efforts should be upgraded to address two of the most common problems in research and evaluation: using valid and reliable measures, and using the appropriate analysis. Some of these studies can be conducted with randomized control designs, but for most employers this will be difficult because,

Table 2-17 Research Ratings for Body of Literature

Research Rating	Definition/Description
Conclusive	Cause and effect relationship between intervention and outcome determined by substantial number of well-designed studies with randomized control groups. Nearly universal agreement by experts in the field regarding impact.
Acceptable	Cause and effect relationship supported by well-designed studies with randomized control groups. Agreement by majority of experts in the field regarding impact.
Indicative	Relationships supported by substantial number of well-designed studies but few or no studies with randomized control groups. Majority of experts in the field believe that relationship is causal, based on existing body of evidence, but view as tentative due to lack of randomized studies and potential alternative explanations.
Suggestive	Multiple studies with consistent relationships but no well-designed studies with randomized control groups. Majority of experts in the field believe causal impact is consistent with knowledge in related areas but see support as limited and acknowledge plausible explanations.
Weak	Research supporting relationship is fragmentary, nonexperimental, and/or poorly operationalized. Majority of experts in the field believe causal impact is plausible but no more so than alternative explanations.

Source: Wilson et al., *American Journal of Health Promotion,* 1996.

Table 2-18 Financial Impact of Workplace Health Promotion: Common Research Methodological Problems

Small number of randomized controlled designs
Small sample sizes
Short duration of the studies
Lack of valid and reliable measurement tools
Inappropriate analysis

Source: S. Aldana, *The Art of Health Promotion,* 1998.

in a comprehensive program that includes organization level changes, the best unit of randomization will be at the organization level. Therefore, multiple organizations will be required to conduct this level of study.

The problems of small sample sizes and short duration of the studies will be difficult to correct at the individual program evaluation level except with the largest employers. In examining medical care costs, we need study samples of at least 10,000 people to overcome the volatility of the data. We also need cost data three years before and three years after the intervention. Ideally, we would like to have a situation in which the intervention is offered, withdrawn, and offered again. This type of research might be possible in a small number of very large organizations that have low turnover. These might include the United States Post Office, the military (focusing on career officers), or some of the twenty or so largest employers. However, this type of evaluation will be very difficult for most employers.

Even with the largest employers, it will be difficult to justify the high cost of high quality research. It is not unusual for a well-conducted study on the impact of a health promotion program on medical care utilization to cost $250,000 or more. Also, structuring a program to comply with research requirements might create significant delays in program implementation, causing resentment from the people not having access to the program. All of these extra problems and costs would serve no direct purpose to the employer . . . they already have sufficient data to show them the program can produce positive financial returns.

Another problem, one not recognized by Aldana, is the absence of a clear temporal mechanism to explain the link between health risks and medical care costs. For example, we would expect that people who have risk factors such as hypertension, excess stress, sedentary lifestyle, tobacco use, poor nutrition, and alchohol abuse to have higher medical care costs. However, there should be a lag of many years between the onset of these diseases and the increase in costs and between the elimination of the risk factor and a reduction in costs. If this lag time does exist, how should we interpret a reduction in medical care costs that occurs immediately after a health promotion program occurs? It would be reasonable to expect rapid cost reductions from programs in medical self-care, seat belt use safety programs, and substance abuse treatment, but not most of the other areas. To fully understand the potential of health promotion programs to reduce costs, we need to conduct longitudinal studies.

To address the problems of study design, sample size, and duration of study, we need to create collaborative efforts among employers, private research foundations, and such government agencies as the National Institutes of Health, Centers for Disease Control and Prevention, Department of Commerce, or Department of Labor to design, implement, and fund large scale research studies. The Health Enhancement Research Organization (O'Donnell, Whitmer, & Anderson, 1999) and the American Journal of Health Promotion (O'Donnell, 2000) have already begun some of these organizing efforts, but much work remains to be done. The results of these proposed studies would help set government policy, not necessarily to advise individual employers. This research might focus on producing standardized outcome measures and identifying a) which interventions are best in producing savings, b) characteristics of the most successful programs, c) how to improve the cost effectiveness of programs, and d) how to reach different gender, ethnic, and income groups. However, the first step in this effort is probably to convene these groups to determine research priorities as part of an effort to develop a national research agenda for health promotion (O'Donnell, 2000).

HOW CAN AN EMPLOYER DETERMINE IF A HEALTH PROMOTION PROGRAM WILL BE A GOOD INVESTMENT?

A process is described below to help a manager determine if the program is likely to produce sufficient returns to justify its cost.

Cost/Benefit Analysis Projections

Like any other program in the organization, the health promotion program should not be a frill. It should pay for itself in terms of the benefits it brings to the organization. Some of these benefits will be tangible and measurable, such as reduced medical care costs or reduced absenteeism. Others will be more difficult to measure but equally valuable, such as improved image. Projecting the financial returns a program may generate is not simple, but it can be done and should be done as part of the feasibility study to determine if the program is a good investment for the organization. A "macro-approach" to cost/benefit analysis is described below (O'Donnell & Harris, 1994). The macro approach has seven basic steps, as listed in Table 2-19 and described below.

Table 2-19 Steps in Determining Whether a Health Promotion Program Is a Good Investment

Step 1: Identify and quantify the areas affected by the health promotion program.

Step 2: Estimate the cost ranges of the health promotion program.

Step 3: Determine the percentage savings required in the areas to be affected in order to pay for the program.

Step 4: Ask if it is reasonable to achieve the level of savings required to pay for the program.

Step 5: Add other nonquantifiable benefits.

Step 6: Compare costs to other expenditures.

Step 7: Decide whether the program is a good investment.

Step 1: Identify and Quantify the Areas Affected by the Health Promotion Program

The first step in the prospective cost/benefit analysis is to determine the areas of the organization that are likely to be affected by the health promotion program, identify sources of information on each of these areas, and quantify these areas. Identifying areas that may be affected by the health promotion program will be relatively easy. A sample list of these is shown in Table 2-20. However, in most organizations, identifying good sources of this information and securing accurate values will be difficult. For example, many organizations track absenteeism at the department level but do not keep central records for the entire organization. Collect-

ing data will often require a physical visit to each department and a manual review of informal paper records. This can be very cumbersome in an organization that has a large number of departments located in multiple geographic sites and can easily result in missing data from some departments. Even this labor-intensive approach will not provide absenteeism rates for previous years because old records are often discarded at each year's end. In some cases, absenteeism is traced for hourly workers but not for salary workers. Other productivity-related data, especially how much high quality work an employee completes per week, month, or year, is just not available in most organizations. Fortunately, this is a new area of focus, and we expect to see this change significantly in the next decade.

Table 2-20 Areas That May be Affected by a Health Promotion Program

Impact Area	Source of Data
Productivity-related	
Absenteeism	Personnel records
Desire to work	Employee satisfaction surveys
Morale	Employee satisfaction surveys
Output per unit of time	Specialized studies
Physical and emotional disabilities	Personnel records
Recruiting success	Interviews with employment representatives
Turnover	Personnel records
Health-related	
Life insurance costs	Benefits records
Medical care costs	Personnel records
Other insurance costs	Benefits records
Type of medical claims	Medical utilization records
Worker's compensation claims	Personnel records
External Image-related	
Community	
—Current client's perceptions	Public relations department
—Potential client's perceptions	Public relations department
—Potential employee's perceptions	Public relations department
Product sales	
—Health promotion programs	Marketing department
—Other products	Marketing department

HOW CAN AN EMPLOYER DETERMINE IF A HEALTH PROMOTION PROGRAM WILL BE A GOOD INVESTMENT?

Collecting information on medical care spending is equally difficult. Surprisingly, even moderately large employers sometimes have trouble determining their annual medical care costs. In most cases they will know exactly how much they have paid a specific carrier, such as Blue Cross/Blue Shield, but their payments may not correspond to a specific calendar year. In other cases they may have additional commercial carriers, different carriers for active employees and retirees, and a number of HMOs, all using different calendar years for collecting premiums. This is not to say that the director of benefits could not come up with an accurate measure of current annual medical care costs if given such a directive by the president of the organization. However, it might be difficult to justify this much effort merely to provide information to facilitate a prospective cost/benefit analysis for a health promotion program. In most cases, the compilation of these figures will be left to the person conducting the study, and it is very easy to make mistakes in such compilations. This problem is compounded when collecting information on past years. Among smaller employers, records on health care expenditures incurred in earlier years may be stored in hard copy but not in computer records. This whole process is very time-consuming and subject to error due to missing or misinterpreted documents.

Collecting information on productivity and image are, of course, far more difficult because most organizations do not keep information on these areas.

Step 2: Estimate the Cost Ranges of the Health Promotion Program

The next step is to determine the probable cost of the health promotion program. This may seem difficult to do before the program is fully defined, but in reality it is not difficult to project general ranges. For example, in the year 2000, the annual costs of an awareness level program would be between $20 and $70 per employee: a behavior-change program $60 to $150, including staffing; and a comprehensive supportive-environment program $150 to $350. During the design process, the principal designers often have a good general sense of the level of program and spending that is likely to be approved.

Step 3: Determine the Percentage Savings Required in the Areas to be Affected in Order to Pay for the Program

Determining the level of spending required for the program to pay for itself can be done by dividing the expenditures in the areas expected to be affected by the program by the cost of the program. For example, if annual medical care costs are $4,000 per employee and the program is expected to cost $150 per employee, the program must reduce medical care costs (or moderate future increases) by 3.75 percent to pay for itself ($150 ÷ $4,000 = .0375). Similarly, if the average employee is paid $15 per hour or $31,200 per year, the program would need to reduce paid staff time by 0.5 percent to pay for itself ($150 ÷ $31,200 = .0048076). (Paid staff time might be reduced by enhancing productivity or reducing absenteeism during hours worked. This is a very simple example used for illustrative purposes only.) Of course, if benefits are realized in both areas, the effect required in each would be reduced.

Step 4: Ask if it is Reasonable to Achieve the Level of Savings Required to Pay for the Program.

Determining whether the level of savings required to pay for the programs is reasonable is not difficult or risky if done right. The key is to ask the question not of the analyst or the health promotion expert but of the person(s) authorizing or paying for the program. This question should be asked twice. First, as part of a feasibility study (see Chapter 3), senior managers should be asked to project in very rough terms how much they expect a health promotion program to affect the three major benefit areas: medical care costs, productivity, and image. Second, after the three steps above have been completed and a basic program plan has been developed, the senior executive should be shown his or her earlier estimate and the amount of savings required and asked if that level of savings seems reasonable at a gut level. The analyst can support this process by supplying research articles and answering any questions asked. The analyst should not be the one to answer the central question about whether the required savings are reasonable to achieve.

Step 5: Add Other Nonquantifiable Benefits

Some of the expected benefits will not be quantifiable yet will be very important. For example, if the health promotion program provides an important publicity angle for the employer that is felt to be an important part of a overall image campaign, the program will provide a benefit that is very hard to quantify but is nevertheless important. Including such non-quantifiable benefits will be "frosting on the cake" if the quantifiable benefits show that the program makes sense; it may provide the necessary additional return if the quantifiable benefits are borderline.

Step 6: Compare Costs to Other Expenditures

Comparing the cost of the health promotion program to other expenditures helps the organization do a comparative cost-effectiveness analysis by considering how much benefit is received from current expenditures compared to those expected from the health promotion program. It is often useful to compare the program costs to each of the other employee benefits, such as paid vacation and holiday time; medical, disability, and life insurance; retirement benefits; and any subsidies for cafeterias, parking, club memberships, and other benefits. Comparing it to in-house training costs, tuition reimbursement, and out-of-town seminars helps to put these costs in perspective with other employee development costs. Comparing it to the cost of preventive maintenance and service for equipment and facilities allows developers to ask how much should be spent keeping employees in good working order as compared to equipment and facilities. Finally, it is often useful to identify all the annual expenditures of similar magnitude to the proposed health promotion program in order to allow direct comparison of the perceived benefits of these expenditures relative to the expected benefits of the health promotion program.

In most cases such comparisons illustrate the relatively low cost of a health promotion program.

Step 7: Decide Whether the Program is a Good Investment

The final step, deciding whether the program is a good investment, is relatively easy if the first six steps are followed.

This macro-approach provides a level of detail and sophistication that is acceptable to most business decision makers. Although it is conceptually simple, it is a challenge to implement due to the difficulty of securing accurate information on the organization's financial expenditures.

CONCLUSION

Keeping employees healthy is very important to most employers, and this is the reason most frequently cited by top managers for developing health promotion programs. Many top managers will fund a program because they want to keep employees healthy and because it is "the right thing to do." However, few programs will survive or thrive on a long-term basis unless they contribute to the mission, long-term goals, and short-term priorities of the organization, or to the special interests of those who approve program budgets AND top management sees data on a regular basis that shows the connection between the program and those organizational outcomes.

The most common justification for health promotion programs is medical care cost containment. A fairly persuasive body of research has emerged that shows that people with unhealthy lifestyles do cost more and that health promotion programs can produce savings in excess of their costs. However, saving money through medical care cost containment will be important to employers only when medical care costs are perceived to be a serious problem.

Returns from productivity related outcomes including enhancing morale, reducing absenteeism, attracting and retaining good employees, and making sure that employees are physically and emotionally able to work are likely to be far greater than returns from medical care cost savings. These areas are also more likely to be closely related to the mission, long-term goals, and short-term priorities of the organization. Research examining the relationship between health promotion programs and productivity is scarce, although a small body of literature does show that programs do indeed reduce absenteeism, and that the returns from absenteeism are greater than the returns from medical care cost containment when compared from a cost/benefit perspective. This is likely to be an area of new research in the next decade.

Research or program evaluation on the impact of health promotion programs on medical care costs or productivity is very expensive to conduct. Therefore, most employers must rely on research conducted in other organizations and extrapolate those findings to their own employees. Furthermore, research or program evaluation on medical care cost containment or productivity enhancement is very difficult to conduct, and few if any studies have been able to eliminate all of the methodological problems.

Nevertheless, for the field in general, the data supporting the claim that health promotion programs can reduce medical care costs and reduce absenteeism is of higher quality than the data most businesses have to support other investments of similar cost and thus is adequate to justify an investment in a health promotion program. A protocol is described in this chapter which shows how employers can decide if a health promotion program is likely to produce a positive return for their organization without conducting expensive research or making precise assumptions about financial returns.

Program managers trying to justify their programs will probably be most successful if they determine the mission, long-term goals, short-term priorities of their organization, and the special interests of those who approve program budgets, THEN design their programs to enhance these organizational outcomes. Next, they should design their program evaluation plan to measure the impact of the program on these outcomes, and make sure top management sees this data on a regular basis.

References

Aldana, S. (1998). Financial impact of worksite health promotion and methodological quality of the evidence. *The Art of Health Promotion.* Keego Harbor, MI.

Anderson, D., Whitmer, R., Goetzel, R., Ozminkowski, R., Wasserman, J., Serxner, S. (2000). Relationship between modifiable health risks and health care expenditures: A group level analysis of the HERO research data base. *American Journal of Health Promotion 15(1).*

Anderson, G. (1998). *Multinational comparisons of health care: Expenditures, coverage, and outcomes.* New York: The Commonwealth Fund.

14th annual national survey of employer-sponsored health plans (2000). Northbrook, IL: William M. Mercer, Inc.

Association for Worksite Health Promotion, U.S. Department of Health and Human Services, William M. Mercer, Inc. (2000). *1999 National worksite health promotion survey.* Northbrook, IL: Association for Worksite Health Promotion and William M. Mercer, Inc.

Bertera, R. (1991). The effects of behavioral risks on absenteeism and health care costs in the workplace. *Journal of Occupational Medicine, 33,* 1119–1124.

Brink, S. (1987). *Health risks and behavior: The impact on medical costs.* Brookfield, WI: Millman and Robertson.

Conrad, K., Conrad, K., & Walcott-McQuigg, J. (1991). Threats to internal validity in worksite health promotion program research: Common problems and possible solutions. *American Journal of Health Promotion, 6,* 112–222.

Edington, D. (1998). *Worksite wellness; 20-year cost benefit analysis and report: 1979 to 1998.* Ann Arbor, MI: University of Michigan, Health Management Research Center.

Edington, D. (2000, March). Changes in costs related to changes in psychological and social support risk factors. Paper presented at Art and Science of Health Promotion Conference, Colorado Springs, Colorado.

Goetzel, R. (1998). Relationship between modifiable health risks and health care expenditures. *Journal of Occupational and Environmental Medicine, 40,* 10.

Goetzel, R., Juday, T., Ozminkowski, R. (1999, Summer). What's the ROI? A systematic review of return on investment studies of corporate health and productivity management initiatives. *Worksite Health,* pp. 12–21.

Green, L., Cargo, M. (1994). The future of health promotion. In M. O'Donnell & J. Harris (Eds.) *Health Promotion in the Workplace* (2nd ed., pp. 497–524). Albany, NY: Delmar Publishers.

Health Care Financing Administration 2000. *National Health Care Expenditures, 2000.* Table 1. Web address: www.hcfa.gov/.

Hoechst, Marion, & Russell, (1999). *HMO/PPO/Medicare-Medicaid Digest.* Chicago, IL: SMG Marketing Group, Inc.

The Interstudy Competitive Edge: HMO Industry Report, 9.1 (1999, April). Bloomington, MN: Inter-Study Publications.

Jee, S., O'Donnell, M., Suh, I., & Kim, I. *Impact of Modifiable Health Risks on Future Medical Care Cost Expenditures: The Korea Medical Insurance Corporation (KMIC) Study.* in press.

Kerwin, K. & Treece, J. (1992, June 29). Detroit's big chance: Can it regain business and respect it lost in the past 20 years? *Business Week,* June 29, 1992, 82.

Koretz, G. (2000, January 17). Employers tame medical costs: But workers pick up a bigger share. *Business Week,* January 17, 2000, 26.

Levit, K. & Cowen, C. (1990). The burden of health care costs: Business, household, government. *Health Care Financing Review, 12(2):* 131.

O'Donnell, M. & Harris, J. (1994). *Health Promotion in the Workplace* (2nd ed.). Albany, NY: Delmar Publishers.

O'Donnell, M., Bishop, C., & Kaplan, K. (1997, March/April). Benchmarking best practices in workplace health promotion. *The Art of Health Promotion, 1,* 1.

O'Donnell, M. (2000). Editor's Notes: Building health promotion into the national agenda. *American Journal of Health Promotion, 14,* 3.

O'Donnell, M., Whitmer, W., & Anderson, D. (1999). Is it time for a national health promotion research agenda? *American Journal of Health Promotion, 13,* 3.

Pelletier, K. (1991). A review and analysis of the health and cost effectiveness outcome studies of comprehensive health promotion and disease prevention programs at the worksite. *American Journal of Health Promotion, 5(4),* 311–315.

Pelletier, K. (1993). A review and analysis of the health and cost effectiveness outcome studies of comprehensive health promotion and disease prevention programs at the worksite. *American Journal of Health Promotion, 1991–1993 Update, 8,* 43–49.

Pelletier, K. (1996). A review and analysis of the health and cost effectiveness outcome studies of comprehensive health promotion and disease prevention programs at the worksite. *American Journal of Health Promotion, 1993–1995 Update, 10,* 380–388.

Pelletier, K. (1999). A review and analysis of the health and cost effectiveness outcome studies of comprehensive health promotion and disease prevention programs at the worksite. *American Journal of Health Promotion, 1995–1998 Update, 13(5),* 66–78.

Sonnefeld, S. (1991, Fall). Projections of national health expenditures through the year 2000. *Health Care Financing Review,* 1–27.

Towers Perrin. (2000). *Health care cost survey report of key findings.* New York: United States Department of Health and Human Services, Public Health Service (1993). 1992 National survey of worksite health promotion activities: Summary. *American Journal of Health Promotion, 7(6)* 452–464.

Wilson, M., Holman, P., Hammock, A. (1996). A comprehensive review of the effects of worksite health promotion on health related outcomes. *American Journal of Health Promotion, 10(6),* 429–435.

Wolf, R., Slack, T., & Rose-Hearn, T. (1993). Factors influencing the adoption and maintenance of Canadian facilities-based worksite health promotion programs. *American Journal of Health Promotion, 7(3),* 189–198.

Yen, L., Edington, D., & Witting, P. (1991). Associations between health risk appraisal scores and employee medical claims costs. *American Journal of Health Promotion, 6(1)* 46–54.

Yen, L., Edington, D., & Witting, P. (1992). Prediction of prospective medical claims and absenteeism costs for 1284 hourly workers from a manufacturing company. *Journal of Occupational Medicine, 34(4),* 428–435.

CHAPTER

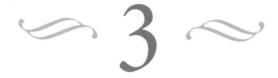

3

Design of Workplace Health Promotion Programs

Michael P. O'Donnell

INTRODUCTION

The purpose of this chapter is to describe a process that can be used by any employer or consultant to design a workplace health promotion program. It draws on a definition of health promotion offered by the *American Journal of Health Promotion* (See Table 3-1).

Table 3-1 Definition of Health Promotion

"Health promotion is the science and art of helping people change their lifestyle to move toward a state of optimal health. Optimal health is defined as a balance of physical, emotional, social, spiritual, and intellectual health. Lifestyle change can be facilitated through a combination of efforts to enhance awareness, change behavior, and create environments that support good health practices. Of the three, supportive environments will probably have the greatest impact in producing lasting changes."

Source: M. O'Donnell, *American Journal of Health Promotion*, 1989.

This suggested design process is significantly influenced by the results of a benchmarking study on the best workplace health promotion programs conducted by the American Productivity and Quality Center (O'-Donnell, Bishop, & Kaplan, 1997). The goal of that study was to identify the best workplace health promotion programs in the United States and determine what made them different from the hundreds of other programs in place. The eight elements unique to these programs are shown in Table 3-2. These elements are organized in a matrix in terms of the impact of the element on program outcome and the level of control a typical program manager would have over building that element into their program. For example, linking the goals of the program to the business goals of the organization has a major impact on the effectiveness of the program and is also something the typical program manager can control. The manager can determine the goals of the organization and align the program goals to support these organization goals. Not surprisingly, another factor that was very important in determining the success of the program was strong top management support. Unfortunately, in the short term, the

Table 3-2 Characteristics of the Best Programs

	Low Impact	Medium Impact	High Impact
high control		• effective communication • communicate evaluation results	• link programs to business goals
medium control		• evaluation component	• incentive program
low control		• strong budget	• supportive culture • top management support

Note: The "low impact" column is empty because the best programs avoid program elements which have low impact.
Source: O'Donnell, Bishop, & Kaplan (1997).

typical program manager has little control over how much support they receive from top management. Interestingly, having a strong program budget was only moderately important in determining the success of a program. Most of the programs studied did have generous budgets, but many of the programs not deemed among the "best" also had strong program budgets. A strong program budget is important, but it is not sufficient to make a program successful.

The striking finding of this study was that management-related factors were more important than programming factors in determining the success of the program. The typical health promotion program manager who is trained as a health expert tends to focus on the health dimensions of a program and often neglects how the program ties into the organization. A team putting together a new health promotion program should build each of these eight qualities into their new program.

The design process described in this chapter has three basic stages: preparing for the design process, collecting data, and determining the program content and management structure for the program. It recognizes the importance of program management and evaluation but refers readers to Chapters 4 and 5 for details on these topics. Short discussions on the

unique needs of workers in industrial settings, and a shift that is likely to occur toward restoring the focus of programs on keeping people healthy versus reducing health risks are discussed in Appendix A and B, respectively.

PHASE I: STRUCTURING THE DESIGN PROCESS

The design process described in this chapter is fairly elaborate and fairly participatory. It assumes that the organization is starting at the beginning, not yet having decided even whether it is ready to develop a health promotion program. Each organization will have to adapt this process to meet its specific situation and the protocols it normally follows to develop a program.

Before an organization starts the design process, it should prepare for the design process by answering four basic questions:

1. How ready is the organization to develop a health promotion program?
2. Are the program outcome expectations realistic?
3. How participative a process does the organization want to follow in designing the program?
4. How extensive a design process does it wish to follow?

Each of these questions is discussed in the paragraphs that follow. See also Appendix A on the Unique Needs of Health Programs Serving Workers in Industrial Settings.

Stages of Readiness

Table 3-3 shows the various stages of readiness in which an organization might find itself and the action it should take for that level of readiness. This is not an exhaustive list of stages, but it covers the full range of situations.

At one extreme, an analyst or program proponent might find that the organization or key decision makers are not at all interested in health promotion. Starting a design process would be a waste of time. Although a feasibility study might uncover some good financial arguments for the program and some pockets of support, it would probably not be taken seriously if no interest exists and would be difficult to complete with a fair degree of cooperation. The analyst or proponent could probably best use his or her time selling the concept.

In another case, the decision makers might be totally sold on the concept and committed to developing a program, but, because of lack of knowledge of program options and benefits, employees might have little interest in the programs. The proponent might de-emphasize the cost/benefit part of the research and follow a design process committed to heavy employee participation.

In some companies, extensive research on feasibility and employee interests may have been completed, and the desired program has been outlined. Additional research can exhaust the companies' patience. The effort might be most successful if it bypasses much of the research and design phases described here and proceeds directly to implementation.

Finally, if the organization is committed to developing a program but resources are inadequate to develop a comprehensive one, the program designer might do additional research to establish the need and attract the resources for a more comprehensive program.

Each organization should determine its stage of readiness within the continuum shown in Table 3 and enter the design process at the appropriate stage.

Setting Realistic Goals

As a discipline, workplace health promotion is in the early adolescent stage. Some significant programs have been in place for almost 40 years, and the vast majority of large workplaces have some form of program (Association for Worksite Health Promotion, U.S. Department of Health and Human Services, & William M. Mercer, Inc., 2000), Health promotion programs are found in all types of large and small, white- and blue-collar, public and private sector organizations. As a science, health promotion is pushing from infancy into its late childhood. The National Institutes of Health finally use the term "health promotion"; major teaching institutions offer health promotion majors; major research institutions are involved in health promotion; over 500 studies have been published on the health impact of programs; and behavior change theory is finally being translated into practical applications. In clinical settings, intensive health promotion techniques have even been able to reduce heart disease (Gould & Ornish, Scher, Brown, Edens, Hess, Mullan, Bolomey, Dobbs, Armstrong, Merrit, Pots, Sparter, Billings, 1995).

Despite this progress, workplace health promotion does have limits. In fact as our science has improved, the limits of our current programs are more clear.

It is realistic to expect program participants to:

- achieve modest weight loss
- stop smoking
- improve cardiovascular condition, muscle tone, and flexibility

Table 3-3 Stage of Organization Readiness

Stage	Action
not interested	sell the concept or wait
interested in concept not sure if it will work	conduct feasibility study
sold on concept	conduct needs assessment
impatient for program	implement quickly

Source: M. O'Donnell, Design of Workplace Health Promotion Programs, 1995.

- reduce stress levels
- develop more nutritious eating habits

It is *not* realistic to:

- expect no relapses to current poor health behaviors
- reverse significantly deteriorated health conditions in less than five years
- expect major improvements in health conditions without major effort
- expect health improvements to continue after a program is discontinued

It is also *not* realistic to:

- expect 100% participation in programs
- see major reduction in health care expenditures within a few years without major investments in the programs
- see absenteeism rates drop off immediately
- see increased job output from all participants in the program
- expect organizational improvements to continue after a program is discontinued

As we perfect our methods, improve our diffusion of knowledge among health promotion professionals, and perfect our execution, we should expect lower relapse rates, greater success in reversing significantly deteriorated health conditions, and higher participation rates in programs. We should never expect major payoffs to the sponsoring organization without a significant investment of resources.

The developer must also be assertive yet realistic about what top management will agree to in the design and implementation of the program. The developer should be assertive by insisting that health promotion be treated as an investment that will benefit the organization, not as an extravagant benefit for employees that can be cut when money is short. The organization may discover through the health promotion program that it should enhance some of its communication practices, refine its organization structure, or do a better job of involving employees in its decision making. Although the need for these changes might be recognized as a result of the health promotion organization, they are changes that will ultimately facilitate the organization's basic goals.

Major shifts that benefit the health promotion program but detract from the organization's basic mission or clash with its culture should not be expected. For example, allowing employees flextime or time off work to participate in programs might have a significant impact on success of the program but may be impractical in many organizations. Flexible (or cafeteria) benefits may generate funds for the health promotion program by allowing employees to apply some of their benefit dollars to programs. However, if the cost of developing and managing a flexible benefit program is greater than the projected benefits of the health promotion program, it has little chance of being implemented.

The ultimate corporate goal of the health promotion program is to make the organization better able to achieve its strategic goals. Therefore the health promotion program must be molded to fit the organization. The organization will not be molded to fit the health promotion program.

Table 3-4 shows the likelihood of achieving various organization goals with each of the different levels of programs. For example, the table suggests it is unlikely that an awareness program will reduce medical care costs but it is probable that a supportive environment program will reduce medical care costs. This table will help the design team and management set realistic goals for the program. The typical struggle occurs when top management wants to achieve a wide range of ambitious organization goals but wants to invest a small amount of money. This chart helps them realize significant programs will be required to achieve significant organization goals. If there is a mismatch between goals and budget, one of the two will have to change. This table should be used during the initial planning stages and later in the process when actual program content is being developed.

Employee Involvement in the Design Process

Participation by employees in the design process is essential to the success of the program. Employees must know that the program is designed to meet their needs and that their involvement is critical to the success of the program.

Table 3-4 Impact of Program Levels on Achieving Organization Goals

Organization Goals	Level 1 Awareness	Level II Behavior Change	Level III Supportive Environment
Enhance Image			
General visibility	unlikely	maybe	very probable
Recruiting	maybe	maybe	very probable
Institutional relationships	unlikely	maybe	very probable
Related product image	unlikely	maybe	probable
Enhance Productivity			
Morale	probable	probable	very probable
Turnover	unlikely	maybe	very probable
Absenteeism	maybe	probable	very probable
Physical stamina	unlikely	probable	probable
Emotional hardiness	unlikely	maybe	probable
Desire to work	maybe	maybe	very probable
Reduce Medically Related Costs			
Medical crises	unlikely	maybe	probable
Medical premiums	maybe	probable	very probable
Disability costs	maybe	probable	very probable
Workers compensation costs	maybe	maybe	probable
Life insurance	unlikely	maybe	maybe

The degree of employee involvement in the health promotion program design process should be significant in all organizations but should fall within the range of employee involvement in other comparable decision processes in that organization. The range of participation levels is listed in Table 3-5.

Table 3-5 Degree of Employee Participation in the Design Process

- top management directs process and makes all decisions
- top management directs process and makes all decisions but seeks input
- top management retains decision making but shares direction of process
- top management shares decision making and direction of process
- employees direct process and decision making

Source: M. O'Donnell, Design of Workplace Health Promotion Programs, 1995.

The employees' level of authority within this design process might be further defined or limited to developing components of the program. For example, top management might have authority to set financial budgets; a consultant or subject-matter expert might have authority to determine specific curriculum and protocols; and the employees on the design committee might have authority to determine specific topics, program components, types of promotional efforts, and operational protocols.

Employee Committee

An Employee Health Promotion Committee can provide a very effective mechanism to ensure employee involvement in the design process. The committee will probably be most efficient if it has six to sixteen members, representing the types of employees listed here.

- Top management spokesperson
- Health benefits manager

- Education and training manager
- Recreation programs coordinator
- Recruiting employment manager
- Medical department coordinator
- Employee association(s) representative
- Union representative(s) (if a large portion of employees is represented by unions)
- Employee(s)-at-large representing various departments
- Middle management representative(s)
- Facilitator
- Communication manager
- Technical expert

A smaller committee is easier to manage; a larger committee may provide better representation of important interest groups.

Committees provide an excellent mechanism for involving employees in decision making, for generating ideas, and for stimulating input from many interest groups. Committees can also be very time-consuming and get bogged down in the decision making process. Committees will be most effective if their purpose and degree of authority in each area

Table 3-6 Topics of Meetings in Typical Design Process

Meeting Number	Topics Covered at Meeting
1	Stimulus for program
	Role and process clarification
	Education on health promotion
2	Education on health promotion
	Presentation of data collected to date
3	Education on health promotion
	Data collection plan
4	Report on data collection findings
5	Synthesis: Organization and health improvement goals
6	Synthesis: Program content and administrative structure
7	Discussion of proposal 1st draft
8	Discussion of proposal 2nd draft
9	Ratification of 3rd draft to be sent to top management

covered is clearly stated and if they are coordinated by an experienced facilitator. Table 3-6 shows the topics of meetings of an actual committee in which the participation level (from Table 3-5) was "Top management shares decision making and direction of the process with employees."

Knowledge and Expertise Required to Design a Health Promotion Program

Employees on the committee should be given authority to set goals and policies to the extent approved by the organization. They should be involved in selecting program topics and developing program protocols, but they should be careful not to exceed their level of knowledge and skill in clinical and organizational areas of health promotion. The individuals responsible for designing the program should have expertise in all of the following areas:

- Organizational theory
- Group process
- Operations management
- Communication and marketing methods
- Motivation techniques
- Design process
- Clinical aspects of health promotion, including
  - health assessment
  - fitness
  - nutrition
  - stress management
  - smoking cessation
  - medical self-care
  - social health

Few organizations will have all of these knowledge areas represented within their existing staff. They can develop or acquire knowledge in these areas by educating existing staff, hiring new staff members with the necessary knowledge, or working with a consultant.

Magnitude of the Design Process

An extensive design process will not be necessary for all organizations. Organizations that have already completed some phases of the process described here can certainly skip those stages. Organizations that know ahead of time that they want a very simple program do not need an extensive process. Organizations working with external vendors can sometimes rely on the vendors' expertise and shorten some of the steps. Each organization must determine the extent of the process appropriate for its needs but err on the side of a more extensive process. The process described in this chapter is probably most appropriate for an organization with 4,000–10,000 employees. Smaller or larger employers or those developing less-comprehensive programs can follow the same framework but adjust the magnitude of the design process accordingly.

Extra time and resources spent on collecting data will provide additional baseline data for later measures of program success. Extra time and resources spent in the design process will increase the opportunity for employee involvement and the likelihood of an appropriate design. Extra time and resources spent on implementation will increase the chances of having a well-introduced program.

Developing and implementing a health promotion program in moderate- to large-sized organizations normally takes 6 to 18 months but can sometimes take years. The typical development timetable is shown in Table 3-7. The time can be on the short side if management is committed to moving quickly and resources are available to design and implement a program. In many cases, however, there is a longer period of "gestation" in which management is becoming familiar with the health promotion concept and is not yet ready to develop a program. In general, the process takes longer in larger organizations, especially if data is required from multiple locations, multiple levels of approval are required, and programs are implemented over time at different locations.

Table 3-7 Development Timetable

Stage of Development	Timetable
Gestation	0–24 months
Assessment	2–12 months
Design	2–12 months
Approval	1–12 months
Implementation	3–36 months

PHASE II: COLLECTING DATA: CONDUCTING A FEASIBILITY STUDY OR NEEDS ASSESSMENT

The second step in the design process is collecting data to gather the information necessary to design the program. This can take the form of a feasibility study or a needs assessment. In some instances, the data collection may be designed to determine if the organization should or should not develop a program. In these cases the data collection might be called a "feasibility study." In other circumstances the decision to develop the program may have already been made, and the data collection may be designed to determine how the program should be developed. This data collection might be called a "needs assessment."

The specific focus and the use of the information derived from these two types of studies will be slightly different, but the tools and process used for both will be very much the same. Moreover, a comprehensive feasibility study can answer both whether or not a program should be developed and how it should be developed. For this reason, this chapter describes how to conduct a feasibility study. Organizations that have already decided to develop a program can make slight adaptions to this approach in data collection.

If an organization expects to evaluate the effectiveness of its program in achieving stated goals, it should expect to collect some data in addition to the basic data collected for the feasibility study. Readers should refer to the chapter on program evaluation (Chapter 5) for guidance in this area.

The feasibility study answers the basic question: Is it feasible for this organization to develop and operate a health promotion program? Five specific questions are addressed in dealing with this basic issue:

1. What are the organization's goals and motives for considering the development of a program?
2. Is a health promotion program a cost-effective investment for this organization?
3. What are the levels of support, need, and interest among employees, middle managers, and top managers?
4. Does the organization have access to the necessary resources within the organization and the community?

If the answers to the first four questions indicate that the program is feasible, the last question is:

5. What are the key factors that should be considered during the actual program design process?

In addition to answering the basic feasibility questions, this study provides much of the background information required for the design process and provides an opportunity to promote the health promotion program among many of the people who will be crucial to its success. It also provides much of the baseline data against which future progress can be measured.

The time and other resources spent on the feasibility study should be determined by the quality of information required and by the impact of that information on the eventual design process. A basic study will take an experienced analyst 40–120 hours over 4–16 weeks if needed data is readily available. If the study is for a large organization, if data are not available, if a major investment may be made in the program, or if there is significant controversy surrounding the prospect of a program, the study can take far more time.

Clarification of Motives and Goals

"We want to have a health promotion program. Let's design one like XYZ Company. The program can reduce our medical care costs, enhance our image, and improve our productivity." This is the typical summary of an employer explaining the concept of and goals for a health promotion program. Unfortunately, if the concept and goals are not further clarified before a program is developed, achieving any of the stated benefits will be almost entirely coincidental.

To be successful, the employer's position should be rephrased. "We want to reduce medical care costs, improve our productivity, and enhance our image. We will develop a health promotion program designed to achieve these goals." With this approach, the employer decides which benefits are most important and then designs a program specifically to achieve them.

It is all right for the organization to:

- think the health promotion concept makes sense and, therefore, to want to develop a program.

- be altruistic and want to improve the well-being of its employees by sponsoring a health promotion program.
- expand the goals of the program after it has had more experience with the program and better understands the potential benefits.

However, in designing the programs, the goals must be clarified and the design process must be directed by the goals. If not, there is much less chance the program will benefit the organization. Major problems in the mismatch of design and goals occur for the following reasons:

- Most managers and executives don't know enough about health promotion programs to realize the time required for the design process.
- Most health promotion program designers don't understand organizations well enough to know the range of benefits that may result from the programs–nor do they understand program design or health promotion well enough to design the program to achieve specific goals.
- Most health promotion program designers don't understand group process well enough to help the organization articulate the goals for the program.
- Many organizations don't adequately clarify the goals of any of their activities.

If the goals of the program are going to be adequately clarified, significant effort will be required to direct the goal clarification process. This will include convincing top management that goal clarification sessions are necessary. The extent of the goal clarification process and the overall program design process will, of course, depend on the extent of the program to be designed.

Most of the goals of the program can be categorized under two headings: management goals and health goals. Management goals will include reduction in medical care costs, enhanced image, and improved productivity. Health goals will address the level of health change desired and the specific area of change, such as nutrition or fitness. Management and health goals will not always be achieved through the same program design, and the relative priorities of the two will certainly impact the focus of the program.

For example, if the management goal of reducing medical care costs were the primary goal, the following process might be followed:

1. Analyze past, current, and projected health care expenditures for patterns and high-cost areas.
2. Determine current and projected future health conditions of employees as they relate to health care expenditures. This is done through health screenings and by reviewing medical insurance and worker's compensation records.
3. Determine which health conditions have the greatest impact on cost and which can be successfully addressed by health promotion programs.
4. Perform a cost/benefit analysis to determine which programs produce benefits that are greater than their cost.
5. Investigate methods to correct or prevent the high-cost health conditions that cannot be affected by health promotion.
6. Develop methods to track the impact of the program on health care costs.
7. Develop health promotion programs that will have the greatest impact on medical care costs. These will probably include special programs for employees with the highest medical care costs, smoking cessation, hypertension control, prevention of lower back problems, auto safety, and general injury prevention programs.

If the goal is a health goal, such as reducing the incidence of heart attacks, the following very different process might be followed:

1. Determine causes of heart attacks.
2. Determine which of these causes can be affected by health promotion programs.
3. Conduct screening of employees to identify cardiac risk factors.
4. Determine which programs are most effective in reducing the cardiac risk factors in the employee population.
5. Investigate methods to correct the cardiac risk factors that cannot be reduced by the health promotion program.

6. Develop methods to track the impact of the programs on cardiac risk factors.
7. Develop the programs that will have the greatest impact on cardiac risk factors. These will probably include nutrition, smoking cessation, fitness, stress management, hypertension control, and social support enhancement.

If the goal is a management goal to enhance the image of the organization, the following process would be followed:

1. Determine the groups and individuals whose perception of the organization is most important.
2. Determine the components of a health promotion program most likely to shape this group's perception and develop these programs.
3. Develop mechanisms to capitalize on the image value of the program.
4. Investigate methods to enhance image other than the health promotion program.
5. Develop methods to track the impact of the program on image.
6. Develop other nonhealth promotion programs that will have the greatest impact on image.

In most cases there will be multiple goals. The challenge to the program designer is to accurately determine the relative priorities of the goals and to design the program to achieve the appropriate balance of benefits in each of the goal areas.

In virtually every case, a third major consideration—in addition to the health and organization goals—will be limits on the human, financial, spatial, and time resources available for the program. These will limit the range of program options considered and will force the programs to be designed in such a way that they achieve the greatest possible return on investment.

The importance of clarifying motives and goals is illustrated by the results of the benchmarking study mentioned earlier (O'Donnell, Bishop, & Kaplan, 1997). The most successful programs tied their program goals to the organization's goals. If the goals are not clarified, the goals cannot be aligned.

It is often difficult for an organization to clarify the goals of a proposed health promotion program. This is true because most executives do not have a precise understanding of the potential benefits of a health promotion program. Also, all large organizations are composed of many decision makers or top managers. It would not be unusual for one manager to expect the health promotion program to reduce medical care costs by 15 percent and another manager within the same organization to expect the program to have no impact on medical care costs. One solution to this problem is to have a clear protocol for clarifying goals. The five-step process outlined here has been used effectively by a number of organizations to clarify goals.

1. Conduct individual interviews with all top managers to determine their goals for the program.
2. After all interviews are completed, review and categorize the goals.
3. Determine which of the stated goals are achievable.
4. Determine the type and cost of programs necessary to achieve the stated goals.
5. Convene a meeting of the top managers. Ask the group to consider the cost and types of programs required to achieve each of the stated goals and to restate their goals in order of priority. Ask the group to reach a consensus on the priority order of the goals.

The goal statement should include a list of organizational, health, and operational goals. It should be as specific as possible. Organizational goals should specify the type and degree of change desired in areas such as image, medical care costs, and productivity. Health goals should include the level of impact desired; the specific health areas of impact, such as fitness, stress management, and smoking cessation; and the specific method used to measure changes, such as surveys, health risk appraisals, or biometric screenings.

Cost/Benefit Analysis Projections

Like any other program in the organization, the health promotion program should not be a frill. It should pay for itself in terms of the benefits it brings to the organization. Some of these benefits will be tangible and measurable, such as reduced medical care costs or reduced absenteeism. Others will be more difficult to measure but equally valuable, such as improved image. Projecting the financial returns a program may generate is not simple, but it can and should be done as part of the feasibility study to determine if the program is a good investment for the organization. A protocol to perform the cost/benefit analysis is described in Chapter 2.

Levels of Support and Areas of Interest

Broad-based and strong support among all levels of employees is critical to the success of the health promotion program. Measuring the level of support during the research phase will show how support figures into the overall design strategy. If support is very strong, that alone may be enough to convince those in power that a program should be developed. If support is very weak but all other measures in the feasibility study indicate that a health promotion program makes sense, program designers should be prepared to allocate a significant portion of resources to promotion of the program. Support should be measured at three levels:

1. Top management
2. Middle management
3. General employee population

Support at all levels is important, but support from top management is probably the most important if the program is going to get off the ground. This support means much more than just agreeing with the concept of the program. Positive answers to all of the following questions would show strong support. For example, will top management agree to the following:

- Will they act as a role model by participating in the program?
- Will they promote the program regularly through formal and informal statements of support?
- Will they provide financial backing for the program?
- Will they provide administrative support through facilities maintenance, financial management,

access to communication channels, and effective supervision?

• Will they be open to reviewing and possibly changing policies that do not encourage a healthy lifestyle?

Table 3-8 shows a set of questions that can be used in structured interviews with top managers. These interviews will also provide an opportunity to deter-

Table 3-8 Questions to Ask Top Managers

1. Program Content
   • What is your concept of a health promotion program?
   • What kinds of programs would work best for this organization?
   • What level of programs (awareness, behavior change, supportive environments) makes the most sense for this organization?
2. Support
   • Would you personally participate in the program?
   • Would you encourage the managers who report to you to participate in the program and to encourage their employees to participate?
   • Would you be available to help in promoting the program to employees in general?
   • Would you be available to troubleshoot if the program needs help?
   • How strong do you expect support for the program to be at each level of the organization?
3. Benefits
   • What do you see as the qualitative and quantitative benefits of a health promotion program for this organization? What percentage improvements would you see in medical care costs and productivity?
4. Budget
   • How much would you budget for the program?
5. Strategy
   • What do you recommend to make the program successful?
   • What do you see as possible obstacles to be aware of and overcome?
6. Organization priorities
   • What is the organization's mission?
   • What are the organization's long-term goals?
   • What are the organization's current priorities?

mine the mission, long term goals, and current priorities of the organization.

Middle managers are the final gatekeepers to the employees' participation in the program. The key question that must be answered about their support is: Will these managers allow, facilitate, and encourage their employees to participate in the programs?

Among the general employee population, the questions of support are simple ones: Do employees want the programs? Will they participate?

As simple as these questions are, measuring support is difficult because most people don't know what a health promotion program is and, worse yet, harbor false impressions. This is evidenced by one senior manager whose young wife was involved in competitive aerobics classes. He said he didn't want to do aerobics because he thought he would look silly wearing tights and dancing to music. He didn't realize aerobics includes a wide range of cardiovascular exercises (like running, swimming, and bicycling) and that none of these programs required wearing skimpy attire. Another middle manager did not want to take a stress management class because she equated this with meditation, which she felt was a form of faddish Eastern religion. She envisioned the group discussions as threatening encounter groups with sexual overtones. Another senior manager was afraid of health promotion programs because he thought he would have to build a fitness facility and talk people into becoming body builders.

Support must sometimes be measured indirectly because of these misconceptions. If a top manager wants to focus effort on reducing medical care costs and has a strong concern for her own well-being and the well-being of her employees, she can probably be counted as an advocate of the program because she supports what it stands for. An employee who wants to exercise more, stop smoking, eat better, or learn to relax and who also feels comfortable accepting guidance from her employer would probably be a supporter of the program even though she does not know what it is.

Personal interviews are probably the most accurate method to measure support in this context. The interview allows the analyst to assess the employees' understanding of the programs and factor that knowledge into the interpretation of their comments. The analyst also has the opportunity to explain the elements of a program and clear up any misconceptions. Unfortunately, interviews take a lot of time. They should be used with members of top management and key nonmanagers, but time usually will not permit extensive interviews with the general employee population.

Questionnaires are the most practical tool to use with large groups of employees, but they do have some limitations. One of the biggest limitations is that the analyst does not know how the employee's understanding of the questionnaire or misconceptions about health promotion programs might bias the answers. Validity and reliability testing can reduce this problem, but most health promotion managers do not know how to perform these tests. Also, response rates to such questionnaires are often less than 30% of the employee population. This is problematic because those who do not respond often have different opinions and practices than those that do respond. Group interviews, called focus groups, can supplement the information provided by questionnaires.

Questionnaires for managers might address the following issues:

- perceptions of levels of specific problems in the organization in areas that may be impacted by the health promotion program
- beliefs on the potential impact of a health promotion program in the organization's specific problem areas
- managers' general level of support for the program
- program content interests

Points to address in questionnaires sent to employees should cover the following:

- current health practices in each health area (e.g., exercise, nutrition, etc.)
- interest in improving health practices in each health area
- interest in participating in programs sponsored by the employer in each health area
- perception of how well the employer is encouraging positive health practices in each health area

Questionnaires to measure employee's health practices, interests, and levels of perceived organizational support can be developed internally or purchased from external vendors. External vendors can also take on the time-consuming task of tallying and summarizing responses. Developing a high-quality questionnaire is difficult and time consuming and should not be attempted unless the developer is skilled in this area. Newly developed questionnaires should be refined for clarity through pilot testing and analyzed for psychometric properties (validity and reliability) through further testing. Without this type of testing, it is not likely that the information collected by the questionnaire will be very useful. Also, it is critical that responses are received from a sufficiently large sample. (See the research methods section of Chapter 5 for information on sample size and psychometrics.)

Vendors selling standardized questionnaires should be asked to demonstrate that their questionnaires have strong psychometric properties. Also, standardized questionnaires should be used only if they include the specific information relevant to the program design effort.

A growing number of vendors can develop custom questionnaires to address for individual needs of different organizations, process the responses, and provide summary reports for a reasonable cost.

Some organizations use a health risk appraisal (HRA) to collect information to design a program. This is a tempting strategy because the HRA does measure employee health risks and provide computer tallies of the results. Unfortunately, this is a more expensive process, and, more importantly, because the HRA requires so much information from employees, the response rate is often low and biased toward people who are interested in making health improvements.

Discussing specific questionnaire content is beyond the scope of this chapter. However, any questionnaire attempting to measure employee health behaviors and interest in participating in programs will be of limited value if it does not measure the employees' readiness to change each health behavior (Prochaska and Velicer, 1997). This concept is discussed in more detail in Chapter 7 on theory-based strategies. Understanding stage of readiness to change is critical to preparing the types of programs most appropriate for the population and for projecting participation rates.

Access to Resources

The resources required to develop and operate the program include money, space, technical knowledge, and staff to run the programs. The organization's ability to finance the program is independent of the cost/benefit value of the program. In addition to recognizing the cost/benefit value, the organization must have access to liquid assets to develop and operate the program. An organization might project it will earn $2 for every $1 it invests in the program; but if it does not have sufficient cash reserves, it may not be able to start the program.

Space is often a problem for organizations located in or close to urban areas, especially when they want to provide fitness facilities. Fortunately, many programs do not require fitness facilities or extensive space.

Technical knowledge on program design, curriculum development, and health assessment–among other areas–is necessary to develop the program. Skilled staff are required to operate it. The organization must have these resources within its employee group or be able to contract for them in the community. Contracting for these services will not be a problem for most organizations in urban settings in the United States but may be difficult for organizations in small towns or in countries that do not have extensive health promotion capabilities.

Program Development Issues

After the organizational goals are clarified, the cost/benefit analysis is completed, levels of interest are measured, and support and access to resources are determined, the organization should be able to determine if it is feasible to develop a health promotion program. If it determines that the program is feasible, it should then address program development issues. The basic program development question it must answer is: If the health promotion program seems to be a good investment of the organization's resources and the organization can draw all the necessary resources from itself and the community, how should it proceed in developing the program? More specifically:

- What departments and individuals should be involved in developing the program?

- What are the various combinations of community and organizational resources that can be used to develop the program?
- Which of the program focus options seem to be most appropriate for achieving the stated organization and health goals?
- What will be the major obstacles to overcome in developing the program?

The answers to these questions give management a clear view of what is required to move to the next step–developing program content.

PHASE III: PROGRAM DESIGN: DEVELOPING PROGRAM CONTENT AND MANAGEMENT STRUCTURE

Program design is the third major phase in developing the program. Although this phase is described as having finite limits–starting after the feasibility study and ending before implementation–the actual design of the program will continue to evolve as it becomes integrated into the organization. This evolution will be visible if the program has a scheduled evaluation and readjustment phase or is implemented on a pilot or phased-in basis. The program will continue to evolve in all cases, even when the evolution is not visible.

Results of the Program Design Phase

Just as the feasibility study produces a guide to lead into the program design phase, the program design phase produces a plan for implementation. The plan should be directed by a clear statement of the health change or lifestyle goals and the organizational goals of the program. Specific descriptions of program contents, program and corporate-level management systems, financing arrangements, use of outside vendors, participant policies, and an implementation schedule are also included. In many cases, specific program curricula will be developed during the design phase. This will be true less often if the program is going or phased in slowly or if course curricula are to be supplied by an outside vendor.

Factors Influencing Program Design

The importance of clearly stating the program's organizational and health improvement goals in such a way that they can guide the design process has been discussed. Unfortunately, it is often very difficult to position the program's goals as the primary factor impacting the design of the program. A myriad of political forces can often skew the focus of the design. A good program designer may be able to recognize these forces and channel them to support, rather than derail, the stated goals of the program in many cases. In other cases, the program designer may be able to recognize but not influence these factors.

Quality of the Design Process

The first challenge will be to ratify stated program goals that reflect the needs of the organization. Top management may have priorities different from managers and employees. The design team's lack of understanding of health promotion programs may further confuse the goal ratification process. The impact of these difficulties can be reduced by education of the design team on the history, operation, and expected benefits of health promotion programs.

Securing Employee Support

The problem of securing employee and middle-management support for programs proposed by top management exists in any large organization. Extensive management processes have been developed to address this problem. The impact of the problem can be reduced if it receives appropriate attention. This is especially important in the design and implementation of a health promotion program because it affects each participant in a very personal way. The most effective strategy is probably to involve employees and managers in all aspects of the design and management of the program, to design the program to meet their specific needs, and to keep them well-informed of program developments.

Impact of the Program on Design Committee Members' Jobs

The development of a program can have a major impact on the jobs of managers operationally linked to the program, e.g., benefits managers, facilities managers, training directors, and managers of employee health. The new program may increase their power base, threaten their turf, increase their work load, or expose the quality of their work. In fact, in most cases a new health promotion program will focus new attention on the management of medical care costs, rates of absenteeism and turnover, and productivity levels. This is one of the spin-off benefits of the health promotion program. The program often provides a non-threatening environment in which to address these problems. Nevertheless, the initial exposure of these problems is often very threatening to the manager(s) in charge of these areas.

Knowledge and Experience of Design Committee Members

The background of the design team members will have a major impact on their input into the design process, especially until health promotion programs are more common. A facilities manager may have an orientation toward fitness facilities, a training director toward classes, a nurse of physician toward screening programs, and a recreation leader toward sports and other fun events. Any exposure team members have had to other programs will further influence their input. If the same group were on a team designing a computer system, their biases would have less impact on their input because they would not feel knowledgeable about computers and would defer to those with technical expertise. However, most people feel they know a lot about health and health habits and can personalize the program to their own situation. Consequently they are more vocal and allow their own personal preferences to affect their input.

Profitability and Organization Transitions

Unrelated cycles of the organization will make a difference in the design of the program. These cycles can postpone the development of the program, speed up the process, or shift its focus. A pending corporate relocation might postpone the program's development until the move is made. However, the construction of new corporate facilities and the initiation of new management programs that usually accompany such a move might facilitate implementation of the program. A high-profit year can free funds to develop the program. A low-profit year can make funds difficult to come by. Ironically an organization in a poor profit situation especially needs to enhance productivity, reduce medical care costs, and correct image problems that health promotion programs address. Further, the cost of a health promotion program is usually not so great that it would be a significant drain on funds. Nevertheless, in tight financial times, new programs and programs not contributing directly to the core business of the organization are often discontinued or delayed.

DESIGN OPTIONS: PROGRAM CONTENTS

Design decisions made during the design phase focus on the contents of the program, the organizational system to manage the program, and the policies governing participation in the program. The three major decisions made about program contents center on (a) the desired level of impact of the program, (b) the desired intensity of the program, and (c) the topics covered by the program.

Level of Impact

The most important decision on program content is the level of impact desired. As discussed in the Preface, awareness programs have the impact of increasing knowledge but have very little impact on behavior. Behavior change programs help people change specific health behaviors, such as quitting smoking, starting to exercise, learning to manage stress, etc. Unfortunately, after people complete these programs, they often revert to their previous unhealthy lifestyles (O'Donnell, 1997). Supportive environment programs are designed to create an environment that encourages people to practice healthy lifestyles on a long-term basis. Supportive cultural environments were one of the

eight characteristics of the most successful programs discovered in the benchmarking study (O'Donnell, Bishop, & Kaplan, 1997). The most successful programs include all three approaches (Heaney & Goetzel, 1997). Also, as shown in Table 3-4, it is important to stress that the supportive environment programs are most likely to achieve the organizational goals that most organizations want to achieve.

Level of Intensity

The level of intensity of the program is determined by the degree of success desired in the health change goal and the level of intensity needed to achieve success. For example, in an awareness program, a weekend health awareness retreat is going to have a greater chance of raising the participants' health awareness than a health fair held at lunchtime. A behavior change course using extensive audiovisuals and a high ratio of staff to participants has a greater chance of success than a self-study course. A supportive environment that includes extensive exercise facilities, frequent incentives to practice healthy behavior, and top management support will have a greater chance of success than a less intensive program. Factors determining the level of intensity include the quantity of resources invested, staff levels provided, and time spent by the participants in the programs. The increased intensity of the program will translate to increased success to the extent that the program is well-designed. The most appropriate level of intensity will also be determined by the health conditions and health practices of specific employees. As discussed in Chapter 2, 10% of the employees are responsible for 70% of the medical care costs. If the goal of the program is to reduce medical care costs or to reach those with the greatest health risks, it will be advisable to provide high-intensity programs to these employees.

Program Topics

Selection of topics will be relatively easy once the program goals are clearly stated and the desired level and intensity of the program are determined. Table 3-9 shows the type of programs that might be

Table 3-9 Programs Most Appropriate for Health Goals

Hypertension
Medical evaluation
and prescription
Nutrition fitness
Weight control
Smoking cessation
Stress management

Obesity
Fitness
Nutrition
Self-esteem training
Stress management
Weight control

Stress
Fitness
Child care
Employee assistance
program (EAP)
Policy review
Stress management

Smoking
Smoking policy
Smoking cessation
Fitness
Weight control
Stress management

Table 3-10 Programs Most Appropriate for Organization Goals

High medical care costs
Medical self-care
Risk rating
Hypertension control
Injury control
Smoking policy
Smoking cessation
Medical coverage

Low morale
Dependent care facilities
& programs
Visible fitness facilities
Employee Assistance
Programs (EAP)
Policy review
Incentive programs
Recreation programs
Other visible programs

Low productivity
Policy review
Fitness programs
Dependent care facilities & programs
Stress management
Comprehensive programs

most appropriate for different organizational goals; Table 3-10 shows the type of programs that might be most appropriate for different health goals. Both of these tables of programs were developed by a health promotion design committee designing an actual program. They are not intended to be the only programs appropriate for the health and organization problem areas shown. In many cases the

program's health goals are not very specific and are instead directed toward improving employees' overall well-being. In those cases a broad range of topics is normally advisable, and program topics might be selected based on what is expected to be most popular.

Also, it is critical to offer programs that are appropriate to each of the major stages of readiness to change. For example, the needs assessment might show that 25% of the employees are smokers, and among the smokers, 40% are in the precontemplation stage, 40% are in the contemplation, and 20% are in preparation. (These would be typical findings.) Only the employees in preparation are likely to join a formal quit-smoking course. In an organization with 1,000 employees, that would mean 250 smokers, 50 of whom are in preparation. If half of them are able to sign up for a quit-smoking course, that would be 25 smokers, enough for one or two courses. Strategies need to be developed for the other 225 smokers. For the remaining 25 in preparation, self-study quit-smoking programs might be offered. The employees in contemplation might be willing to read information on the health hazards of smoking. The employees in precontemplation will probably be unwilling to listen to quit-smoking messages and may even "tune out" on this issue to the extent they will not even be aware of quit-smoking programming efforts. Table 3-11 shows strategies that might be appropriate for each of the stages of readiness to change. These strategies can be adapted to each of the health behavior areas.

Modeling Best Programs

Another factor to consider in developing program topics is to model the programs found in the best practice programs in the benchmarking study (O'-Donnell, Bishop, & Kaplan, 1997). Each of these "best practice" programs included incentive efforts, effective communication efforts, and supportive cultures. (Supportive cultures were discussed above.)

Effective communication programs should include awareness programs to reach the employees in precontemplation and contemplation. They should also include effective marketing programs to com-

Table 3-11 Stage-Appropriate Strategies for Smokers

Precontemplation to Contemplation
- unconditional acceptance of the smoker as a person
- high information, low pressure
- indirect messages on outcome efficacy
  - –health risks of smoking for other people
  - –health, financial, social benefits of quitting for other people
  - –importance of being a healthy role model for children/students
  - –health impact of secondhand smoke on other people
- use fear with caution: get attention, don't immobilize
  - –requests from children to quit
- incentive programs: a different reason to think about quitting
- recruit into other health promotion programs

Contemplation to Preparation
- direct messages
- enhance outcome efficacy (benefits of quitting)
- enhance self- (behavioral) efficacy

Preparation to Action
- set quit date and visualize not smoking
- enroll in quit-smoking course
- realistic review of challenges of quitting
- enhance behavioral self-efficacy
- ex-smoker support networks

Action to Maintenance
- participate in quit-smoking course
- enhance self- (behavioral) efficacy
- enhance outcome efficacy
- ex-smoker support networks

Maintenance to Termination
- reinforce self- (behavioral) efficacy and outcome efficacy
- maintain ex-smoker support networks
- train as quit-smoking leader

municate program offerings to all employees. The key here is not just to have a communication effort but to have a communication effort that is professional in appearance and effective in reaching all employees.

The primary impact of incentive programs is to enhance participation. This is critically important because, as discussed above, only the employees in preparation will be ready to join actual programs, and this typically represents only 20% of the employees. Incentives may be an effective way to attract the attention of the other 80% of the employees. Incentives can be simple small-prize giveaways to people who complete a health screening or class or rebate programs for those successful in making behavior changes. They can also be more elaborate ongoing systems. To date, incentive programs do not seem to have much impact in actually changing health behaviors (Matson, Lee, & Hopp, 1993). Also, as discussed in Appendix B, the relative priority of keeping healthy employees healthy, versus making high-risk employees healthy, needs to be considered.

Finally, all programs should be consistent with behavior change theory, which is discussed in the Chapters 6, 7, and 8 on strategies and in the intervention chapters, 9 through 17.

Developing a Management Structure

Important management decisions to be made during the design process include where to place the program in the organization structure, how much staffing is required, how to build strong top management support, how to finance the program, how often to use vendors and consultants, who will be eligible to participate, what will be the necessary operating procedures, and how to evaluate the program.

Location in the Organizational Structure

The placement of the health promotion program in the organization will depend on the focus of the program and the related organizational goals; rank within the organizational hierarchy; and personalities, images, and work loads of various departments.

Program Focus and Goals

It makes sense to pair the program with the department most closely responsible for achieving the health or organizational goals the program is designed to achieve. If the program goal is educational, the training and development department might be most appropriate. A program centered on health screening and risk reduction might fit best in the medical or employee health department. A fitness facility with very little programming could be supervised by the facility's management department. The benefits department might be appropriate if the program is designed to reduce health care expenditures. A recreation-centered program might fit well within the employee association. If the program focus is broader and is designed to improve the overall well-being of the employees, direct management by the human resources department probably makes the most sense.

Organizational Hierarchy

The health promotion program should be at a level high enough in the organization that the manager has direct access to top management when necessary and is on the same level as line managers supervising the employees who will be enrolled in the programs.

Personalities, Images, Work Loads of Managers and Department

A new health promotion program is in a precarious position. Because it is a new concept that is sometimes not very well-understood, much of its long-term success will depend on how well it is positioned at its inception. Ideally, the department responsible for the health promotion program should have a positive image. The manager supervising the program director should be well-respected, very supportive of the concept, a good role model, and have sufficient time to give strong support for the program during its inception.

Linkages with Other Departments

The health promotion program will normally be designed to achieve numerous organizational goals, including reducing health care expenditures, improving the corporate image, reducing absenteeism, and increasing work output. In most cases, specific departments in the organization are responsible for each of these areas. Therefore, each of these departments should be linked to the health promotion program. Additionally, other departments–such as communications, public relations, and plant management–will be important to the successful day-to-day operation of the program and should also be linked to the program. Finally, the participation of the employees from all departments in the organization is critical to the growth and survival of the program. Linkages to all of these staff support departments and to line managers in other departments should therefore be established.

The optimal mechanism for the linkage to each of these groups will be different in each case. Committees are appropriate in some cases; however, in order to be effective, they should have clear tasks and be well-managed. Recruiting key managers and employees to serve as volunteers in responsible operational roles in the program can also work.

If the program is managed by a support department such as human resources, additional links should be made directly to top management. One method is to appoint a top line manager as a figurehead leader of the program. The program manager would be responsible for all administrative functions, but the figurehead top manager would be available for troubleshooting and public relations efforts. This is analogous to the city manager/mayor form of government used in some cities or the executive director/honorary national chairperson of a national campaign.

Staffing Levels

The benchmarking study determined that the best programs have approximately one full-time professional staff person for every 1800 employees (O'Donnell, Bishop, & Kaplan, 1997). This figure is also consistent with the staffing ratio recommended by a number of major program management companies. See Chapter 4 on program management for more details.

Modeling Best Programs to Build Top Management Support

Having strong top management support is one of the characteristics of the best health promotion programs. Which came first? In most cases, the former preceded the latter. Many programs become excellent because they have strong top management support. Despite this fact, program developers should focus on this point as they develop their program. First, they should tell top management that strong support is one of the eight ingredients for a successful program. This may motivate some top managers to become more involved. Second, developers should ask top managers what they need to do to insure strong support from top management, make sure those things are done, and make sure top management knows these things are being done. As discussed earlier, the important factor in developing top management support is probably linking the program to the organization's goals and making top management aware of how the program is supporting those goals.

Financing the Program

The employer should not assume that all financial support for the program must come directly from the company's general operating fund. However, the company should be prepared to support the program if other sources are not secured and to provide most of the support in all cases. Some sources of support include the following:

- Direct contribution from the employer
- Direct cash support from participants (memberships or fee-for-service)
- Cafeteria-style benefits (for example, trading some vacation days for participation in the program)
- In-kind contributions from health insurance companies, managed care organizations, or pharmaceutical companies

The ultimate source of support for the programs will come from the savings they produce. However, recognizing and securing these savings will require significant effort, time, and cooperation from such supporting industries as insurance carriers and medical providers. In the short term, these savings cannot be counted on to fund the program. In determining how to fund the program, the employer should consider the following issues:

1. The program is being developed because it is believed to be a cost-effective method of achieving the organization's goals. The goals will be achieved only if the program is adequately funded.
2. Charging program participants may motivate some employees to maintain health improvements achieved in the programs but may discourage others from participating.
3. The magnitude of the employer's benefits will be in proportion to the number of employees in the program. Any charges to participants should be structured in such a way that they do not discourage initial or long-term participation in the program.
4. Contributions to a health promotion program available to all employees are currently considered "welfare benefits" by taxing authorities. Like health insurance, workers compensation, and vacations, the employee is not taxed for the benefit. This is in contrast to company cars, dinner club memberships, and other benefits that are considered a form of income for the employee and thus are taxed.
5. Some insurance companies and managed care organizations offer health promotion programs to their client organizations at no charge. Most of the time these programs are offered for marketing purposes, with the goal of attracting new employer clients or retaining existing clients. Sometimes, the programs are offered with the expectation of improving health and thus reducing medical care costs. In both cases, these programs can be an excellent augmentation to an employer's health promotion programs and should be accepted if they are compatible with the organization's health promotion program. However, the employer should not depend on such programs to continue to be free on a long-term basis and should always be prepared to fund the full cost of the program.
6. Some pharmaceutical companies offer health promotion materials to employers at no charge. These materials are often high quality and should be accepted if they are compatible with the organization's health promotion program. However, the pharmaceutical company's goal will always be to sell their medications, so employers should always examine materials closely for medication sales messages.

The benchmarking study (O'Donnell, Bishop, & Kaplan, 1997) found that the average annual budget among the best programs was approximately $200 per eligible employee (not per participant) in 1996 dollars. This is consistent with the author's experience that an internally managed comprehensive program that includes awareness, behavior change, and supportive environment programs costs approximately $135 per employee (not per participant) in an organization with at least 4,000 employees. These figures include staff salaries but do not include office space, employee benefits, overhead benefits, staff recruitment, initial training costs, or the cost of top management's supervision of the program. If fitness facilities are included, this will add an additional $100 to $200 per employee (not per participant), including amortization of construction costs over 15 years but not including land acquisition or space costs. Fitness facility costs can often be reduced by charging employees a modest membership fee.

Use of Vendors and Consultants

In the United States, vendors and consultants are available to serve virtually all the employer's needs related to the health promotion program. They can design the program, hire staff, build facilities, manage programs, present courses, supply materials and equipment, and evaluate programs. They can do this on a turnkey basis or piece-by-piece.

The criteria and methods used to determine whether to use vendors, how much to use them, and how to select them should be the same as those used in evaluating the use of vendors for other projects. The employer's experience in going through the same questions in developing the organization's health insurance plan, its computer capabilities, or its facilities can be helpful models. The individual responsible for these decisions should have some knowledge of health promotion and be skilled in dealing with vendors. If vendors or consultants are involved in the design or management of programs, the arrangement should be structured in such a way that the employees feel that they, and not the vendor, own the program.

Table 3-12 shows estimated program costs from two companies that provide health promotion program management services. Outside management companies also normally have a wide range of experience and other support services that can be drawn upon as needed. When all the hidden costs of an internally managed program are considered, the costs of managing a program internally and externally are comparable. Working with an outside management company also has the advantage of being able to start a program quickly and terminating it when the contract period has passed. It is not surprising that a large portion of workplace health promotion programs are now managed by external management companies.

Table 3-12 Estimated Program Costs (1999 dollars)

	Author's Experience	Stay Well[a]	American Corporate Health Programs[b]
Home delivered programs	$45	$35–$50	no estimate
Basic program	$10–$50	$50	$50
Comprehensive onsite program (without fitness center)	$135	$125–$175	$75
Fitness center			
operating costs	$80	$125–$175	$100–$150
amortized capital expenditures (no swimming pool)	$40	$30–$50	no estimate

[a]Provided by David Anderson, Vice President, Programs and Services, The Stay Well Company.
[b]Provided by Dick Robson, President and CEO, American Corporate Health Programs.

Eligibility for the Program

The size of the program and the method for selecting employees eligible to participate in the program should be determined during the design phase.

The program can be made available to all employees or only to selected employees. It can be offered to spouses, children, unmarried partners, and retirees. The eligibility policy should be determined by the goals for the program and the resources available to develop it. The program might start as a small pilot project and grow on a phased-in basis until it becomes available to all employees. In other cases, it might start small and stay small. It might be offered to employees in one division or location; to top management; to employees with specific health conditions; to a random cross section of all employees; or on a first-come, first-served basis.

Regardless of which employee groups are eligible to participate in the program, spouses and dependents should be eligible for the program if the program hopes to enhance health or reduce medical care costs. Family participation is important if the goal is improving health habits because it is very difficult for an employee to change a health habit without the support of key family members. This is especially true for smoking and nutrition. Similarly, the family is important if the goal is to reduce medical care costs because spouses and dependents account for up to three-quarters of all medical claims.

Operating Procedures

Procedures for operating the program should be outlined during the design phase. These procedures will include staffing plans, scheduling, promotional methods, facilities maintenance, budgeting, materials and equipment management, and evaluation methods. Some of the details of these procedures will be refined during implementation and initial operation. These are discussed in Chapter 4.

Evaluation Plan

An evaluation effort is an important part of every health promotion program. The bench-marking study (O'Donnell, Bishop, & Kaplan, 1997) showed that the best programs have evaluation efforts in place and, equally important, that they communicate their evaluation results. In addition to measuring the impact of the program on health outcomes, the evaluation effort should measure the extent to which it addresses the organization's long-term goals and current priorities. Of course, these findings should be communicated to top management.

The evaluation plan–including what will be evaluated, when it will be evaluated, how, by whom and for what purpose–should be specified as the program plan is developed. If the evaluation plan is not developed and approved as part of the basic program plan, it will be very difficult to start the evaluation once the program is up and running. Also, some baseline measures will need to be recorded before programs are launched so that progress against these values can be assessed. If the evaluation plan is not developed, it will be difficult to know which baseline measures need to be taken.

Five to 10% of the budget should be allocated to program evaluation.

Details on how to develop an evaluation plan are in Chapter 5.

CONCLUSION

One of the biggest challenges facing all health promotion professionals is adapting their content training in exercise, education, psychology, nutrition, nursing, or any other clinical area to work settings. Very few of these professionals receive training in management procedures. This becomes very evident when they attempt to design a workplace health promotion program. Fortunately, protocols like those described in this chapter have been developed that work. Our challenge in health promotion program design is not so much to develop better design techniques but to make health promotion professionals aware that they exist and to improve their ability to follow them.

Note: This chapter is partially excerpted from the workbook, *Design of Workplace Health Promotion Programs,* also written by the author (O'Donnell 2000).

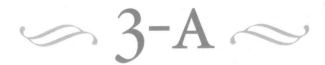

Tim McDonald and John Harris

UNIQUE NEEDS OF HEALTH PROMOTION PROGRAMS SERVING WORKERS IN INDUSTRIAL SETTINGS

Historically, health promotion programs have been more common in office and high tech settings than industrial settings, but this is starting to change. Health promotion programs have been developed in many industrial settings including Detroit Diesel, Ford Motor Company, Daimler-Chrysler, and many others. For the past four years, General Motors has been implementing the largest workplace health promotion program in the world. The purpose of this section is to describe the unique needs of health promotion programs in industrial settings and to recognize the elements that are very similar in industrial and office settings.

There are a number of factors that influence the approach to health promotion that will be most effective at any location. Some of these factors include the size of the worksite, the type of work performed, the demographics of the workers, and the hourly/salaried mix of the population. "Industrial Settings" are usually thought of as having some or all of the following characteristics:

- a predominately hourly workforce
- a unionized environment
- located away from the corporate headquarters
- a sizable physical plant
- the performance of heavy work such as manufacturing or assembly

Table 3A-1 identifies factors that are often unique in industrial settings and provides specific information on serving industrial workers effectively. While the objectives of health promotion programs are often the same regardless of the setting, the opportunities, barriers, and processes of delivery can be very different.

The following table provides general information on the unique health promotion needs of workers in the "industrial setting." From a public health perspective, their needs are not unusual, but how health promotion is delivered to this population is. The factors described above should be taken into consideration when programming in the industrial setting, but each site is different and will have its own specific issues to consider. Sensitivity to the uniqueness of the industrial setting will allow health promotion professionals to maximize their success in programming for this sector.

Table 3A-1 Unique Factors Affecting Health Care Programs in Industrial Settings

Factor	Unique Needs of the Industrial Setting
Proximity to the corporate headquarters	Industrial settings are often far removed from the corporate headquarters. As such, they have autonomy but often feel a lack of support for programming efforts from senior leadership. Thus, evidencing corporate support, as well as generating visible local senior leadership support, is essential.
Facility size	Often the size of the industrial setting physical plant is immense. Additionally, few workers have direct access to such productivity tools as computer terminals, e-mail, and personal telephones. Few common areas exist, and even those that do (conference rooms, cafeterias, break areas, etc.) can be a distance from the worker's work location. To be effective, both program promotion and delivery must be taken to the people.
Demographics	While industrial demographics are changing rapidly, many industrial settings have a predominance of males and are often skewed toward older ages. Some industrial settings also have disproportionate percentages of minority groups, such as African-Americans, Hispanics, or Asians. Programming for multiple ages, genders, languages, and cultures will maximize the level of success.
Income level	Income levels can be disparate. Some industrial settings pay high wages with time-and-a-half for overtime pay. In these situations, the wages earned by industrial workers can be considerable. In other industrial settings, wages can be low. Thus, income level must be considered on a location-by-location basis and recognized as a variable in health promotion programming.
Education level and learning style	A majority of industrial workers are not college educated. While this is the case, the number of industrial workers who have pursued college degrees or are well-read should not be underestimated. Health promotion programs in industrial settings must reach a bell-shaped curve of education levels, reading abilities, and levels of intelligence. They should also recognize that many workers have alternative learning styles not well suited for the classroom and should seek to accommodate them with creative programming, such as self-guided modules.
Work culture	Like corporate office environments, work culture influences how health promotion programs must be delivered to be effective. Programming is easier in supportive environments, regardless of the setting. In general, many industrial settings are less cohesive and more contentious than the average corporate office environment. Communication is more difficult, and more distance exists between the constituencies (hourly/salaried, union/management, supervisors/workers, etc.). For health promotion programming to be effective, all constituencies must be reached and supported. Equal and visible support from all constituencies results in the greatest program success.
Work environment	Many industrial workers have little flexibility in work schedules or when they may attend programming. The nature of their work (e.g., an assembly line) or bargaining agreement restrictions require that they stay actively engaged, other than at lunchtime or for regularly scheduled breaks. Having workers relieved from work to participate in health promotion programming is often an expensive (i.e., loss of productivity) or logistically difficult task for management and therefore is hard to accomplish. Thus, programming must accommodate these factors, or adequate support and justification must be garnered to have workers relieved for specific programming efforts.

(continued)

Table 3A-1 Unique Factors Affecting Health Care Programs in Industrial Settings—*continued*

Factor	Unique Needs of the Industrial Setting
Work schedule	Many industrial workers perform shift work. Often they are on fixed shifts (consistently working 1st, 2nd, or 3rd shift), but some workers are on swing or rotating shifts, meaning that their shifts can vary from week to week. Shift work creates challenges for health promotion programming. Programs must be delivered around the clock and recognize that not all workers will be available at a consistent time for ongoing health promotion classes, such as weight loss. Effective health promotion programs also address the fatigue that often accompanies shift work.
Health needs	Often workers in industrial settings have a higher incidence of high blood lipids, smoking, being overweight, and having poor nutrition and sedentary lifestyles. Disease incidence rates have also been found to be higher in this population for diabetes, hypertension, musculoskeletal injury, and heart disease. While health care benefits are often good for industrial workers, compliance with therapeutic protocols is often lower than in corporate populations. Thus, focusing health promotion programs on lifestyle improvement, preventive examinations, and surveillance and treatment compliance is essential.
Health interests	Industrial workers have traditionally been difficult to reach and change with health promotion programs. Their current habits are ingrained, and their support for or interests in change are generally lower. To be effective in this population, health promotion professionals must come to understand and meet the interests and motives of the people. Often incentives and other inducements can be used to facilitate change. Packaging programs in ways industrial workers understand and trust is also essential (i.e., exercise programs to prepare for hunting season; stress management for shift workers, etc.). Multiple program options that meet the wide interests and profiles of industrial workers will also facilitate greater penetration of this population. Finally, gaining credibility with industrial workers and sustaining trust is essential.
Resources	The resources available at the industrial setting are often more limited than at corporate headquarters. For instance, conference rooms, fitness centers, and cafeterias are far less prevalent. Food services that do exist are often limited in scope, with little wherewithal to provide nutritious meals. The health promotion program must recognize these limitations and overcome them. Mapping safe walking areas around the plant, seminars on nutritious brown bagging, and use of break areas for mini-seminars have all been done effectively. Communications resources must also be considered. While e-mail or desk-to-desk communication may not be available, often plant-wide video communication, bulletin board, or paycheck messaging is possible. Large industrial settings have already discovered the best ways to communicate with workers. The health promotion program can use these channels to communicate health information.
Worker representation/ involvement	Unionized worksites or worksites where employees use self-guided work teams or other empowered work arrangements pose both opportunities and challenges for the health promotion program. On one hand, the greater the number of representative groups that are supportive of health promotion efforts, the greater are the chances of success. On the other hand, convincing multiple groups to agree on direction is difficult. This adds a political factor that becomes paramount to planning and delivery. All parties must be given equal respect and say in the process to maximize support and ownership and to eliminate any barriers to success.

(continued)

Table 3A-1 Unique Factors Affecting Health Care Programs in Industrial Settings—*continued*

Factor	Unique Needs of the Industrial Setting
Confidentiality	Nowhere is confidentiality more important than in the industrial setting. A level of suspicion has traditionally existed between workers and management, and thus privacy is a major issue. Successful health promotion programs not only ensure that all personal information is kept confidential but also eliminate all possible perceptions that information could be disclosed. Of specific importance is making sure that concerns about confidentiality do not create convenient excuses for workers not to participate.
Ability/willingness to pay	Given the disparate pay scales that exist across industries, it is impossible to generalize about "ability" to pay for health promotion programs. This will vary from industry to industry. However, "willingness" to pay is another matter. Many employees in industrial settings have enjoyed first dollar coverage for health care benefits, and thus are not used to paying for health-related services. This is not to say that asking some workers to pay for health promotion services in some industries is not possible or appropriate but that rather it has been a less accepted norm in industrial settings.

APPENDIX

3-B

Michael P. O'Donnell

A PARADIGM SHIFT: KEEPING PEOPLE HEALTHY VERSUS REDUCING HEALTH RISKS

Our thinking as to whom health promotion programs should be directed has evolved significantly in the last few decades. During the 1970s and early 1980s, most programs were offered to the general population. Those who were interested in participating joined voluntarily. We discovered that many programs attracted people who were basically healthy, people who already exercised, ate nutritious foods, and practiced other healthy lifestyle habits. Our programs reinforced their positive efforts and helped build these healthy practices into their daily routine, but as long as these programs did not attract the least healthy employees, these programs did not seem to be reducing health risks substantially. When the stages of change concept was introduced in the mid 1980s (Prochaska & DiClemente, 1986), we realized that the people we were attracting were those in the maintenance and action stages and sometimes those in preparation. As such, many of these early programs were criticized because they were perceived to have little impact as long as they attracted people who were already healthy.

This criticism of early programs grew stronger as we learned more about the relationship between health risks and medical care costs. It became clear that the vast majority of medical care costs were concentrated among a very small percentage of people. For example, in a typical employee group, 50% of employees have annual medical care cost under $245, while 10% have costs over $3,387 (Edington, 1999). When it became clear that the U.S. economy was entering a recession at the end of the 1980s and beginning of the 1990s, financial pressures increased and health promotion programs were forced to document their financial impact to better justify their existence. Some programs could not do this and were discontinued.

This combination of circumstances forced programs to concentrate on high-risk employees, and this focus has persisted through the 1990s. The reasoning is that the most severe health risks and the highest medical care costs are concentrated among a small portion of a typical employee population. If more intensive program resources are concentrated on helping this high-risk group learn how to exercise, quit smoking, eat nutritious food, manage stress, etc., this will have the greatest possible impact on improving the organization's health and on reducing medical care costs. This thinking spawned new methods to identify and recruit these high-risk employees, counseling efforts to help them set goals, and intensive programs to help them form new health habits. These new efforts were successful from the perspective that more high-risk employees were recruited into programs, and some of these employees were motivated to make significant changes in their lives. Unfortunately, most high-risk employees did not join the programs, and those that did required intensive support and still often suffered relapses. When viewed through the perspective of Prochaska's stages of change, we now realize that most of these high-risk employees were in the precontemplation or contemplation stages and thus were not ready to make health behavior changes. Those in preparation could be persuaded to join but, because of their often severe health risks and years of practicing unhealthy habits, required extensive support to make changes. Few programs could offer this level of support, and once again, programs were criticized, this time for low participation rates among high-risk employees and high failure rates for those who did participate.

In early 2000, Dee Edington introduced a concept called "Changing the Natural Flow" (Edington, 2000). After observing data on health risks and health costs collected during a span of over 20 years on almost 2,000,000 individuals, Edington observed that there is a natural flow of people from high risk (or multiple risks) to medium and to low risk (or few risks), from low risk to medium and high risk, and from medium risk to low and high risk. Some people stay in the same risk category. (See Figure 3B-1.) In the absence of a health promotion program, aging of the population, or a major crisis, the flow between risk groups tends to offset each other so that the percentage of the population in each risk category remains fairly constant over time. He also observed that medical care costs were highest for people with the most health risks and lowest for those with the fewest health risks. He found that an individual's medical care costs increased as health risks increased, that medical costs decreased as health risks decreased, and that medical care costs were basically stable when health risks were stable. This is consistent with what we would expect to discover. However, Edington discovered that cost increase associated with an increase of one health risk was greater

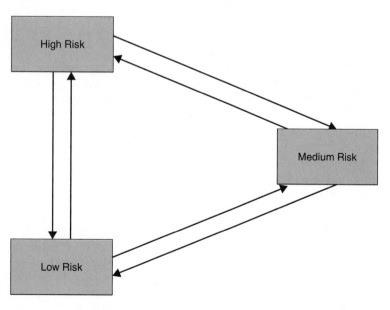

Figure 3B-1 Natural Flow of Employees by Health Risk Category Over Time

than the cost reduction associated with a decrease of one health risk. Annual medical costs associated with one decreased risk averaged $153 per person, compared to $350 associated with one increased risk. This finding was NOT expected and forced Edington and his team to question the strategy employed by most health promotion programs of focusing on reducing existing health risks rather than working to prevent future risks. In fact, if the goal of a program is to reduce medical care costs, it may be more cost effective to focus resources on helping healthy people stay healthy rather than on helping high-risk people reduce their risks. If we can disrupt the natural flow of people from the low- and medium-risk categories to the high-risk category, this is probably the most effective way to increase the portion of the population in the low-risk category and thus to control medical care costs.

This realization is a conceptual breakthrough that will probably reshape our field in the first decade of the twenty-first century. It will probably stimulate programs to invest a significant portion of their resources in efforts to keep healthy people healthy. These programs will focus on those in the maintenance and action stages to help them CONTINUE to exercise regularly, not smoke, eat healthful foods, manage their stress, maintain a healthy weight, etc. These programs will include on-site fitness centers and discounts in local off-site centers, additional recreation and activity programs, and support groups. This will be a very positive development for two major reasons. First, it seems to be a very effective method to control medical care cost increases. Second, it is much easier to recruit and retain people who are already healthy than it is to recruit people who are not healthy, and it is probably easier to help people maintain these behaviors than it is to help unhealthy people adopt new behaviors.

Does this shift in focus mean that we should stop our efforts to recruit and help high-risk people? Some programs will probably drop their high-risk programs for cost containment reasons, but the best programs will continue to serve both groups. These programs will offer stage-based options which are designed to move those in precontemplation to contemplation, those in contemplation to preparation, and those in preparation into action. Programs will be most effective if they focus additional resources on high-risk individuals who are in preparation by providing individual counseling to help them set goals and develop and maintain a plan to achieve these goals.

References

Association for Worksite Health Promotion, U.S. Department of Health and Human Services, William M. Mercer, Inc. (2000). *1999 National worksite health promotion survey.* Northbrook, IL: Association for Worksite Health Promotion and William M. Mercer, Inc.

Chapman, L. (1997). In search of program models for health promotion. *The Art of Health Promotion, 1*(5), 8.

Edington, D. (1999). *Worksite wellness: 20 year cost benefit analysis and report, 1978 to 1998.* Ann Arbor, MI: University of Michigan Health Management Research Center.

Edington, D. (2000, March). Changes in costs related to changes in psychological and social support risk factors. Paper Presented at *Art and Science of Health Promotion Conference.*

Gould, L., Ornish, D., Scher, W., Brown, S., Edens, R., Hess, M., Mullan, N., Bolomey, L., Dobbs, E., Armstrong, W., Merrit, T., Pots, T., Sparter, & S., Billings, J. (1995). Changes in myocardial perfusion abnormalities by positron emission tomography after long-term, intense risk factor modification. *Journal of the American Medical Association, 274*(11), 894–901.

Heaney, C. & Goetzel, R. (1997). A review of health related outcomes of multi-component workplace health promotion programs. *American Journal of Health Promotion, 11,* 290–307.

Matson, D., Lee, J. & Hopp, J. (1993). The impact of incentives and competitions on participation and quit rates in worksite smoking cessation programs. *American Journal of Health Promotion, 7*(4), 270–280.

Prochaska, J. & DiClemente, R. (1986). Toward a comprehensive model of change. In W. Miller & N. Healther (Eds.), *Treating Addictive Behaviors,* New York: Plenum.

Prochaska, J. & Velicer, W. (1997). The transtheoretical model of health behavior change. *American Journal of Health Promotion, 12*(1), 38–48.

O'Donnell, M. (1989). Definition of health promotion: Part III: Stressing the impact of culture. *American Journal of Health Promotion, 3*(3), 5.

O'Donnell, M. (1994). Employer's financial perspective on health promotion. In M. O'Donnell & J. Harris (Eds.) *Health promotion in the workplace* (2nd ed., pp. 54–57). New York: Delmar Publishers.

O'Donnell, M. (2000). Design of workplace health promotion programs (5th ed.), *American Journal of Health Promotion.*

O'Donnell, M. (1997). Health impact of workplace health promotion programs and methodological quality of the research literature. *The Art of Health Promotion, 1*(3), 1–8.

O'Donnell, M., Bishop, C., & Kaplan, K. (1997). Benchmarking best practices in workplace health promotion programs. *The Art of Health Promotion, 1*(1), 1–8.

CHAPTER

4

Program Management of Workplace Health Promotion Programs

William Baun

INTRODUCTION

During the 1990s there was a profound shift in the management focus of health promotion program managers. This shift followed the large flow of programs moving from activity-centered approaches to results-oriented ones (Hunnicutt, Deming, Baun, & Buffett, 1998). Program managers now face a new set of rules and requirements for measuring, maintaining, and reporting program success. Offering activities that track health observance calendars and maintaining participation levels has lost its "protective value" in sustaining senior managers' support. Senior managers have begun to question the relevance of program activities to the organizations' mission and bottom line.

This chapter will review the current program management practices that are being used to manage results-oriented programs. It will focus on the essential program management processes necessary to initiate, maintain, and expand these programs. The chapter will start with a discussion of the need for the integration of the health promotion manager's leadership roles and management functions. Following the integration discussion, the five functional areas that guide a program manager's working life will be defined. The majority of the chapter will be spent discussing each of the five areas in depth. Throughout the chapter, models and processes will be provided to enhance the problem-solving, creative, and innovative abilities of program managers. Programming examples will be utilized to demonstrate specific ideas and to provide practical solutions for managing small, large, single site, multi-site, and remote- or headquarter-based programs.

Integration of Leadership Roles and Management Functions

The difference between leadership and management is a debate that theorists have waged for many years. In the 2nd edition of this book (O'Donnell & Harris, 1994), the program management chapter provided very specific management functions. Program managers were expected to plan, organize, coordinate, implement, and maintain the major program tasks. Major program tasks were defined as human resource management, programming management, marketing management, financial and budgeting management, and facility and equipment management. But with the shift to results-oriented programming, program managers have been called into roles requiring a new set of skills. Managers now must be individuals who have both authority and responsibility for the actions of their departments but also are expected to informally coordinate and influence the actions of other managers and stakeholders in order to improve the health of individuals and the company culture. This new role is challenging health promotion managers to be leaders. Bennis and Nanus (1985) provided a clear difference between leaders and managers when they suggested that managers are people who do things right and leaders are people who do the right thing. Taking this a step further, a manager could be defined as an individual who has responsibility and accomplishes, conducts, and makes things happen. In contrast, a leader is an individual who influences and guides the direction of opinion and the course of action within a group or organization.

Successful program managers have increased their potential and the potential of the program by integrating these two roles. The synergistic relationship between leadership and management provides a balance in the program that increases the opportunity for continued program success and growth. Gardner (1990) in his book on leadership suggests that integrated leader/managers will:

- act as visionaries and futurists who always consider the effects of their decisions in both the short and long term
- look toward the larger organization in understanding how their department's actions fit into the larger picture and avoid becoming narrowly focused
- influence others beyond the boundaries of the organization's bureaucratic boundaries
- emphasize vision, values, and motivation
- deal with the many different expectations and conflicts that arise from their customers/clients

- think in terms of change and renewal to help the organization keep pace in an ever-changing world

Successful leaders/managers create and communicate a vision that provides a health promotion plan strongly aligned with the mission and goals of the organization and the wants and needs of employees. The plan should complement both the management and customer service philosophy to insure the program fits the corporate culture. These leaders not only provide a health vision for the organization but help transform it and its employees into health visionaries. Health visionaries are individuals who are willing to take risks for health behavior change and understand the necessity and importance of building a culture strengthened by the values of support and community.

Five Functional Areas Guide Health Promotion Manager

Program Administration

In the early 1900s, Henri Fayol, a trained engineer in a senior executive position at a large French coal-mining company, was concerned with efficiency and effectiveness of the entire organization. His concern gave birth to the development of management theories that focused on coordinating the internal activities of an organization. The basis for the program administration functional area that will be discussed in this chapter is Fayol's administrative management theory (1925). His theory first identified the management functions of planning, organizing, commanding, coordinating, and controlling. The best practice health promotion programs are based on program administrative models that have a strong infrastructure, have effective and flexible operational plans, and strategic plans that focus on consistent program quality and growth.

Program Marketing

The American Marketing Association (Sandhusen, 1993) has defined marketing as a process of planning the conception, pricing, promotion, and distribution of goods and services to create exchanges that satisfy individual and organizational objectives. This suggests that the purpose of marketing is a matching process between an organization's capabilities and the wants and needs of customers. The matching process takes place in what has been referred to as the "marketing environment" (McDonald, 1995). In a health promotion program the marketing environment is composed of organizational and interpersonal support and health norms that surround employees (Ribisl & Reischl, 1993). Marketing is based on marketing research that has evaluated program capabilities and employee needs. It also has a marketing audit process that provides a view of both external and internal factors affecting the health of employees. Successful marketing requires a clear understanding of market segments, targets, and positioning. These three approaches help define groups of employees who will benefit from specific health programs or interventions. What increases the opportunity of success in these three approaches is the marketing mix. Marketing mix is the combination of marketing tools that a health promotion program manager attempts to control and orchestrate in order to maximize the opportunity for success. Marketing mix is what drives the marketing plan forward. In traditional marketing, these tools are referred to as the Four Ps: product, place, promotion, and price. In this chapter, these have been changed to reflect specific health promotion program challenges relative to health behavior change and compliance. The Four new Ps will be packaging, place, price, and promotion. The last marketing component that will be discussed is strategy and will reflect the "bigger picture" of the marketing environment facing health promotion programs.

Program Delivery

The focal point of a health promotion program is its programs and activities. The third functional area of a health promotion manager's working life is program delivery. This section will provide an in-depth view of making program mix decisions and will describe the programming tools that have been borrowed from marketing and management principles and processes. It will introduce the concept of an eighteen-month program calendar managed with winning project management techniques. One of the most critical times in program delivery is program implementation, and this section will detail the implementation steps necessary in successful programming for the three levels of interventions-awareness, lifestyle change, and supportive environment (O'Donnell & Harris, 1994).

Financial Control & Budgeting

There are many reasons that programs grow, and one of the most important factors is the growth of necessary resources. The financial and budgeting responsibilities are crucial to the success of programs. Through financial budgeting controls and processes, program planning is forced to be realistic and performance can be measured in various values relative to cost. This section will describe the budgeting process and the different types of budgets and budgeting tools utilized to monitor progress. It will also provide tips to growing a budget for both the short and long term.

Facilities & Equipment

Facilities are not always a component of health promotion programs, but when a facility is included, its impact on the program's success is directly related to the effectiveness of its management. Facilities that work in support of health promotion programs and activities are those that are an integrated component of the health promotion strategy. The goals and objectives found within the program strategy dictate the facility space necessary for specific programs. Unfortunately, many programs accept rooms or areas that are inappropriate for the activities required by management. These inadequate spaces can detract from the quality of programming being offered. This section will discuss space guidelines, standards, and planning components. It will also provide information concerning risk management and the liability issues surrounding a facility and its equipment. Innovations that are being driven by technology and enhance the opportunity for successful behavior change have increased. The health promotion manager of the 21st century must be ready to add technology-based equipment to the programming mix and manage it effectively. This section will also address some of the preventative maintenance issues related to facilities and equipment.

PROGRAM ADMINISTRATION

It has been shown that organizational-level variables, such as management support, social environment, and organization resources, influence the implementation process and program outcomes (Crump, Earp, Kozma, & Hertz-Picciotto, 1996). Gottlieb, Lovato, et al (1992) studied the implementation of a restrictive smoking policy in a large state agency and found interaction between program implementation organizational-level variables significant. These studies support the need for an administrative model that is built on a strong infrastructure and for operation planning driven by a dynamic policy and procedural manual. But behind the consistent day-to-day operations in these programs is a strategic plan that provides the visioning that insures program and participant growth.

This section will provide the tools and processes necessary to successfully administer a health promotion program. We will start with the core elements of a strategic plan: mission, infrastructure, and goals and objectives. Strategic planning leads to the need for staff, and a detailed description of the processes involved in initiating and maintaining a program staff will be reviewed. Staff success depends on its ability to develop into a high performance team and initiate partnership alliances that move the program forward. Teaming and partnering ideas will be presented, along with concepts concerned with operations management and the basics of how a team and its partners must work together.

Strategic Planning—The Basics

Strategic planning is the process that a department uses to envision its future and develop the necessary procedures and operations to achieve that future (Goodstein, Nolan, & Pfeiffer, 1993). Health promotion planners sometimes mistake long-range plan-

ning for a strategic plan. Long-range planning generally spans from one to three years and serves as a bridge between the operation plan (day-to-day plan) and the strategic plan. The big difference between long-range planning and strategic planning is that long-range planning is based on an expected outcome predicted through extrapolation of current and historical data. Strategic plans are based on trends, threats, opportunities, and events that help you push further out in the future. If strategic planning is completed successfully, daily operating decisions improve, new focus toward the future better aligns delegation of authority and responsibility, and internal and external communication is now driven with new purpose. Strategy is not about predicting the future but making decisions today that will create a future (Quigley, 1993).

Coca-Cola's health promotion program is a good example of a strategic plan that over the years has transformed the program from its "silo" system of corporate departments working independently to a "non-silo" system. The non-silo system has linked the health promotion, fitness, medical, risk management, and benefits departments in concept, delivery, data management, and outcome analysis. Coca-Cola conducts business in more than 200 countries, and the concept of employee health management has successfully gone global with a strategic plan that created a future (Landgreen, 1999).

Strategic planning requires creativity, analysis, honesty, and a level of soul-searching that is not required in long-range and operation planning. When the planning process has been completed, three basic questions will be answered.

1. Where are we going?
2. What is the projected environment?
3. How do we get there?

These three questions will drive the strategic planning process and help move it through the self-examination, confrontation of difficult choices, and setting priorities that all will be faced throughout the process. There are many possible strategic planning models that can be used as guides. Table 4-1 provides a planning model that has been has been adapted from

Table 4-1 Strategic Planning Model

Step	Title	Description
1	Pre-Planning	Answers questions critical to the planning process: Who should be involved? How will absent stakeholders be involved? How long will it take? What information is needed? Who needs to develop the data?
2	Environmental Monitoring	What is happening outside the organization that might affect them?
3	Values Scan	What are the personal and organizational values found in the team? What is the department's philosophy of operation? What is the culture? Perform an analysis of stakeholders.
4	Mission Formulation	What functions does the department perform? For whom are the functions performed? How are the functions performed? Why does the department really exist?
5	Strategic Process Modeling	This is the first attempt to spell out in detail the paths by which the department's mission is to be accomplished. Included should be critical success indicators, strategic thrusts, and program lines.
6	Performance Audit	Once the future has been envisioned, the current position must be clear. This will include analysis of forces inside and outside of the department.
7	Gap Analysis	What gaps are present between the current performance and future expectations?
8	Integrated Action Plans	This is the grand strategy that offers a comprehensive approach to guiding the department to its future by integrating the various parts of the plan.
9	Contingency Planning	It is always helpful to develop several alternative futures, each based on the trends, threats, and opportunities being analyzed. Contingency planning provides scenarios for each major possibility.

Source: adapted from Leonard Goodstein's Applied Strategic Planning Model, in L. Goodstein, T. Nolan, & J. Pfeiffer, *Applied Strategic Planning: How to Develop a Plan That Really Works,* 1993.

Leonard Goodstein's Applied Strategic Planning Model (Goodstein, Nolan, & Pfeiffer, 1993). Let's look at a few of the important strategic planning variables.

Infrastructure–Visioning

Infrastructure does more than just answer the questions of who will be responsible for the program and how the program will be administered. It provides more than just a description of the different teams or committees that are involved in guiding the programs. It first must answer the "why" and "what" questions that provide a vision for program design and planning. How important is the visioning process in organizational success? Joel Barker, a well-known futurist, suggests that organizational success is a function of having a dream of future success and leaders that can share and inspire others within the organization (Goodstein, Nolan, & Pfeiffer, 1993). So the first step in building a strong infrastructure is to develop a vision or image of the desired future. This image will provide a word picture and set the overall direction of the program. A good vision will help staff and participants set program goals—but remember that good program visions are not to be written on colorful brochures used for many years or painted on the health promotion resource room walls. Good program visions are fluid and always evolving, and they represent a desire from the "heart" that is shared by people of different functions within the organization (Senge, Kleiner, Roberts, Ross, & Smith, 1994).

Core Values

The next step in infrastructure development is to agree on a set of values that will guide the thoughts and actions of individuals and groups within the program. Values have been referred to as the essential and enduring tenets of an organization that are truly central and can stand the test of time (Collins & Porras, 1996). Recognizing what core values individuals bring to work is one of the first steps in value development. The Disney Company values of imagination and wholesomeness or Hewlett Packard's value of respect for the individual all came from deep personal beliefs of the founders. Values should be decided independently of current management fads, environment, and market competition. Some management teams confuse core values with operating practices or business strategies. When trying to decide a program's core values, it is helpful to ask the following question: What are the values that we would like to see guide the behaviors that will help move our program closer to the program vision? A good example of core values that support an institution's vision to be the "premier cancer center in the world" is The University of Texas M. D. Anderson Cancer Center core values of caring, integrity, and discovery. After agreeing on core values, a health promotion team should work on the program's mission.

Mission

Mission has been defined as the organization's reason for being, or what we aspire to be (Quigley, 1993). The mission of The University of Texas M. D. Anderson Cancer Center is to eliminate cancer in Texas, the nation, and the world through outstanding integrated programs in patient care, research, education, and prevention. This is a good example of a mission statement because it provides deeper reasons for the organization's existence. Goals and business strategies will change many times, but the program mission may never be completely fulfilled. It serves as a guiding star on the horizon that captures the soul of the program and continually inspires change and progress. Not only does it provide the purpose for the program and quality standards but also provides a description of the groups eligible for the programs.

Good mission statements are customer-driven and also sensitive to environmental and cultural forces.

A powerful method to discover the true mission of a program is to use the "five whys". This starts with a statement that describes the program and then asks "Why is it important?" five times. For example, for the mission statement, "Our program provides health risk assessments to all employees", the answer to each why will bring the mission fundamentally closer to the true purpose of the program (Collins & Porras, 1996). Linking mission statements to the company or business strategy seems obvious, yet many program managers realize too late that their inability to garner management and employee support is directly related to their program's mission and goals. Short-term acceptance and long-term survival of a worksite program depend on its ability to meet the basic mission and goals of the organization it serves. O'Donnell and Harris (1994) suggest three reasons organizations invest in health promotion programming (see also Chapter 2).

1. To enhance the company's image
2. To increase productivity
3. To reduce medical care costs.

These three motives can help better focus efforts in formulating a mission statement that is aligned with the company's mission and underscores the value of the health promotion department. After a team has written a mission statement, they must address the program goals and objectives.

Goals and Objectives

Goals are the envisioned future. Goals have been defined as a specific and measurable accomplishment that can be achieved within a specified time and under specific cost constraints. Goals should complement the fulfillment of the stated mission and require a personal commitment and effort of individuals and team members. It is important that the individuals who will be involved in goal achievement are also active participants in the goal-setting process. Active participation produces an ownership that is very important in instilling the motivation and commitment to reach the goals that have been set.

Four steps should be included in a goal-setting process to maximize the opportunities for active participation.

1. Define the accomplishment to be achieved.
2. Determine the specific, measurable outcomes.
3. Create a timeline and deadline for completion of goals.
4. Identify the resources to accomplish the goal (finances, time, staff, etc.).

These four steps will help answer the questions of "Who? What? When? How? and How much?", which are the raw materials of goal setting.

Goals can be divided into three different categories: essential, problem-solving, and innovative goals. Essential goals are those that are necessary for continued and ongoing progress. An example of an essential goal in a worksite program might be to complete an HRA program intervention on 25% of the workforce by the end of the third quarter using existing staff and staying within budget. A problem-solving goal outlines the necessary activities needed to improve performance. An example would be to reduce the number of individuals who drop out of prenatal classes from 50% to 30% during the second quarter class offerings without adding to staff or budget. The last goal category is innovative goals, and it is focused on making something better or improving the current condition. It is not focused on a problem but on ways to get things done faster, better, cheaper, easier, or safer. An example of an innovative goal would be to change the current class registration system so individuals can register using an online system by the end of the third quarter (Rouillard, 1998).

Well-defined goal statements are crucial to goal achievement. It formalizes the Who? When? and How? questions into a statement that is clear and motivating. Many teams use the S.M.A.R.T method (Rouillard, 1998) to ensure that all the necessary elements are included in goals statement:

S – specific
M – measurable
A – action oriented
R – realistic
T – time and resource constrained

Once goal statements have been written, objectives can be developed that become the tactics or methods that are used to reach and achieve the goals. Once the vision, mission, goals, and objectives have been determined, staffing levels can be projected.

Staffing
Job Audits/Workforce Planning

The major program opportunities, projected activities, and size of employee population will influence the level of staffing. Job audits or workforce-planning processes that evaluate the current and future staffing needs help determine the need for staff positions. Management teams will use these processes to determine the minimum number of people needed to accomplish the program mission. The next step is to establish the type of positions that will be created.

The two types of positions that can be found in a staffing model are full-time employees and part-time employees. Full-time positions also have two categories. The first is a career path position that is composed of sequential jobs that are interrelated and lead to higher positions within the program (Montana & Charnov, 1993). A good example would be an entry-level specialist who next could move to a health promotion coordinator, then to health promotion administrator, health promotion manager, and finally to health promotion director. These five jobs are all interrelated but require different levels of professional experience and skill. The other full-time position categories are those positions that are not part of any career path. In some large hospital-based sites there is an epidemiologist or research positions that generally do not belong to a clear career path. Part-time staff in a health promotion program might include class teachers, intervention leaders, student interns, or clerical help that only work several days or fewer than 20 hours a week.

In many programs, the part-time staff is larger than the full-time staff because this provides an effective way to gain the professionalism necessary to offer a comprehensive program without the financial burden of a large full-time staff. In most programs salary represents 35–40% of the operating budget (Grantham, Patton, York, & Winick, 1998), and program managers are looking for effective ways to use these dollars. Once the job audit or workforce plan has been completed, it is time to develop job descriptions and/ or position descriptions.

Job Descriptions and Position Descriptions

A job description outlines the purpose, duties, responsibilities, relationship with other staff, physical condition required, and salary range. In some organizations, the job description serves as a general description of a general position, and the position description describes specific tasks and responsibilities of a particular job (Evans, 1995). These are very important to the next stage of staffing, which is recruitment.

Recruitment

The major objective in recruitment is to inform well-qualified candidates that job vacancies exist. Large organizations will have set policies and procedures for broadcasting job vacancies. Some of the more common recruitment methods used include recruiting from within the organization, professional referrals, classified advertising, employment agencies and search firms, professional association career centers, computerized databases, and school internships. The list below provides some of the associations that prepare individuals for careers in health promotion, and many maintain job banks that are helpful in searching for new employees (McDowell, 1999).

- American Alliance for Health, Physical Education, Recreation and Dance (AAHPERD)
- American College of Sports Medicine (ACSM)
- American Council on Exercise (ACE)
- American Dietetic Association (ADA)
- American Massage Therapy Association (AMTA)
- Aquatic Exercise Association (AEA)
- Association for Worksite Health Promotion (AWHP)
- Association of Hospital Health and Fitness (AHHF)
- Idea, The Health & Fitness Source
- International Health, Racquet & Sportsclub Association (IHRSA)

- International Spa Association (ISPA)
- Medical Fitness Association (MFA)
- National Intramural-Recreational Sports Association (NIRSA)
- United States Water Fitness Association (USWFA)
- Wellness Councils of America (WELCOA)

A recruitment process will bring letters of application, résumés, and phone calls. It is important that an effective system for screening these items be developed.

Screening, Interviewing, and Selection

It is important that either the immediate supervisor of the position being hired or a search and selection committee complete the screening. It is helpful to develop a checklist or rating system that is applied to each résumé and application received to help reduce the initial field of applicants. The first screening might be a telephone interview that insures the person is still interested in the job and can help validate the candidate's qualifications. Once a short list of the most qualified and those that have the best fit for the job has been developed, it is important to check the applicant's credentials and references before the interview. This provides the interviewer an opportunity to ask relevant questions during the interview. It is not uncommon to have an applicant teach an exercise class or deliver a health education seminar to further reduce the number of applicants before in-depth interviews are held. In many health promotion settings, the in-depth interviews also include meetings with employees or employee committees. Job offers can be made at the in-depth interviews or after these interviews through formal negotiations. After an individual has been hired, it is important that a new employee orientation be held to familiarize newly hired employees with company policies, procedures, objectives, and work expectations.

Orientation

Generally, new employees are oriented in a class, or an employee handbook is used that describes the company and explains benefits. This is usually followed by a discussion of the dress codes, hours, chain of command, and a program and equipment review. Most programs will have a process to help the new employee become productive members of the health promotion team. Some departments set up mentoring relationships, which are an excellent way to help new employees begin to understand the organizations' culture. Other programs will set up formal on-the-job training to insure that the new staff are exposed to and understand the professional and technical aspects of their job. It is not unusual for a new staff person to be given a probationary period from 60–180 days. During the probationary period a new employee can be terminated at will.

Performance Evaluation

Performance evaluation is a process in which the immediate supervisor of an employee reviews and assesses the employee's progress, performance, results, and sometimes expected behaviors. Expected behaviors might include things like communication, leadership, teamwork, respect, and competent performance. A performance evaluation system should include formal, regularly scheduled assessments mixed with informal spontaneous feedback. Evans (1995) suggests that an effective performance system will have four components:

1. a standard or yardstick used to judge performance
2. a careful measuring of performance relative to time on the job, variety of projects, and individual and team skills
3. assessment of both favorable and unfavorable performance from pre-set standards
4. full description of the actions necessary to eliminate the unfavorable performance and show improvement

The final process in a performance evaluation is for the supervisor to test how accurately the message has been received. One method of checking the accuracy is to have employees describe their understanding of what has been discussed and then for them to propose an action plan to insure growth and accomplishment of goal statements.

With the significant surge of team growth in the past decade, there has been a need for new feedback and evaluation innovations. Three hundred sixty-degree feedback programs have been implemented in a number of companies. These programs involve feedback for targeted employees and/or managers from four sources: (a) downward from the target's supervisor, (b) upward from subordinates, (c) laterally from peers or coworkers, (d) inwardly from the target themselves. It is important to remember that, in any evaluation system, it is what gets measured and rewarded that can drive behaviors. In order for a 360-degree feedback system to be successful, the measures must be closely tied to the accomplishments of department goals. This feedback system will require training of all individuals involved because most participants have never been involved in rating a fellow employee. The benefits of a 360-degree feedback system can be seen in organizations and teams that have increased their productivity and teamwork through opening communications between all levels on core issues relative to goal accomplishment (Waldman & Atwater, 1998).

Employees also need to reflect upon their performance as a team. Quarterly team performance evaluations provide team members an opportunity to review the program purpose and goal statements in relationship to the work that has been accomplished. By holding a team review every three months, adjustments can be made when necessary to insure accomplishment of annual goal statements. Another means of insuring individual and program productivity is staff development.

Staff Development

Staff development has been shown to be a cost-effective method to increase productivity (Marquis & Huston, 1996). The two components of staff development are training and education. Training is an organized method to insure that staff members increase the knowledge and skills necessary to perform their duties. It is structured, content-focused, solution-oriented, and directed at individuals. Managers use training to help staff members acquire new skills that will increase individual and team productivity.

Education is usually more formal and is designed to develop an individual in a broader sense. If the employees of a health promotion team are expected to participate more in the management of the team and share responsibility for the potential program impact and outcomes, then development and training programs must be established to provide incentives and opportunities to learn. Training and education should not be "done to" or "for" people but organized to support employees' needs in attaining their personal goals and objectives. They should help employees gain knowledge and skills necessary to insure growth, achievement, responsibility, and recognition (Myers, 1991).

One approach is to have each employee design an annual development and training strategy with his or her supervisor. It should include courses, conferences, workshops, and also work-related learning experiences. A health promotion specialist who has just begun a worksite career might list several planned programming experiences for the coming year as development opportunities. They might include developing the awareness portion of a marketing effort for a major intervention, developing the registration form for an upcoming walking program, and being a member of the new participant evaluation team. An individual who has worked in health promotion for three to five years might consider a statistics class or a research project with a local university as staff development. Many organizations have internal policies concerning the budget and time that can be allocated for training and education on and off the job. Staff development policies within the department can provide the manager with guidance about job rotation and assistant positions to provide skill acquisition and new learning opportunities.

If health promotion teams are to continue to grow and meet the needs and interests of the worksite, then team development must also be considered. There are many ways team members can train together through educational and training programs or through informal learning experiences. Team learning requires communications, trust, and the willingness to work together in the development of the team skills.

Health Promotion Team

Much has been written about the ability of a team to outperform other groups and individuals (Katzenbach & Smith, 1994; Scholtes, 1998). Teams can combine multiple skills, experience, and judgement in real time better than a collection of individuals forced to work together. When a staff is organized and managed as a high-performance team, characteristics like innovation, quality, cost effectiveness, and customer service can be sustained and provide a competitive advantage that is hard to match. Health promotion teams can range from 2–25 individuals; but, remember, large teams can be harder to manage. Larger teams should be broken into subteams rather than try to function as one team. A team's capacity to be successful is its mix of complementary skills that are committed to common purpose, performance goals, and mutual accountability. The health promotion manager must insure that the team has a good mix of complementary skills that include the necessary technical and functional expertise, problem-solving and decision-making skills, and interpersonal skills. It is surprising how many teams are assembled primarily on the basis of compatible personalities and not skill requirements. Teams must work at team discipline and processes that pull them together. This collective responsibility and accountability must be experienced and learned through health promotion programming as a team. There is no replacement for doing things together.

Management of A High Performance Work Team

Rees (1991) provides a simple four-step model for developing and maintaining an efficient work team. The first step is to lead with a clear purpose. This should be a purpose that everyone understands and that can serve as the core for team and individual goal statements that motivate high performance. If these goal statements are visible to all team members, they can serve as guides for decision making. The second step is to empower employees to participate in achieving their individual and team goal statements. The term empowerment in this context is used to describe a process that enables or permits staff members to actively become engaged in stretching toward the goal statements. The third step is to push the team toward consensus throughout the life of the team. This does not mean that there will not be conflict, but when there is conflict, it can be used to bring forth new ideas and opinions that will strengthen the team's performance. Always pushing for consensus that meets the needs of the team and the individual team members will increase overall team effectiveness. The last step is to direct the process by using methods that maintain the team's focus on purpose and accomplishment of goal statements. Successful team leaders are good listeners and are able to provide clarity to what has been discussed. They intervene when the group is getting off track, making suggestions to help the team refocus on results. The team leaders' energy and enthusiasm should help maintain the team process, providing greater opportunity for high performance and accomplishment of the goal statements. In today's results-oriented program environment, a good health promotion manager must also be effective at building partnerships and alliances with stakeholders.

Partnerships and Alliances

Stakeholders have been defined as those persons who have a vested interest in a problem, opportunity, process, or common issue. They become stakeholders because they are either affected by the "common item", can affect it, or a combination of the two (Svendsen, 1998). Stakeholder groups in health promotion programming can be found inside and outside of the parent organization. Some of the common internal stakeholders found in a health promotion environment are departments of health services, benefits, employee relations, health and safety, and ergonomic teams. External stakeholders might include the American Red Cross, American Heart Association, American Cancer Society, American Lung Association, and the YMCA. An alliance is generally viewed as an agreement to cooperate to insure a specific outcome. A partnership is a relationship between "partners" to share the risks and benefits of working together. The difference between the two in health promotion might only be semantics, but it is important in setting up

these relationships that each member fully understands their meanings. Partnerships have been viewed as the work version of a marriage in which all parties derive adequate gain from the relationship. In their book, *Dance Lessons: Six Steps to Great Partnerships in Business and Life,* Bell and Shea (1998) suggest six steps to achieve successful partnerships:

1. prepare to partner by insuring that you are committed to a purpose that can best be expressed through a partnership
2. choose the right partner by an "auditioning" process that allows you to test the fit
3. rehearse, rehearse, and rehearse so that the first steps of being partners will help put together the plans and processes needed to move it forward
4. focus on the processes that keep the partnership going and growing
5. learn what it takes to manage through the pain of adversity
6. recognize when it is time to call it quits

There are many good examples of programs that have effectively managed multiple stakeholder models and grown their programs into truly comprehensive and integrated systems. Such partnerships enhance the opportunity for improved employee health status through programming with support, empowerment, self-efficacy, and motivational qualities that are hard to maintain and manage in a nonpartnered model.

Operations Management

Operations management is management of the day-to-day activities and is the backbone of a health promotion department. These are the daily activities that insure program consistency and quality for management, employees, and staff. Weak operational plans or poorly executed plans are a major reason for worksite program failure and termination. For most participants and stakeholders, the day-to-day program activities provide them their only view of the program. Unfortunately, a good programmer does not necessarily make a good operation's manager.

Operations management is about the balance of effective resource allocation and satisfactory customer service. The strengths and weaknesses of the department influence the balance of these objectives as do the push and pull of management, employee, and staff. The scope of operations management encompasses many of the topics that will be discussed individually in this chapter (financial control and budgeting, quality control, facility and equipment management). Two key systems to operations management are capacity management and scheduling (Wild, 1996).

The usable resources of a system are defined as its capacity. Capacity management is concerned with matching the capacity of the department with the demands placed on it by the needs and wants of management and employees. The first step in capacity management is to put together a capacity plan that determines their current capacity level and the level of resources necessary to be successful. The gap between current levels and what is necessary provides an opportunity to initiate a plan that will insure appropriate capacity levels can be reached. Many times capacity requirements can only be based on forecast, which rely on sound qualitative methods to insure accuracy. The four better known qualitative forecasting methods are Expert Opinions, Delphi Method (group technique in which a panel of experts are individually questioned about their perceptions of future events. They do not meet as a group, but send in their forecasts and arguments to an outside party for summary. This process continues until consensus is reached), Staff Polling, and Customer Surveys (Shim & Siegel, 1999).

A work schedule will provide the manager with an effective tool to direct the accomplishment of the program goals and objectives. Work schedules are organized to maximize staff ability to meet the needs of participants and the program goals and objectives. Schedules should be designed so individual staff members have opportunities to rotate into different tasks. Job rotation increases staff opportunity for a variety of health promotion experiences. This is important for individual training and development of staff while increasing the opportunity for job satisfaction. The schedule should reflect the work of the whole health promotion team to help increase the interconnectedness of the individual tasks into a group task. Work defined as a group task increases the in-

trinsic value of the work and increases the potential for team success.

Individuals who manage fitness or health education learning facilities will have schedules to open, monitor, and close these areas. It is important in designing routine task schedules that adequate control processes and tools are established that provide high standards and mechanisms that promote communications between staff members on the different shifts. Schedules that have a master checklist of the necessary tasks involved in opening or closing a facility can be used to insure that proper procedures are followed and that safety and maintenance needs are noted. These forms can also be used to pass on information about individuals, events, and activities that need special attention.

PROGRAM MARKETING

Health promotion marketing will be defined as the process of planning the conception, pricing, promotion, and distribution or delivery of programs and interventions that satisfy individual and organizational health objectives. Marketing is composed of activities and strategies that have been systematically designed to communicate with and direct individuals toward the programs and services. It is the matching of a program's capabilities with the wants and needs of employees.

This section will provide the tools and processes necessary to successfully market a health promotion program. The section will start with the development of a market plan and an in-depth discussion of the steps necessary to complete the planning process. Marketing research and the four components of a market mix will be discussed and worksite examples will be provided. A section will follow this on market segments, targets, and positioning which are all part of the market planning process. The final section will be on strategic marketing and provide insight into program growth strategies.

Market Plan

Market planning is a logical series of activities that lead to setting marketing objectives and forming a plan to achieve them. Health promotion departments should have a systematized process for developing a marketing plan. Conceptually, it should be a simple process that first involves marketing research that provides a review and analysis of the four basic components of the marketing mix (packaging, place, price, and promotion). The second step involves identifying the market segments or subgroups that have similar behaviors, health needs, or reactions to the marketing efforts. The third step is to quantify the data collected and formulate marketing objectives that are consistent and aligned with the overall departmental goals and objectives. The last step is to schedule and determine costs of specific marketing activities that are most likely to bring about achievement of the objectives (McDonald, 1995).

Marketing Research

The first step in developing a marketing plan is to use a systematic approach to collect relevant data and information about the marketing mix, segments, targets, and position that are relevant to developing a planning document. The objectives of the research process will help identify the issues and questions that need to be addressed during the research step. For example, a common marketing research objective is to explore employees' needs, interests, and prior participation in health promotion programming. Another key objective could be to describe the market readiness of an employee population. The marketing research objectives that will be identified and defined for the start-up of a health promotion program will be complex and require more information be collected than for an annual review of an ongoing program. Once objectives have been clarified, the research design and data collection and analysis procedures can be decided. How the information and data is to be collected is determined by the type of information desired, the degree of validity and reliability required, and the respondents' abilities to provide the necessary information (Sandhusen, 1993). A good deal of the information required in the marketing research step will concern the market mix components and come from needs and interests surveys, health risk assessment instruments, cultural audits, and other

internal and external resource appraisals. This information will help programmers make decisions concerning the market mix.

Market Mix

The market mix is a combination of the four tools that a programmer uses in order to maximize the opportunity for marketing success. In traditional marketing, the four P's include product, price, place, and promotion. The four P's have been modified to specifically address the challenges found in a health promotion program and, as such, are program packaging, price, place, and promotion. The first of the four P's is program packaging, which includes all the activities, programs, interventions, and products that are used in a program. What has been added to the traditional product "P" is the element of "packaging" programs that meet the different needs and interest of employees or groups. The second element in market mix is price, and it refers to everything a person needs to spend or give up in order to receive the service or participate in the program. This includes out-of-pocket fees they must pay, time required to attend the program or complete assignments, and travel time. Location, flexibility, effectiveness of the program, and specific requirements defining individual success can also affect the price. The third element is place and refers to the location at which the product or service is available. In health promotion programs, the location of facilities (office, classrooms, and/or resource rooms) and the distribution points for materials and other services represent place. The last element is promotion, which refers to the strategies undertaken to persuade the market segment or target to participate in the programs and/or services. Promotion is about finding the best means to get a message to employees so that in the short-term they choose to participate, and in the long-term they choose to comply with behaviors that will help change and maintain health.

Program Packaging

Packaging refers to different programs, interventions, products, and services that are being offered and packaged in multiple ways. When packaging programs, it is very important to consider different employee populations, behaviors, and feelings toward the program packages. On-site worksite health promotion programs capitalize on the "convenience" of their offerings. Many employees will initially participate in activities because they are so accessible.

One behavior to consider is "shopping," which is a prime reason why programs that are being packaged in multiple ways are offered within a major product line. An example would be the use of multiple smoking cessation options, such as classes, support groups, computer aids, self-help packages, and counseling, before a company enforces a smoke-free policy. Offering a variety of options allows those who want to try to quit smoking an opportunity to "shop" for the approach that fits their needs. It provides them choices and places them in control of this decision. Another behavior that is successfully used in health promotion is that of "specialty", unique activities or events that are of high value to employees. For example, many health and fitness centers have mileage clubs in which individuals are given mugs or T-shirts for walking or jogging certain distances each year. These self-paced awards become personal accomplishments but also gain value as they are shared with fellow employees. The last behavior deals with employee attitudes toward program packages. There is always a segment of the population that is not seeking health through health programs, and their behavior can be described as "unseeking." Employees who demonstrate this behavior might be unaware of the programs or interventions being offered or could have a low readiness level. Low readiness for many individuals is a major factor discouraging participation. We also find that unseeking individuals are the hard-to-reach employee or segments of the population with low self-efficacy. Successful marketers understand program packaging, emphasize the benefits derived from program participation, and utilize different program packaging to make the program accessible and realistic for all individuals.

Price

Price is the most flexible of all the elements in the market mix. It allows health promotion program-

mers the ability to make changes to a program package that could mean the difference between program success and failure. Extending the registration period of a weight management program to allow more individuals to sign up for the activity is a price change. Lowering the required mileage so that a specific segment of walkers can be successful in a program is also a price change. The price employees are willing to "pay" shows how much they value the program. Lowering the price decreases the value a participant needs to place on the program in order to participate. A lower price can serve as a registration or program completion stimulator, as in the program examples described above. But lower prices can also have a negative affect on a program by decreasing the value of a program to participants by being inconsistent with the program position. For example, a cholesterol screening program might be promoted as being "the best deal in town", and to the staff's surprise, participants become concerned about the accuracy of the test. Since price can be changed on short notice, it is the most flexible of the marketing mix elements. It plays a significant role in influencing the employees' perception of the program packaging because it translates into "value". A "back to basics" weight management program marketing campaign will elicit a different response than a "total weight management system" campaign. Perception of the price that must be paid for each program is the difference.

Place

In a health promotion program, the place portion of the market mix answers the question of where the programs or services will be offered. Place decisions also determine the time the programs or services will be offered. The objective of a good marketing mix is to offer the right programs, interventions, services, and products at the right place and time. Deciding on an appropriate location will involve distribution decisions that insure the right quantities of materials or programs are being offered. For example, during National Employee Health & Fitness Day, many worksites set up health fairs offering employees a wide assortment of screening opportunities. A recent cardiovascular sudden death in an employee population can motivate many employees to take advantage of a free electrocardiogram. The long lines, and unhappy employees, at the single electrocardiogram station teach the staff a quick lesson about timing and distribution.

Promotion

The communication-persuasion strategies and tactics that help make the program packages familiar, acceptable, and even desirable to employees has been defined as promotion (Sandhusen, 1993). The promotional mix consists of four basic elements. The first element of the promotional mix is advertising. In health promotion programs, newsletters, program flyers, displays, bulletin boards, and other printed and broadcast media directed toward the population as a whole represent advertising. The second element of the promotional mix is personal selling. This is the person-to-person process that is sometimes called counseling and coaching in health promotion programs. A third element of the promotional mix is sales promotion and can be used with advertising and personal selling. These are activities that offer incentives to persuade participation. Incentives are used in health promotion programs to stimulate enrollment by creating a sense of urgency and excitement (Hunnicutt, Deming, Baun, & Buffett, 1998). The overuse of sales promotions or program incentives can affect the program by overshadowing the need for employees to develop intrinsic reasons for participation.

The last element in the promotional mix is public relations, and its primary focus is to foster a positive image to participants and individuals outside the internal market. Successful public relation programs will help participants focus on the high quality of their program experience. During National Employee Health & Fitness Day, many employee populations will be involved in large efforts to get everyone walking or doing some fitness activity. Stories in employee newspapers summarizing the success of these programs are examples of public relations. Participant stories in employee newsletters that model positive health changes are also examples of public relations. These stories help other employees focus on the program and its potential.

Market Segments, Targets, and Positioning

A major objective of the market research process is to identify potential market segments. Market segments are groups of individuals with similar wants, needs, or characteristics. For example, in a worksite health promotion program, market segments might be broadly defined as managers and nonmanagers, men and women, young, middle-aged, and older employees. They might be based on such health characteristics as smokers and nonsmokers, exercisers and nonexercisers, etc. Finally, these characteristics might be combined to identify smaller segments, such as women nonmanagers who smoke cigarettes. The reason for describing employees in terms of market segments is to help determine the best way to reach them. For example, different marketing efforts might be used to reach young women with high-school educations who are slightly overweight than to reach women who are middle-aged senior secretaries. Young women might be attracted by messages related to fashion and social benefits, while older women might be receptive to messages related to increasing energy levels and managing ongoing health problems related to aging.

Market Segments

The marketing literature (Sandhusen, 1993) defines four market segments that can be helpful in categorizing an employee population. They are geographic, demographic, psychographic, and behavioristic. The geographic segment focuses on location and the characteristics that distinguish each location. Health promotion programs that have multiple sites find that different regions of the United States have cultural differences that can be addressed in the market mix. The different demographic segments are also important in identifying employee populations. Important demographic characteristics are age, gender, family size and type, occupation, race and nationality, and education level. At Tenneco, the first HIV informational programs initiated during the mid 1980s found that 95% of their first meeting participants were young women. For many programmers, this was a surprise because they expected young males to attend these programs. A different market mix was required for these programs to appeal to the young male population.

The psychographic base is the most widely used in health promotion programming. A psychographic base is concerned with lifestyle, social class, and personality. Programs that utilize health risk assessments gather lifestyle information that can be used in a segmentation process. Social class might be gathered in the same instrument and has been shown to have a significant effect on health knowledge, skills, and status (Glanz, Lewis, & Rimer, 1997).

The last segmenting characteristic is the behavioristic base. In a health promotion program this includes participation behavior. Employees might be classified as facility members, non-members, participants, nonparticipants, and program dropouts. Skilled programmers are sometimes able to project which market segments or targets will show interest in their program or products. For example, right before annual physicals, many hard-to-reach employees become interested in fitness and losing weight. Specific programs that offer information, guidelines, and new skill acquisition processes that promise results can be packaged and targeted to these individuals.

Another important behavioristic segmenting characteristic is readiness. It deals with participant awareness, acceptance, and past-participant satisfaction and success in lifestyle change efforts. Most important, it refers to readiness to participate or make a behavior change. Readiness is an important clue in properly positioning program packages. For example, in 1989 the Tenneco program had successfully decreased the number of employees who smoked from 31% to 10%, but the remaining smokers were hardcore smokers (Tenneco Internal Data, 1989). The data also showed that only a small percentage of these smokers were willing to try to quit smoking. For the majority of these smokers, personal readiness was low, but interest in information they could give their children concerning reasons not to start smoking was high. Readiness is also affected by employees' knowledge of what programs, interventions, and services are available, combined with their perception of how popular current lifestyle changes are. Cholesterol screening and testing programs have been very popular the past few years because of the large amount of information communicated in the lay press, radio, and television about the importance of knowing cholesterol level. People have signed up for cholesterol screenings but are not prepared to make the necessary lifestyle changes required to lower their cholesterol. A programmer's understanding of all the readiness factors involved in specific program packaging is important if behavioristic segmenting is to be used correctly.

In program initiation, immediate program success is critical to the image of the total program, and market segmentation strategies play an important role in maximizing opportunity for program success. Focusing the initial smoking cessation activities on those smokers who are in a high readiness state is smart programming and uses what has been termed a concentrated segmentation strategy (Sandhusen, 1993). In a concentrated segmentation strategy, programmers select a single market segment and develop a market mix that will focus on that one segment. The alternative to a concentrated strategy is a multisegment strategy that develops multiple market mixes for multisegments. A multisegment is a more realistic strategy for a health promotion program that has passed its initial program test and has the resources to expand without lowering program quality.

Target Market

A concentrated segmenting strategy would target specific employee groups for certain programs, interventions, products, and services. These groups are called target markets and are chosen for a variety of reasons. Some of the common reasons for target market dispersion are location, group size, and, most important, readiness to participate in specific programs. For example, men over the age of 50 represent the target market for a PSA (prostate specific antigen) prostate cancer-screening program. This is the employee group that the screening test has been designed to serve, and the lay press has done an excellent job of increasing the readiness of men in this age group to take the test. Target marketing increases the opportunity for program success and can lower the promotion cost because of the limited group that receives the marketing message.

Positioning

Positioning is created over time, and the associations that create program position are derived from an assortment of sources. Positioning should be considered strategic because it takes years to create, is difficult to change, and can have a significant effect on marketing success. A good example from the business world is the Macintosh computer that has been positioned for those individuals needing high quality graphics. There are many ways to position a program package, some of the core strategies are:

1. use or application–weight lifting is positioned to turn a male weakling into a man who can defend himself and has an improved self-esteem
2. product class–flexibility and stretching exercises have been positioned to be good alternatives for relaxation programs
3. place of origin–Swedish massage or Chinese magnetic ball massage promise something we cannot get from just a regular massage
4. product user–free weights offer a "roughness image" for its users
5. competition–the new glide machines combine both the advantages of a treadmill and a stairclimber

Strategic Marketing

Strategic marketing is concerned with setting strategies to insure market growth. Market growth strategies can be classified into three categories: intensive, integrative, and diversified.

Intensive Growth Strategies

Intensive strategies focus on cultivation of current markets. They use penetration approaches to aggressively persuade present participants to participate more and to persuade nonparticipants to participate. A second approach involves developing strategies that attract new members to the market. The final approach develops new program packages that attract new participants to existing markets.

Integrative Growth Strategies

Integrative strategies are usually used in strong programs in which the marketing strategy allows it to gain participants by moving backward, forward, or horizontally in the market. Backward integration might involve a program that partners with a vendor to create a new program targeted at a specific employee group. An example of backward integration is the client-vendor development of diabetic program materials created to impact the cost of diabetes. Forward integration would be a program that increases control over the health risk assessment process by purchasing software that analyzes the data and generates reports. Horizontal integration would be used when a health promotion program takes control of the company recreational program. In horizontal integration a department increases its control over competitors.

Diversification Growth Strategies

Diversification strategies are utilized when few opportunities exist in current markets but many appear to exist in markets outside the current mission. The first approach is horizontal and entails adding program packages unrelated to the current product lines. These programs will be designed to appeal to existing targets but will represent different packages. A good example would be adding a behavioral counselor who could deal with some of the employee assistance issues (drug and alcohol abuse, parenting, etc.). Another approach is concentric diversification, which introduces new program packages bearing technological or marketing similarities to existing programs. An example might be a hypertension program that utilizes a palm-pilot recording device that has been successfully used to manage diabetes (Sandhusen, 1993).

PROGRAM DELIVERY

The major purpose of a worksite health promotion program is to deliver quality programming that supports the mission and goals of the department. Programming has been called both an "art" and a "science" because of the mix of skills and experience required in planning and implementation. Program delivery is divided into three stages: program design and planning, implementation, and closing.

Program Design and Planning

During this initial stage of programming, the wants and needs of individual employees, employee groups, and organizational stakeholders uncovered in the market research step are formulated into programs and services. During the program design stage, a sketch of the program (or, what is termed in product design books, a service definition) will be produced (Bobrow, 1997). This sketch should provide a three-dimensional definition that answers the following questions:

- Who is the target for this program or service? Who will be most interested in it? Who will probably use it the most?
- What are the program features? What are its benefits? What is its value? What design requirements (time, frequency, social learning principles, etc.) are necessary to insure success?
- Why should this program or service be offered?

The "how" and "by whom" questions will be answered in the planning step and will complete the initial stage of the program delivery process. During the design and planning steps, there are several tools that have been borrowed from the marketing and management literature that will help complete this initial stage more effectively.

Benchmarking

Benchmarking is defined as "finding and implementing best practices that lead to superior performance" (Camp, 1995). In worksite health promotion, we face many programming challenges that can be better met with the information gained through benchmarking. What is the best approach to blue-collar smokeless tobacco use? How do you provide a

nursing population with the knowledge and skills necessary to cope with stress when they are not given any training time or flex time? How do you motivate a middle-aged white-collar male population to take advantage of annual medical exams. These are the types of questions that can be answered with a benchmark process.

Step One:

The first step is to identify what will be benchmarked. In this step, factors you consider critical to program success will be noted and become the process or program components that will be benchmarked. For example, in a smokeless tobacco program the development of materials that have value to the employees, or the incentives utilized to promote registering for the program. Benchmarking works best on specific program details and not broad programming issues.

Step Two:

The second step is to select benchmarking partners. Partners might come from inside your organization. Some of the best incentive programs have been built from successful incentive programs already existing inside the organization. The first thought of many programmers is to partner with the world-class leaders in worksite health. But this might not yield sufficient information to be helpful. They might have more resources, more senior manager support, or have more years of experience. Actually, some of the best benchmark partners are those who come from outside the health promotion industry. Companies that have excellent training departments might provide programmers lessons in gaining and maintaining senior management support. A benefit department that packages materials to thousands of employees and daily answers hundreds of questions would be an excellent partner for packaging ideas. When Southwest Airlines wanted to benchmark the time spent on the ground fueling, cleaning, and catering between destinations, the team met with racing car pit crews because these teams represented the world's best at similar tasks.

Step Three:

The third step is to collect the data. This step is not initiated until a set of questions has been prepared in advance to insure consistency among the different benchmarking partners. Tenner and DeToro (1996) suggest that a good approach to reach penetrating questions is to first list the topics on which information is desired and then prioritize the lists. This prioritization will provide a "short list," which can further be prioritized to a list of "vital few". They also suggest taking advantage of different forms of questions (open-ended, multiple choice, scaled) to extract many different answers. Data should be collected from a number of different sources (world-class partners, literature reviews, and professional association contacts) to increase the breadth of information being collected.

Step Four:

Once the data has been collected the fourth step is data analysis. In this stage the differences between what is being done at your organization and the benchmark partners' is analyzed for gaps. Are you ahead of your partners, behind them, or at parity to their practices or processes? It is important in this stage to define some of the key performance indicators that can be used to represent the overall bottom-line results. Examples in health promotion would be the average registration rate expected in smokeless tobacco programs or the average compliance or completion rates. These key indicators will help you analyze performance and processes that can lead to better practices. Gap analysis provides the momentum necessary to develop new market strategies, give birth to new program ideas, and improve programs that have lost their shine.

Step Five:

The lessons learned from the benchmark process are used to develop plans and actions that will integrate and/or innovate these practices into your programs (Mears, 1995).

SWOT Analysis

Another management tool that can be used to help make decisions concerning appropriate actions to fill

Present Operation	Future Operation
Strengths	Opportunities
Weaknesses	Threats

Figure 4-1 SWOT Matrix
Source: adapted from P. Montana & B. Charnov, *Management: A Streamline Course for Students & Business People,* 1993.

the gaps discovered in the benchmarking process is called SWOT analysis. In this approach the strengths, weaknesses or faults, opportunities, and threats to the program are analyzed. These data are gathered through interviewing selected individuals within the company. In a health promotion program, it is useful to interview individuals of diverse job categories because the program services all employees. Once the data has been collected, it can be organized into a SWOT matrix (see Figure 4-1) that can help staff decide what should be done to safeguard the strengths of the current operation or to overcome weaknesses. It will also illuminate what must be done to take advantage of future opportunities or to avoid future threats.

Product Life Cycle (PLC)

Product life cycle (see Figure 4-2) is a marketing theory that suggest that every market goes through a series of phases that are analogous to the biological

Biological Phase	Product Life Cycle Phase
Birth	Market Development
Growth	Market Expansion
Adolescence	Market Turbulence
Maturity	Market Maturity
Old Age	Market Decline

Figure 4-2 Product Life Cycle
Source: Taylor, J. W. (1996) *Marketing Planning: A Step-by-Step Guide.* 1996. Used with permission.

phases of life (Taylor, 1996). As in business, the PLC can be utilized in health promotion programs to help programmers better understand the engine that is driving their programs.

In health promotion, a product life cycle usually extends over a period of several years and can be affected by both the adoption and diffusion of innovation processes described by Rogers (1983). Adoption describes the series of stages that an individual goes through in deciding to get involved in a program. Rogers identifies these stages as awareness, interest, evaluation, trial, and adoption. The Stages of Change process developed by Prochaska (Prochaska, Norcross, & DiClemente, 1994) is a complementary concept that defines five stages that individuals go through in behavior change (Precontemplation, Contemplation, Preparatory, Action, Maintenance). Diffusion is the spread of a program or program idea through an employee population or culture. Diffusion is defined by five categories of adopters: (a) innovators, (b) early adopters, (c) early majority, (d) late majority, and (e) laggard. Programmers can collect information on their participants that will help them understand who is getting involved, why they are getting involved, and where people fall within these various stages. When these three questions are answered, both the adoption and diffusion processes can be better understood and product life cycle tracking can begin. There are many data points that can be tracked in health promotion programs. Important to programmers are total number of participants, repeat participants, new participants, par-

ticipants who complete half of the program, participants who complete the total program, successful participants, and total dropouts. Figure 4-3 illustrates how a health promotion program can be tracked using the concept of PLC.

A program that has experienced low participation or success in the development stage but showed good promise in pilot programs might be considered for a program recharge. A program recharge strategy would change one or several components of the program design to raise the program's potential for success. Programs in the maturity stage that are experiencing high dropout rates during and after the program might add new relapse strategies to their program design. These strategies will lessen the backsliding and help employees learn effective coping responses (Marlatt & Gordon, 1985). Using the product life cycle concept helps programmers extend the life of good programs and can identify an appropriate time to terminate or suspend programs. Wise programmers will offer some programs every other year in order to extend their maturity stage and head off a rapid program decline.

Program Mix

Program mix has been borrowed from the product management literature and can help programmers learn to stretch their markets, plug programming gaps, and initiate campaigns to help build traffic for specific programs, an entire line, or the whole program (Sandhusen, 1993). The program mix refers to

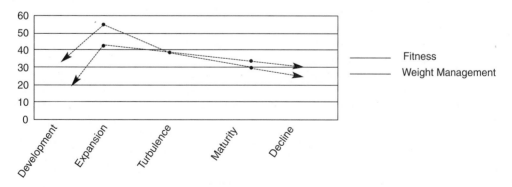

Figure 4-3 Comparison of PLC for Fitness, and Weight Management Programs

Table 4-2 Program Mix

Depth (options available)	Breadth (program lines available)	
	Narrow	Broad
Shallow	Few program lines and few options in each line	Several program lines but few options in each line
Deep	Few program lines but many options in each line	Several program lines and many options in each line

all program opportunities offered to employees in a health promotion program and is defined by the mix of program breadth and depth. Program lines represent program breadth. Examples of program lines are the various health promotion activities that can be offered like nutrition, fitness, pre/postnatal, weight management, stress reduction, ergonomic, parenting, self-care, and many other activities and services offered in a worksite program. Program depth refers to the number of intervention levels employed in offering the different program lines. O'Donnell and Harris (1994) define three levels of intervention: awareness, behavior change, and supportive environments. Table 4-2 illustrates the concept of program mix.

New worksite programs usually have a narrow program breadth and shallow program depth. This allows programmers to concentrate their efforts on learning the basics in an employee population that has not experienced health promotion programming. A shallow program depth suggests that employees have few program options in each program line being offered. An example of a narrow shallow program would be one that only offers the American Cancer Society "Freedom From Smoking" self-help materials and organizes a group that utilizes the nicotine patch.

A mature health promotion program will have a variety of program lines supported by several different intervention options. An example of a mature program would be one that offers several different fitness classes, including different weight management classes for the obese and for those needing to lose less than 10 pounds. It might also offer classes to teach the different skills necessary for parenting or to handle life stress. In a successful program, the mission and goals are strongly reflected in the program mix. Program mix is one of the most powerful programming tools because it allows the successful tailoring of different health promotion lines at various intervention levels.

Program Calendar

Developing a program calendar is the last step in the planning stage. It places the program mix in a time line for program development, preprogram promotion, program registration, program implementation/delivery, and program evaluation. The first step in developing a program calendar is to decide the period of time that will be utilized. Comprehensive programs can be complex and offer many different program opportunities during a month, which will require a calendar format that aids program staff in managing the many activities. These calendars provide a layout that includes dates for task completion, deadlines, and checkpoints. Smaller, less intense programs might utilize a quarterly calendar format that has grouped months together and tracks only program titles. Program calendars help staff coordinate and manage the many tasks involved in programming, thus it is important that a time frame be chosen that insures program consistency and growth.

Many programs now utilize 15- or 18-month program calendars to insure that programming becomes a better long-range vision and not just 12 months of programming. A year-plus calendar also insures that the program mix provides for programming assortment. Successful health promotion programs vary program length, intervention level, and intensity. Intensity refers to required participant effort. Programs requiring participants to only pick up self-help materials are less intense than programs requiring return of a feedback form after reading materials. When utilized, a year-plus program calendar will become the major focus for staff task assignments and insures that the programming efforts are balanced throughout the year for both participants and staff. Program activities should be staggered throughout the calendar so that different staff members can shift between being the primary and secondary staff responsible for programming efforts. It is this shifting that allows staff to rest, be challenged, and grow throughout a programming cycle.

Programmers have found that it is useful to weave national or state health themes throughout a programming cycle. Using these national events to help support programming efforts provides credibility and enhances the marketing efforts. For example, April is National Cancer Control Month and is a good time to offer information on cancer screening or offer cancer-screening programs. Table 4-3 provides a calendar of national programs and events segmented by O'Donnell's (1994) three levels of intervention (awareness, behavior change, and supportive environments).

Table 4-3 National Health Observances Calendar 2000

Month	Awareness Activity	Behavior Change	Supportive Environment
January	March of Dimes Birth Defects Prevention Month (914) 428-7100 • Information table	First Step To Health • Buddy Incentive– Program supporting health behavior change	Mom's To Be • Initiation of prenatal support groups
February	American Heart Month–AHA (800) AHA-USA1 • CPR Training	First Step to Health • Continue incentive program	Healthy Menu sponsored in cafeteria
March	National Nutritional Month–ADA (800) 622-9010 • Brown Bag Series on Nutrition & Choices	First Step To Health • Close of incentive program and celebration of success	Employee cook book of healthy ideas put together and sold
April	Infant Immunization Week–CDC (404) 639-8226 • Information table	National Cancer Control Month–ACS (800) ACS-2345 • Several cancer screenings offered	Mammography and testicular plastic hanging screening material provided
May	High Blood Pressure Month–HLB Institute (301) 251-1222 • Balloons and BP cards given to employees	Blood pressure screenings offered, and a walking club is started with National Physical Fitness Week as the kick off–Governor's Council (317) 237-5630	Automatic blood pressure cuffs placed on each floor for checkout Start of summer family newsletter packed full of ideas for a safe and fun summer of family activities
June	Cancer in Sun Month • Suntan lotion given to employees at cafeteria	Walking Club meets for a community walk	National Men's Health Week • Men's support groups started for post cardio-vascular disease (CVD) Second summer family newsletter

Table 4-3 National Health Observances Calendar 2000—*continued*

Month	Awareness Activity	Behavior Change	Supportive Environment
July	Summer Safety Seminars	Kids Camp • Week of day camp activities	Third summer family newsletter
August	World Breast Feeding Month–La Leche League (847) 519-7730 • Information Table	Employee Picnic and Back-to-School Blues	Initiation of postnatal support group
September	National Cholesterol Month–HLB Institute (301) 252-1222 • CHO screening offered	Back-To-School Stress Groups • Start group to address how to cope with stress	800 Stress Line initiated
October	National Breast Cancer Awareness Month–ACS (800) ACS-2345 • Information table	Second push for breast cancer screening	Vegetarian Aware Month–(800) USA-VEGE • Vegetarian menu items added in cafeteria
November	National Hospice Month–Hospice Organization (703) 243-5900 • Information Tables	Great American Smoke Out–ACS (800) ACS-2345 • Buddy program	Tie One On For Safety Campaign–MADD (214) 744-6233 • Red ribbons available to tie onto cars
December	Annual Health Goal Challenge • What are your health goals for the new year?	Annual Health Goal Challenge	Counselors and coaches helping people with health goals for new year

When developing a program calendar, it is also important to note the different seasonal cycles that will have both positive and negative effects on programming. For example, many employees are highly motivated to lose weight right before summer so they can once again fit into their bathing suits. Health promotion programs can take advantage of this seasonal motivation to promote realistic/safe weight loss programs that encourage eating right and exercise. It is just as important to remember that in the fall many organizations are preparing budgets, and this is not a good time for intense programming efforts–but it is a good time to provide awareness and self-help materials on stress reduction and how to take a much-needed five-minute vacation at work.

Winning Project Management Techniques

Early adoption of project management techniques in the design and planning stages by the programming team will increase the opportunity for program success. One of the first lessons that must be learned by the programming team is how to decide program prioritization. A program priority worksheet (adapted from Baker & Baker, 1998) can be utilized that:

1. Lists all current and potential programming ideas
2. Determines the need or opportunity for each project
3. Establishes rough delivery dates and budgets
4. Judges feasibility of each program
5. Establishes risk (potential for failure) associated with each program

6. Review these lists with programming team, employees, and management
7. Eliminates programs that are inappropriate or unfeasible and prioritizes the rest
8. Selects the most important

This worksheet will help staff move past the program prioritization step that so many find is a major barrier to creativity.

Another programming staff challenge that arises in the program design and planning stage is the need to develop a work plan. A work plan is a document that organizes and summarizes the task to be completed in a document that will insure the work moves forward. It could be as simple as a sequential list that provides: description of the task to be completed, estimated time required to complete the task, team member responsible for task completion, target start date, potential milestones (clearly identifiable points in a project), and target end dates.

Ultimately, a work plan will also include a schedule and a list of the resources necessary to complete each task. The first step in developing a work plan is to define the independent task that can be sequenced, assigned, and scheduled. The complexity and length of the program being planned will determine how complex a work plan needs to be. A blood pressure program that will last for six months and involves various behavioral interventions will require more detail than an eight-week weight management program. What makes a work plan different from a list of tasks to be completed is the integration of tasks into a total system that improves staff understanding of the project and communications between staff members. Work plans provide the team leader a tool to manage both weak and strong staff members and build team spirit and pride. Other project management tools (Brassard, 1994) used in conjunction with a work plan are:

* Critical path–a sequence of tasks that determines the minimum schedule for a project.
* Network diagram–logical representation of tasks that defines the sequence of events in a project.
* Tree diagram–systematically maps out in increasing detail the full range of paths and tasks that are required.

Program Implementation

The second stage of program delivery is implementation and is concerned with maintaining participation and compliance and reaching the outcome and impact goals that have been set in the design and planning stage. Implementation is concerned with following the steps outlined in the program plan for the various programs that are to be implemented. Various programming techniques will be used in this stage to insure program success. The following programming techniques will be briefly discussed relative to implementation:

* Registration
* Program orientation
* Goal setting
* Incentive systems and motivation
* Support systems
* Program momentum
* Program tracking

Program Registration

Program registration is the first step in program implementation and allows employees to sign up for programs. The process should be kept simple and require only necessary information critical to participant success. If the process is cumbersome, it will be hard to administer and deter sign-up. A registration form might include basic demographic information, initial screening and assessment results, or benchmark data from knowledge and behavioral surveys. Complex programs might require registration packets with multiple forms to be completed, while simple programs could use an all-purpose registration form.

Companies with networked computers and electronic mail should allow employees to register by computer. Another simple registration method is to use the company phone mail system. This allows a large number of individuals to enroll for a program without having to complete a registration form. Key components of a successful registration process include starting the enrollment period at the peak of preprogram promotion, keeping procedures simple, and collecting only information that is absolutely necessary.

Program Orientation

Many programs will start with a program orientation or kickoff meeting to insure participants understand the participation rules or guidelines and the expected outcomes. These could be one-on-one sessions in which the results of screenings and assessments are provided and a program plan is negotiated with participants. In-group programming becomes team meetings in which participation schedules and team support strategies are discussed and planned to insure team and team-member success. Young programmers sometimes eliminate program orientation steps in order to save staff time, but it is a very important step for both individual and group programming. For in-group programming, this step initiates the team process; and in programs involving individuals, the important coaching/counselor relationship is initiated with a staff member.

Goal Setting

Goals provide individuals and groups involved in behavior change with a program focus that is very important to forward progress. They provide a clear understanding of a specific target and serve as a frame of reference for decision making and performance feedback. Goals are shared conceptions of intention and place value on the processes and outcomes involved in daily tasks. Locke's (1978) research into goal setting has shown that establishment of, and working toward, goals by employees provide motivation for higher performance. Team goals should be reviewed and tracked at team meetings that provide a continued focus on results. Weekly and monthly reviews of employee personal goals provide opportunities for feedback and revitalization. During both team and personal goal reviews, the individuals involved should be ready to adapt or re-write goal statements to fit the current problems, issues, or challenges.

Figure 4-4 provides an example of a goal-setting behavior change contract that can be used in a variety of programs. It emphasizes the need for both a long-term goal that is challenging and short-term goals that provide the small steps that are reachable along the way. Individuals who are focused on running their first marathon will use 5 and 10k races as the small steps before they begin to master the half marathons and 20+ mile runs. The other elements that are necessary in a goal-setting plan are action steps, such as the specific 5 and 10k races to be run in marathon preparation. Feedback and reinforcement strategy should follow the action steps. Feedback and reinforcement will be discussed in both the incentive and motivation and the program tracking sections.

Incentives and Motivation

Maintaining participant motivation throughout the program is a core responsibility of the programmer. Good programmers will help participants measure their motivation during different program milestones and use a variety of motivation techniques to keep them involved and moving forward. A combination of self, buddy, team, or staff monitoring can provide an individual the attention that is necessary to maintain successful participation.

Incentive systems should be a balance between extrinsic and intrinsic rewards. Extrinsic incentives (rewards obtained externally) should be things that the individual is interested in receiving. Successful health promotion programs will survey employees annually to see what types of extrinsic incentives they are interested in receiving. Some of the best extrinsic systems are part of another reward system within the company. A good example would be individual health goals being part of the health and safety bonus reward system. Intrinsic incentive (rewards obtained internally, feeling of fulfillment, self-worth) structures must be built into a program. This provides participants opportunities to "honor" themselves. An example of an intrinsic structure might be a chart that provides participants the value of quitting smoking. It might be a table that allows individuals who have lost weight or inches around their waist a way to understand the number of pounds of pressure that is no longer pulling down on their back. The balance between extrinsic and intrinsic motivation is important for it is what keeps participants moving forward during the lapse (slips) and relapse (backsliding) that will most likely occur during behavior change efforts.

Name _____

Staff Coach _____

Long-term Goal (Realistic, challenging, measurable, and set for a specific time period)

I will _____

_____

Short-term Goals (Goals that will help me achieve my long-term goal)

I will _____

I will _____

I will _____

Action Steps (Rules I will follow to reach my short-term goals)

I will _____

I will _____

I will _____

Feedback Strategy (Ways to help me monitor my success)

I will _____

I will _____

I will _____

Reinforcement Strategy (Ways I will support the short-term goals & action steps)

I will _____

I will _____

I will _____

Figure 4-4 Goal-Setting Behavior Change Contract

The mechanics of rewarding extrinsic incentives needs to be well-planned. Insure that the rules governing incentives are fair and that the pickup process is realistic both for the staff responsible for administering the pickup and for the participant. Unfortunately, many happy participants have been turned into dissatisfied participants after becoming angry over their inability to pick up a $4.63 T-shirt. Insure that the pickup date and time window is large enough for all participants and an alternate pickup option is available for those who travel or are sick during the pickup time.

Support Systems

Programs need to have support strategies incorporated into their design. They could involve the buddy system or teams that group individuals into natural support systems. It is important to remember when forming teams or buddy systems that guidelines and rules need to be provided in order for these groups to effectively work together. Many individuals have tried to change a behavior with someone else, but most of these experiences do not end in success. So it is important that these teams be provided instructions on the characteristics of a successful group.

The family is the major support system in worksite programs, yet most programmers fail to give individuals ideas on how to get the family to be a positive support system. Programmers should provide individuals with information sheets that can be given to family members so they better understand their role. Other support systems could be the formal or informal support groups that are found in worksites. Some of the most popular support groups are informal groups that meet in the lunchroom to discuss a variety of topics. These groups can be formed with placement of a placard on a lunchroom table announcing that a "parenting support group for 2–4 year olds" is meeting every Tuesday from 11:30–12:30pm. These groups are very popular in many settings. There is also environmental support. An example might be healthy snacks in vending machines or ergonomic computer programs that remind individuals to take breaks and stretch every hour. Support is an imple-mentation strategy that can make the difference, not only in program success but also long-term program compliance.

Program Momentum

Program momentum deals with keeping participants focused and involved with the concepts of health and well-being. Even if employees do not register and get involved in specific programs, program momentum that has been generated can keep nonparticipants focused on making healthy choices. It's the program momentum in a worksite that becomes a very strong cultural value pushing and pulling individuals to participate in programs and/or to maintain health without participation. Experienced programmers will develop a program mix that builds program momentum in a variety of offerings and intensities. Program momentum is an art that must be practiced differently at each worksite and each stage of program maturity.

Program Tracking

Goals provide the measures that will track individual, group, or organizational programming. A good tracking system is built so that individuals can follow themselves without the need for staff involvement. Skinfold calipers have been used for years to measure body fat, but they require a skilled staff person to provide the measure. Body Mass Index (BMI) is a much better measure, not only because of the health-related data correlated to its measurement but also because it can be measured by the participant without the need for help. By providing participants with an index to measure their own success, they become empowered differently.

Technology has increased the possibilities for tracking systems, but it is important that the value of such systems be measured before advanced systems are engaged. In small to medium worksites, it might be more cost-effective to maintain a team tracking system on a large bulletin board in the cafeteria. With 75% of the workforce eating in the cafeteria every day, the bulletin board is more effective than multiple screens on the company computer system. Stair-walking challenges pull people into stairwells because of tracking systems that are maintained at the first floor, middle levels, and the top floor. These bulletin boards become badges of honor that provide an immediate sense of accomplishment. This sense of immediate accomplishment is lost when a participant must return to their desk, open up a tracking program, and enter their data. Programmers need to carefully evaluate the need to move their entire tracking system into a computer system that might not allow them to reach all employees. Many hospital systems claim to have their entire workforce on computers, but many of the employees involved in direct patient care (nurses, technicians, nurses' aides) do not have the time during their workdays to use the computer except for patient care.

Technology does offer effective ways to reach remote sites and individuals that travel. There are now tracking programs being set up on Palm Pilots that have increased the potential variables that can be monitored and enhance immediate feedback. The number one rule in setting up a tracking system is to insure that you have picked variables that can be realistically monitored and that the measure will result in feedback important to individual or group participants.

Program Closing

The last step in program delivery is program closing. It is in the closing stage that individuals, groups, and organizations are given opportunities to understand what they have learned or gained. Program endings need to be as strategic in their planning and execution as program startup or kickoff. It is in the closing stage that staff will ask participants questions and collect data that will be used to complete process, outcome, and impact evaluations. The debriefing of participants and reporting of appropriate findings to stakeholders is what moves the programming process forward. During this stage, program relapse prevention strategies are better defined, new program ideas are developed, and many weary programs are recharged.

FINANCIAL CONTROL AND BUDGETING

Health promotion managers often pride themselves in their knowledge about working with people and marketing and delivering high quality programming. They are often not as confident about their financial control and budgeting skills. The financial and budgeting responsibilities in every health promotion program are crucial to the success of programs. Through the budgeting process, planning becomes realistic, expected performance can be articulated, and feedback from achievement is possible (Marquis & Huston, 1996). The budgetary process is an opportunity for staff members to become involved, familiar, and gain ownership in a crucial quality-control system. Identifying the different cost and profit centers within the department is a necessary step in developing and administering a quality-control system. Understanding the monthly financial statements allows the manager to perform analytical budgetary techniques that enhance understanding and the ability to better manage the relationships of cost, participation, and individual, group, and program success.

Budget Planning

A budget is the formalized financial plan of the goals and objectives of the organization. It is generally expressed in schedules of expenses, surplus or deficits, and product or service volume for a predetermined period. The budget is a realistic way of obtaining the most productive use of the department's financial resources. Many program budgets are drawn from a larger departmental budget, such as Human Resources, Medical Department, or Facility Management, and thus are initiated by a combination of a top-down and bottom-up budgeting procedures. The process begins with the health promotional team reviewing programming, marketing, and promotional plans for the coming year. Each component of the plan is described in terms of costs, revenue, and potential participation or services to be delivered. The manager then adds appropriate administrative costs (such as salaries, facility rent and upkeep, and revenues) to complete the plan. This completed plan is then submitted to the next budgetary level for review. Once the review process has been completed, the health promotion budget becomes part of a collective budget document that, when finally approved, becomes the comprehensive budget.

Budget Types

There are several different types of budgets, but most health promotion programs will be asked to submit personnel, operating, and capital budgets. A personnel budget reflects all the costs related to "staffing" and is generally the largest budget type. An operating budget reflects the "operations" of the department and focuses on the major areas on which expenditures are made (equipment, programming, preventive maintenance, materials, supplies, etc.). There are various formats that can be used to display and manage an operating budget. The most common is the line-item budget that groups different categories of expenditures.

A capital budget generally reflects expenditures that are associated with equipment, facility, or new technology development projects. These expenses are sometimes centralized into a single administrative account for the entire organization or could be specified for each major budgetary unit. Capital expenditures often are divided into categories of capital improvements and equipment. An example of a capital improvement might be additional space requirements for new classrooms or office space, special electrical wiring for a new sound system or audiovisual center, and painting or carpeting. Equipment is customarily classified under the capital budget if its cost is over $100.00 and has a life expectancy of more than five years. In fitness centers, the constant wear of aerobic fitness equipment in a successful health and fitness center usually requires replacement of this equipment after three to five years to keep safety high and downtime to a minimum. Strength equipment is generally replaced every seven to ten years because of both high replacement cost and constant technology developments increasing safety and increasing participant strength training success rates. An innovative replacement strategy staggers replacement of equipment so that some of the equipment is replaced almost every year. This provides participants with variety and keeps interest high. This also provides the department a reason to be a part of the annual capital budgetary process.

O'Donnell & Ainsworth (1984) suggest two other budgetary formats. The functional-area and the intervention-area budget formats are more effective in illustrating the impact that expenditures have on program success. Functional-area budgets allocate expenditures according to the areas in which they are used. An example of a functional-area budget is the categorization of expenses into marketing, programming, delivery, administration, personnel, and facilities and equipment areas. In an intervention-area budget, expenditures would be allocated according to the specific impact focus. An example of an intervention-area budget would be allocation of expenses to fitness, stress management, nutrition, weight management, cancer screening, parenting, and hypertension control.

Implementing a Budget

A budget serves as a quality control. The document helps the team identify budgetary priorities and justifies decreasing or increasing programming expenditures. For example, it might be standard policy for all promotional flyers to be three colors, but a quick review of the budget shows a deficit in the reprographics budget line. This would require staff to design cheaper promotion pieces that would help reduce the reprographics deficit. All programming decisions are based in part on budgetary performance standards. A budget also provides a common denominator for communicating the goals of the department by integrating the different impact or functional areas. Efficient record management techniques and use of computer spreadsheet and accounting programs help coordinate and implement a budget.

Record Management

Competent record management requires specific procedures and methods for controlling and documenting expenditures and revenues. Health promotion departments should have formal procedures for paying contract services, salaries, rent, and ordering/paying for supplies and materials. These procedures will insure that proper records are maintained to provide a paper trail history of each action. One method to manage records is to maintain a separate folder on potential expenditure or revenue-generating items. For example, for each health education vendor there might be a separate file that contains all requests for purchases, purchase order forms, and material received forms–all with the signature of an authorized person. Proper record management of supporting documents is vital to a successful budgetary process.

Computer Spreadsheet and Accounting Programs

There is a wide assortment of computer software programs that provide budget management and analysis capabilities. Computer spreadsheet programs can be used to track the budget and provide a variety of financial analysis techniques that can be used to make future budgetary projections. Most of these programs have built-in graphic capabilities that create graphs and charts that can be used to enhance budget presentations. There are also accounting software programs that provide similar functions but offer more statistical and financial functions. A good example would be Quicken.

Maintaining and Growing a Budget

The financial control of a health promotion team is often left up to a secretary or clerk who has the time or business inclination and has always maintained the support documents. When a health promotion director relinquishes this responsibility, it weakens the potential efficiency and growth of the program. Only by observing and understanding the departmental expenditures and revenues that parallel the volume of participation will the manager insure budget efficiency and growth.

Budget Variance Report

A budget variance report shows budgeted amounts compared to actual amounts spent. The report uses a multicolumn format that has an "actual" column,

"budget" column, and "variance" column. The variance column represents the difference between actual dollars spent and the dollars budgeted. Typically the report provides a dual set of dollar values representing data from the current period (month) and year-to-date data. Erroneous variations between the budgeted allowances and actual results should be corrected and explained. If, for example, the contract labor line of the summary report shows that actual is larger than budgeted, it is important to backtrack through this specific account to find the cause. Company policy often dictates when variance explanations are required, but it is good management to review each summary report and insure actual expenditures have been accurately recorded.

Budget Efficiency

The health promotion manager has the responsibility not only for planning a budget but also for insuring that the assigned amounts are monitored and used for the specified resources. Budget efficiency is computed by making a ratio of the difference between the actual expenditure and budgeted amount, divided by the budgeted amount:

$$\text{Efficiency Ratio} = \frac{\text{Difference Between Actual \& Budgeted Amounts}}{\text{Amount Budgeted}}$$

The budget efficiency ratio provides information about the performance of each line item and provides comparisons for budgetary periods. Budget efficiency is influenced by many factors; but, in health promotion programs, participation is the major determinant of expenditures and revenues. Three types of costs are defined as fixed, variable and semi-variable (Chenoweth, 1998). Fixed costs are those that remain constant over the reporting period. An example of a fixed cost would be rent. Variable costs would be those that rise and fall in relation to changes in program participation or other activities that change during the reporting period. An example of a variable cost would be the rise in health education material expenditure during a health fair offering many different types of pamphlets, brochures, and fliers. Semi-variable costs are those that are partially fixed, and partially variable. In fitness centers, there is an expected participation level that sets the amount of soap and shampoo that will be purchased. When participation level increases over a certain range, then a variable amount of soap and shampoo must be ordered to meet the rise in activity. Managers can plot the performance of fixed, variable, and semivariable costs and revenues to have a clear view of the variability to be expected in the budgetary process.

Budget Growth

The monthly variance report, computed budget efficiency equations, and the charting of expenditure variability gives the manager helpful information in building a case for budget growth. Budget growth in health promotion is tied to current program success and the potential increase in future activity level. If the worksite population is increasing, then the program budget must also grow to insure that the same level of programming can be maintained as the population grows. If a new program or activity is added without the termination of a current program, the budget must grow to support the new effort. Crucial to budgetary growth is the understanding and delivery of what is expected by senior management. Programs cannot seek new budget resources for a new program that is at odds with the organization's goals and objectives.

Several budget growth strategies are important when considering this challenge. First it is important to emphasize how effectively and efficiently the budget has been managed. Managers have a greater opportunity for increasing their budgets if they have displayed the skill and understanding necessary to manage the budget. The second strategy is to maneuver the reviewers so that they recognize the need for budget expansion and mandate the necessary actions. This requires creating a win-win position for the reviewers so that they receive personal or organizational gain. The last strategy is to present the facts that stress the uniqueness of the department and its role in carrying out management's expectations. No other department performs services that tell employees "the company cares" and helps employees care for their own health and well-being. Budget growth is

not a necessity for program growth. Programs can grow and be successful by switching their financial resources between different activities and events in different program years. In providing variety, managers increase their opportunity to spread their financial resources and still maintain successful programs.

FACILITIES & EQUIPMENT

Facilities are not a component of all health promotion programs; but, when a facility is included, the effectiveness of its management is directly related to program success. The health promotion program plan will dictate the facility and equipment needs. Each program component included in the program mix must be reviewed for facility and equipment requirements. Facility requirements must be reviewed for functional space requirements, participant accessibility, signage, and safety and emergency procedures. There are several sources in the literature that provide extensive information about facility planning. This information will range from the initiation of space planning with an architect to the selection and supervision of the contractor. If facility planning is a necessary component of a director's role, then Grantham, Patton, York, & Winick (1998) and Tharrett and Peterson (1997) should be reviewed.

Facility and Equipment Plan

Many health promotion programs are initiated with the understanding that they will receive no new space. The training or facility departments maintain the space they must use for programming. These programs will have space needs but will not be concerned with an extensive facility plan. They will review their space and chair and table requirements, along with any special equipment needs. Educational programs need a variety of special pieces of equipment, including audiovisual, computer hardware and software, health assessment tools, and possibly portable cooking appliances. A small program that offers fitness programs in training rooms will need chairs and tables that can be easily stacked to clear room for the class. These classes also need exercise mats and fitness class accessories that are portable and can be easily stored. Exercise or health education equipment that works effectively in the space provided is a major factor to the success of a small program.

Programs that have dedicated exercise or health education space will have comprehensive facility and equipment plans. These plans will maximize efficient use of space with the minimum number of pieces of equipment that will meet the goals and objectives of the program. Two key ideas in planning a facility and equipment plan are, first, to insure the safety of participants and staff in the space design and equipment selection; second, facility and equipment decisions need to be made on the potential success of individual participants and the total program. For example, the decision to turn a closet space into a lactation room should be based on the demographics of the employee population and the immediate and long-term needs and goals of the program. Once the facility and equipment needs have been documented, a plan is developed and proposed to senior management. This plan is very important to the success of the program because program space and equipment decide the mode, format, and accessibility of the activities and events.

Coordination and Implementation of a Facilities Plan

After a facilities and equipment plan has been accepted, it must be coordinated and implemented. This could result in the building of a learning center, resource room, or fitness center. It might mean the renovation of existing space into a new lifestyle change area or into testing and assessment rooms. The coordination and implementation of these plans involves a management opportunity that rarely happens in the life of a program but can have significant impact on future success.

The architect or contractor is not responsible for insuring that the facility and equipment plan meets the goals and objectives of the program. This responsibility belongs to the health promotion team. These responsibilities include site inspections to insure design, governmental code, and material requirements have been met and that the set construction time schedules are being followed. During this phase of facility and equipment management, many issues will

arise that will require equipment and structural changes be made. It is important that the health promotion team be organized and ready to accept this responsibility.

Equipment Receiving

It is also during this stage that equipment is delivered. Equipment purchasing records and receiving statements are very important for they show that the expected equipment pieces arrived on time, in the proper quantity, in working order, and are what was ordered. Purchasing records should have a delivery date documentation about the item and seller information (phone, fax, etc.) to reconcile any potential problems. The entire staff should be alerted to the potential daily delivery of items and understand the specific requirements necessary to document that the proper equipment was received and signed for. Also, instructions on safe use of equipment are usually provided at delivery and should be reviewed to insure they are complete and will serve to help design participant equipment orientation sessions. Equipment should not be accepted unless the seller has provided a day and time that the health promotion team members can be shown how to use and perform the proper preventive maintenance on the new pieces of equipment.

Computers, Software, and the Internet

Health promotion, like many other industries, has experienced incredible growth because of the power of technology. The ability to provide multiple cost-effective screening options, tailored intervention programming, and sophisticated tracking systems has made computer systems an integral component of worksite programs. These systems also provide a health promotion team the ability to coordinate the many different processes occurring between participant, staff, and management. Basic data management and spreadsheet programs are used to manage a wide range of data, from participant information to the inventory of books and videocassettes. The need for these systems has increased the availability of specialized software (fuelware) programs that have been

written for health promotion and fitness environments. A list of companies that offer fuelware applications to these environments can be found at
http://www.fitnessworld. This list includes facility
management, member management and billing, front
desk operation, employee activity log-in, and report
generation.

Computers provide health promotion teams an advantage in managing large amounts of data and integrating complex programs. The Internet gives the
health promotion staff a window to unlimited opportunities in professional networking and information
retrieval, which can significantly expand their creative and innovative abilities. However, surfing the
Internet can be time-consuming, and individuals
should find and use those search engines and websites that serve them best. New programming opportunities have also been opened in multiple-site and
remote-site environments where a computer system
now allows the cost-effective coordination and communication of activities and events. Computer systems, fuelware programs, and the Internet are tools
that can be used to help make a program more effective. Good strategic planners make them a core
strategic tool that is woven into the program plan to
help increase the opportunity for program success.

Risk Management

Regardless of the definition that is used to define risk,
it is always bad. It is always associated with an event
that could happen in the future and is undesirable. In
health promotion programs, there are three components that interact as risk contributors in the programs. The three basic risk contributors in worksite
programs are people, equipment, and facilities. Each
must be managed so that the opportunity for an undesirable event occurring is minimized. A health promotion staff person should be well-aware of the disease risk factors that should guide individual and
group exercise programs. Many staff people do not
understand the increased risk involved in using
equipment or facilities that have not been maintained.
Good risk management programs maintain the
proper documentation on participants, equipment,
and facilities. Facility and equipment inspections and

screening of members and potential members are performed on a regular schedule. Safety equipment and
supplies are essential to responding to an emergency
situation, but staff also must be trained and consistently tested on response capabilities.

Planning for Special Populations

Many employees who have disabilities are not getting
the exercise and wellness programming they need.
Why? It's a fact that most worksite health promotion
programs do little to make people with disabilities
feel welcome in their programs. Accessibility is a major problem in fitness centers for people with disabilities, but the same problems exist in some of the
crowded health education resource rooms or demonstration areas. Early in the facilities and equipment
planning stages, staff should review the Americans
With Disabilities Act (ADA) and consider how to
provide access to all their programming regardless of
disabilities. It is estimated that by the year 2010 the
number of 55–74-year-olds will outnumber the 25–34-
year-olds by 18 million (McGough, 1999). As this
"graying" of the population occurs, workplace programs have begun to feel the impact of this phenomenon on program participation and special program
requests. Successful programs have segmented out
these special populations and developed program
offerings that service these special needs. Good examples are the osteoporosis programming in worksites that provide screening, along with organized
nutritional and exercise programs. Another good example would be on-site physical therapy programs
that not only service company sprains and strains but
also help individuals who are facing a variety of bone
and joint challenges due to diabetes, arthritis, bursitis,
or just normal aging. In the American College of
Sports Medicine's *Health/Fitness Facility Standards and
Guidelines* (1997), there are several recommended
sources for more ideas about making exercise and
health education facilities more accessible. The following items are adapted from that list:

- Architectural and Transportation Barriers Compliance Board
(800) USA-ABLE

- Barriers Free Environments, Inc.
  (919) 782-7823
- Mainstream, Inc.
  (301) 654-2400
- National Center for Access Unlimited
  (312) 368-0380

Facilities & Equipment Preventive Maintenance

The last function in successfully managing a facility and its equipment is preventive maintenance. This function keeps employees feeling comfortable in a health and fitness program because the center is clean, and in an educational program it insures that the audiovisual equipment functions properly. Effective preventive maintenance requires that the owners' manuals and warranty papers are catalogued for future use, and a listing of manufacturer representatives is maintained.

It also requires an up-to-date staff manual that collects the policies and plans necessary to operate a safe and successful program in an easy-to-understand and useful format. Policies are statements and instructions that provide important direction to a staff member on activities that require an action. A good example would be ordering supplies or requesting an all-employee e-mail. Policies would address who on staff could sign for specific budget levels or areas. They would define the procedures necessary in order to justify an all-employee e-mail. Procedures provide the sequence of steps required in performing specific actions. What are the steps required in reporting an injury during a walking club program? What are the steps required to run the end-of-the-month batch membership evaluation program?

Policy and procedure manuals address key issues involved in the operation of a health promotion program. These manuals document the administrative actions expected in a variety of situations, from program planning and new member orientation to emergency procedures. These manuals can be organized in a variety of ways but generally are arranged into key areas with appropriate subsections. Table 4-4 provides a sample of potential categories found in a policy and procedures manual in a worksite program.

Table 4-4 Example of Table of Contents for a Policy and Procedure Manual

Key Area	Subsections
Staff management	Hiring Termination Work schedule Temporary workers Annual employee evaluation Travel request Training request Vacation request Media inquiries Internship
Facility management	Opening and closing procedures Emergency procedures Preventive maintenance schedule Key control Purchasing procedures Inventory control procedures Lost and found Cleaning schedule Equipment checkout procedures (testing, audiovisual, computers)
Member management	Program enrollment/registration Program termination Fee collection procedures Screening and assessment schedule Guest and associate memberships Activity registration Participant data reporting Inactive member follow-up Material checkout (videocassettes, resource books, etc.)
Program management	Screening and assessment procedures Annual and quarterly calendars Promotion request Program development worksheet Program evaluation Annual staff planning event Committee charters

This manual provides proper documentation, but documentation is not enough to insure that facility space and all equipment is well-maintained.

Small Problems That Create Big Headaches

The facility and equipment issues that can create huge participant perception problems many times are very small problems. Staff members who do not know the basics on use of certain pieces of equipment will lose their credibility fast when they cannot answer participant questions about basic instruction. This problem can easily be managed by requiring all staff members to attend new equipment orientations and equipment use updates as part of staff training.

Participants can be thrilled to be losing weight or gaining control of their hypertension through a stress management program but quickly forget their behavioral successes with one bad lost-and-found experience. Lost-and-found forms should be maintained in a notebook recording the name, date, and item found or lost. The lost-and-found policy should provide infrequent program users an opportunity to retrieve lost items. Holding found items for a two-month period makes allowances for vacations, extended company travel, and the infrequent participation of some users. Lost-and-found areas should be designed to hold shoes, clothing, bags, briefcases, books, and personal toiletries. Items of value should be turned in to the building security office and recorded in a lost-and-found ledger book.

Equipment that is broken or a facility area that needs cleaning should be recorded on a maintenance record form. These forms provide staff the ability to follow up on maintenance problems. The forms will be used to record the nature of the problem, area in which the problem has occurred, date of occurrence, and staff member and employees who can be contacted for more information. These forms should be collected daily from suggestion boxes and staff daily logs. Prompt corrective action is a necessity, and this requires that a single staff person manage the process. Once action has been taken and completed, the manager should inspect and sign off the work as completed and then file the form for future reference.

Every member of a health promotion team must feel responsible for the upkeep of the facility and equipment. Good programming is the result of a team effort, and good preventive maintenance must also be a team effort. As a team matures, opening and closing procedural forms may be discarded as the team takes pride in insuring the facility and equipment look their best, but a good program manager understands the need to continue documentation that insures tired staff will not forget important steps or make bad decisions in emergency situations. Team pride is very important to a successful health promotion program and a successful team understands the importance of preventive maintenance.

CONCLUSION

The Association for Worksite Health Promotion identified four core strategies to improve health within work environments (AWHP, 1999).

1. targeting health risk and encouraging behavior change
2. mobilizing inner resources for health improvement
3. mobilizing social support for health improvement
4. developing organizational support for health improvement

Programs use these strategies in developing and maintaining their programs. Effective management is the key component in successfully operationalizing these strategies.

The program director designs the workforce plan that ultimately becomes the health promotion team. Hiring the right people that can be molded into a strong health promotion team provides the leadership necessary for successful programming. Health promotion teams evolve through group and individual employee training experiences that provide incentives and the opportunity to learn. This learning process should be managed so that team members are challenged to reach beyond their dreams. The people side of program administration management is made easier with well-developed plans. Nevertheless, it is the day-to-day people experiences and willingness to fail and learn through our failures that enable program leaders to become successful people managers.

The key to good program management is having a realistic mission statement or purpose, and goals that are results orientated. Program goals represent a balance between management's expectations, employees' needs and interests, and the program mix. A key factor in successful program management is prioritization of program goals which requires the staff to focus on distinct elements of the program mix. Goals are further defined by objectives and task assignments that provide the steps necessary for goal accomplishment.

One of the more exciting challenges of health promotion programming is defining the program mix. The number of program line and intervention level combinations is immense and offers programmers a wide variety of programming opportunities. Programming is an art that requires many tries, near misses, and some failures that requires strong leadership which helps guide the team to success. Program leaders should surround themselves with individuals who have strong potential and good skills in a variety of different program areas and who are committed to teamwork. It is through effective teamwork that new program ideas are developed, used programs are recharged, and relapse prevention strategies are maintained effectively.

The marketing process is initiated when the employees' wants and needs are first defined. It is important during the market research stage that employee readiness is reviewed and the price in time and dollars the employee is willing to pay be understood. Many good program ideas have failed to be implemented successfully because of a failure to understand the importance of location. Fitness facilities built too close to office space can experience low participation levels, because no one wants to be seen by management in the gym. On-site cholesterol testing is viewed in some locations as just another way for management to test for drugs. Place decisions must be made with the customer in mind so that program timing and distribution issues can be targeted appropriately. A clear understanding of how the components of the marketing process interact is crucial if a successful marketing effort is to be implemented.

Market segmentation adds to both the efficiency and effectiveness of health promotion programming. The division of an employee population base into broad markets allows programmers to better tailor programs to the employees' needs and interests. When these broad segments are further divided into specific market targets, the most successful health promotion programs are implemented.

The administration of a successful health promotion program also includes proper management of the budget. A budget is a control tool for the program director. It is the common denominator for all program events and activities. It can effectively communicate the departmental goals and objectives, and is one of the major items to be reviewed when trying to prioritize the program mix for a new programming year. A major challenge for any new health promotion program is establishing a budget that management is willing to support and one that provides flexibility in programming and staffing. Once an acceptable budget has been established, only good record keeping and appropriate ongoing budget analysis will maintain management's support of the current budget level.

It is usually not the large programming issues that irritate senior management, but the small maintenance problems. In a fitness facility, mold on a shower curtain can become an item that a senior manager will inspect on every trip to the facility. Facility and equipment maintenance can be successfully managed only when each member of the health promotion team feels responsible for high maintenance standards.

Managing a health promotion program is no different than managing any other department in a company. Individuals in these positions have a wide variety of educational backgrounds and worksite programming experience. However, people who know very little about health promotion usually supervise these positions. Consequently, the challenge of managing a successful program can largely depend on an individual's communication skills. Most supervisors do not understand the time it takes to plan programs or marketing efforts. They generally have a one-dimensional view of health promotion that fails to appreciate the detail necessary to organize, coordinate, and implement programs. Therefore, a program director's major job becomes one of educating their supervisor about worksite health promotion.

References

Aaker, D. (1988). *Strategic market management* (2nd ed.). New York: John Wiley & Sons.

Association for Work Site Health Promotion (1999). *Creating a healthy workforce: Health promotion programs at the work site.* Northbrook, IL: AWHP.

Baker, S., & Baker, K. (1998). *Project management: The complete idiot's guide to project management.* New York: Alpha Books.

Bell, R., & Shea, H. (1998). *Dance lessons: Six steps to great partnerships in business and life.* San Francisco, CA: Berrett-Koehler Publishers, Inc.

Bennis, W., & Nanus, B. (1985). *Leaders: The strategies for taking charge.* New York: Harper & Row.

Bobrow, E. (1997). *New product development.* New York: Alpha Books.

Brassard, M. & Ritter, D. (1994). *Memory jogger.* Methuen, MA: GOAL/QPC.

Camp, R. (1995). *Benchmarking: The search for industry best practices that lead to superior performance.* Milwaukee, WI: Quality Press.

Chenoweth, D. 1998. *Work site health promotion.* Champaign, IL: Human Kinetics.

Collins, J., & Porras, J. (1996, September/October). Building your company's vision. *Harvard Business Review,* 65–76.

Crump, C., Earp, J., Kozma, C., & Hertz-Picciotto, I. (1996). Effect of organizational-level variables on differential employee participation in 10 federal worksite health promotion programs. *Health Education Quarterly,* 23(2), 204–223.

Evans, D. (1995). *Supervisory management: Principles and practice* (4th ed.). New York: Cassell.

Fayol, H. (1925). *General and industrial management.* London: Pittman and Sons.

Gardner, J. (1990). *On leadership.* New York: The Free Press.

Glanz, K., Lewis, F. M., & Rimer, B. K. (1997). Health behavior and health education: Theory, research and practice. San Francisco, CA: Jossey-Bass, Inc.

Goodstein, L., Nolan, T., & Pfeiffer, J. (1993). *Applied strategic planning: How to develop a plan that really works.* New York: McGraw-Hill, Inc.

Gottlieb, N., Lovato, C., Weinstein, R., Green, L., & Eriksen, M. (1992). The implementation of a restrictive worksite smoking policy in a large decentralized organization. *Health Education Quarterly,* 19(2), 77–100.

Grantham, W., Patton, R., York, T., & Winick, M. (1998). *Health fitness management: A comprehensive resource for managing and operating programs and facilities.* Champaign, IL: Human Kinetics.

Hunnicutt, D., Deming, A., Baun, W., & Buffett, W. (1998). *Health promotion: Sourcebook for small businesses.* Omaha, NE: WELCOA.

Katzenbach, J., & Smith, D. (1994). *The wisdom of teams.* New York: Harper Business.

Landgreen, M. (1999). Employee health management goes global. *Work site health,* 6(4), 12–16.

Locke, E. (1978). The ambiguity of the technique of goal setting in theories of and approaches to employee motivation. *The Academy of Management Review,* 3(3), 594–601.

Marlatt, A., & Gordon, J. (1985). *Relapse prevention.* New York: The Guilford Press.

Marquis, B., & Huston, C. (1996). *Leadership roles and management functions in nursing: Theory & application* (2nd ed.). New York: Lippincott.

McDonald, M. H. (1995). *Marketing plans: How to prepare them, how to use them* (3rd ed.). Jordan Hill, Oxford, Great Britain: Butterworth-Heinemann, Ltd.

McDowell, S. (1999, August). Associations: are they worth it? *Fitness Management.*

McGough, S. (1999, July). Strength equipment for special populations. *Fitness Management,* 30–32.

Mears, P. (1995). *Quality improvement tools & techniques.* New York: McGraw-Hill, Inc.

Montana, P., & Charnov, B. (1993). *Management: A streamline course for students & business people* (2nd ed.). Hauppauge, NY: Barron's Educational Series, Inc.

Myers, M. J. (1991). Every employee a manager, 3 ed. San Diego, CA: University Associates, Inc.

O'Donnell, M., & Harris, J. (1994). *Health promotion in the workplace* (2nd ed.). Albany, NY: Delmar Publishers, Inc.

O'Donnell, M. P., & Ainsworth, T. H. (1984). *Health promotion in the workplace, 2nd ed.* New York, NY: John Wiley & Sons.

Prochaska, J., Norcross, J., & DiClemente, C. (1994). *Changing for good.* New York: William Morrow and Co., Inc.

Quigley, J. (1993). *Vision: How leaders develop it, share it, and sustain it.* New York: McGraw-Hill, Inc.

Rees, F. (1991). *How to lead work teams: Facilitation skills.* San Diego, CA: Pfeiffer & Company.

Ribisl, K., & Reischl, T. (1993). Measuring the climate for health at organizations. *Journal of Occupational Medicine, 35*(8), 812–824.

Rogers, E. M. (1983). *Diffusion of innovation, 3rd ed.* New York, NY: Free Press.

Rouillard, L. (1998). *Goals and goal setting.* Lanham, MD: Crisp Publications, Inc.

Sandhusen, R. (1993). *Marketing: A streamline course for students & business people* (2nd ed.). Hauppauge, NY: Barron's Educational Series, Inc.

Scholtes, P. (1998). *The leader's handbook: A guide to inspiring your people and managing the daily workflow.* New York: McGraw-Hill.

Senge, P., Kleiner, A., Roberts, C., Ross, R., & Smith, B. (1994). *The fifth discipline fieldbook: Strategies and tools for building a learning organization.* New York: Bantam Doubleday.

Shim, J., & Siegel, J. (1999). *Operations management: A streamline course for students and business people.* Hauppauge, NY: Barron's Educational Series, Inc.

Svendsen, A. (1998). *The stakeholder strategy.* San Francisco, CA: Bennett-Koehler Publishers, Inc.

Taylor, J. (1996). *Marketing planning: A step-by-step guide.* 1997. Englewood Cliffs, NJ: Prentice Hall.

Tenneco Internal Data (1989). [Tenneco health program]. Unpublished.

Tenner, A., & DeToro, I. (1996). *Process redesign: The implementation guide for managers.* Menlo Park, CA: Addison-Wesley.

Tharrett, S., & Peterson, J. (1997). *ACSM's health/fitness facility standards and guidelines* (2nd ed.). Champaign, IL: Human Kinetics.

Waldman, D. A., & Atwater, L. E. (1998). *The power of 360° feedback.* Houston, TX: Gulf Publishing Co.

Wild, R. (1996). *Essentials of production and operations management* (4th ed.). New York: Cassell.

CHAPTER

Program Evaluation

Ron Z. Goetzel and Ronald J. Ozminkowski

INTRODUCTION

Do worksite health promotion programs really work? Can they improve employee health, lower absenteeism, save health care dollars, and improve productivity? These are the questions typically asked of health promotion program evaluators. As these programs become more prevalent in the workplace, a growing body of literature has emerged that is focused on evaluation of these initiatives. However, a formidable challenge faces program evaluators: how to design and implement a scientifically credible evaluation in "real-life" worksite settings.

How is health promotion evaluation research performed? How can program managers gather documentary evidence that proves these programs have impact? Is such research, in fact, doable? What evaluation studies can program managers do on their own, and when should they bring in outside experts? These are some of the questions that are addressed in this chapter.

During the 1990s, a growing number of organizations introduced or enhanced worksite health promotion programs (Hewitt Associates, 1996; Fielding,

1991; Fielding, & Piserchia, 1989; Hollander and Lengermann, 1988). The movement is partly attributable to an increased emphasis on worker productivity and a belief that keeping employees healthy, both physically and mentally, will enhance their on-the-job performance. Additionally, health promotion has expanded its focus beyond primary prevention to include demand for medical treatment and disease management interventions that address the needs of individuals who may be ill and who may already be using health care services.

Unlike more traditional "wellness" programs developed in the 1970s and 1980s, today's programs offer secondary and tertiary prevention targeted at high-risk and high-cost workers. For example, a contemporary health management program might provide exercise, nutrition, immunization, and stress management programs, which are generally considered primary prevention activities. Additionally, the program may offer breast cancer screening, hypertension management courses, and smoking cessation programs, all of which provide secondary prevention. Finally, the program may include asthma, diabetes, and cardiovascular and other disease management interventions that are considered tertiary prevention. All of these activities may be supported by self-care guides, nurse hotlines, proactive mailings, and telephone communications. In many ways, health promotion programs have become broader and deeper in their scope, and the boundaries between prevention and treatment have become more blurred.

As health promotion programs mature and assume a more comprehensive focus, the need for effective program evaluation has assumed a higher priority. Very often, program sponsors are challenged to prove that health promotion programs work and save money.

Today, a greater number of organizations are seeking to document a clear business purpose for health promotion program introduction and continuation. Decision makers require data to support the view that investment in employee health is a wise business decision in addition to being "the right thing to do."

At the same time, health promotion program managers understand that if their programs are to survive and thrive, their programs must be subjected to rigorous program evaluations that determine their impact on the furtherance of corporate objectives. Consequently, the need for data collection, analysis, and evaluation have emerged as key priorities for those establishing and maintaining worksite health promotion programs. Often, evaluators garner data from insurance claims databases to support an economic justification for corporate programs.

Similarly, once a health promotion program has been approved and funded, program administrators and decision makers seek additional reassurance that the program is being well-managed and is achieving anticipated results. Thus, there is a need for regular reporting and monitoring to document program success and allay decision makers' anxieties about the program's efficacy.

PURPOSE, SCOPE, AND FORMAT

This chapter provides a practical measurement and evaluation guide for health promotion program managers and outside program evaluators. The purposes of the chapter are multifold. For program managers not trained in advanced statistical methods and evaluation research, the chapter illustrates the complexity of conducting evaluations. It is hoped, however, that specific measurement tasks and procedures can be undertaken by the novice program manager using this chapter as a guide. As an example, a program manager with little background in measurement theory might adapt the sample employee survey, found in the appendix to this chapter, to measure several key program success factors. The sample assessment relies upon participants' self-reported satisfaction with the program, improved health habits, behavior change, and other outcomes that are of interest to the program manager and sponsor.

For individuals with advanced training in program evaluation, the chapter illustrates how techniques and principles used in other applied research studies can be adapted to worksite health promotion evaluations. In conducting worksite health promotion studies, a multidisciplinary team of experts, who possess a variety of skills and backgrounds, often needs to be assembled. It is not unusual, for example, to include as part of the team experts in the fields of epidemiology, behavioral medicine, public health, statistics, social science research, employee benefits, economic analysis, health education, human resources, and computer science. Whereas the "typical" program manager might not ever consider assembling such a diverse and talented team of experts, the manager might consider calling upon any one or several such experts as advisers or consultants to the evaluation project. The manager may also be able to identify individuals within the organization who possess the skills necessary for such studies and draw upon their expertise in an evaluation effort.

Unlike the prior evaluation chapter published in the second edition of O'Donnell and Harris' *Health Promotion in the Workplace* (1994), the current text places a greater emphasis on the economic evaluation of worksite programs. Specifically, the chapter discusses the detailed data analysis requirements for financial analyses and methods employed in the conduct of cost/benefit and cost/effectiveness studies.

The beginning of the chapter poses and answers eight questions that help guide the development of an evaluation plan. The bulk of the chapter then discusses basic research principles, including design, sampling measurements, and analysis. The chapter is not written as a cookbook or step-by-step manual on how to conduct health promotion evaluation research. However, in an effort to make this material tangible, theoretical discussion is combined with examples drawn from "real life" program evaluation efforts.

DEVELOPING AN EVALUATION PLAN

Just as it is important to develop an effective, state-of-the-art health promotion intervention, it is equally important to develop a high-quality evaluation of that program. In developing an evaluation plan, the program manager should be prepared to answer the following questions:

- Why should programs be evaluated?
- Can research results be generalized from one program to another?
- Why do health promotion programs fail?
- Are there good arguments against performing program evaluations?
- What should be evaluated?
- How is an agreement on the program objectives achieved?
- Should the focus be on a few or many outcome measures?
- What are the basic questions that need to be answered when conducting evaluation studies?

Each of these questions is discussed in this section.

Why Should Programs Be Evaluated?

Program evaluations and tracking studies serve four basic functions.

First, *program evaluations support a business case for program introduction.* In a sense, program evaluation begins even before a program is put into place. In deciding whether to initiate a new program, the program champion often needs to compile evidence of "problems" or needs within the organization that a health promotion program can solve. Thus, evaluation involves gathering data to justify investment in such a program. The program is then "sold" to senior management by using a variety of data sources to cost-justify the investment. Often a cost/benefit model is developed, whereby costs associated with initiation of the program are compared to the potential benefits that will be realized from the program. This analysis is often referred to as a prospective return on investment (ROI) study, whereby current investment is evaluated vis-à-vis future return.

Second, *program evaluations provide ongoing monitoring and measurement of program performance in order to fine-tune or renew program elements.* Here, the focus is on "process" measures that assess the reactions of participants and how well the program is being implemented. Data gathered from these measures are used by program planners and administrators in the same way that standard program metric reports (often referred to as dashboards or report cards) are used to monitor program progress. In addition, problems in the design and implementation can be identified early in the process and corrected. This stream of data provides reassurance to program sponsors that their investment is being well-managed and results will be forthcoming.

Third, *program evaluations offer evidence of whether the right decision was made and whether the program has been successful in achieving its objectives.* At this point, the focus shifts from process to outcome measures–the extent to which specific program objectives are achieved. At certain milestones, the evaluator convenes the decision-making group and presents evidence that the program has, or has not, been successful in meeting its goals. At the conclusion of such a meeting, the decision makers determine whether the program is an overall benefit or cost to the organization.

Fourth, *program evaluations contribute to the science of organizational and individual change.* As individuals and groups develop exemplary programs, knowledge of these programs should be passed on to others through scientific articles and public presentations of program results. These communications of program achievement are most convincing when credible results accompany the description of the program's design and implementation. Thus, the credibility of program achievements often hinges upon the strength of the evaluation design.

Can Results Be Generalized from One Program to Another?

Often, program managers are asked: "Why should we spend the money to prove that health promotion works if others have already shown that to be true?" An appropriate response might be: "If you wish to assume that our program is similar in design and implementation to others that have preceded us, and you are willing to also assume that our results are identical to theirs, then, indeed, spending time and money on a new evaluation would be wasteful." However, few decision makers are willing to accede that the above assumptions apply to their own situations.

Thus, in thinking about evaluation of health promotion programs and the generalizability of results from any one evaluation to other situations, program administrators should take into account the enormous variability in program design and intensity. It would be erroneous to assume that any one health promotion program is like any other. Consequently, evaluations of alternative program designs need to consider the effect that these various approaches may have on specific outcomes of interest and overall program impact.

For example, some companies make programs available to all employees, while others limit these programs to certain sites, high-risk groups, or executives. Still others may extend the program to dependents and retirees.

Staff and facilities for health promotion programs may be worksite-based, community-based, program vendor-based, or any combination of the above. Programs may be run by professionals or by volunteers. Program components may be integrated under a central program management staff or run as independent efforts. Program offerings may be comprehensive or limited in scope. Singular topic areas may be offered in a variety of formats; for example, classroom instruction, self-paced study guides, interactive sessions, through telephone delivery, or via computer learning. Conversely, a singular presentation mode (e.g., classroom lecture) may be employed in which various topics are discussed.

A variety of incentives for participation and behavior change may be offered by organizations. These include individual prizes, team awards, and, most recently, cash or insurance premium rebates. In one organization, senior and middle management may be supportive of the health promotion initiative, while in others they may be cynical and obstructive. Some companies may allow their employees time off for participation, while others may offer programs only on employees' own time. Companies may require employee contribution (cost-sharing) or make programs available free of charge.

In short, there are many organizational and programmatic factors that either facilitate or hinder implementation. These need to be considered when attempting comparisons between program outcomes and in planning an evaluation effort.

Why Do Health Promotion Programs Fail?

There are many examples of successful health promotion initiatives and probably as many examples of unsuccessful ones. The reasons for failure often fall into one of the following three categories (adapted from Weiss, 1972, as cited in Sloan, Gruman, & Allegrante, 1987).

1. The *theory* underlying the program design was inappropriate or inadequate. The approach to behavior or attitude change might have been flawed. Interventions may have been constructed based on the program managers' intuition or "feel" instead of scientific evidence of program effectiveness or a widely-accepted theory of behavior change. The intervention may not have addressed underlying motivations for behavior change. The intervention may have been too narrow. The program may not have been sufficiently comprehensive, integrated, synergistic, or rational. In short, the structural underpinnings and theoretical foundation for the program may have been so shaky that no matter how hard the staff tried, they could never have achieved success.

2. While the theoretical framework for the program may have been adequate, and perhaps even elegant, the individuals charged with the task of *program implementation* may have performed poorly. For example, resources may not have been

adequate to do the job properly; the staff may not have been well-trained and -supervised; the essential equipment may not have been provided; or senior management may not have been supportive of the effort. In short, the theory was fine, but the implementation was poor.

3. Finally, in some programs, program design and execution are excellent, but inadequate efforts are made to **document the program's success.** Improper measurement may have taken the form of poor instruments or tools to record program accomplishments. The overall design of the evaluation might have been flawed. Consequently, the program may have been terminated because administrators lacked the proper information with which to evaluate it. This experience may be likened to the tree in the forest that crashes to the ground and is "not heard" because listening devices (ears) are not in place to record the event.

Are There Good Arguments Against Performing Program Evaluation?

Despite the many good reasons to perform program evaluations, the reader should be aware of why an evaluation component is often left out (adapted from Chapman, 1991).

1. *Evaluation may be viewed as a low priority activity that is expensive and distracting* from the actual intervention. When decision makers purchase health promotion programs, they may conjure up a vague picture of what they hope to accomplish (e.g., reduce costs, improve productivity, or heighten satisfaction).

   However, once a conscious decision has been made to invest in health promotion, their attention is almost entirely directed at determining how to put the program into place. The details of implementation, therefore, often drown out concerns about evaluation. In addition, since the investment in the intervention is often substantial, asking the decision maker to consider an additional expense for evaluation (which is classified as administrative rather than programmatic) is often problematic.

Finally, many companies believe that program evaluation is unnecessary due to an inherent faith in the probable benefits of health promotion programs. They may have reviewed studies that have discussed evaluations of similar programs and are satisfied that the same outcomes will apply to their situation. Consequently, they choose to invest in high-level programming rather than evaluation. As noted earlier, this involves a leap of faith that may not always be justified; one never really knows how well (or poorly) a program performs without evaluating it, and surprises are fairly common.

2. *Negative results may undermine the program.* The decision maker, as well as the program administrator, is naturally worried about what might happen if the results are not as they would like. Program administrators may feel that if an investment is made in measurement, the evaluator and decision maker are obligated to release the results of that evaluation, even if those results are negative. For those uncomfortable with entering into situations in which the outcome is ambiguous, deciding to conduct an evaluation that may produce negative results may be difficult. On the other hand, continuing a program that is not achieving positive outcomes is not defensible. The alternative to discarding a poorly performing program is to modify it so that it does achieve positive results. In either case, one should evaluate programs to identify their pluses and minuses, learn from their mistakes, and build on their accomplishments.

3. *An evaluation may require archival data that are often either difficult to access or unavailable.* The evaluator may discover that historical data are only available from specific sources and in unusual formats. The effort needed to unearth the available data and preparing them for analysis may be formidable. Historical, as well as contemporaneous, data may be unavailable simply because they are not routinely collected by the organization. Alternatively, data may only be available in an inconvenient form, such as hard copy, individual-level information, or weekly absenteeism reports. Facing the prospect of locating and collecting these data may

frustrate a prospective program evaluator. Here is where consultants or outside experts can help. Assembling a talented team within or outside the organization to address these problems can avoid frustrations facing program managers.

4. Executives have neither the time nor interest to carefully review a description of complex methodology and accompanying lists of limitations and caveats. If they don't understand how results are obtained, these decision makers may be reluctant to support the study and its conclusions.

   Thus, *evaluation is often viewed as overly academic, complex, intellectual, and "ivory tower-oriented."* Decision makers may be used to one-page executive summaries with accompanying conclusions and action steps.

   This point is well taken in that it is crucial to explain the objectives, methods, results, and implications of the evaluation in a way that motivates creative and productive corporate policy. In short, if the evaluation would be avoided because of the failure by evaluators to produce a useful product, it is better to obtain the services of a better evaluator, as opposed to scrapping the evaluation altogether.

5. *It takes time and resources to conduct studies.* Many U.S. corporations focus on quarterly results. An organization's economic climate, workforce composition, and strategic focus may change frequently. When told that they may have to wait several years for evaluation results on some measures, decision makers are often reluctant to commit resources. A response to this argument is that the evaluation may result in a better long-term corporate outlook that should not be avoided entirely. Alternatively, the evaluation should be crafted in a series of shorter steps that produce actionable recommendations in the short-run, as well as the ultimate overall answer, which may take longer to find.

6. *The evaluation may be viewed as intrusive or disruptive.* Assessment of program results should be accomplished by gathering the necessary data with the minimum amount of disruption and intrusion. Nonetheless, the decision maker may be reluctant to allow proactive data-gathering from individuals

engaged in the program and more so from individuals who are not directly affected by the intervention, that is, a control or comparison group. Disruption can be minimized or avoided by letting outside experts gather the data.

7. *The economic buyer who decides to conduct the evaluation may commit to doing so at only a very minimal level and with limited funding.* Even though the company and personnel in the health promotion department may lack the expertise to design and implement an appropriate evaluation program, the decision maker may elect to use internal resources to save costs. Consequently, little effort is directed toward the evaluation project, and the result is a sketchy and inconclusive analysis. At worst, an inadequate evaluation may lead to misleading results. Economic realities are important, but conversations about the potential costs and benefits of a good program evaluation that occur early on may help avoid penny-wise but pound-foolish strategies.

In sum, while the initial bias of many decision makers developing a new, high-quality health promotion program is to support a high-quality evaluation effort, this bias often fades when they realize the cost and complexity of conducting such an evaluation. Before a decision is made, much thought should be given to the consequences (both positive and negative) of having limited or misleading information about the value of a relatively costly corporate program.

What Should Be Evaluated?

Assuming the organization overcomes all of the obstacles cited above, there are three broad areas (see Table 5-1) that should be evaluated in a health promotion program (adapted from Wagner & Guild, 1989):

1. *Program Structure:* The program structure is the basic framework of the program–the "inputs" into the program. The purpose of a structure evaluation is to determine whether the program's design and critical components are in place according to plan. This evaluation is often referred to as an audit of

design plan compliance. Questions asked about the structure include: What is the intervention? How many program areas are covered? How is the program delivered to participants? How many classes are offered? How often are they offered? Where does the program take place? Who administers the program? What are their credentials? What equipment is used? What presentation techniques are used? Who is eligible for the program?

While these are not evaluation issues, per se, these need to be addressed when describing the program features, design, and content (often as the program description section of a research paper). Also, these issues are often addressed in administrative reports rather than evaluation or outcome studies. One way of thinking about a structural evaluation is as an assessment of the extent to which the program meets requirements for design and execution.

2. *Program Process:* Evaluating the program process is the same as asking how well the program is run. The purpose of a process assessment is to determine whether the execution of the program is progressing according to plan and whether the operation of the program is smooth. Questions addressed by process evaluations include: How many people participate? How satisfied are they with the course content? How do they feel about the instructors, facilities, and administrators? Which programs are best attended? How many individuals successfully complete programs?

3. *Program Outcomes:* Evaluation of program outcomes allows program managers to demonstrate the extent to which specific program objectives are achieved within a given time frame. Essentially, the purpose of an outcomes study is to determine whether the program's goals and objectives have been met according to plan.

The reason for focusing on all three areas, structure, process, and outcome, is that desired outcomes can only be achieved or maximized if structural and process features are sound. Bad outcomes can result from either bad structure or bad process. It is the evaluator's job to find out if either is problematic, and, if so, how to fix it. If it turns out that the program

Table 5-1 What should be evaluated?

Examples of Commonly Asked Questions

Structure
- What is included in the program? What is the intervention?
- Where does the program take place?
- How is the program delivered?
- What content is included?
- Who manages the program?

Process
- How many people participate?
- Do participants complete the program?
- Are participants satisfied?
- Which aspects of the program are best attended?

Outcome
- Does the program improve knowledge about health issues?
- Does the program change behavior?
- Does the program save money?
- What is the return on investment (ROI)?

achieves positive outcomes, it may be exportable to other settings and replicated. Thus, a complete evaluation can illustrate the good and the bad, leading to better programmatic decisions, structures, processes, and outcomes.

How is Agreement on Program Objectives Achieved?

Historically, companies institute health promotion programs for a variety of reasons (O'Donnell & Ainsworth, 1984). However, within any one organization, individual decision makers may have different criteria for program success based upon their area of expertise and responsibility in the organization. For example, the benefits director may wish to reduce health care or other costs; the personnel director may wish to curtail absenteeism; the human resources vice president may wish to reduce turnover and attract the best possible employees; the medical director may wish to improve employees' health; and the president may wish to improve the company's image to its employees and the community as an employer who cares about employee health and well being.

Consequently, program evaluators may find that there is no one company spokesperson who effectively verbalizes a consensus opinion regarding the organization's health promotion goals and objectives.

One of the most important initial tasks for those who are developing an evaluation program is to help the key decision makers form a consensus opinion on conceptual and operational definitions of program success. Among those who need to be polled, and who often play a role in defining the requirements for a successful program, are the:

- Economic buyer (the chief executive officer, chief financial officer, or vice president of Human Resources)—often this individual is, or is close to, the "visionary" of the organization, whose job it is to create a link between programmatic and organizational strategic objectives;
- Program administrator—the individual responsible for running the program and who may be most knowledgeable about what a health promotion program can achieve;
- Medical or health science professional—the physician (medical director) or occupational health nurse who provides clinical supervision of the program;
- Human resources executive (benefits director, quality manager, or training professional) who provides corporate level management and often funding of the program; and
- Other interested parties, who may include the fitness center director, general manager, company consultant or someone who has taken an active interest in the program and is willing to become its champion.

In building consensus among this diverse group of individuals, the facilitator must first understand the reasons each has for introducing health promotion programs into the workplace and how each hopes the program will benefit the organization or, for that matter, the individual who is advocating the program. This process culminates in those assembled, articulating, specific, quantifiable, and measurable outcomes for the program.

One way of building consensus for program outcomes is to expose each of the interested parties to the views of the others on this issue. Once individuals understand their colleagues' reasons for introducing the program, they may decide to focus on a limited number of outcomes that reasonably can be accomplished and measured.

For example, if the benefits director, whose chief aim is to reduce medical care costs, accepts the idea that an effective way to achieve this is to reduce the number of people at high risk for specific diseases, then documenting health risk reduction for the population may be adequate in proving program success. As added ammunition, the program champion may present recently performed research by the Health Enhancement Research Organization that links modifiable risk factors and increases in health care expenditures (Goetzel & Anderson, et al., 1998). These data can be used to make a compelling case for the cost burden of risk factors in the employee population and the potential cost reductions that can be realized if that risk profile is improved. If, on the other hand, the link between risk and cost is not accepted, then a more expensive and complicated medical claims analysis may be warranted.

Aligning Health Promotion Goals with the Company Mission

Experience in the field, supplemented by reports on "best practice" companies, highlights the need to clearly connect health promotion programming with the corporate mission and vision statements (O'Donnell, Bishop, & Kaplan, 1997; O'Donnell, 1999; M. P. O'Donnell, personal communication, July 5, 1999; Goetzel, Guindon, Humphries, et al., 1998). Best-practice health promotion teams start by reviewing their organizational mission and then translating that mission into easily understood health promotion goals and objectives that are core to the organization. These teams are careful to connect health promotion outcome metrics to organizational mission metrics. Best-practice health promotion teams are explicit about how accomplishment of their goals and objectives directly benefits the achievement of organizational goals and objectives.

Those responsible for health promotion programs recognize that they do not need to connect all they do to organizational objectives. However, they do understand the need to establish a direct link between their health promotion efforts and a bottom-line productivity metric, which the team can directly influence. Oftentimes, that link is found by focusing on the safety of the work force as a significant factor affecting organizational success (Goetzel, Guindon, Newton, et al., 1999).

Best-practice organizations translate their health promotion metrics into easily understood human terms; for example, productivity loss can be measured as:

- number of workers missing from work each day;
- daily and annual organizational expenses associated with absent workers; or
- annual direct and indirect costs attributable to employees suffering from a chronic disease, such as depression, allergy, back pain, asthma, obesity, or coronary heart disease.

When feasible, program advocates attempt to monetize key health promotion measures and present them in dollar terms. Further, they attempt to calculate the savings opportunity resulting from influencing a change in a health promotion metric. Demonstrating that health promotion can positively influence employee safety often gets the attention of key officers in the organization. As noted above, safety concerns can provide the linkage between health promotion and the organization's mission. Usually, it does not take much convincing for a CEO or a CFO to realize that worker safety is a business imperative.

If health promotion metrics are reviewed regularly by high-ranking executives, the program remains fresh and a high-priority activity relevant to business success. If these measures are linked to incentive compensation or employee bonus plans, they become even more relevant. The astute program administrator is therefore urged to develop easy-to-understand performance metrics that are central to the health promotion program's success, as well as to overall business success.

Should the Focus Be on a Few or Many Outcome Measures?

In general, it is recommended that as many measures as are reasonable should be considered in a comprehensive evaluation project. Since the intervention is likely to affect many outcomes simultaneously, it is advantageous for the program evaluator to gather data in multiple areas rather than relying upon measuring success in one key outcome. In that way, a rich story can be told regarding program effects on a variety of issues of interest to various audience members. If a more limited list of success factors is earmarked for evaluation purposes, the evaluator must take special care to ensure that the outcomes identified directly coincide with program goals and that they are indeed measurable.

The disadvantage of a comprehensive evaluation approach is that scarce evaluation resources are then distributed across several outcomes rather than concentrated in any one area. Thus, a situation may emerge in which the program's effects on many outcomes are evaluated inadequately because of insufficient investment in any given evaluation.

However, the advantage of a multiple measure evaluation approach is that different individuals' agendas are addressed simultaneously, and the reasons behind program success or failure can more easily be determined. This, in turn, helps shape future program designs and implementation strategies.

How much should be spent on health promotion program evaluation? Respondents to a survey administered by Johnson & Johnson Health Management, Inc., to its client companies (Johnson & Johnson Health Management, Inc., 1989) suggested that five to eight percent of a program's budget should be devoted to measurement and evaluation. The authors offer as a rule of thumb that approximately five percent of the total program budget be earmarked for evaluation research. However, it is likely that more dollars will be spent in early years of the program to establish a valid reliable baseline database, gain agreement on evaluation design, and report short-term outcomes.

O'Donnell (1999) offers the following guidelines for developing an evaluation budget: one percent for basic process measures, five percent for tracking detailed participation in the program, and ten percent if a number of outcomes are tracked in addition to qualitative measures. These guidelines include staff time to collect the data and the costs of hiring outside experts. The key forces in establishing an evaluation budget are the overall size and intensity of the intervention program (i.e., is it a $50,000 or $5,000,000 program) and the requirements of program funders (i.e., general descriptive information or an evaluation worthy of publication in a peer-reviewed journal).

The Basic Questions of Research

In developing an evaluation plan, the researcher may get lost in the details of design options, sampling procedures, operational definitions, statistical techniques, and so forth. It is useful, therefore, to step back from the minutiae and ask some basic questions relevant to the overall design. The following eight questions can be useful in the formulation of a final evaluation plan for the project:

1. *What do I want to* know? What is the question that I hope to answer? What problem am I trying to solve? What hypotheses am I testing?
2. *What will the answer or solution to the problem* look *like?* What measures of effect will be estimated? For example, if health care cost reduction is the goal, what level of reduction is anticipated?
3. *How will I see it?* What are the operational definitions of the constructs of interest?
4. *How will I* record *the data?* How will the data be collected? What instruments will I use? What methods for recording phenomena will be employed?
5. *How will I* categorize *and analyze the data?* What categories of data will be developed? What coding schemes will be used? What analytic models will be employed? What potential confounders will be controlled? What statistical techniques will be applied? How will I group the data? What will the final tables/charts look like?
6. *How will I* affect *the data?* Will I, as the evaluator, introduce systematic bias into this project simply because I have a stake in its outcome? What can I do to minimize this effect? Should an outside, independent evaluator be brought in to conduct the studies?
7. *What will I* infer *from the data?* What interpretations can I make once the results are prepared? What actions can be taken, given alternative study outcomes?
8. *What will I ultimately* find *out that I didn't know before I started?* What will I have learned that I didn't know beforehand? "So what?" Is this effort worth it?

The final question, similar to the first question, forces the evaluator to reexamine the importance of getting the answer to the initial question given the amount of effort necessary to perform the study in a valid fashion. It is remarkable how often these fundamental questions are not asked, and hence not answered, before an extensive and resource-consuming evaluation project is begun. In particular, the first question, asked quite innocently, may still trip evaluators who have spent much time and effort conjuring elaborate designs and statistics that are directed at issues not easily operationalized and often unanswerable.

RESEARCH PRINCIPLES

This section reviews some general principles of applied research and how these are considered in health promotion evaluations. As part of this review, alternative research designs are described and their relative merits discussed, especially as they relate to study validity. Next, methods of identifying target populations for studies, recruitment of participants and sampling techniques are addressed. A discussion of ways to measure specific outcomes of interest follows. The section concludes with some recommendations on possible evaluation timetables and ways to present results to decision makers.

The section begins with a discussion of some general research principles and why these are important to consider in any evaluation effort.

General Principles of Applied Research

In performing health promotion program evaluations, the evaluator is attempting to apply scientific methods to assess program effect. Scientific methods differ markedly from less rigorous methods of evaluation that are often erroneously referred to as common sense approaches (Kerlinger, 1973).

Scientific methods of evaluation rely upon the development of hypotheses based on theoretical models that are internally consistent and, in turn, that give rise to testable predictions. Specific procedures are used to systematically and empirically test predictions resulting from the theory.

A common sense approach, on the other hand, relies upon a "person in the street" or conventional wisdom interpretation of reality. This approach tests hypotheses selectively, by only including data that confirm hypotheses or preconceived ideas.

Scientific methods attempt to control for competing explanations of observed phenomena; in other words, they attempt to take into account other possible causes for what is perceived as an outcome or effect. Using common sense, the evaluator doesn't actively seek out other explanations for events, nor does the evaluator actively attempt to control extraneous sources of influence.

Most importantly, the scientific method seeks to determine a cause and effect relationship between events (i.e., what event causes what other event). The common sense approach may observe two events that occur simultaneously and infer that one causes the other. For example, a young child may accidentally spill a bowl of cereal on the floor and hear a doorbell ring. The child may erroneously infer that spilling the cereal causes the doorbell to ring, then not-so-accidentally try that trick again. The poor parent is left with the task of cleaning up the mess and answering the door at the same time.

The reason for expending space on this topic in a text devoted to health evaluation is at first not obvious. Why should decision makers be concerned with scientific methods when all they wish to determine is whether the program was effective? They may, in fact, draw a distinction between evaluation and research, noting that the former need not be as rigorous or "scientific" as the latter.

When discussion proceeds as to how these studies should be performed, the methods applied in conducting scientifically valid studies, and the cost of performing the analyses, decision makers may advocate a less rigorous approach. They may make such statements as, "We don't need a study that is of publishable quality," or "We just need some results–not a scientifically valid study." This is a common dilemma faced by program evaluators; and, in practice, a less rigorous evaluation methodology is often employed as a consequence. This will produce results, but these may be at best misleading and at worst quite wrong.

A review of literature by Heaney and Goetzel (1997) illustrates this point quite vividly. The authors examined 36 studies reporting health and productivity outcomes attributable to multicomponent worksite health promotion programs. As the research design for these studies increased in rigor, the findings became more equivocal. For example, 11 studies used a less rigorous preexperimental design, and all of their results (100%) were encouraging. However, of the nine studies employing a more rigorous experimental design, only two (11%) found encouraging results, five (56%) had mixed findings, and two (22%) had discouraging results. If the aim of the evaluation is to get as close as possible to the true impact of the program, then more rigorous scientific methods should be considered and, if feasible, applied.

Having stated the obvious, many studies are still conducted that do not follow the rules of scientific inquiry. From a pragmatic standpoint, it is clear that these types of studies need to be performed in order to justify programs and assure their continued existence. In some cases, the cost of scientifically rigorous studies would exceed the cost of the intervention. Nonetheless, evaluators need to be aware of differences in study designs that impact study validity and how compromises in the application of scientific principles hinder the ability to make useful decisions about the programs being evaluated. At the very least, evaluators need to explicitly state the limitations of their studies in both oral and written presentations of findings. In designing program evaluations, they should, whenever possible, recommend performance of excellent scientific research that carefully and empirically examines the effects of the program on key outcomes of interest.

Design

Purpose of Study Design

In formulating an evaluation project, the research design must come first. A research design is "the plan, structure and strategy of investigation conceived so as to obtain answers to research questions and to control 'variance' " (Kerlinger, 1973). More precisely, the design forces the evaluator to carefully plan what will be done to test specific hypotheses. This involves selecting a structure for the theoretical model under investigation and developing a strategy for gathering and analyzing the data.

The first objective in selecting an appropriate design is to provide answers to specific questions. In order to achieve this first objective, a secondary objective needs to be addressed, which is the control of variance. Research design helps the evaluator to determine what observations to make, how to make them, and how to analyze the data collected. In addition, the design forces the evaluator to confront the issue of extraneous factors that may influence outcomes and how these might be controlled through appropriate design.

The most effective means of controlling for extraneous variables is through random assignment of individuals or groups of individuals to intervention and control conditions. However, it is recognized that randomization is rarely practiced in health promotion evaluations because top management generally decides which groups of employees are eligible to participate in programs and individuals decide whether or not to join.

Another method for controlling the effects of extraneous variables is use of appropriate analytic techniques. For example, if the evaluator suspects that age and sex may play a role in the outcome of interest (e.g., health care costs), then a design may be formulated in which the age and sex of participants is considered and controlled through such statistical techniques as stratification of individuals into discrete age and sex bands or through multivariate analysis. The problem with stratification and multivariate techniques is that it is difficult to identify and control all extraneous variables. What if, for example, attitude toward one's health or health insurance benefits is an important determinant of health care utilization and costs? If that variable is not considered in the design, then appropriate control for participant attitude may not easily be accomplished. Therefore, a randomized approach is the most effective way of controlling for alternative explanations for study results.

The advantages and disadvantages of alternative designs are presented below, with a discussion of how these might be applied to worksite health promotion evaluations. For the interested reader, a thorough review of statistical and design issues discussed here can be found in Kerlinger (1973) and Campbell & Stanley (1963). Additionally, a more rigorous and technical review of methods that can be used to adjust for unmeasurable factors like attitudes can be found in Heckman and Robb (1985).

Designs of Studies

Nonexperimental (Observational) Studies

Nonexperimental, observational studies are the simplest and least expensive to perform and the most widely used in health promotion evaluations. The most common among these is a design referred to as *one group, posttest only*, which is diagrammed as follows:

$$X \qquad O_2$$

where X is the "intervention" and O_2 is simply the "observation" or recording of some phenomenon following the intervention.

The most frequently used example of this approach is the participant satisfaction or behavior survey that asks individuals to report on their satisfaction with program components and self-reported behavior changes. These surveys are administered at appropriate milestone points and the results summarized for those responding to the survey.

The advantages of this approach are its low cost and ease of administration. Results are readily gathered and reported back to decision makers. The biggest disadvantage of this design is lack of baseline information or information gathered for a control group against which results can be compared. When this design is used, the evaluator must assume a baseline condition in order to determine whether the program has had an impact. Where such assumptions are clearly justified, as in the evaluation of program satisfaction, this design is appropriate.

Feedback from this form of design can provide valuable information from program participants on their perceptions of program performance that, in turn, can be used to improve its functioning. However, this design is of limited usefulness in evaluating whether a change has occurred since the design does not include a comparison group to indicate what might have happened in the absence of the intervention. When this design is used, especially in survey research, special effort should be made to obtain opinions from the majority of program-eligible individuals and from those who typically do not complete survey instruments.

A second nonexperimental design is the *one group, before-and-after or pretest-posttest-only* design. This is diagrammed as follows:

$$O_1 \qquad X \qquad O_2$$

Here, a pretest (O_1) is administered to a group of individuals, the intervention (X) takes place, and a posttest (O_2) is then performed. This evaluation design is the second most common form of evaluation in worksite settings. The prime example of this approach is the administration of a baseline health risk appraisal (HRA) as a first intervention in a comprehensive program. The HRA is subsequently readministered after an appropriate time interval has elapsed, usually 12 to 24 months after the program is implemented. Other common applications of this design are evaluations of smoking cessation, exercise, nutrition, or other behavioral change programs.

Key factors necessary for the success of this approach include a high initial participation rate in the survey or HRA and a very high (80–90%) follow-up rate for participants. (Being realists, the authors acknowledge that high participation rates in surveys or HRAs are difficult to reach and that a 50% or more response rate is often the best that can be obtained.) While this design allows comparisons before and after the program, it is also limited in its ability to support conclusions about program impact because there is no comparison group. This is a problem because many people change their behaviors even without entering into a program. For example, Shipley, Orleans, Wilbur, Piserchia, & McFadden (1988) found that 17% of control subjects, as compared to

23% of intervention subjects, quit smoking in a two-year study examining the effects of the Johnson & Johnson LIVE FOR LIFE® program. Even though repeated health risk appraisals may have influenced the high quit rates among controls, some employees are likely to have quit on their own for personal, organizational, or societal reasons. Warner, Smith, Smith, & Fries (1996) cite a 2.5% "background" chance of quitting each year, independent of any other external factors.

In a meta-analysis conducted by Fiore et al. (1990), the authors concluded that most cigarette smokers who try to quit do so on their own and, in fact, are more likely to be successful than those who seek help in quitting. Thus, when assessing the success of a program, it is important to compare outcomes for individuals in the program with those not offered the program or, at the very least, with general trends in the population. In some instances, the aging process may work against positive outcomes, especially in health measures such as weight, cholesterol, and blood pressure values.

Another nonexperimental design is the *longitudinal or time-series* analysis, which is diagrammed as follows:

$$O_1 \quad O_2 \quad O_3 \quad O_4 \quad X \quad O_5 \quad O_6 \quad O_7 \quad O_8$$

With this design, a series of observations or measures (O_1, O2, . . .) are taken prior to the intervention (X) in order to establish a baseline. These are followed by another series of observations ($O_5, O_6, \ldots$). Ideally, the baseline measures are relatively stable so that any deviations from the baseline measures are attributed to the effects of the intervention.

For example, following a series of baseline measures, a stable absenteeism rate is established. The program is introduced, and absenteeism is reduced. Then the effects of the program are noted for specific outcomes of interest.

However, alternative explanations for these reductions are plentiful. These may be classified as changes related to "history," changes attributable to other events, or combinations of events occurring simultaneously with the study. For example, reductions in absenteeism rates may be associated with changes in absenteeism policies; changes in overall economic conditions that make jobs harder to find and make those employed more likely to work harder to keep their jobs; and company layoffs that result in the least productive employees (those with the most absenteeism) being dismissed.

A variation of this evaluation design is the *multiple time series* design diagrammed as follows:

$$O_1 \quad O_2 \quad O_3 \quad O_4 \quad X_1 \quad O_5 \quad X_2 \quad O_6 \quad X_3 \quad O_7 \quad O_8 \quad O_9$$

Here, as above, a series of baseline measures are collected, an intervention takes place, and follow-up observations are conducted. Additional interventions $(X_2, X_3, \ldots)$ may be introduced at varying intensities to determine whether these create incremental changes in the observed outcomes.

For example, following a series of baseline measures, a stable aerobic exercise frequency measure is established at a given worksite. A fitness program is then introduced and aerobic exercise frequency is increased. The program is intensified (or modified), and aerobic exercise frequency is further increased. The program is then withdrawn, and exercise frequency returns to its original baseline level. As a result of these alterations in the program, effects are noted for specific outcomes of interest. Ideally, a "dose-response" relationship is observed in which the more intensive the program becomes, the more positive the outcomes. As above, alternative explanations for improvements or decrements need to be considered when interpreting study results.

Quasi-Experimental Design

One of the chief limitations of the above designs is that they lack appropriate comparison groups. It is, therefore, difficult to answer the question, "What would have happened if we did nothing?" To answer this, changes in the participant group must be compared to changes in a nonparticipant group. The key task, therefore, is to secure an appropriate group of nonparticipants who are sufficiently similar to the participant group to allow valid estimates of what would have occurred in the experimental group without the intervention.

Ideally, a segment of the population is randomly assigned to the intervention while another segment functions as the control. This random assignment constitutes an experimental design. When random assignment is not possible, the next best choice is to select a comparable site or location where employees are not offered the program. Alternatively, the evaluator compares the experience of participants and nonparticipants at the same site.

This nonrandom assignment to intervention and nonintervention (i.e., comparison) groups constitutes a quasi-experimental, or controlled observational, design. Baseline differences among groups (demographic characteristics or other baseline measures) can often be controlled through statistical means. However, some unmeasured differences among these groups (e.g., motivation to change, residence in a unique organizational culture, specific work assignments) may still confound the estimate of the effect of the health promotion program intervention. Heckman and Robb (1985) describe how to deal with these unmeasurable factors to minimize their influence.

The category of research designs termed "quasi-experimental" (somewhat experimental or, more commonly, preexperimental) offer distinct advantages over the nonexperimental approaches. The evaluator, faced with the reality that it is extremely difficult to conduct randomized studies, should take steps to identify a comparison group with as many similar attributes to the intervention group as possible and then to further control differences between these groups through statistical analysis. These steps increase, but do not guarantee, the likelihood of achieving valid study outcomes.

The most common quasi-experimental approach in health promotion evaluation is the *pretest and posttest with comparison group* design (also known as the nonequivalent control group design).
This is diagrammed as follows:

$$\frac{O_1 \quad\quad X \quad\quad O_2}{O_2 \quad\quad\quad\quad O_2}$$

With this design, baseline measures are taken for two groups, one of which is subject to the intervention. Follow-up measures are also recorded for these groups.

An inferior variant of this model, but one that is quite common and frequently encountered in evaluation studies, is the *ex post facto* design, which is diagrammed as follows:

$$X \quad\quad\quad O_2$$
$$O_2$$

Here, no pretest measures are taken. Instead, two groups are compared to one another at posttest only. The obvious limitation of this design is that it does not measure the impact of the intervention.

The factor that distinguishes these approaches from a true experimental design is the lack of random assignment of subjects to study and control conditions (the dashed line denotes lack of random assignment). In a worksite environment, one group of individuals might voluntarily enroll in the health promotion program while another group might elect not to join. Most often, participants are compared to nonparticipants across a number of dimensions. Differences in the two groups are then attributed to the program.

However, a clear issue not addressed by this comparison is the initial motivation of individuals to participate in the program. The social science literature refers extensively to stages of change, the first of which is an acknowledged readiness for change (Prochaska, DiClemente, Velicer, & Rossi, 1993). Since participants are volunteering to take part in the health promotion program, they have, on their own accord, initiated the change process by indicating readiness. This acknowledgment separates the group from those who have not as yet decided that they wish to change. (This scenario assumes all participants in the program are at one worksite.)

One way to address the problem of self-selection into a health promotion program is to classify all employees who are offered a health promotion program at a site as treatment subjects. As such, all employees at that site who are eligible for the program can be compared to another group of employees at another site who are not offered an opportunity to participate. While this approach can help avoid problems related to different motivational levels between program participants and nonparticipants, it still has its shortcomings. There may be several reasons why any given site is selected as the health promotion pilot site. The site may be led by a visionary general manager; employ-

ees may demand the program as part of their labor contract; the employees may be more highly compensated and willing to contribute to the cost of the program; the site may have a history of high benefit costs that senior management is attempting to moderate; and so forth. Thus, selection bias at the site level is also problematic.

The approach in which sites receiving a program are compared to those without the program, also known as ecological studies, has been employed in several large-scale evaluations of health promotion programs, including those by Johnson & Johnson (Bly, Jones, & Richardson, 1986) and Blue Cross/Blue Shield of Indiana (Conrad, Reidel, & Gibbs, 1990). The design which is termed *pre- and posttest with control group without random assignment* is probably the best design that most health promotion program evaluators will be able to achieve, outside of large government- or university-sponsored research efforts.

Dealing with Self-Selection Bias in Research Design

Regardless of whether the control subjects come from a comparable site or from the same site, the lack of randomization increases the chance that some unmeasured factors will confound or bias the estimate of the impact of the program of interest. If highly motivated people are more likely to participate in the intervention, for example, those people may engage in other unmeasured activities that enhance their health status. How can we differentiate between these other factors and participation in the program when the evaluation is conducted?

In many cases, sophisticated statistical analyses (e.g., multiple regression analyses) are used to account for as many factors as possible when the evaluation is conducted. Through statistical processes, researchers control for measurable differences between program participants and nonparticipants that might influence their health status and program outcomes. Examples of common control variables are age, gender, insurance type (e.g., managed care vs. fee-for-service), job type, length of exposure to the program, stage of readiness to change, or other factors likely to influence results. Applying controls for these factors leads to better estimates of program impact.

But what about factors that cannot be measured (e.g., motivation to take care of oneself)? How can we account for these? In the absence of successful randomization, this is quite difficult.

Fortunately, in the last twenty years, more sophisticated regression analysis techniques have been developed to control for unmeasurable factors, as long as these factors are also associated with measurable decisions to participate in the health promotion program and in the outcomes of that program. These techniques have been developed by Heckman (1979), Olsen (1980), Rosenbaum and Rubin (1984), and Heckman and Robb (1985), all of whom offer highly technical explanations of how to adjust for unmeasurable factors. Such explanations of statistical methods are beyond the scope of this chapter, but it is worth noting that a common thread exists in all of these works. Specifically, if a list of factors that influence decisions to participate in the program can be measured, this information can be used to estimate the probability of participating in the intervention.

Heckman (1979), Olsen (1980), & Rosenbaum and Rubin (1984) showed how this probability can be used to control for unmeasurable factors, thereby limiting self-selection bias. In a successfully randomized study, the probability of participating in the intervention is the same for everyone, participants and nonparticipants alike, so there is no selection bias. Within a quasi-experimental design, methods developed by the authors noted above may allow the researchers to postexperimentally control for differences in the probability of participating in the intervention. Factors that influence the probability of participation in an intervention might include ease of access to a program (e.g., distance to a fitness facility or relationships between work hours and facility hours), one's health beliefs or attitudes, or one's social affiliation tendencies. To obtain measures of these variables, specialized surveys may be required.

In the context of a social experiment, Heckman and Smith (1995) recently showed that results obtained from his self-selection bias approach may equal the results that would have been obtained from a purely experimental, randomized study. Again, the key is knowing which factors people use in order to decide to participate in the intervention, measuring these

factors, and then statistically subtracting the probability of participating in the intervention from the overall program effects. This information can be capitalized upon using advanced statistical techniques to arrive at a better estimate of the impact of the program of interest.

A concrete example of this approach is best illustrated in a case study in which program evaluators were attempting to measure the savings derived from participating in a fitness center program. The challenge was to identify a variable that predicted fitness center participation but had no effect on health care costs or absenteeism. For statistical reasons noted by Heckman (1979), such a variable helps generate a valid measure of the probability of participating in the intervention of interest. This in turn allowed the researchers to control for differences in the probability of participation when comparisons were made between fitness center participants and nonparticipants.

In this example, a key variable found to predict participation in the fitness center program was the distance between worksite and the fitness facility. The employee's distance measure predicted his or her use of fitness center facilities but did not predict health care costs or absenteeism. Thus, the researchers were able to use the sophisticated methods developed by Heckman (1979) to statistically account for the likelihood of participating in the program independent of program outcomes. The analysis found that the fitness center program still produced a positive return on investment, albeit a slightly more subdued ROI than originally reported. However, the additional selection-bias adjustments increased the credibility of the analysis and deflected anticipated critiques directed at quasi-experimental research designs.

Experimental Designs

While the above approaches are widely employed and are easier to implement than true experimental designs, they may evoke biased results due to nonequivalence of the intervention and comparison group. This would be true even with the approaches promoted by Heckman (1979), Olsen (1980), and Rosenbaum and Rubin (1984) if the list of factors that influenced the decision to participate in the program is not fully known or measurable. Conrad, Conrad, & Walcott-McQuigg (1991) provide an excellent discussion of the threats to internal validity in worksite health promotion research when designs other than *true experimental designs* are used. Diagrammatically, experimental design is configured as follows:

$$[R] \quad \frac{O_1 \qquad X \qquad O_2}{O_1 \qquad \qquad O_2}$$

Here, subjects are randomly assigned into a control or experimental group, and observations are made before and after the intervention. The [R] and solid line employed in the paradigm indicate that subjects have been randomly assigned to experimental and control groups above and below the line, respectively.

A common argument used against this approach is that to randomly assign individuals is unfair or unethical since a program that is likely to benefit all individuals is withheld from some. If good evidence is available that a program is beneficial, the rationale for the evaluation is indeed questionable. Randomized trials are ethically justifiable only when considerable uncertainty exists as to the effects (both positive and negative) of an intervention or when budgets for program participation are limited. In the latter case, it is not financially feasible to apply the intervention to everyone who would be eligible, so a lottery-based or randomized approach may be viewed as the fairest way to choose participants and nonparticipants.

A more difficult issue relates to the way in which health promotion programs are typically introduced at a worksite. Most often, the program is introduced to the entire worksite rather than to specific individuals therein. Consequently, the worksite itself may be viewed as a unit of interest since the aim of the intervention is to alter the culture and norms of that site.

Thus, an effective evaluation design of worksite health promotion programs calls for the comparison of sites with and without the program, rather than a comparison of participants and nonparticipants at any given site with the program. Since companies are reluctant to expend enormous resources to test the efficacy of a program by offering that program to some randomly assigned sites while withholding the program at other sites, experimental designs are rarely employed in evaluations of health promotion programs.

An alternative approach calls for the assignment of volunteers for a program at a given site into treatment and "waiting list" groups on a random basis. Hence, outcome measures are assessed for equally motivated individuals–some of whom participate in the program and the balance of whom are asked to wait until space becomes available. Unfortunately, this evaluation approach does not work for single-site interventions that are environmentally- or culturally-based, since these often include introduction of no smoking policies, removal of "junk food" vending machines, or extensive marketing campaigns. All of these changes might also change the behaviors of those in the waiting list groups.

An additional problem of using the waiting list approach is the collection of data from the nonintervention group. If the data collection effort is directed at archival data (e.g., absenteeism or health care records compiled routinely and stored historically), then comparisons of intervention and comparison groups are possible and uncomplicated. However, if the analysis calls for a comparison of data that need to be collected directly from employees (e.g., health status, biometrics, satisfaction, attitudes, etc.) then potential contamination may occur. For example, if health measures are to be compared across sites, then the collection of these measures may be viewed by the participants as an intervention, especially if, as in the case of an HRA, individual feedback is provided to both study and comparison group populations.

These testing effects can be controlled by a study that randomly assigns individuals into four possible conditions: groups that receive pre- and posttests, with and without intervention, and groups that receive either pre- or posttests alone, without intervention. This design is diagrammed below:

$$[R] \quad \begin{array}{c} \dfrac{O_1 \qquad X \qquad O_2}{O_1 \qquad \qquad O_2} \\[2ex] \overline{\rule{4cm}{0pt}} \\[1ex] \dfrac{O_1 \qquad \qquad}{\qquad \qquad O_2} \end{array}$$

This design, known as the Solomon Four Group Design (Solomon, 1954), allows comparisons across multiple conditions in order to determine the independent (true) effects of the program. To date, health promotion programs have not been evaluated using this design, perhaps because it requires a heavy emphasis on data collection from multiple sites, which can be difficult to administer and quite expensive.

Table 5-2 summarizes the various evaluation designs discussed in this section and offers a reference guide to health promotion program evaluators.

Using Multiple Designs in Evaluation Studies

When assessing multiple outcomes in health promotion evaluations, it is inevitable that several research designs will be used. For example, satisfaction, interest, and awareness surveys are frequently administered to the population offered the program. The intent is to gauge the thoughts, feelings, and opinions of those exposed to the program and a one-group, posttest-only design is most often applied.

In assessing the impact of the program on health behaviors and biometric measures, a quasi- or true

Table 5-2 Evaluation Designs

Nonexperimental designs
- One Group Posttest Only

  $X \quad O_2$
- One Group, Before and After (Pretest-Posttest Only)

  $O_1 \quad X \quad O_2$
- Longitudinal or Time Series

  $O_1 \quad O_2 \quad O_3 \quad O_4 \quad X \quad O_5 \quad O_6 \quad O_7 \quad O_8$
- Multiple Time Series

  $O_1 \quad O_2 \quad O_3 \quad O_4 \quad X_1 \quad O_5 \quad X_2 \quad O_6 \quad X_3 \quad O_7 \quad O_8 \quad O_9$

Quasi-experimental designs
- Pretest and Posttest with Comparison

  $O_1 \quad X \quad O_2$

  $O_1 \qquad\quad O_2$
- Ex Post Facto

  $X \quad O_2$

  O_2

Experimental designs
- True Experimental

  $[R] \dfrac{O_1 \quad X \quad O_2}{O_1 \qquad\quad O_2}$
- Solomon Four Group

  $O_1 \quad X \quad O_2$
  ───────────────────
  $O_1 \qquad\quad O_2$

  $[R] \quad$ ───────────────────
  O_1
  ───────────────────
  O_2

Note. $O_1, O_2, \ldots$ = Observations or recording of behaviors, test scores, or other phenomenon. X = Health promotion intervention. --------- = Lack of random assignment to treatment and control conditions. [R] ——— = Random assignment of subjects to treatment and control conditions.

experimental design is preferred in which volunteers are assigned into either comparison or experimental conditions. When testing the effectiveness of a new program modality or intervention, there is no substitute for this rigorous approach. However, for routine studies of program effects on health outcomes, a one-group pretest/posttest-only design is most often used. The validity of such a design is enhanced when high initial participation and high follow-up rates are achieved and when several iterations of the evaluation are conducted that allow evaluators to monitor changes periodically over a long time.

Financial impact studies typically rely upon pretest/posttest designs with comparison groups or time series designs. These studies often use statistical techniques in attempts to control for possible confounders. When multiple sites are available for study, those with the program are often compared to those without it. The larger the number of comparison groups and the greater the extent to which sites are arbitrarily assigned to treatment and comparison conditions, the stronger the design may be, and the more valid the results may be.

Threats to Validity

The credibility of study results will be based on the extent to which factors that threaten internal and external validity have been carefully considered. Consequently, the responsible evaluator will acknowledge any shortcomings or limitations inherent in the study design and point to potential threats to internal and external validity.

Validity is straightforwardly defined as the extent to which you are measuring what you think you are measuring (Kerlinger, 1973). Internal validity refers to the extent to which the measured effect of the program reflects the true program effect in the study group. External validity refers to the extent to which the effects observed among those involved can be generalized to other situations with different populations and under different conditions.

Campbell (1957), Campbell and Stanley (1963), Cook and Campbell (1979), Rossi and Freeman (1999), and others have published guides for establishing internal and external validity. Conrad et al. (1991)

provide a review of these threats as they apply to health promotion research. The most important ones are summarized below.

Selection Bias

When volunteers (or participants) for a health promotion program are compared to nonvolunteers (nonparticipants), a questionable assumption is made that the outcomes being measured would be the same in these groups in the absence of intervention. Since program participants self-select into health promotion programs, are they equally likely to change behaviors, improve their health outcomes, and reduce their health care service use when compared to their nonparticipant counterparts? The methods by Heckman (1979), Olsen (1980), Rosenbaum and Rubin (1984), and Heckman and Robb (1985) were developed to minimize selection bias. These methods require estimation of the likelihood of participating in the intervention, for both participants and nonparticipants. Once these probabilities are known, differences between participants and nonparticipants can be reduced even further (in a statistical sense), and more valid results can be obtained from the evaluation.

Attrition

This is the effect of loss of subjects during the course of interventions due to dropout from the program. Those who drop out may be individuals who are least successful in making the desired behavior change. High attrition rates may reflect poor program design and implementation.

Maturation

The effect that subject aging has on any of the values or measures recorded is known as maturation. For example, as people age they are likely to gain weight and increase their blood pressure.

History

Factors in the environment, such as changing laws, cultural trends, or adaptation of worksite policies that may affect behaviors or attitudes of subjects comprise the history.

Instrumentation

This involves changes in the way data are recorded; for example, self-report versus biometric readings or changes in recording equipment or measurement tools.

Regression toward the mean

The tendency of extreme values to move toward the average is the regression toward the mean. For example, people with very high values or scores in blood pressure, cholesterol, or stress might have lower values or scores on retesting, even without participating in the program. This is because individuals with extreme scores often tend to report scores or measures closer to average levels when tested a second time. As another example, an individual reporting high stress at time 1 may be in the midst of a stress-inducing life crisis. Getting through that crisis will likely result in a lower stress score at time 2 when that individual is retested. This may not apply in some areas, such as weight loss or smoking cessation, where high values (pounds or cigarettes smoked) tend to remain stable over time.

Treatment fidelity

Variation in the ways in which the program is delivered across sites/locations that might cause differences in the outcomes is described as treatment fidelity.

Diffusion of treatments

A spillover of effects from site to site or within sites may occur where control site individuals might have access or exposure to intervention materials or programs being offered to treatment subjects.

Testing

The effect of taking readings or measures from the control group might cause a change by itself. A special case of the testing effect is known as the "Hawthorne Effect," in which any change in the work environment, even simply increased attention to a group of employees, will lead to a temporary increase in productivity.

In many cases, the impact of these validity threats can be reduced by choosing a high-quality experimental or quasi-experimental design to conduct the evaluation. Applying sophisticated statistical testing approaches help as well.

In either case, the phrase "high-quality" deserves note. Randomized designs generally address most validity threats, but randomized designs require a great deal of effort and constant monitoring. While an excellent randomized trial is superior to quasi-experimental designs, poorly conducted randomized trials can be just as invalid as poorly controlled quasi-experimental studies. At times, poorly conducted randomized trials can be inferior to well-conducted quasi-experimental studies. Quasi-experimental retrospective studies have the advantage of reporting what actually takes place in a real-life naturalistic setting as compared to a more sterile, and at times contrived, experimental laboratory environment.

Sample

Most evaluations focus on a distinct sample of the total population. The population may be as broad as workers in U.S. companies, blue-collar workers, teachers, or municipal employees. Since it is typically impossible to assess an entire population, or the universe of individuals belonging to a given broad class, a sample of that universe is selected and studied. For example, a study sample may consist of teachers in a given municipality who elected to participate in a health promotion program and who voluntarily completed a health risk appraisal instrument. Several rules and guidelines apply for selecting a target population, developing an appropriate comparison group, recruiting subjects, establishing adequate sample sizes for the study, and sampling from the universe of potential study participants in order to be able to generalize results to the larger group. These are described below.

Target Population

In establishing an evaluation plan, there must be a well-defined target population. This group may include all potential recipients of the program in addition to those employees who actively participate. For example, in an ecological study, all employees at a given site might constitute a target population.

Even when the evaluation only focuses on program participants, it is important to be precise in defining the total eligible population so that accurate success rates are determined. For example, when considering the quit rate for a given smoking cessation program, all attendees at the *first* program session should be included as the target population rather than only those who completed the course and were present at the final session. Further, quit rates should be assessed at varying time periods following program completion (e.g., at 3, 6, 12, and 18 months). In each follow-up assessment, as many initial program participants as possible should be identified and tracked.

To obtain a more complete estimate of the impact of the program, the analyses should also account for the amount of time that participants spend in the program (e.g., for the number of sessions attended). This allows the evaluator to calculate a "dose-response" relationship between the program and its outcomes. In the process of conducting such analyses, information is often obtained on why some participants choose to complete a program and others do not. Such information can be useful when fine-tuning programs to make them more appealing to their intended audience.

Comparison Group

In quasi-experimental evaluation studies, the evaluator needs to identify a suitable comparison group against which the experience of the treatment group can be compared. An ideal comparison group is composed of similar employees who are not offered the program. Other possible, but less attractive, options for comparison groups include employees at other companies or published normative data (e.g., data on changes in smoking rates for the U.S. population, health care utilization trends for different industries, employee absence rates derived from the Bureau of National Affairs, etc.).

A common method for evaluating health promotion programs is to compare participants to nonparticipants even when both groups are situated at the same site or location. This approach certainly has its limitations. Nonparticipants generally have poorer health habits and are at higher risk (Lovato and Green, 1990). They are generally less motivated to change unhealthy lifestyle habits. They may be less educated and be at lower income levels than participants. There may be a greater proportion of females and younger males among participants. In short, participants may differ in a variety of ways when compared to nonparticipants.

As noted earlier, multiple regression techniques can be used to adjust for differences in age, gender, and other factors that are known and recorded for both groups. In addition, the techniques developed by Heckman (1979), Olsen (1980), Rosenbaum & Rubin (1984), and Heckman & Robb (1985) can be used to control for unmeasured factors that influence the likelihood of participating in an intervention and its outcomes. These approaches limit the impact of self-selection bias and produce better estimates of the true effectiveness of the intervention.

Recruitment

Recruiting program participants is an art in itself. Picking the subpopulation to be studied can be done in either of two ways. The evaluator can either select the entire population being offered the program (and an appropriate comparison group) or a sample of the larger population. When sampling, aggressive efforts need to be made by the evaluator to recruit study participants in order to achieve a representative view of the larger population. The evaluator should also be cognizant of issues related to informed consent, that is, the extent to which study subjects need to be made fully aware of the study purpose and its implications for participants. Often, a signed consent form is required for participation in the intervention as well as the evaluation.

Sample Size

Successful evaluations often require data to be collected from or about intervention participants and nonparticipants. Depending upon the magnitude of the differences in outcomes one expects from participants and nonparticipants, researchers may wish to collect data from hundreds or even thousands of subjects.

There are two reasons why large samples may be desirable. First, the larger the sample, the more likely the evaluation will produce results that can be generalized to other settings or populations. Second, standard statistical techniques used to estimate the impact of the intervention may require large samples in order to achieve results that can be accepted with greater confidence (see Table 5-3).

Several possible methods to estimate the appropriate sample size for a program evaluation are described below. It should be noted, however, that recently several approaches have been developed that greatly enhance the power (and therefore the usefulness) of evaluations conducted with very small samples. These approaches are known generically as computer-assisted randomization tests and are described by Eddington (1995).

There are two common circumstances requiring sample size determination: a) estimating the preva-

Table 5-3 Sample Size Requirements for Health Profiles and Employee Surveys

Total Eligible Population	Sample Size
50	44
100	79
200	132
300	168
400	196
500	217
700	248
1000	278
2000	322
5000	357
10000	370

Note. The sample size estimates assume an error of 5% (e = 0.05) and an alpha level of 0.05; in other words, the results achieved will be within 5% of the true value at least 95% of the time. For example, when assessing smoking rates for a population of 1,000 individuals, the evaluator finds that 30% of the 278 randomly surveyed individuals smoke. The sample prevalence (in this case 30% smokers) will be within five percentage points (25% to 35%) of the population value, 95% of the time.

lence of risk factors in a population, and b) comparing changes in risk factors for treatment and comparison groups. For the serious student, a much more detailed discussion of sample size theory and calculations can be found in the writings of Cohen (1977).

Sampling to Estimate the Prevalence of Risk Factors

In the first application of sampling methods, the evaluator wishes to estimate the prevalence of a risk factor in a population using a random sample from that population. The question asked is how many individuals should be selected at random from the larger population in order to achieve a reliable and valid estimate of the behavior or risk factor in the population as a whole.

In determining the sample size needed to estimate a proportion, the evaluator must make several assumptions regarding the larger population studied. The formula used in selecting a random sample is (Kahn & Sempos, 1989):

$$n = \frac{NPQ}{((N-1)(e^2/z^2) + PQ)}$$

For larger populations (over 50 people), the following formula may be substituted for the above:

$$n = \frac{NPQ}{((N)(e^2/z^2) + PQ)}$$

where n is the sample size required or the number that the evaluator is solving for. The symbol P is the true proportion in the population of the behavior or risk factor studied. Since this proportion is unknown (for example, the proportion of the population who are smokers), a value of 0.5 can be used as the most conservative estimate (i.e., it may be assumed that half of the population smokes). If, on the other hand, the evaluator has a sense that the true proportion is closer to 30%, then P would be set at 0.3. The symbol Q is the proportion who do not have the risk factor, or simply, $1-P$. This would be 0.5 in the first example and 0.7 in the second. N is the entire population from which the sample is drawn.

The symbol e denotes the error that is acceptable, most often plus or minus five percentage points, or

0.05. The symbol z denotes the standard normal deviate corresponding to the acceptable Type I error, a situation in which the evaluator thinks that a difference is detected between two groups when such a difference really does not exist (Konrad & DeFriese, 1990). A choice of 0.05 for this value would mean that the estimated proportion would fall within the designated acceptable error (e.g., five percentage points) of the true value 95% of the time, or $p \leq 0.05$.

For example, if $e = 0.05$, $z = 1.96$ (corresponding to an alpha level, or Type I error level, of 0.05) and $N = 1,000$, the resultant sample size requirement is 277. Increasing N to 3,000 results in a sample size requirement of 340. The sample sizes listed in Table 5-3 were calculated for various populations using these equations.

How Sample Size Can Affect Study Conclusions

If a large enough sample is not drawn initially when undertaking an evaluation study, then the conclusions drawn from that study may be tenuous. This is especially true when conventional (and more familiar) statistical tests are used in the analysis.

For example, an evaluator may be charged with the task of evaluating a smoking cessation program using a time 1/time 2 cohort group design without comparison group (referred to earlier as "the one group, before-and-after or pretest-posttest-only design"). The initial population of 500 employees includes 150 smokers (30% of the total population). If the organization loses ten percent of their employees a year through attrition or turnover, this will leave 122 individuals from the original smoker group after two years ($150 \times 0.90 \times 0.90 = 122$).

If the evaluator now remeasures the remaining cohort group of 122 employees and determines a certain quit rate, then an error factor will need to be calculated for that quit rate. The error is estimated with the following formula:

$$e = \sqrt{\left(\frac{z^2(PQ)}{n}\right)\left(\frac{N - n}{N - 1}\right)}$$

A shorthand formula for this is:

$$e = 100 \times \sqrt{1/n}$$

where n = the number of individuals who remained in the cohort group, in our example, 122. (This shorthand formula assumes that $P = 0.5$ and that a 95% confidence interval is used.) The error factor for this example is therefore nine percent, which means that the evaluator is 95% confident that the true quit rate after two years is plus or minus nine percent. Thus, if 50% of the remaining 122 individuals quit, then the evaluator can say with a 95% level of confidence that between 41 and 59% of the population truly quit.

The only way to decrease the error estimate and more precisely estimate the true quit rate would be to increase the population sampled. If n is increased, then the error factor will decrease.

Sampling To Compare Proportions Between Two Groups

Another circumstance in which sample sizes would need to be determined is in comparing the changes in two groups. For example, in a smoking cessation program, the evaluator wishes to know if the quit rates are different for treatment and control groups. Determining the sample size in this case utilizes a statistical concept called *power analysis*.

Statistical power is the extent to which we are confident that a nonstatistically significant difference between two groups does indeed reflect a lack of difference between those groups, as opposed to the nondifference being attributable to an insufficient sample size. Just as significance levels are typically set at 0.05, power is typically set at 0.80, meaning that we are confident that a difference that is not statistically significant is indeed a nondifference in 80% of the cases.

The formula for calculating a required sample size is as follows:

$$N = ((1.96 \times SE \times (1 - SE))/\Delta^2) \\ + ((1.96^2 \times SP \times (1 - SP))/\Delta^2)$$

where N = required sample size, SE = the sensitivity estimate, SP = the specificity estimate, and Δ = the width of the confidence interval (Dobson, 1984).

Since formulas for calculating sample size are complicated, evaluators normally draw figures from tables such as those in Fleiss (1981). For example, let's assume we expect 25% of smokers in the treatment group and 10% in the comparison group to quit smoking. Next, we set our significance levels at 0.05, and power at 0.80. Under these conditions, we would need 113 subjects in the treatment group and 113 subjects in the control group to detect differences in quit rates between groups, assuming the program will be successful.

Newell, Afaf, Sanson-Fisher, & Savolainen (1999) note that in a worst-case scenario in which both sensitivity and specificity are set at 50%, a sample size of 192 subjects in treatment and an equal number in a control group would be required to estimate sensitivity and specificity at a 95% confidence interval of width ± 10%.

Estimating power and sample size requirements prior to initiating research is important because the small intervention group sizes common to health promotion programs, combined with the relatively low rates of change frequently observed, often make it difficult to detect true differences between treatment and comparison groups. For additional discussion on this topic, the reader is referred to Konrad & DeFriese (1990) and Cohen (1977, 1988).

Sample Sizes With Archival Data

As the sample size formulas noted earlier show, the larger the variance of an outcome of interest, the larger the sample size must be to study that outcome. When using archival or administrative data, we are often interested in studying outcomes such as medical expenditures, days of work lost due to illness or short-term disability, or work time lost due to workers' compensation or other accident claims. In general, these outcomes tend to have very large variances and consequently large samples are required to study them.

The need for large samples is expected because the severity of illness often differs among employees. In addition, underlying health risks and behavioral habits may vary significantly among individuals, resulting in a large variance in health care costs between those who take poor care of themselves and those who are more health conscious.

Doctors can often be heard lamenting that no two patients are exactly the same. It is true that differences in patient case mix or illness severity often

lead to wide variations in health expenditures, absence days, or other work loss. The wide range of values for these outcome variables means that the average values do not always reflect what is typical. As a result, a large number of subjects may be required for evaluations that use archival or administrative claims data.

While studies of "more stable" outcomes (e.g., program satisfaction, employee attitudes, changes in health risks) may require that only *hundreds* of subjects are needed, studies of medical claims or other administrative data often require that *thousands* of subjects are needed. Thus, the reader is cautioned that the final sample size for an evaluation should be governed by the sample size requirements *for the most variable* outcome measure. In our experience, it is common for analyses of medical expenditures, absenteeism, or work loss to require a minimum of 1,500–2,000 subjects for the intervention group and an equal number for the comparison group.

How to Randomly Sample

Random sampling is a technique for picking research subjects in such a way that each person has an equal chance of being selected. This technique is distinguished from one in which every fifth, tenth, or "nth" name or number is picked, a technique known as systematic sampling. Most often, a computer program is used to select a random group of individuals from the total eligible population. Alternatively, most statistical textbooks include a table of random numbers that may be used for random selection of names or social security numbers from a list comprising the total population.

In general, the evaluator is encouraged to recruit as many subjects as possible from the random sample list in order to achieve the most representative sample possible. However, if budgets are limited, smaller random samples (e.g., 40–50% of the population) may still adequately represent the population of interest. Unfortunately, there is no single rule of thumb that applies. Under the best of circumstances, in order for the random sample to be considered representative of the larger population, a *very high* participation rate among those sampled is required (80–90%).

Achieving High Survey Response Rates

Evaluations often rely upon survey instruments to collect information about participants and nonparticipants in an intervention program. Examples include satisfaction and attitude surveys and health risk appraisal questionnaires designed to measure health habits and other risk factors.

High response rates are more likely to be achieved when questionnaires are short (one to two pages) and primarily composed of closed-end questions (checklists, yes/no, rating scales), management is supportive of the survey process by allowing time off to complete the instrument, and completion is rewarded with incentive items. Further, participants are more likely to offer opinions when surveys are anonymous or when confidentiality is assured. (For a discussion of ways to achieve high response rates in health promotion programs, see Thompson, Bowen, Croyle, Hopp, & Fries, 1991.)

When low response rates are anticipated because of general antipathy against survey instruments or low literacy rates for the population, the evaluator might consider structured interview protocols that are administered either by telephone or in person. These techniques are also effective as follow-up measures to elicit responses from erstwhile nonrespondents. Often response rates can be greatly enhanced through person-to-person solicitation as opposed to written communications.

When response rates are low despite the best efforts to maximize them, survey analysts often use regression-based weighting techniques to assure that the responses to the survey data adequately represent the population as a whole. With these techniques, more weight is given to people who responded to the survey even though their underlying propensity to respond was low. The rationale for this approach is that these individuals are more likely to represent nonrespondents than are others who typically respond to surveys with little hesitation.

Kalton and Kasprzyk (1986) describe the methods used to estimate the likelihood of responding to surveys and associated weighting techniques. Generally, the evaluator collects information on factors expected to influence response rates. For example, very low-income workers tend to respond less often to surveys.

Sometimes survey response varies by job type, educational level, gender, or by such factors as worker morale. The evaluator's job is to collect information on as many of these factors as possible so that they can be controlled in the analysis of data.

Armed with these data, the evaluator then conducts a logistic regression analysis designed to estimate relationships between factors influencing response rates and whether or not the survey was completed. The logistic regression results are used to estimate each person's probability of completing the survey. These probabilities are then inverted (i.e., the ratio of 1/probability is calculated) and the inverted probabilities become the survey weights. The weights assign more importance to those who were expected not to respond to the survey based on their demographic profile (i.e., the weights are higher for those least likely to respond).

More importance to low-probability responders is assigned by multiplying the actual value of each observation by its associated weight before analyses are conducted. If these low-probability responders are similar to non-responders, using the weighted observations in the analyses helps account for the impact of those who did not respond to the survey.

Measurement

Data Sources for Evaluation Research

It goes without saying that in order to measure program success, the evaluator first needs to gather the data. There are, fortunately, no shortages of some forms of data in corporate computers. However, there are limited resources at most companies to extract the needed data and to compile them into meaningful reports.

Often, program administrators are burdened with the task of cajoling database keepers into releasing information necessary for analytic studies. Quite frequently, corporate attorneys who are brought into discussions express reservations regarding the release of data because of concerns for employee privacy and confidentiality. Such scenarios reinforce the need for a clear data analysis plan that is communicated to corporate officials. These should include specific safeguards against potential abuse of confidentiality and employee privacy.

When collecting data for health promotion program evaluations, three principal methods of data aggregation are used:

1. *"Paper and Pencil" measures* that might include sign-in or attendance sheets; health risk appraisal instruments; employee or participant questionnaires; and tests, quizzes, or knowledge questionnaires.
2. *Observation techniques* that might include staff attendance forms; data collected from biometric measures (such as blood pressure readings); and unobtrusive observations by parking lot security personnel who record the number of seatbelt wearers.
3. Retrieval of data from *archival files* such as health care insurance claims databases; personnel records; disability and workers' compensation claims; computerized attendance files; medical records; class enrollment records; tuition reimbursement records; and normative databases.

Each of these data sources can be analyzed independently or integrated with other sources. Before expending time and effort in building integrated or relational databases, organizations should ask and answer the "so what" question, that is, how will the data be used in making decisions about program design and implementation?

To avoid the cost of designing customized data acquisition systems, off-the-shelf statistical computer packages such as SAS, SPSS, or BMDP can be used to link these databases. These software programs are very powerful analytic packages while being quite straightforward to use. Most questions of interest to the evaluator can generally be addressed through such software programs. If, however, ongoing inquiries are required and regular monitoring reports and systems are necessary for program management, a customized health management information software system may be more appropriate.

Measurement Instruments

Validity and reliability of measurement instruments are of foremost concern in the development of survey questionnaires, health risk appraisals, observation or interview protocols, and protocols for accessing archival data. This section describes some of the basic issues related to the development and use of measurement instruments. The rationale for establishing instrument reliability and validity is discussed since these are critical elements in the reporting of credible study findings.

Social science research texts (for example, Kerlinger, 1973) devote considerable attention to ways of improving validity and reliability in measurement systems. To review, validity refers to the extent to which the measurement instrument is measuring that which the evaluator intends to measure. Reliability, on the other hand, refers to consistency of such measurement. Surveys that do not adhere to the rigors of scientific assessment are likely to yield data of questionable value.

Validity

Scientific instruments are generally subject to the following types of validity evaluations:

1. *Face validity* is determined by a panel of content experts who review the instrument to determine whether it includes all relevant issues and that they are written in an understandable and appropriate manner. Essentially, these experts determine whether the instrument, on its surface, measures the trait or quality that it is supposed to measure. Face validity considers the question: Does the instrument adequately address the core issue under study?
2. *Content validity* considers another question: Does the instrument address *all* of the relevant content areas (subcategories of the core issue) under study? Thus, if a concept or trait that is to be measured encompasses many different areas, a content validity analysis determines whether all of these areas are addressed by the instrument. This analysis is typically done by experts in the field who know the theoretical underpinnings of a concept or trait and can determine whether each relevant component is considered in the instrument's design.
3. *Construct validity testing* subjects the instrument to a more rigorous analysis by experts and/or computer analysis to determine whether theoretical elements of the construct under assessment are captured by the measure. For example, if an in-

strument is designed to measure a construct such as "general well being," then a panel of experts and a computer analysis will be employed to determine whether key component elements of this general concept (e.g., ability to cope with anxiety, overall depression, coping skills, social support network, etc.) are included in the construction of the measure.

4. *Predictive or criterion validity* determines the extent to which the instrument can be used to predict certain outcomes or behaviors. This is done by comparing scores on the newly developed instrument to those of other already-validated instruments or observation techniques. For example, if a new fitness questionnaire is developed asking people about their fitness levels, scores on this measure can be compared to direct measures of strength, flexibility, and aerobic capacity. Similarly, skinfold thickness test results (measures of body fat) can be compared to such established body fat measures as underwater weighing.

5. *Discriminant validity* tests the extent to which the instrument can discriminate (distinguish between) certain groups of individuals with known differences in the area assessed by the measure. For example, the anxiety scale mentioned above might be administered to a group of psychiatric patients who have been diagnosed as anxious and to a control group of nonpsychiatric patients. The instrument, if valid, should be able to distinguish between these two populations on the basis of their scores.

Reliability

In addition to assessing instrument validity, evaluators need to concern themselves with its reliability. *Reliability* is the extent to which an instrument is stable, dependable, consistent, and predictable in its scoring of a given trait or behavior for any given individual over a period of time (Kerlinger, 1973).

For example, test-retest reliability is the extent to which an instrument captures similar responses over time when no real change has occurred. It may be determined by retesting a group of individuals using the instrument shortly after the first measure is taken, ideally within one or two days. Reliability of the instrument is measured as the degree to which results of the first test are similar to those on the second test.

Another technique for assessing instrument reliability is to develop two equivalent forms of the instrument and administer these forms to two similar populations (randomly assigned to either group A or B). Once again, a reliable instrument (versions A and B) would yield comparable results for both groups.

Finally, in order to determine the internal consistency of the instrument for any given respondent, responses to similar items on the instrument are compared to one another to test whether they are correlated. A high internal correlation (alpha coefficient) determines that the instrument is internally consistent in assessing the trait or behavior of interest.

Inter-rater reliability (i.e., consistency of data-collection being performed by different data collectors) is necessary when observational data such as biometric measures are collected from multiple professional assessors. Before starting, these individuals need to check their level of agreement on measures of blood pressure, body fat, height, weight, etc. Multiple measures by these individuals of the same subjects should be conducted until data collection protocols are made uniform, and consistency in measures across professionals is obtained.

If budgets preclude the use of multiple testers to assess inter-rater reliability or the use of multiple tests to assess test-retest reliability, internal consistency measures such as the alpha coefficient can be used to assess reliability. These are far more efficient and less costly. Also, they are remarkably accurate. For example, Cochrane (1978) showed that high levels of internal consistency often relate to high levels of other reliability measures, such as inter-rater reliability.

However, internal reliability measures are only relevant to survey instruments with multi-item scales that measure theoretical constructs. They are less relevant to biometric screenings or other observational measures that rely upon multiple observations by the same person or on independent observations of a given phenomenon by two or more persons.

Why Use Valid and Reliable Instruments?

When possible, existing measures with known and acceptable levels of validity and reliability should be used in evaluation studies focused on health promotion programs. These are not merely academic concerns. If the questionnaire or test used is not a valid and reliable measure of the area of interest, the results reported will be misleading and, in many cases, worse than having no information at all.

For example, if an invalid instrument is used to measure emotional stress and the measure underestimates the true stress experienced by the employee, program designers might conclude that a stress management program is not needed when in fact it is. Erroneous conclusions can also be drawn about the need for fitness, alcohol management, driver education, and nutrition programs if measures used are inadequate.

Similar concerns emerge when evaluating program success. If the measurement instrument is unreliable or invalid, then actual improvement may remain unrecognized when in fact it occurred. This could result in discontinuing a very effective program. Conversely, an ineffective program may be expanded even though actual improvement is suspect, given the measurement tools used.

Results

Outcome Measures

Outcome evaluation generally begins with the basic question, "What effect did the intervention have?" Hopefully, the answer is tied to program objectives. Examples of objectives include general goals such as to improve employee health, reduce the rate of increase in health care costs, and improve worker productivity. Objectives may be stated in more specific terms, such as "reduce by ten percent the number of employees with high total cholesterol levels (240 mg/dl cholesterol and above) within one year" or "reduce the rate of increase in inpatient costs for lifestyle-related illnesses for active employees by 25% over a three-year period."

In addition to focusing on outcome variables, evaluators also measure specific process variables that lead to program outcomes. If, for example, health improvement is the goal, what activities, structures, participation rates, human facilitation factors, and organizational norms led to goal achievement? A discussion of various process and outcome variables commonly assessed in health promotion programs is offered below.

Which Outcomes Are Most Important?

Two separate surveys conducted by Johnson & Johnson Health Management, Inc. (JJHMI), one in 1989 and the other in 1992, asked decision makers to rate the relative importance of various health promotion program outcomes. The survey conducted in 1989 involved 28 JJHMI clients (representing a 48% response rate). The companies queried, mostly from Fortune 500 firms, were asked to identify the reasons for investing in health promotion. The reasons given are listed below in order of importance:

1. To enhance the organization's image as caring for its employees
2. Improve employee health
3. Improve productivity
4. Improve attitudes and morale
5. Reduce health care costs

Additionally, respondents were asked to assess some key process measures. Their responses are listed below in order of importance.

1. Reach those at greatest need
2. Achieve high participation
3. Have satisfied participants
4. Reach different demographic groups
5. Achieve high completion rates

In 1992, 30 corporate decision makers, some of whom were Johnson & Johnson clients and some not, were asked to rank a list of process and outcome variables (JJHMI, 1992a). These variables were ranked in the following order of importance:

1. Improve health habits of high-risk employees
2. Achieve high awareness
3. Achieve high satisfaction with the program

4. Improve the health habits of all employees
5. Improve the company's image
6. Improve morale
7. Reduce health care costs
8. Improve productivity
9. Reduce absenteeism
10. Reduce turnover
11. Improve employee recruitment

Recently, William M. Mercer, Inc. (1999) surveyed its clients about the factors that contributed to the decision to implement a health management program. Reasons cited by 248 respondents included the following factors which influenced their decisions:

- high health benefit costs   57%
- need to enhance corporate image or morale   54%
- to attract and retain employees   28%
- management pressure to cut costs   25%
- employee demand for services   19%
- management pressure to improve productivity   9%

As shown, the relative rank ordering of issues differs between surveys. However, common themes do emerge. Companies are most concerned about reaching and improving the health of employees who are at greatest risk. There is a recognition that this outcome can be clearly linked to health promotion programming and implementation strategies.

Companies also express interest in improving what are traditionally considered "softer" outcomes, including satisfaction, morale, and image. The "harder" outcomes related to reduction in costs, in particular health care costs, are noted as program goals but not as the highest ranked goals. This may be because decision makers are aware of some of the difficulties involved in measuring cost outcomes and are therefore content with establishing health improvement or program satisfaction results.

In a survey of Colorado businesses, Davis, Rosenberg, Iverson, & Bauer (1984) found that, among companies with existing health promotion programs, the leading reason for having these programs was to improve employee health (cited by 82% of the firms). Other nonfinancial goals included improving em-

ployee morale (59%); responding to employee interest or demand (33%); to be part of an innovative trend (32%), or to improve the company's public image (20%). Financial objectives included reducing health care costs (57%); reducing turnover and absenteeism (51%); and improving productivity (50%).

Interestingly, when Davis' group asked companies who were contemplating introducing health promotion programs, the relative weighting of objectives shifted. Improving employee health remained the number one motivation (68%). However, three financial objectives (reducing health care costs [68%], improving productivity [64%], and reducing turnover and absenteeism [57%]) were close behind the lead objective. Possible explanations of these discrepancies might include more realistic expectations on the part of existing program sponsors on what are reasonable short-term outcomes from these programs and recognition of the value of nonmonetary benefits that are gained from health promotion.

What are the lessons learned from these decision maker surveys? First, there is great diversity in the types of outcome measures necessary for documentation of program success. Second, economic outcomes are important, but they may not be of primary importance to some decision makers, especially after they have been made aware of other outcome options. Finally, it may be illuminating for decision makers to know that their compatriots may be focusing on issues other than economic return on investment and that the softer measures may be as relevant as some of the harder measures. The astute evaluator will use these data to point out the variety of outcomes of interest to others investing in health promotion and force choices regarding the relative merit of alternative outcome measures.

Although some outcomes are perceived as more important than others, all of the issues cited above are viewed as important by decision makers. As such, measurement of many, if not all, of these issues may be necessary. Despite the apparent priority placed on soft measures, decisions related to continuing and expanding a program may be more dependent on the overall financial condition of the company and the extent to which health promotion programs are viewed as supportive of economic growth.

Methods to assess these multiple outcome variables as part of a comprehensive health promotion evaluation are discussed below. The outcomes are organized from most easy and economical to assess to those that are more complex that may require outside expertise.

Awareness of the Health Promotion Programs

Health promotion programs may be viewed as large-scale communication or advertising initiatives by the organization. The company is attempting to "sell" changes in individuals' behavior and employee management of their health and productivity. This may be likened to modifying individuals' buying practices in the area of health behaviors or habits. Thus, for a health promotion program to be successful, it must demonstrate its ability to effectively market its wares and, at the very least, increase the potential buyer's awareness of the product. Since engaging in health promoting behaviors can be linked to a buying decision made by consumers several times a day (i.e., whether to exercise, not smoke, eat nutritiously, drink excessively, etc.), then the consumer of health promotion services needs to be continuously "sold" on the value of the health promoting behavior.

Assessing consumer awareness and the programs' product "reach" is, therefore, an essential first step in evaluating health promotion programs. The questions asked by an awareness assessment are: a) To what extent are potential consumers aware of the product and its offering? b) More specifically, do they know how to enroll in the program, participate in its activities, and benefit from program incentives?

To test program awareness, or reach, a simple consumer survey can be administered to address the questions above. If an adequate response rate is achieved, the validity of the results can be confirmed and appropriate conclusions drawn, that is, the program is or is not well-communicated to or understood by the population.

Assessment of employees' awareness of the program is often tied to other process measures such as satisfaction. One way to determine whether the program has been adequately communicated to employees is to ask those who have not participated why

they have not done so and to determine how many were simply unaware of the program.

Participation in Health Promotion Programs

Another key component of program success is its ability to attract and retain participants. Participation is most often defined as engagement of unique individuals in one or more health promotion activities. Reported participation rates in health promotion programs have ranged from 20–40% for on-site programs and 10–25% for programs offered outside the workplace (Fielding, 1984, cited in Lovato & Green, 1990). Johnson & Johnson has achieved participation rates that range from 25–95%, depending upon program intensity and participant solicitation efforts. In a study performed by Johnson & Johnson (1992b), participation rates were found to be significantly correlated to the level of investment by the sponsoring organization.

In assessing participation, several key issues need to be addressed. The first is how participation is defined. At one extreme, a participant is defined as anyone who engages in any health promotion activity (e.g., a health risk appraisal) in a given year. At the other extreme, a participant may be defined as one who regularly or routinely engages in health promotion programs; examples include exercising regularly, attending health education classes, completing weekly activity cards that record health promoting activities performed at home, etc. The former definition, while more liberal and inclusive, allows greater flexibility in counting participants and acknowledges that even minor attempts at behavior modification may have impact.

Some organizations differentiate between *any* participant and one who is an *active* participant. An example of active participation may be attending at least 75% of the sessions in a smoking cessation program or exercising aerobically for 20 minutes at least three times a week.

The rationale for adopting the more liberal definition of participation (i.e., engagement in one or more health promoting activities) is simple: program evaluators do not know whether any one intervention or combination of interventions will achieve the desired effect.

For example, an individual who participates in only one activity in a given year, a health risk appraisal, is told that she has high blood pressure and should immediately be seen by a physician. The individual might follow the advice of the report or counselor, and get a prescription for blood pressure medication which, in turn, controls her high blood pressure. That individual's outcome would be successful, even though her participation in the health promotion program was limited.

Another individual may participate in several elements of the health promotion program but do so as a passive observer rather than as an active participant. That individual, while classified as a participant, might realize little (if any) behavior change and consequent positive health effects.

In addition to assessing "any" and "active" participation in a program, it is also helpful to flag participants in specialized high-risk intervention programs since these have been shown to have a significant impact on program results (Heaney & Goetzel, 1997). Further, it is useful to assess the intensity of program participation (e.g., number of visits to fitness centers, number of assessment materials returned, number of educational sessions attended, etc.), as these have been shown to be correlated with program success; in other words, the more intensive the participation levels, the better the outcomes. This "dose-response" relationship was recently shown in the evaluation performed for Chevron Corporation that focused on its Health Quest fitness program (Goetzel, Dunn, Ozminkowski, Satin, Whitehead, & Cahill, 1998). In that evaluation, individuals who participated in the program more frequently achieved the greatest cost savings.

In assessing participation rates, it is important to ascertain a correct estimate of the eligible population. The eligible population includes all those who are eligible to participate at any given point in the program's history. If terminated employees are to be counted as participants, then their number needs to be added to the eligible count as well.

Most health promotion administrators find it difficult to keep accurate and complete eligibility information since this requires almost daily updates of personnel records. One solution to this problem is to use an accurate midyear count as the estimate of the eligible population from which a participation rate is calculated. This technique is appropriate when an organization experiences relatively low turnover rates over the course of a study period. If, on the other hand, employee population levels fluctuate during the year, an alternative technique that estimates "person-years" (the actual number of months, divided by 12, for which person-specific data are available for any given individual study subject) could be applied to determine the eligible population.

Beyond capturing overall participation rates for the program, sophisticated tracking and management information systems combine participation and eligibility data with health risk appraisal and screening data. Inputs into the system might include:

- Personnel or human resource files that help determine program eligibility
- Health risk appraisal data
- Participation data from a variety of sources, including:
  - Computerized "sign-in" or "log-in" stations
  - Hard copy "sign-in" or attendance sheets
  - Self-report participation logs (activity or nutrition records)
  - Payroll deduction, fee payment, or reimbursement records
  - Mail-in materials, forms, cards

Ideally, each contact with the participant is captured efficiently by the management information system and integrated with other databases. Time stamps on each participation entry are essential for tracking participation and for linking to other relevant databases.

A system can be designed that provides invaluable process and impact data across a number of dimensions. For example, the program can be designed to elicit information on participation in various topic areas, such as smoking, exercise, or nutrition. Participation across various delivery modalities (e.g., multiple-session courses, brief one-time seminars, health risk appraisal or screening programs, incentive systems, contests, games, or telephone delivery) can also be assessed in order to determine whether certain modalities are more popular than others.

In addition, other useful pieces of information can be ascertained from such a system. These might include the demographic characteristics of participants, usage patterns for various programs (e.g., time of day, frequency of usage), whether first-time users are being engaged in the program, differential participation rates across time periods, and so forth. Finally, by combining health risk appraisal and participation data, the evaluator can determine the extent to which the population at greatest risk is being reached by the program. This is achieved when the vast majority of the eligible population complete an HRA so that high-risk status can be ascertained. The analytic function of identifying high-risk individuals and determining the extent to which they are participating in the program is critical in developing and evaluating a high-risk program.

The ideal tracking system records the level of program participation (e.g., whether programs are completed once initiated) and appropriate knowledge, health, and satisfaction measures of participants engaged in the program. These, in turn, allow the program administrator to monitor individual, group, and overall program progress across a number of dimensions. Several software programs are available from health promotion vendors to accurately track key participation metrics.

Satisfaction with the Program

An important process measure in health promotion programs is the extent to which participants are satisfied with program content, administrators, instructors, materials, logistic arrangements, and other program components. While satisfaction may be viewed as a soft measure, it may have significant impact on the perception of program quality and, ultimately, on program outcomes. It may also have an indirect influence on employee morale and productivity.

Since customer satisfaction is a key factor influencing the purchasing decisions of consumers, it is critical that this component of the program be evaluated. Customer or participant satisfaction will not only influence the individual's decision to participate in the program but is likely to have an impact on the individual's decision to follow through on program recommendations and behavior change attempts.

There are numerous instruments that measure satisfaction (for example, those developed by Chapman, 1991). In selecting the right instrument, it is important to determine which aspects of the program need to be assessed. Such a determination should be driven by an assessment of which aspects are most important to the success of the program and which can be modified in response to consumer opinion.

It is also important that the participant not be bombarded with satisfaction measures after each encounter with the program. Such an approach may elicit apathy or even resentment on the part of the participant. If changes take place in response to widespread opinions and recommendations expressed by program participants, then respondents will be more likely to feel that they are being heard and, consequently, more inclined to complete such surveys.

Feedback of results to program administrators and group leaders is critical. Such feedback aids program improvement and identifies areas requiring immediate modification. It is important that the recipients of study findings understand how to interpret the results and how to use them in ways that improve program and individual performance. Using customer satisfaction results to gauge the program administrator's job performance is yet another way to use data to continuously and incrementally improve the program.

Attitudes Toward Management

One rationale for introducing health promotion programs is that they project an image of caring about employees' health and well being. Offering health promotion programs is expected to instill a greater sense of loyalty toward the employer who has demonstrated a willingness to invest in the physical and mental health of the workforce. Positive sentiments toward the employer are expected to eventually achieve lower turnover, lower absenteeism, and overall increased productivity.

Management is therefore concerned that the program, which represents a human resource expense, is viewed positively and improves morale. To test that assumption, an employee survey may be administered as part of the evaluation process to test program effects on employee attitudes, morale, and self-assessed productivity. These may be measured using a pretest-posttest approach in which the same attitudinal statements are examined before and after program introduction. Alternatively, employees may be asked *post hoc* about the effects of the program on their productivity, morale, and attitudes toward management after the program has been in place for a given time period (such as a year).

In developing questionnaires that assess program effects on satisfaction, morale, attitudes, and productivity, the evaluator should structure questions that are unbiased and worded so that respondents are not guided toward a socially desirable response. For example, an unbiased question might ask: "What effect has the health promotion program had on your . . . morale, productivity, attitude, etc.?" Participants are then offered the following response options: "no effect," "negative effect," or "positive effect."

Figure 5-1 provides a graphic example of a report showing program effect on employee attitude. The example report is for Notable Enterprises, a fictitious company, although the data provided in this and other graphics below are actual results from company reports.

Behavior Change and Health Improvement

Ultimately, besides gaining high participation rates, the most important and relevant aim of health promotion practitioners is to improve the health and well-being of their target populations. In order to achieve this aim, a significant portion of employees with poor health habits who are at high health risk need to be engaged by the program. Additionally, they need to attend to the behavior change messages sent and to respond positively to these messages.

Thus, an important test of program effectiveness is its ability to modify unhealthy habits and improve the risk profile of the highest risk population. Additionally, the program can be judged on its ability to keep low-risk people from becoming high-risk. In short, both improvements and decrements in risks should be evaluated when measuring behavior

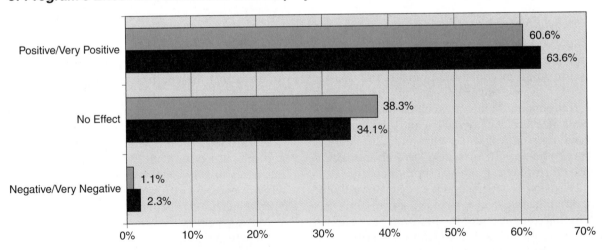

Customer Satisfaction Survey (Random Sample) of Program's Effect on Satisfaction with Employer

Positive/Very Positive: 60.6% / 63.6%
No Effect: 38.3% / 34.1%
Negative/Very Negative: 1.1% / 2.3%

Figure 5-1 Sample graphic showing a health promotion program's effect on employees' satisfaction with their employer at fictitious Notable Enterprises.

change and risk reduction efforts. If high-risk individuals improve while low-risk individuals worsen in their risk profiles, the net effect is zero, and the program should be judged as lacking impact.

To test program effectiveness in achieving health improvement and risk reduction aims, the evaluator needs to collect valid and reliable baseline data on the target population's health habits and characteristics and to reassess these after an appropriate time interval. It is important to emphasize that in order to demonstrate an environmental impact for the program, the majority of employees (or a representative sample) need to be assessed at both baseline and at follow-up. Since the decision maker is most interested in improving the health and well-being of the total workforce at a given site, demonstrating significant changes in a minority of the population (i.e., those who elect to participate in a screening program) will often not satisfy a requirement to demonstrate overall program impact.

As with other survey methods, a high participation rate is desirable and achievable through intensive one-on-one solicitation and through creative marketing approaches that include the use of incentives for participation.

Follow-up assessments should be performed during the same season as the baseline assessment (12 or 24 months following the baseline study) to avoid the problem of a seasonal effect on reported health habits and biometric measures.

For example, at the request of a program administrator, the lead author of this chapter conducted a baseline HRA study in the spring and a follow-up study right after the Christmas holiday period. Not surprisingly, right after Christmas, biometric and self-report measures indicated that subjects were more overweight, consumed more alcohol, practiced poorer eating and driving habits, and in general were in worse physical health compared to baseline data.

It is best to use similar techniques for collecting measures at both baseline and follow-up screening. A recent analysis by Newell et al. (1999) compared the accuracy of self-reported and objectively gathered data relating to cardiovascular and cancer risks. They found that reliance on self-report data consistently underestimated the true proportion of "at-risk" populations. Thus, if biometric measures of weight, cholesterol levels, and blood pressure are recorded by a health professional at baseline, then at follow-up it is best to have health professionals record them again (as opposed to relying on self-reported measures). This also applies to the different methods of collecting biometric data. For example, when collecting serum cholesterol data, the same method (e.g., venipuncture or finger stick) should be used at both baseline and follow-up assessments.

In assessing health improvements, how is change defined? Even small changes in biometric measures when recorded for a large population can elicit statistically significant results. When assessing change, it is desirable to compare the proportion of the population "at need" or "at high risk" at Time 1 versus Time 2. This approach provides uniform reporting across measures, which is readily understood by nonsophisticated audiences. As a matter of course, need and high risk must be operationally defined prior to the study; in many cases, these definitions are well-established and represent the consensus of the health education professional community.

For example, "need" for cholesterol management programs may exist for individuals with total cholesterol readings of 200 mg/dl or greater. "High-risk" individuals, on the other hand, may be those with total cholesterol levels of 240 mg/dl or greater. Similarly, "at need" smokers may be defined as individuals who smoke any amount of cigarettes, while "high-risk" smokers may be those who smoke more than one pack of cigarettes a day. A sample follow-up health profile group report is shown as Figure 5-2.

An extensive review of articles focused on documenting improvements in health and reduction in risk can be found in Heaney and Goetzel (1997). More recently, an evaluation of Citibank's health management program by Ozminkowski et al. (1999) provided an excellent description of how to measure health improvement for program participants as a group and for high-risk program participants.

Is the demonstration of improvement in health habits and biometric measures of a population

Number and Percent of Health Promotion Participants at High Risk at First and Last HRA, by Risk Category

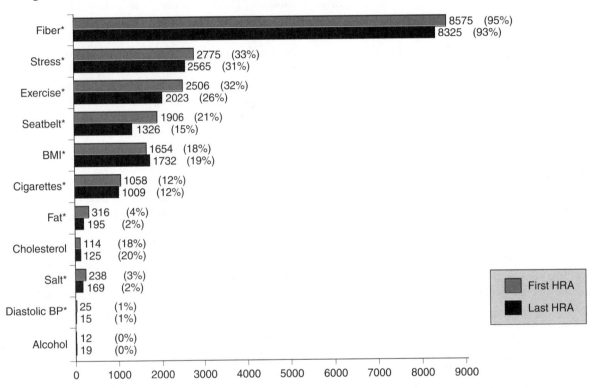

Figure 5-2 Sample follow-up health profile group report showing number and percent of health promotion program participants at high risk at Time 1 and Time 2.

Percentages represent the proportion of total participants for whom data are available, by category. BMI = Body Mass Index; BP = blood pressure.
*statistically significant at the p<0.05 level (McNemar Chi-square).

sufficient evidence that the program is effective? In many cases it is. Many employers may, over time, reach the conclusions that improvement in the health and well-being of their population will lead to improvements in productivity and reductions in insurance benefit costs and that those financial benefits don't need to be measured directly. These conclusions are beginning to be supported by research that links health risk levels to medical expenditures (Goetzel, Anderson, Whitmer, Ozminkowski, Dunn, & Wasserman, 1998) and changes in risk to improvements in an organization's health care experience (Edington, Yen, & Witting, 1997).

Financial Measures

Recently, several literature reviews have been written focused on the financial and productivity-related outcomes associated with worksite health promotion programs (Fielding, 1982, 1990; Warner, Wickizer, Wolfe, Schildroth, & Samuelson, 1988; Goetzel, Danaher, et al., 1990; Pelletier, 1988, 1991, 1993, 1996; Edington, 1992; Aldana, 1998; Heaney & Goetzel, 1998; and Goetzel, Juday, & Ozminkowski, 1999).

In spite of several studies on the subject (see Chapter 2), skepticism remains regarding the financial impact of health promotion programs. The conventional wisdom expressed by many corporate benefits directors is that these programs are worthwhile be-cause they improve morale and 'probably' reduce health risks. However, they, and their benefit consult-ants, continue to express doubt about the economic re-turns attributable to these programs. Part of the skep-ticism is derived from a lack of knowledge concerning the state of research findings in this area, especially the newer methods employed in evaluating financial re-turn on investment studies for these programs (for example, Goetzel, Dunn, et al., 1998; Ozminkowski et al., 1999; and Goetzel, Juday, et al., 1999).

The problem is not the lack of research efforts at documenting cost savings from such initiatives; there are many studies, some large scale, that have taken on the challenge of documenting savings. The prob-lem is that these studies often contain methodologi-cal flaws in their design that call into question some of the conclusions presented (Conrad, et al., 1991). These design flaws are common in "real-life" re-search because of the many problems related to achieving internal and external validity noted above. Nonetheless, evaluators are encouraged to continue to design and implement financial analyses focused on health promotion programs that improve upon previous efforts by better addressing issues of valid-ity and reliability.

To paraphrase Warner in his discussion of work-site wellness (Warner, 1990), it is ironic that the same level of proof demanded of health promotion pro-grams (that they document their effectiveness, cost-effectiveness, and cost savings) is rarely applied to medical treatments that are far more costly and in general less cost-effective from a societal standpoint, than health promotion programs.

Today, program administrators are often chal-lenged to prove that their programs are saving money or, at the very least, paying for themselves. Economic markers that are commonly tracked in corporate en-vironments include costs associated with health care insurance programs, absenteeism, turnover, workers' compensation, short- and long-term disability, and employee productivity. These indicators are usually tracked differently by different organizations or dif-ferent departments within the same organization, and the quality of data associated with each program is sometimes questionable.

Table 5-4 Financial Measures Assessed in a Health Promotion Evaluation

Measures	
Absenteeism	Turnover
Disability	Workers' compensation
Productivity	Medical care utilization and cost
Possible Data Sources	
Personnel records	Human resource files
Payroll files	Supervisory ratings
Disability	Medical records
Insurance claims data	Benefits consultant reports
Self-report data	

Source: adapted from J. E. Fielding, unpublished manuscript, 1986.

A wide range of financial outcome measures and data sources for these measures are discussed below and listed in Table 5-4 (adapted from the work by Fielding, 1986). When displaying the range of human resource expenditures for an organization, the eval-uator may wish to diagram these as shown in Figure 5-3 in order to draw attention to the large numbers of health and productivity programs already in place and the potential of saving dollars by better coordi-nating intervention programs across organizational functions (see DeJoy and Southern, 1993).

Financial Outcomes of Interest

In assessing program effects on *absenteeism*, it is im-portant that a consistent definition of absenteeism be used. Prior to the assessment, agreement should be reached as to what constitutes absenteeism attributa-ble to health and lifestyle factors (i.e., absenteeism for illness but not for jury duty, military leave, family medical leave act (FMLA), etc.). Quantifying absen-teeism usually involves estimating the prorated pay-roll cost for each category of employee (e.g., wages for hourly employees), excluding fringe benefits (such as insurance costs) for each hour lost to absen-teeism.

It is also important to recognize that absenteeism rates may be influenced by a variety of factors other than employees' own illnesses or injuries. Job satis-faction, general employee morale, changes in com-

Your HPM Results and Opportunities:
Health and Productivity Management Totals

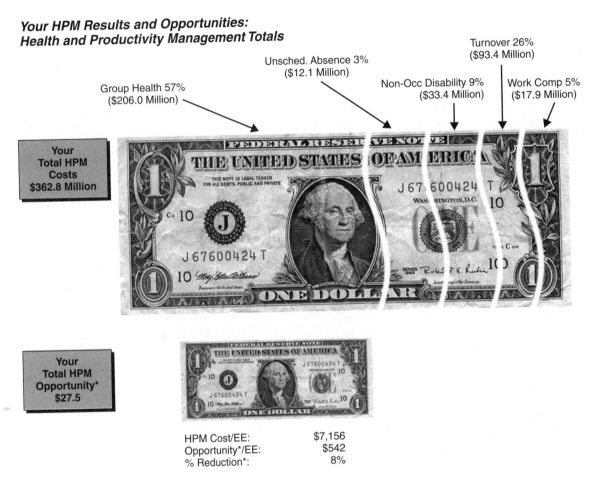

Group Health 57%
($206.0 Million)

Unsched. Absence 3%
($12.1 Million)

Turnover 26%
($93.4 Million)

Non-Occ Disability 9%
($33.4 Million)

Work Comp 5%
($17.9 Million)

Your
Total HPM
Costs
$362.8 Million

Your
Total HPM
Opportunity*
$27.5

HPM Cost/EE:	$7,156
Opportunity*/EE:	$542
% Reduction*:	8%

* Based on comparisons to HPM costs at the 25th percentile of survey participants for each program.

Figure 5-3 Sample aggregate financial analysis showing relative costs and opportunities for savings in five human resource areas falling under the heading of Health and Productivity Management (HPM).

pany policies toward absenteeism, and outbreaks of adult and children's illnesses in the community are all factors that affect absenteeism rates. Use of comparison groups who are exposed to similar social and environmental conditions is, by far, the best way to control for potential confounders.

The evaluator should be aware that groups with higher than average absenteeism rates at baseline are most likely to exhibit reductions and subsequent cost savings as a result of a health promotion intervention.

Groups with low rates may already have eliminated unnecessary days absent and may show little additional improvement. An example of a baseline absenteeism analysis, in which the company's experience is compared to norms, is shown in Figure 5-4.

Turnover, particularly of well-trained employees, can be expensive (Goetzel, Guindon, Humphries, et al., 1998; Saratoga Institute, 1999; Pinkovitz, Moskal, & Green, 1999). Expenses associated with recruitment, training, and initial reduced productivity can

Your HPM Results and Opportunities:
Total Dollars per Employee

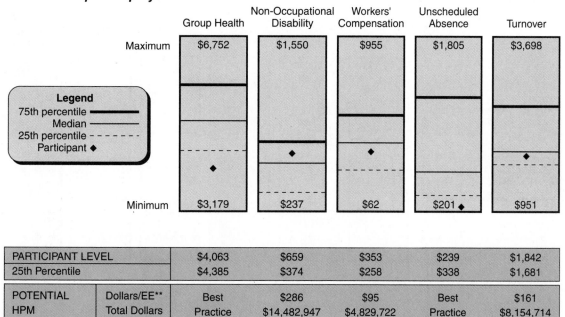

	Group Health	Non-Occupational Disability	Workers' Compensation	Unscheduled Absence	Turnover
Maximum	$6,752	$1,550	$955	$1,805	$3,698
Minimum	$3,179	$237	$62	$201	$951

Legend
75th percentile ▬▬▬
Median ───────
25th percentile − − − − −
Participant ◆

PARTICIPANT LEVEL		$4,063	$659	$353	$239	$1,842
25th Percentile		$4,385	$374	$258	$338	$1,681

POTENTIAL HPM OPPORTUNITY*	Dollars/EE**	Best Practice Company	$286	$95	Best Practice Company	$161
	Total Dollars		$14,482,947	$4,829,722		$8,154,714
	% Reduction		43%	27%		9%

* Based on comparison to 25th percentile of survey respondents within individual HPM programs.
** Dollars/Employee

Figure 5-4 Detailed analysis of five human resource areas that fall under the heading of Health and Productivity Management (HPM) showing norms and best practice values.

oftentimes be estimated. A conservative estimate of turnover costs often used by employers is 40% of first year salary (R. Sample, personal communication, 1992). Others (Goetzel, Guindon, Humphries, et al., 1998; Drakeley & Smith, 1999) estimate turnover costs as high as 50–150% of an employee's annual salary. However, in some industries, for example retail or fast food, turnover costs are far lower and may, in fact, be "negative" since newly hired employees for relatively low-skill positions often accept lower starting wages than more senior employees.

Tracking turnover may be difficult since organizations do not always record reasons for termination (e.g., voluntary, layoff, dismissal). As in absenteeism, the evaluator needs to be aware of other conditions that may have changed during the course of the study

that may influence turnover rates; examples include improved job security measures introduced into labor contracts; introduction of profit sharing or stock option benefits; future prospects for the company or industry; and overall employee morale related to views of senior management. In some sectors of the economy in which turnover is traditionally very low, it is difficult to detect reductions in turnover regardless of the effectiveness of health promotion programs. An example of a baseline turnover study graphic comparing the company's experience to norms is shown in Figure 5-5.

Organizational compensation for *short- and long-term disability* is determined in different ways for different organizations, making cross-company comparisons of rates and costs difficult. Most companies

Your HPM Results and Opportunities: Employee Turnover

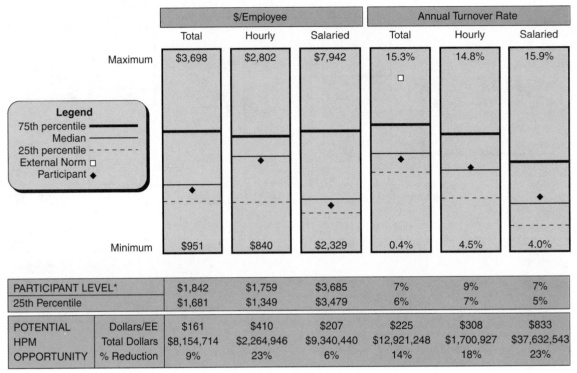

	$/Employee			Annual Turnover Rate		
	Total	Hourly	Salaried	Total	Hourly	Salaried
Maximum	$3,698	$2,802	$7,942	15.3%	14.8%	15.9%
Minimum	$951	$840	$2,329	0.4%	4.5%	4.0%

Legend
75th percentile ——
Median ——
25th percentile - - - - -
External Norm □
Participant ◆

PARTICIPANT LEVEL*		$1,842	$1,759	$3,685	7%	9%	7%
25th Percentile		$1,681	$1,349	$3,479	6%	7%	5%
POTENTIAL	Dollars/EE	$161	$410	$207	$225	$308	$833
HPM	Total Dollars	$8,154,714	$2,264,946	$9,340,440	$12,921,248	$1,700,927	$37,632,543
OPPORTUNITY	% Reduction	9%	23%	6%	14%	18%	23%

* Participant level metrics are calculated independently for Hourly, Salaried, and Total Employees.

Figure 5-5 Sample baseline turnover analysis of employee versus norms and best practices.

differentiate between short- and long-term disability, but company policies as to when short-term disability ends and long-term disability begins vary from three months to more than one year. Employers also offer different benefit packages for disability. For those employers who have a flexible benefit structure, employees can choose the desired benefit level each year when enrolling in the program. There is also no standard system of reporting causes or types of disability. Some systems report specific ICD-9-CM codes, while others report broad categories of disability (such as "back problem" or "cardiovascular disease").

In spite of these limitations, it is beneficial to track utilization of disability benefits and costs across time to determine whether the health promotion program is having any demonstrable effect on this program. Once again, comparison group studies are preferred over time series analyses when tracking disability costs because of the numerous factors cited above that may influence a company's disability experience.

Workers' Compensation claims, often referred to as occupational disability or safety incidents, are important outcome measures for tracking the effectiveness of health promotion programs. Often, worker safety is of great concern to senior management and therefore high on the priority list of benefit program management (Goetzel, Guindon, Humphries, et al., 1998). This concern can be used as a leverage point for health promotion program managers and evaluators.

Where possible, program evaluators should report workers' compensation costs and incidence rates as indicators of the company's focus on prevention activities. However, it is often difficult to report these measures since laws differ from state to state and even within states for different occupational groups, such as police and fire department employees. There is also variability in the coverage provisions for different categories of claims. For example, stress-related claims may be considered valid in one jurisdiction but not another. For workers' compensation studies, when longitudinal studies are employed, it is best to compare groups who have stable turnover rates and stable work assignments for the types of work performed. Further, stability in state statutes, company policies, and insurance carriers are important in these types of assessments.

When workers' compensation and safety studies are performed, it is best to focus on specific illness or disability areas that are targeted by the intervention programs. For example, the incidence of back problems, carpal tunnel disorders, strains, and sprains should be impacted by programs emphasizing proper lifting techniques, exercise, weight management, and ergonomic modification of the physical space. Surprisingly, health promotion programs that ally with other initiatives that aim to improve the organizational climate and work environment may also significantly impact workers' compensation claims and costs (Bigos, Battie, & Spengler, 1991).

There is a wide range of definitions and measures of *productivity*. The evaluator should consider tapping into existing quality and efficiency measures already used in the organization. Some of these may include internal measures of productivity (e.g., widgets produced per unit of time) or external measures of productivity (e.g., acceptance of widgets by customers expressed as revenues or profits per employee). Often, customer and even employee satisfaction can be used as a proxy for productivity, especially when these have been shown to be correlated with shareholder value.

Quality and productivity indicators are easier to track for some occupational groups than for others. For example, productivity can be measured for production typists, telephone operators, computer data entry workers, insurance claims processors, and for individuals paid for individual output (e.g., garment or agricultural workers). For white-collar workers, sometimes referred to as knowledge workers, measurement may involve the administration of validated self-report instruments, "beeper" studies in which workers record what they are doing (on- or off-task) whenever they are "beeped," and simulation studies in which workers are asked to perform real-life tasks in a laboratory environment that simulate their real jobs. Some recent examples of research focused on health and productivity can be found in the works of Claxton, Chawla, and Kennedy (1999), Burton, Conti, Chin-Yu, Schultz, and Edington (1999), and Cockburn, Bailit, Berndt, and Finkelstein (1999).

In measuring productivity, more than with any other outcome variable, multiple internal and external confounders will affect the data. These include market conditions; availability of capital and raw materials; quality of leadership and management practices; presence of economic incentives for increased productivity; overall morale; and labor-management relations. While productivity indicators can theoretically be compared across groups, over time, and in real-life situations, such convenient comparison groups are rarely available.

In the area of *medical care costs*, many of the problems discussed above are even more pronounced. Companies may change their benefit plan provisions from year to year. They may switch claims administrators. The administrator may change the way in which data are collected and stored; for example, the administrator now may require detailed diagnosis coding whereas that requirement was not present previously. Employees may migrate from indemnity plans into HMOs in which claims administration and data storage is far less precise. The company may institute cost control measures such as utilization review systems or preferred provider networks.

Another concern in working with health care data is the wide variation in utilization among different segments of the population. Some employees may utilize a great number of medical services while others may not. Traditionally, a small minority of the total covered population uses a disproportionate amount of health care resources and consequently consumes a major portion of resources devoted to health care benefits. Usage of resources may vary from year to year as the health status of individuals fluctuates. Thus, performing year-to-year studies on a cohort group may present analytic problems simply because of the disparate nature of claims data.

Illnesses attributable to lifestyle practices, such as heart disease and cancers, may have evolved over a very long period of time. Improvement in the company's health care experience may take several years once habits are changed. In many cases, health care costs may increase in the first year of program introduction as employees become aware of problematic conditions such as hypertension or high cholesterol and seek medical attention. On the other hand, the company may realize short-term savings if certain lifestyle practices are improved, such as not drinking and driving, wearing seatbelts, taking actions to correct home safety problems, and seeking treatment for drug and alcohol abuse problems.

Most studies of the relationship between health promotion programs and medical care costs have used overall or inpatient health care experience as outcome variables. Whenever possible, it is useful to focus attention on specific lifestyle-related diagnoses within the context of overall medical care expenditures. An obvious example of costs that should not be included are those resulting from normal obstetric care in which a healthy newborn is delivered without complications. In such circumstances, demographics of the workforce, fertility of the female population, and individual choice, as opposed to adverse lifestyle practices, will determine costs.

On the other hand, the rate of complicated deliveries (e.g., those resulting in premature or low-birth weight infants) will be affected by lifestyle practices of the mother (e.g., poor nutrition, smoking, or drinking alcohol) and should, therefore, be considered in evaluations of lifestyle-related medical care utilization and cost. Therefore, improving the lifestyle practices of the population should reduce the rate of adverse pregnancy-related outcomes and associated costs.

Some other medical conditions have no known relationship to lifestyle habits and characteristics. Lifestyle issues may, however, affect the course of treatment and severity of illness for conditions that are not directly associated with health habits. For example, the individual with good lifestyle habits who enters a hospital for appendicitis may be less likely to experience complications than one with poor habits.

Framework for Selecting Outcome Measures

Which of the above measures should be considered in an evaluation effort? That decision will hinge upon the importance of each measure to the decision maker; the availability of data in a "clean" and usable format; the availability of expertise to analyze and interpret the data; and funding for both program and evaluation efforts. Further, when requesting individual-level personnel or medical claims data, sensitivities regarding employee confidentiality often emerge. Finally, the time required to realize economic impact may be a factor to consider when deciding which area of financial analysis is worth undertaking.

For example, if immediate results (i.e., within 12 months) are required in order to maintain or enlarge a program, the evaluator should put in place measuring systems to track program awareness, satisfaction, participation, health improvements, and morale or attitude shifts. Within 24 months, improvements in absenteeism and disability rates (both occupational and nonoccupational) are likely to be noticed. Within 36 months, health care cost savings should become available.

Returning to the issue of evaluation costs as related to overall program costs, it was noted earlier that evaluation budgets should equal at least five percent of total program budget. For a $100,000 intervention program, this translates to $5,000 devoted to evaluation. Such a budget can most often accommodate measures of participation, awareness, or satisfaction using survey research techniques.

Studies that examine health improvements among program participants require that a follow-up health risk assessment be conducted. In general, it is most efficient to randomly sample from the baseline population to obtain an appropriate follow-up group, and to diligently pursue this sample for a follow-up assessment. The costs of doing this type of study include those associated with retesting or rescreening, as well as the analysis and interpretation of data. If the rescreening costs are classified as programmatic costs, since such rescreening is itself an intervention, then the costs of study preparation and data analysis can often be accomplished within a $5,000 budget (assuming the availability of internal staff expertise to design the measurement instruments, distribute the survey, code the responses, analyze the data, and prepare a final report).

Financial impact studies are generally more elaborate and therefore more expensive to conduct. Typical absenteeism and medical claims studies can cost between $50,000 and $100,000 (excluding database development costs). More elaborate evaluation efforts that examine and relate multiple databases may cost hundreds of thousands of dollars. Thus, when discussing evaluation activities directed at financial impact measures, program sponsors and evaluators need to be educated regarding the complexity of such studies and concomitant cost implications.

Analysis Timetable

Once all of the groundwork has been completed in planning the program, a plan for reporting results needs to be developed. It is imperative that decision makers be shown periodic results to track program performance and identify possible problems.

In preparing the groundwork for a health promotion program and its evaluation, it is important to emphasize that some program effects are likely to be seen almost immediately, while others will take longer. Immediate results are likely to be realized in self-reported morale and attitudes toward management.

Health improvement will take longer to document and will often occur in the following sequence. The participant will enter a psychological state of readiness to change; educational materials and behavior change information will be reviewed and incorporated; new behaviors will be attempted; and, finally, the new behaviors will become integrated as part of the individual's behavioral repertoire. While some of these steps may be observed in the short term, the assessment of whether new behaviors are integrated and maintained may take several years.

Effects on rates of cardiovascular and cancer disease prevalence may take years to discern. Concomitant medical care cost savings associated with the reduction of disease in the population will require additional years of analysis.

Nevertheless, from a practical point of view, a 12-month period is a useful milestone for reporting back to management on program accomplishments to date and on anticipated outcomes expected in the near term. Since companies generally plan and budget programs over a 12-month cycle, providing program achievement data at a point sufficiently in advance of the budgeting cycle is recommended.

A sample evaluation plan for an organization interested in a wide range of process and outcome measures is shown in Table 5-5.

The timetable shown in Table 5-5 reflects an early effort at collecting baseline data. These data often evaporate over time as files are purged or archived (i.e., put into "cold storage", often offsite), so the advice to the program evaluator is to gather all of the relevant data that are available in each area of evaluation focus in order to take advantage of a window of opportunity.

The timetable also underscores the need to collect and report follow-up measures as quickly as possible. Year one results can be reported to management in such areas as: program awareness, participation, satisfaction, attitudes, self-reported improvements in morale, and health improvement. In year two, improvements in absenteeism should become available, provided baseline values were not below normative levels. In years three to five, improvements in the company's health care experience should become apparent (assuming the study has been properly designed—with appropriate comparison sites—and that a sufficiently large population is assessed). Establishing a realistic evaluation timetable for management tempers their expectations for program performance and lessens the pressures on program administrators.

Presentation of Results

When reporting results of evaluation efforts, the presenter must be cognizant of the audience's interests and level of sophistication. High-level presentations

Table 5-5 Sample Evaluation Timetable

Project Milestone	Outcome of Interest	Instrument/Technique
Before the program begins	Health care utilization/cost	Baseline claims analysis, including a focus on lifestyle-related illnesses
Baseline measures	Human resource expenditures	Baseline analysis of human resources expenditures covering the following areas: absenteeism, overall health care, turnover, workers' compensation, disability and productivity–Human Resources Cost Analysis (HRCA)
	Interest/attitude	Baseline employee interest and attitude survey
At program initiation	Employee health status	Health risk appraisal/health profile–group report
Year 1	Employee health status	Follow-up health profile–
	Biometric measures	group report
	Participation results	Quarterly/annual participation reports
	Human resources cost trends	HRCA
	Employee satisfaction/attitudes	Employee satisfaction survey
Year 2	Employee satisfaction	Employee satisfaction survey
	Human resources costs	HRCA
	Participation results	Quarterly/annual participation reports
Year 3	Employee satisfaction	Employee satisfaction survey
	Human resources costs	HRCA
	Participation results	Quarterly/annual participation reports
	Return on Investment (ROI)	Medical care, absenteeism, disability, workers' compensation, and productivity study

to senior management should focus on overall conclusions presented in "bullet" format or as simple graphs. Typically, 15-30-minute presentations are adequate.

In contrast, presentations to middle managers and program administrators should be more comprehensive. A two- to three-hour review of the data and the methodology used to gather the data is not unusual. This format allows sufficient time for discussion. The presenter should know ahead of time the questions foremost in the audience's mind—for example, whether the focus should be placed on economic or health care outcomes. Are there specific questions of interest that need to be answered? Which charts or graphs will have the greatest impact?

Use of audiovisual aids is recommended. Typically, results are presented using overheads, slides, or computer projection devices. Overheads have the

advantage of being easily and quickly modified. The evaluator should consider a variety of media in the presentation of results. For example, audio or videotape testimonials by employees (or managers) on how the program has affected these individuals' quality of life is a very powerful presentation tool. Similarly, engaging managers in the health promotion process through individualized health risk appraisals or "personal training" with feedback can be a useful way of educating the decision makers on the relevance of the program on an individual basis.

It is imperative that all of the data, both positive and negative, be presented to decision makers. The credibility of the evaluation team and the results they present hinges on their openness and honesty in presenting program results. If it is determined at a later date that misinformation was presented or that critical information was omitted, then not only is the credibility of the evaluation team at stake but also that of the staff managing the intervention program.

In presenting results, the evaluator needs to help the audience interpret the results and reach conclusions. To the evaluator, the conclusions may be obvious, only because he or she has been working with the data for some period. To the audience members who are being exposed to the potentially voluminous and complex findings for the first time, results may be confusing and even contradictory. Thus, the evaluator should summarize and draw conclusions from the data to help the audience verbalize possible implications for action. Finally, the evaluator should prepare the audience for future results by speaking about ongoing research activities, other studies that are planned, or follow-up studies to those currently presented.

A Closing Note and a Touch of Reality

Throughout this document, the authors have presented guidance and recommendations that may appear contradictory at times to the reader. As a general theme, we have attempted to emphasize the need to perform evaluation research using the most rigorous methods available. We have underscored the need to profile representative samples, conduct studies with suitable comparison groups, control for confounders using advanced statistical methods, achieve very high follow-up rates, and so forth. These are the requirements for excellent scientific research. These are also the expectations of scientists who review evaluation research and whose pronouncements relative to the value of such research is highly esteemed. In short, much of the chapter describes what *ought* to be done in an almost perfect world when performing evaluation studies focused on worksite health promotion programs. When these rules and guidelines are followed, the final product will be more accurate and consequently more valuable.

But, the authors are also realists. We understand that what should be done in real-life research is not always what is done. We know that the audience for evaluation studies is often unsophisticated and has far lower expectations for scientific rigor than an audience with academic credentials. We understand

and appreciate that budgets for these studies are often limited or, in some cases, nonexistent. We realize that the necessary expertise to perform rigorous evaluation studies is not always resident in-house and that often there are no budgets for hiring outsiders. We understand all this. That is why in several sections of the chapter we discuss "low-cost" and "easy" ways to gather outcome data. For example, we reference the Employee Satisfaction Survey instrument found in the appendix as a quick and easy way to gather outcome in five different areas.

So, what should the "typical" program evaluator do? The answer is: be pragmatic. If the requirements for documentation are low and the budget is limited, perform the minimum amount of studies to fulfill requirements. However, perform these studies using the most credible methods and resources available. Most importantly, when performing "quick-and-dirty" studies, be honest and forthright about the inherent limitations of such research. Specify the methods that would have to be employed to overcome those limitations and how the study could be improved.

What if the sophistication of the audience is low and the budget is tight, but the expectations are still high? What do you do when the decision maker requests that you "document ROI using medical insurance claims data, absence history, disability and safety data, and measure productivity—all for under $5,000." Here, the evaluator is faced with an ethical and practical dilemma: should he or she "fake it" or communicate honestly to the decision maker that the requirements do not match the resources available. Our recommendation is to do the latter— to communicate to the decision maker that the expectations are not realistic and that he or she should either temper those expectations or provide additional resources.

The program evaluator should keep in mind the rule of thumb advanced above regarding budget for evaluation—that is, evaluation costs should equal approximately five percent (or more) of the intervention costs in any given year. Such budget constraints should help form the boundary and scope conditions for the evaluation and establish more realistic expectations.

In short, the program evaluator is encouraged to design an evaluation protocol that achieves the evaluation goals in the most cost-effective manner and within the resource constraints established by the program funder (O'Donnell, personal communication, 1999). This discussion also accentuates the need to clarify program goals at the project's initiation before expectations regarding outcomes are crystalized. If the goal is to publish results in a first tier scientific journal, the highest level of rigor is required. If, on the other hand, the goal is to provide sufficient data to senior management regarding program accomplishments so that they can make an informed decision about future funding, then a far lower level of rigor is required.

CONCLUSION

For health promotion programs to succeed, they need clearly formulated action plans that are based on sound scientific theory and that are subject to thoughtful measurement and evaluation. Support for the program needs to come from the "movers and shakers" of an organization. In order to maintain their support, the evaluator needs to clearly understand their motivations for introducing and maintaining the program and the types of results they expect of the program. Since there are often multiple customers within an organization, each of whom has different requirements of the program, it is recommended that multiple measures be applied to assess program achievements across different indicators. To the extent possible, program objectives and measures focused on those objectives should be clearly aligned with overall company mission and vision statements.

It is recommended that the evaluator provide the customers of health promotion programs with results as they become available, either individually or in a group. Keeping the program current, listening to the customers and their shifting requirements and emphases, continuously collecting and reporting data on program results in each area of customer interest, using a variety of measures and reporting strategies, and varying presentation techniques and styles are some of the approaches used to insure that the program will continue to receive the attention and support of senior management.

Finally, evaluators need to recognize that they may not be able to do it all alone. Effective program evaluation requires the combined skills and talents of a variety of individuals who may include professional evaluators, statisticians, computer programmers, epidemiologists, econometricians, health policy analysts, benefit specialists, physicians, and public speakers. Very few individuals in our society have all of these skills and talents. Experienced evaluators know that they need to seek the opinions of experts in the field and gain peer review of their designs and evaluation results. It is recommended that second opinions be secured at every stage of the evaluation process.

In closing, while health promotion program administrators, and the decision makers who fund these programs, have a need for data that support their investment decisions, they may not be very knowledgeable about ways to secure those data. They may feel that the data should be easy to obtain and may feel frustrated when their expectations are not easily fulfilled. It is the responsibility of evaluators to inform and educate their customers on issues discussed in this chapter and to support their efforts to obtain good information on program results. Working in partnership, evaluators, program managers, and decision makers can gather quality data that support continued investment in employee health.

References

Aldana, S. G. (1998) Financial impact of worksite health promotion and methodological quality of the evidence. *The Art of Health Promotion*, 2:1, 1–8.

Bigos, S., Battie, M., & Spengler, D. (1991). A prospective study of work perceptions and psychosocial factors affecting the report of back injury. *Spine*, 16(1), 1–6.

Bly, J., Jones, R., & Richardson, T. (1986). Impact of worksite health promotion on health care costs and utilization: Evaluation of Johnson & Johnson's LIVE FOR LIFE program. *Journal of the American Medical Association, 256*, 3235–3240.

Burton, W. N., Conti, D. J., Chin-Yu, C., Schultz, A. B., & Edington, D. W. (1999). The role of health risk factors and disease on worker productivity. *Journal of Occupational and Environmental Medicine, 41*(10), 863–877.

Campbell, D. (1957). Factors relevant to the validity of experiments in social settings. *Psychological Bulletin, 54,* 297–312.

Campbell, D., & Stanley, J. (1963). *Experimental and quasi-experimental designs for research.* Skokie, IL: Rand McNally.

Chapman, L. S. (1991). *Evaluation: The key to wellness program survival.* Seattle, WA: Corporate Health Designs.

Claxton, A. J., Chawla, A. J., & Kennedy, S. (1999). Absenteeism among employees treated for depression. *Journal of Occupational and Environmental Medicine, 41,* 605–611.

Cochrane, W. G. (1978). *Sampling techniques* (3rd ed.). New York, NY: John Wiley & Sons, Inc.

Cockburn, I. M., Bailit, H. I., Berndt, E. R., & Finkelstein, S. N. (1999). Loss of work productivity due to illness and medical treatment. *Journal of Occupational and Environmental Medicine, 41* (11), 948–953.

Cohen, J. (1977). *Statistical power analysis for the behavioral sciences.* (Rev. ed.) New York: Academic Press.

Cohen, J. (1988). *Statistical power analysis for behavioral sciences.* Hillsdale, NJ: Lawrence Erlbaum Associates.

Conrad, K. M., Conrad, K. J., & Walcott-McQuigg, J. (1991). Threats to internal validity in worksite health promotion program research: Common problems and possible solutions. *American Journal of Health Promotion, 6*(2), 112–122.

Conrad, K. M., Reidel, J. E., & Gibbs, J. O. (1990). Effect of worksite health promotion programs on employee absenteeism. *Association of Operating Room Nurses Journal* 38(12), 573–580.

Cook, T. D., & Campbell, D. T. (1979). *Quasi-experimentation: Design and analysis issues for field settings.* Boston, MA: Houghton Mifflin Company.

Davis, M. F., Rosenberg, K., Iverson, D. C., & Bauer, J. (1984). Worksite health promotion in Colorado. *Public Health Reports, 99,* 538–543.

DeJoy, D. M., & Southern, D. J. (1993). An integrative perspective on worksite health promotion. *Journal of Occupational Medicine, 35*(12), 1221–1229.

Dobson, A. J. (1984). Calculating sample size. *Trans Menzies Foundation, 7,* 75–79.

Drakeley, C. A., & Smith, A. M. (1999). Here today and gone tomorrow. *California Computer News.* [On-line]. Available: www.ccnmag.com (April 1999 issue)

Edington, E. S. (1995). *Randomization tests.* New York, NY: M. Dekker.

Edington, D. W. (1992). *Worksite wellness: Cost/benefit analysis and report* (Vol. 3). Ann Arbor, MI: University of Michigan, Fitness Research Center.

Edington, D. W., Yen, L. T., and Witting, P. (1997). The financial impact of changes in personal health practices. *Journal of Occupational and Environmental Medicine, 39:*11, 1037–1046.

Fielding, J. E. (1982). Effectiveness of employee health improvement programs. *Journal of Occupational Medicine, 24,* 907–916.

Fielding, J. E. (1986). *An overview of existing evaluation designs and issues in the measurement of the effectiveness and efficiencies of worksite health enhancement programs.* Unpublished manuscript, Research Triangle Institute. Research Triangle Park, NC.

Fielding, J. E. (1990). Worksite health promotion programs in the United States: Progress, lessons and challenges. *Health Promotion International, 5*(1), 75–84.

Fielding, J. E. (1991). Preventive services as a health management tool; Occupational health physicians and prevention. *Journal of Occupational Medicine, 33*(3), 314–326.

Fielding, J. E., & Piserchia, P. V. (1989). Frequency of worksite health promotion activities. *American Journal of Public Health, 79,* 16–20.

Fiore, M. C., Novotny, T. E., Pierce, J. P., Giovino, G. A., Hatziandreu, E. J., Newcomb, P. A., Surawicz, T. S., & Davis, R. M. (1990). Methods used to quit smoking in the United States: Do cessation programs help? *Journal of the American Medical Association, 263*(20), 2760–2765.

Fleiss, J. (1981). *Statistical methods for rates and proportions.* New York: John Wiley & Sons, Inc.

Goetzel, R. Z., Anderson, D. R., Whitmer, R. W., Ozminkowski, R. J., Dunn, R. L., Wasserman, J. and the HERO Research Committee (1998). The relationship between modifiable health risks and health care expenditures: An analysis of the multi-employer HERO health risk and cost database. *Journal of Occupational and Environmental Medicine, 40*(10), 843–854.

Goetzel, R. Z., Danaher, B. G., Fielding, J. E., Hillman, J., Knight, K. K., Wade, S., & Wilson, A. (1990). *Worksite health promotion: Review of the literature and state of the art analysis.* Santa Monica, CA: Johnson & Johnson Health Management, Inc.

Goetzel, R. Z., Dunn, R. L., Ozminkowski, R. J., Satin, K., Whitehead, D., & Cahill, K. (1998). Differences between descriptive and multivariate estimates of the impact of Chevron Corporation's Health Quest Program on medical expenditures. *Journal of Occupational and Environmental Medicine, 40,* 538–545.

Goetzel, R. Z., Guindon, A., Humphries, L., Newton, P., Turshen, J., & Webb, R. (1998). *Health and productivity management: Consortium benchmarking study best practice report.* Houston, TX: American Productivity and Quality Center International Benchmarking Clearinghouse.

Goetzel, R. Z., Guindon, A., Newton, P., Turshen, J., & Webb, R. (1999). *Health and productivity management: Consortium benchmarking study best practice report.* Houston, TX: American Productivity and Quality Center International Benchmarking Clearinghouse.

Goetzel, R. Z., Juday, T. R., & Ozminkowski, R. J. (1999, Summer). What's the ROI?—A systematic review of return on investment (ROI) studies of corporate health and productivity management initiatives. *AWHP's Worksite Health, 12*–21.

Heaney, C. A., & Goetzel, R. Z. (1997). "A review of health-related outcomes of multi-component worksite health promotion programs. *American Journal of Health Promotion, 11*(4), 290–307.

Heckman, J. J. (1979). Sample selection as a specification error. *Econometrica, 47*(1), 153–161.

Heckman, J. J., & Robb, R. (1985). Alternative methods for evaluating the impact of interventions. In J. J. Heckman & B. J. Singer (Eds.), *Longitudinal analysis of labor market data.* New York, NY: Cambridge University Press.

Heckman, J. J. & Smith, J. A. (1995). Assessing the case for social experiments. *Journal of Economic Perspectives, 9*(2), 85–110.

Hewitt Associates (1996). *Health promotion initiatives/ managed health provided by major U.S. employers in 1996: Based on practices of 1,050 employers.* Lincolnshire, IL: Hewitt Associates LLC.

Hollander, R. B., & Lengermann, J. J. (1988). Corporate characteristics and worksite health promotion programs: Survey findings from Fortune 500 companies. *Social Science and Medicine, 26,* 491–501.

Johnson & Johnson Health Management, Inc. (1989). *Customer advisory board survey results.* Unpublished manuscript, Santa Monica, CA.

Johnson & Johnson Health Management, Inc. (1992a). *Customer satisfaction requirements project report.* Unpublished manuscript, Santa Monica, CA.

Johnson & Johnson Health Management, Inc. (1992b). *Relationship between participation and cost: Results of LIVE FOR LIFE program results.* Unpublished manuscript, Santa Monica, CA.

Johnson & Johnson Health Management, Inc. (1992c). *Lifestyle related utilization and cost: Results of 30 lifestyle claims analyses.* Unpublished manuscript, Santa Monica, CA.

Kahn, H., & Sempos, C. (1989). *Statistical methods in epidemiology.* New York: Oxford University Press.

Kalton, G., & Kasprzyk, D. (1986). The treatment of missing survey data. *Survey Methodology, 12,* 1–16.

Kerlinger, F. N. (1973). *Foundations of behavioral research.* New York: Holt, Rinehart and Winston, Inc.

Konrad, T. R., & DeFriese, G. H. (1990). Primer on evaluation methods: On the subject of sampling. . . . *American Journal of Health Promotion, 5*(2), 147–153.

Leviton, L. (1987). The yield from worksite cardiovascular risk reduction. *Journal of Occupational Medicine, 29,* 931–936.

Lovato, C. Y., & Green, L. W. (1990). Maintaining employee participation in workplace health promotion programs. *Health Education Quarterly, 17*(1), 73–88.

Newell, S. A., Afaf, G., Sanson-Fisher, R. W., & Savolainen, N. J. (1999). The accuracy of self-reported health behaviors and risk factors relating to cancer and cardiovascular disease in the general population. *American Journal of Preventive Medicine, 17*(3), 211–229.

O'Donnell, M. P. (1999). How well do your programs contribute to the mission, long-term goals, and current priorities of the organization? *American Journal of Health Promotion, 14*(1), IV.

O'Donnell, M. P., & Ainsworth, T. (1984). *Health promotion in the workplace.* New York: John Wiley & Sons.

O'Donnell, M. P., Bishop, C., & Kaplan, K. (1997). Benchmarking best practices in workplace health promotion. *The Art of Health Promotion, 1*(1), 1–8.

O'Donnell, M. P., & Harris, J. S. (1994). *Health Promotion in the Workplace* (2nd ed.). Albany, NY: Delmar Publishers, Inc.

Olsen, R. J. (1980). A least squares correction for sensitivity bias. *Econometrica, 48,* 1815–1820.

Ozminkowski, R. J., Dunn, R. L., Goetzel, R. Z., Cantor, R. I., Murnane, J., & Harrison, M. (1999). A return on investment evaluation of the Citibank, N.A. health management program. *American Journal of Health Promotion, 14,* 31–43.

Pelletier, K. R. (1988). Database: research and evaluation results. *American Journal of Health Promotion, 2*(4), 52–57.

Pelletier, K. R. (1991). A review and analysis of the health and cost-effective outcomes studies of comprehensive health promotion and disease prevention programs. *American Journal of Health Promotion, 5*(4), 52–57.

Pelletier, K. R. (1993). A review and analysis of the health and cost-effective outcomes studies of comprehensive health promotion and disease prevention programs, 1991–1993 update. *American Journal of Health Promotion, 8,* 50–62.

Pelletier, K. R. (1996). A review and analysis of the health and cost effective outcomes studies of comprehensive health promotion and disease prevention programs, 1993–1995 update. *American Journal of Health Promotion, 10,* 380–388.

Pinkovitz, W. H., Moskal, J., & Green, G. (1999). *How much does your employee turnover cost?* [On-line]. Available: www.uwex.edu/ces/cced/publicat/turn.html.

Prochaska, J., DiClemente, C., Velicer, W., & Rossi, J. (1993). Standardized, individualized, interactive and personalized self-help programs for smoking cessation. *Health Psychology, 12*(5), 399–405.

Rosenbaum, P., & Rubin, D. (1984). Reducing bias in observational studies using subclassification on the propensity score. *Journal of the American Statistical Association, 79*(387), 516–524.

Rossi, P. H., & Freeman, H. L. (1999). *Evaluation: A systematic approach* (4th ed.). Newbury Park, CA: Sage Publications, Inc.

Saratoga Institute (1999). *Human resources financial report* [On-line]. Available: www.HR2000.com/saratoga/ad.html.

Shipley, R., Orleans, C., Wilbur, C., Piserchia, P., & McFadden, D. (1988). Effect of the Johnson & Johnson LIVE FOR LIFE program on employee smoking. *Preventive Medicine, 17,* 25–34.

Sloan, R. P., Gruman, J. C., & Allegrante, J. P. (1987). *Investing in employee health: A guide to effective health promotion in the workplace.* San Francisco: Jossey-Bass Publishers.

Solomon, R. (1954). An extension of control group design. *American Journal of Psychology, 67,* 573–589.

Thompson, B., Bowen, D. J., Croyle, R. T., Hopp, H. P., & Fries, E. (1991). Maximizing worksite survey response rates through community organization strategies and multiple contacts. *American Journal of Health Promotion, 6*(2), 130–136.

Wagner, E. H., & Guild, P. A. (1989). Primer on evaluation methods: Choosing an evaluation strategy. *American Journal of Health Promotion, 4*(2), 134–144.

Warner, K. E. (1990, Summer). Wellness at the worksite. *Health Affairs,* pp. 64–79.

Warner, K. E., Smith, R. J., Smith, D. G., & Fries, B. E. (1996). Health and economic implications of a work-site smoking cessation program: A simulation analysis. *Journal of Occupational and Environmental Medicine, 38*(10), 961–992.

Warner, K. E., Wickizer, T. M., Wolfe, R. A., Schildroth, J. E., & Samuelson, M. H. (1988). Economic implications of workplace health promotion programs: Review of literature. *Journal of Occupational Medicine, 30*(2), 106–112.

William M. Mercer, Inc. (1999). *Mercer's Fax Facts Survey: Health Management.* Mercer's USA Resource Center: News Releases. [On-line]. Available: www.wmmercer.com.

Employee Satisfaction Survey

General Information

Date of Birth		___/___/___					
Sex	☐	(1)	Male	☐	(2)	Female	
Employment Status	☐	(1)	Salaried	☐	(2)	Hourly	
Department	☐	(1)	4000	☐	(3)	5300	
	☐	(2)	4600	☐	(4)	Other	
Business Unit	☐	BU#1		☐	BU#3		
	☐	BU#2		☐	BU#4		

Participation in the Health Promotion Program

1. Have you participated in any aspect of the Health Promotion Program? (For example, Health Profiles, Health Improvement Programs, Lunch 'N' Learn Seminars, or Exercise Programs.)

   ☐ (1) Yes (Go to Question 3)   ☐ (2) No

2. Which of the following would explain why you have <u>not</u> participated in the Health Promotion Program? (Check all that apply.)

   ☐ I was not aware of the program

   ☐ Lack of motivation or interest on my part

   ☐ Programs are not scheduled at convenient times

   ☐ Program locations are too far from my work area

   ☐ Tight commuting schedule/car pooling arrangements

   ☐ Other (please specify) _____

Evaluation of the Health Promotion Program

3. Which of the following health improvements have you made since September 1998? (Check all that apply.)

Topic Area	Improved	I did not improve	This was not a problem for me
Weight management			
Exercise			
Eating habits			
Cigarette smoking			
Alcohol consumption			
Seatbelt use			
Stress management			
Blood pressure management			
Cholesterol management			
General well-being (e.g., nervousness, anxiety, depression)			
Other			

Comments: _____

_____

_____

4. As a result of your participation in the Health Promotion Programs, how satisfied are you?

1	2	3	4	5
Very Dissatisfied	Dissatisfied	Neither Satisfied nor Dissatisfied	Satisfied	Very Satisfied

5. What effect has the Health Promotion Program had on your. . . (Circle one number per item)

	Very Negative Effect	Negative Effect	No Effect	Positive Effect	Very Positive Effect
Morale	1	2	3	4	5
Productivity	1	2	3	4	5
Satisfaction with your job	1	2	3	4	5
Satisfaction with your employer	1	2	3	4	5
Health, lifestyle and level of fitness	1	2	3	4	5

6. Please write any additional comments that you have about the Health Promotion Program.

_____

_____

THANK YOU FOR TAKING THE TIME TO COMPLETE THIS SURVEY
Please return this form in the envelope provided to:
The Health Promotion Program Office–Building 147
no later than September 30, 1999.

CHAPTER

6

Awareness Strategies

Larry S. Chapman

INTRODUCTION

This chapter provides an overview and discussion of the traditional and nontraditional awareness strategies used in most worksite health promotion programs. In addition to an examination of the role of such strategies in programming activity, newer technologies and a model for maximizing the behavioral impact of awareness activities is also presented. As one of three major conceptual elements of all worksite-based programming, awareness strategies, as a collection of activities, have played a significant role in past worksite programming and will likely play an important role in future worksite efforts. It is highly likely that awareness strategies, along with behavior change and cultural change efforts, will continue to constitute the conceptual and technical troika of worksite health promotion.

THE ROLE OF AWARENESS STRATEGIES IN HEALTH PROMOTION PROGRAMS

Awareness strategies usually represent a major portion of most worksite health promotion program ac-

tivities. Their role has evolved over the past decade to embrace emerging technologies and a growing pressure to demonstrate their contribution in achieving relevant improvements in health behavior, health status, and key organizational gains. The role of awareness strategies will likely remain at center stage in the years ahead as worksite health promotion programs continue to mature and undergo more rigorous evaluation and resulting refinements.

Overview of Awareness and Information

Awareness strategies are defined as . . .

> a variety of communication dissemination and information transfer activities that are intended to enhance the knowledge levels of individuals, help catalyze and reinforce behavior change, while intentionally leading to improved individual health and productivity.

This definition reflects the somewhat open-ended nature of awareness and the somewhat global role that it plays in human interaction and discourse. In a general sense, the transfer of information or knowledge is an integral component of all human systems. Specifically, awareness strategies represent the mainstay of information transfer activity within the context of worksite-based health promotion programs.

The roles of awareness strategies and activities in health promotion programs are generally threefold. First, awareness is intended to function in communicating relevant information that helps prepare the individual for health behavior change. Second, awareness activities are intended to help empower and enable the individual to formulate a personal application of the information that is transferred. Third, awareness is intended to enable the individual to gain practical access to the applicable technology or services that can aid or assist in the reinforcement or initiation of a specific health behavior. In short, awareness provides information, helps empower individuals to change, and helps connect the individual with services and resources to facilitate and maintain the change.

In this view, awareness represents a major pathway and technology for the exchange or transfer of information that can assist or catalyze the initiation and reinforcement of behavior. In order for these roles to be fulfilled, the awareness activities must be utilized by the recipient and must be perceived as relevant or desirable in relation to a felt need.

Theory Related To Awareness Strategies

Health promotion programs are intended to help people adopt and maintain healthy lifestyles and health behavior changes. One of the primary purposes of awareness programming is to provide information to specified individuals in defined populations in a manner that helps facilitate health behavior change and changes in underlying attitudes and values. The need for information, and the need to actively inform, are inherent in any circumstance in which a purposeful change in behavior is desired.

A second purpose of awareness programs is to help activate the individual to change his/her behavior, attitudes, and values. This activation implies that the individual receives personally relevant information that produces the desire and initiation or activation of change in a specific behavioral area. Awareness without some degree of activation is of limited value other than as preparation for later potential activation. Other related concepts linked to this function of awareness include empowerment, self-efficacy, self-responsibility, and self-determination. Each of these related concepts is an important part of the personal dynamics of health promotion programming.

A third purpose of awareness programming is the reinforcement of existing desirable behaviors, attitudes, and values. For those individuals who have already adopted healthful living practices and thought patterns, it is important to use awareness programming to encourage and enhance continued adherence, retention, and repetition of helpful activities.

A fourth purpose of awareness programming is to help catalyze change in personal beliefs. A desirable outcome of health promotion programming is to help create change in personal beliefs that enable the individual to enhance the length and quality of his/her life. Where these specific objectives guide health promotion program activity, it seems entirely appropriate that awareness programming can contribute in a positive way by catalyzing change in beliefs such as unlearning "learned" helplessness; overcoming inertia, resistance, and apathy; revising self-destructive intentions; and overcoming self-deprecation and social alienation.

In a similar vein, awareness programs typically function to enhance the individual's perceptions of susceptibility to disease, impairment, or dysfunction by exploring lifestyle and health risk factors and their differential contribution to increased disease and injury occurrence. Lately a major challenge to this traditional risk-driven dynamic of awareness programming has emerged around the area of holistic-oriented wellness or health promotion programming (Robison, 1997; Ornstein & Sobel, 1989; Carlyon, 1984; Lyons, & Burgard, 1990). This view questions the wisdom of reinforcing personal perceptions of susceptibility due to its adverse effects on motivation; ancillary production of guilt, fear, and more negative emotional components of behavior; and personal empowerment. The emerging research and evaluation on this approach will help to further identify its utility and value in broad-based health promotion programming. Regardless of the outcome of these research and evaluation efforts, some form of awareness activity will presumably always be a core component of health promotion programming. The content and emphasis may shift as the research findings corroborate the need for new approaches, but awareness programming will likely always be a major component of all worksite health promotion activities.

Another purpose of awareness programming is to enhance the sense of empowerment that the individual feels about his or her ability to successfully change personal behavior at will. Much has been written about this concept over the years under such concepts as locus of control, self-efficacy, self-mastery, self-determination, and self-responsibility (McGinnis, 1990; Miller, Ellis, Zook, & Lyle, 1990; Pierce, McCaskill, & Hill, 1990; Rudd & Glantz, 1989; Gooder & Welberg-Ekvall, 1989; Bandura, 1978; Heller & Krauss, 1991; Graninger, 1990). More will likely be written on these topics due to their importance in the realm of voluntary behavior change. An increased sense of empowerment is supportable through awareness programming and is likely to be an even more important function of awareness programming efforts in the future. The concept of readiness to change is another key element of health promotion and of awareness programming. Awareness activities are usually designed to help create a readiness to change in a particular target population. This underlying purpose of awareness effort requires a consistency and perseverance in all programming efforts and the recognition of collective and individual cycles of increased readiness to change. Active recruitment and a proactive orientation to programming are also emphasized under the Transtheoretical Model™ (Prochaska & DiClemente, 1989). Often informal awareness efforts may focus on individual health events, such as heart attacks of key employees, seasonal preparation for change (e.g., preparing for summer swimsuit opportunities), back-to-school patterns of autumn, participation in major sporting events, or facilitation of New Year's changes. This fluctuating series of collective and individual cycles can be aided with a sound approach to awareness programming.

An additional purpose of awareness programming is to market program offerings to eligible employees. Without some level of core awareness efforts, how are employees going to know what activities, assistance, or resources are available? This essentially reflects the marketing and/or promotional function of programming. The associated purpose of awareness programming is an important component of any organized worksite health promotion program.

A well-balanced awareness program will likely address all these purposes while providing a consistent avenue of communication with various program constituencies and target groups. The various potential program purposes identified above will likely ebb and flow over the life of the worksite health promotion program.

Some of the classical theories related to awareness programming are reviewed below.

Social Cognitive Theory

One classical model of individual behavior change was postulated originally by Lewin (1951) and then further refined by Bandura (1971). This model of behavior change is usually referred to as Social Cognitive Theory. The core of the model is the identification of restraining forces and supporting forces for a defined behavior, such as cigarette smoking. This model is further described in this book by Wallston and Armstrong in Chapter 7.

Awareness in the social learning model of behavior change was to be instrumental in raising knowledge and understanding of the counterpositioned factors from the individual's perspective regarding a specific behavior change. Awareness programming functioned under the model as the vehicle for communicating the dynamics of the potential change and as a necessary tool for unbalancing the restraining and supportive forces at the level of individual decision making. Awareness functions as a catalyst, carrier, or insight-producer in unbalancing the various forces involved in maintaining or catalyzing behavior change.

Health Belief Model

The health belief model, originally developed by Hochbaum (1979) , and modified by Becker and associates (1974), represents another major classical model for viewing health behavior change and is also discussed in Chapter 7. The health belief model is based on the core concept that perception of personal susceptibility to an adverse health outcome, risk, or condition provides the principal motivational force behind a potential health behavior change. The role awareness plays in the health belief model is similar to the role it plays in the social cognitive theory of behavior change. Awareness programming functions again as a primary vehicle for internalizing a sense of susceptibility that helps provide the motive force for selected behavior change. This functional purpose of awareness under the health belief model is that of a vehicle, or methodology, for communicating information that confirms and deepens the individual's sense of susceptibility to an undesirable end. As a corollary, awareness activity can function to impart positive information about the development of alternative responses and behavioral options once the decision to change has been made.

Transtheoretical Model

The Transtheoretical Model™ developed by Prochaska and associates is also described in Chapter 7 and represents a very useful construct for affecting health behavior. Awareness strategies are also key elements in bringing about movement from one stage to another and provide a theoretical construct for the tailoring and personalization of information to affect health behavior. Stage-sensitive information contained in awareness activities offers an effective tool for health promotion professionals who are developing programs for worksite settings. These applications can be made at the population level and the individual level.

MAJOR AWARENESS METHODS

A variety of awareness methods and strategies can be used to develop programs for employee and spousal populations. These methods and strategies can be grouped into traditional, nontraditional, and newer technology types of interventions.

Traditional Awareness Intervention Methods for the Worksite

The traditional methods of awareness programming have been familiar components of all organized educational and informational activity conducted in the American workplace. These traditional methods have generally become part of the fabric of most work cultures. The frequency of use and actual format of the method usually reflect the size of the work force, the degree of geographic dispersion of the work group involved, the budgetary commitment to awareness and communications, and the sophistication of the employer in conducting formal and informal communication programs.

The following awareness and communications methods represent traditional methods and vehicles used in the American worksite to educate and inform employees and their family members. It is not unusual to find several of these methods used in the communication of specific information to working populations. Table 6-1 contains a list of the traditional awareness communications methods for use in worksite settings.

Announcements During Meetings

One of the more effective methods is to make an informational announcement as part of a meeting with employees or with key staff. This awareness/

Table 6-1 Examples of Traditional Awareness Communication Methods

Announcements during meetings
Written individual notices
Bulletin board notices
Printed pamphlets
Payroll inserts
Marquees and electronic billboards
Face-to-face individual information sessions
Group information sessions
Audio presentations
Audiovisual presentations
Video presentations

communication method, as is true of all methods, does not assure 100% retention or even familiarity. However, individuals who are exposed to informational messages in this way are likely to have a fairly high degree of retention of the information.

Written Individual Notices

The individual notice, memo, or letter is a typical approach used by the vast majority of work organizations. This approach can be embellished with distinctive art styles, colors, and desktop publishing attributes to enhance readership and retention. Unfortunately, a significant percentage of employees do not read written correspondence, usually because of illiteracy, apathy, or outright resistance. Penetration of awareness programming into spousal and dependent populations is also hindered by gatekeeping that occurs for many different reasons.

Bulletin Board Notices

Another very traditional awareness/communication method involves the use of employee bulletin board notices. Prescribed as a required communication method in many state and federal laws, it is almost universal in all but the very smallest worksites. In relation to bulletin board use, the unfortunate reality is that announcements that are placed on bulletin boards, even if they are moved periodically and not crowded together, often do not get read. In addition, it is likely that many employees will not look at employee bulletin boards unless there is a compelling reason to do so.

Printed Pamphlets

A very traditional component of most awareness programs is the use of printed pamphlets that focus on specific health and health promotion topics. Typically, these vehicles are maintained in specified locations and can be picked up at will by employees. Other methods of distribution include mail request cards or memos that allow the individual employee to request a limited number of pamphlets on specific health topics of interest. The best strategy with pamphlets is to provide them only when they are desired by the individual, primarily when he/she is interested in making a behavior change or is concerned about his/her own behavior or a loved one's risks and needs.

Payroll Inserts

Payroll inserts are written materials that are included in paycheck envelopes and are used to distribute selected information to employee populations. This method has been declining in usefulness as the number of employees with direct electronic deposit of paychecks increases. In addition, frequent speculation has been made about the quick discarding of everything but the paycheck by the employee upon its receipt, further undermining this method's usefulness. This limitation can be partially overcome by adopting a policy that prohibits electronic bank deposits and by using payroll check inserts to communicate well-advertised and important items of information. This would hopefully further develop a sense of the importance of written materials received with employee paychecks.

Marquees and Electronic Billboards

This method involves the use of centrally located marquees or electronic billboards with a looped or repeating message. These are frequently used in building foyers, elevators, reception areas, lunchrooms, break rooms, waiting areas, and meeting areas.

Face-to-Face Individual Information Sessions

Undoubtedly one of the most effective methods for raising awareness involves the face-to-face encounter. The information exchange is usually two-way and capable of enhancing retention and understanding. From informal observation by the author, it appears that the most effective form of this method is the question-and-answer approach involving challenge questions and specific knowledge goals.

Group Information Sessions

The use of group meetings for delivery of information is another traditional communication method and is reasonably effective, depending on the style of delivery and the nature of the information conveyed. Brief meeting "inserts" on health promotion topics can become a routine part of periodic meetings with employee work groups.

Audio Presentations

Audiotape media are used increasingly in most working populations. The use of personal headsets and audio and CD recorders is widespread, although limited use is made of this awareness method in most worksite health promotion programs. The span of content that audiotapes address is very wide, and more resources are becoming available. Professional education in many of the technical areas of concern in health promotion and wellness includes a large number of audiocassette resources.

Audiovisual Presentations

The use of audiovisual technology is also a fairly typical approach used by employers. The options include 35mm and overhead slide presentations, film media, LCD screens, computer projection devices, and audiotape combinations. These approaches are typically integrated with other communication and awareness methods and are used in orientation, employee training, and waiting areas.

Video Opportunities

Video-based communication methods appear to be widely used. The use of videotapes, television monitors, and VCRs has greatly extended this awareness and communication method with employee populations. Continuous loop presentations, user-initiated or -controlled operation, and miniaturization of video recorders and monitors have greatly enhanced the potential of this method and its use by employers.

Nontraditional Awareness Intervention Methods for the Worksite

The following awareness and communication methods are generally considered more innovative and more in keeping with changes in the way that adult learners are prone to understand, assimilate, and retain information. These methods are considered nontraditional but may be combined with traditional methods in the design of awareness or employee communication programs. Table 6-2 highlights the major nontraditional awareness and communication methods that can be used in the worksite.

Table 6-2 Examples of Nontraditional Awareness Communication Methods

Information-based puzzles, acrostics, or limericks
Self-quizzes
Health risk appraisals
Mail-request vehicles
Trigger cards
Electronic bulletin boards
Fax networks
Online telephonic support

Information-Based Puzzles, Acrostics, or Limericks

A creative option in awareness programming is to use information puzzle devices or limericks with questions to attract the adult learner's interest. An example of this type of awareness method is a crossword puzzle that asks questions which require knowledge concerning the topic addressed. An example is a crossword puzzle labeled "Fat is always bad. . . Or is it?" Questions are then posed for the crossword puzzle that produce words that fit in the puzzle and help answer the question raised. Limericks or acrostics that use health promotion knowledge are also an example of this kind of nontraditional awareness method.

Self-Quizzes

Self-quizzes on health promotion topics are another nontraditional awareness tool that can be used to engage the adult learner. The questions can be connected to incentives, used as a qualifying requirement, or placed in a Jeopardy-type game format. Self-quizzes can include answers or can require an additional step or action to provide access to the right answers.

Health Risk Appraisals

This method involves the use of self-scored or computer processed questionnaires that provide opportunities for the individual to answer questions concerning health behaviors, health risks, perceptions about health status, use of health resources, medical history, and other information and then to receive an assessment of the health implications of their responses. Initially, these instruments provided feedback on mortality risk and now they typically provide information on morbidity and quality of life issues.

Mail-Request Vehicles

This method involves providing employees and/or their family members a written form that can be used to request a limited number of pamphlets or materials on health promotion topics. These materials are then sent to the address indicated by the requestor. If a limited number of materials (i.e., no more than two or three written items per request) is used, it will tend to focus the individual on the information that is most relevant for decision-making needs. This method tailors information requests to individual needs. Periodic distribution of such a request vehicle is advisable.

Trigger Cards

This awareness method involves the use of small wallet or pocket cards with health and wellness-related information specifically focused on behavior change. These materials can be made available in human resource or occupational health offices or disseminated through routine distribution or contact channels. The types of topics they can address include questions for your doctor, consumer health skills, cholesterol reduction tips, stress management techniques, etc. Each card can contain 250–300 words if front and back surfaces are used.

Electronic Bulletin Boards

Another awareness technique or method involves the use of computer or electronic bulletin boards. This method is used in heavily computerized organizational settings or where there is relatively high access to computer networks and equipment. A wellness or health promotion electronic bulletin board can contain listings of information about community-based programs and resources, as well as topic-specific information.

Fax Networks

Facsimile transmission equipment offers another more innovative methodology for the dissemination of health information. The widespread distribution of fax technology makes this a particularly useful tool for remote worksites and locations. Many fax machines provide simultaneous, preprogrammed multisite transmission.

Online Telephonic Support

The use of inbound health advice lines and the provision of toll-free access to health and wellness professionals for advice represents a newer nontraditional approach to awareness programming. Providing an opportunity for asking questions of a health professional through a telephone advice and support system will likely increase in an effort to bring useful information to employees and dependents who are geographically dispersed among relatively small worksites (Chapman, 1998a).

Newer Technology Interventions for the Worksite

The newer technologies that are emerging for use in awareness programs are identified in Table 6-3 and explained in the discussion that follows (Chapman, 1998b).

Electronic Mail

Another computer-based communication technique involves the use of electronic mail. A sender can program and transfer information via computer networks or through modem linkages. The types of information transferred in this way can include health information as well as program promotional informa-

Table 6-3 Examples of Newer Technology Awareness Communication Methods

Electronic mail
Proactive telephone contact
Computer-based multimedia presentations
Interactive voice response
Tailored messaging
Interactive informational kiosk
Internet websites
Virtual reality applications
Adaptive survey technology

tion. With many remote worksites, health promotion coordinators can utilize electronic mail to notify program contacts of upcoming activities, conduct informational polls, or provide program cues or reminders for follow-up.

Proactive Telephone Contact

Unsolicited telephone contact by specially-trained health and wellness professionals with high risk individuals represents another newer approach to awareness programming. The provision of an opportunity for unsolicited coaching interventions, encouragement, and support for behavior change will likely increase in worksite populations.

Computer-Based Multimedia Presentations

A newer technology option involves the expanded role of computers in multimedia presentations. These typically include text, sound, and picture capability linked to monitors or large-screen equipment. This technology is a recent development, and it is likely that more health promotion-related applications will become commercially available as the data transmission capabilities of computer systems are enlarged.

Interactive Voice Response

Another newer technology involves the use of telecommunications linked to voice synthesizing and recognition capability. These applications have been growing significantly in the benefits field and particularly in the open enrollment process for cafeteria or flex plans. This technology has application for health information and can be linked to a variety of health behavioral issues.

Tailored Messaging

Pioneering work has been completed over the last decade for asking a limited series of questions of the individual seeking information on health behavior change, then to provide messages that are tailored to the individual's responses. Special question sets and linked text response blocks are used in health risk appraisals and kiosk-based health information stations. These tailored messages utilize health belief model constructs or Transtheoretical Model™ perspectives.

Interactive Informational Kiosk

Another awareness method that is usually linked to internet or intranet/CD-ROM technology is the provision of computer information capability for consumers that allows them to enter diagnoses or health topics of interest. Personalized information, as well as abstracts and full articles, then comes up on the screen. Messages can be tailored or provided in standard forms. These informational sources can then be printed, providing on-demand health information for the individual user.

Internet Websites

There has been significant growth of internet websites that provide health information, products, and support and that are being accessed by a very large segment of American workers. These websites frequently provide a medical self-care component, a behavioral change support, an information research capability, a newsletter type of function, and a component that provides "chat room" type information and/or referral functions. This particular awareness intervention method will likely see significantly greater growth in the years ahead.

Virtual Reality Applications

The use of virtual reality glasses and headgear provide a potentially powerful technology for learning. Within the headgear, the individual perceives images and sound, creating a "virtual" sense of reality. Much of this technology is also interactive and subject to high levels of individual control.

Adaptive Survey Technology

The linkage of health risk appraisal (HRA) technology with advanced computer and printing technology will open the way for each subsequent HRA an individual fills out to be modified according to previous survey answers, producing increasingly tailored personal reports and leading to an even more tailored follow-up survey. This increasingly tailored and personalized approach may eventually make standardized HRAs somewhat obsolete as awareness tools.

Major Challenges and Limitations of Awareness Strategies and Interventions

There are a variety of challenges ahead for awareness intervention efforts in worksite health promotion programs. Some of the more significant ones are as follows:

Illiteracy

It is estimated that somewhere between 6 and 20 percent of the United States work force is significantly affected by illiteracy (Hammad & Mulholland, 1992). With the increasing cultural diversity of the United States work force, this challenge will likely increase in the years ahead. The challenge will require creative use of graphics and visual images and the use of multimedia approaches to information transfer. Language options other than English are likely to become even more important.

Gatekeeping

Gatekeeping is a serious challenge to the diffusion of information through work-based populations. This is particularly true when considering the transfer of information from employees to dependents. Other forms of gatekeeping include supervisors who can selectively withhold information on health promotion programming efforts in order to minimize work performance disruptions of employees. These activities constitute a challenge to effective awareness programming as well as overall health promotion programming.

Receiver Overload

Overloading of the individual receiver of communication and/or information is another major challenge to programming efforts. Workshops that provide excessive amounts of information without opportunities to personally process or apply the information are an example of this kind of challenge. A parallel exists in the area of bulletin boards that contain dense and highly packed messages. In these situations, the density of informational messages often produces avoidance behavior rather than exposure and retention. The overloading phenomenon is likely to reduce participation, retention, and satisfaction among employees who are unwittingly exposed to its excesses.

Scotomas

A scotoma is a blind spot in a visual field. This challenge is reflected in the selective perception of susceptibility or risk inherent in an individual's view of his/her own health and well-being (Adams & Victor, 1985). This "blind spot" phenomenon represents a challenge to risk-based or holistic-based awareness education and reduces the effectiveness of awareness communication. When people choose to view their health and lifestyle in an unrealistic way, they can lose the ability to be motivated or concerned. With the expansion of genetic interventions, such as targeted gene repair, it is possible that this challenge may increase in importance, particularly as individuals perceive that "magic bullets" for health improvement are available.

Prejudicial Avoidance

The existence of prejudicial beliefs that cause personal avoidance is another major challenge to awareness programming (Applebaum, 1974). Often those individuals with the strongest prejudicial set of beliefs concerning health and personal well-being exhibit the highest occurrence of personal health risks. The types of prejudice may include very distorted views of the risk of exercise, futility of weight control, and impossibility of becoming a nonsmoker, as well as many others.

Inappropriate Timing

Another major challenge to awareness programming is inappropriate timing of information transfer. Frequently this can take the form of health promotion information that is provided at a time when the individual has little or no interest in the topic or issue or when the information is of limited value to the population involved due to its lack of timeliness, relevance, or utility. Information that is provided with limited purposefulness or perceived interest on the part of recipients is likely to be of limited value and therefore limited effectiveness.

Lack of Redundancy

Another major challenge in awareness programming is the absence of redundancy in awareness and communication efforts. Redundancy or repetition is important in penetrating the conscious awareness of recipients. Some redundancy is important in the design of promotional information concerning program activity. This is primarily due to the selective perception of employees and the fact that a significant portion of employees do not read or review the major communication methods used in the worksite.

Overreliance On Singular Communication Methods

Associated with a lack of redundancy is the overreliance by program staff on single communication methods, such as only using a newsletter to distribute program promotional information. This overreliance usually results in relatively low levels of participation and behavioral response to promotional activity.

Computer Illiteracy

With the continual growth of computer communication and Internet-based applications, those without access to computers will experience a growing disadvantage in many realms. High-tech companies that are moving into "paperless office" status represent the extreme case but are likely to reflect an emerging trend that deserves serious attention, making this challenge more significant over time.

Major historical developments are continuing to shape awareness programming in the field of health promotion. Many of these technological developments clearly represent watershed events. Some of the more important developments affecting awareness programming are listed in Table 6-4.

Copy Capability

A very significant historical development in awareness has been the development of the capability to make low-cost and high-resolution copies that appear very credible. This technologic development has made a great deal of communication and diffusion of information possible in virtually every work

Table 6-4 Major Developments Affecting Awareness Activities

Copy capability
Increased communicative competition
Increased use of video technology
Tele- and videoconferencing
Personalization of communication
Cultural diversity of the work force
Flexibility of work schedules

organization. This copy capability also has had significant impact in reducing the cost of programmatic communication. However, on the negative side, due to its almost universal access, it also allows the transmission of unsound health information on topics such as unproven herbal remedies, untested nontraditional therapies, hazardous health practices, etc.

Increased Communicative Competition

An additional development has been the vast increase in pressure from communication activities that are in direct competition for the attention of the individual. The significant increase in alternative forms of communication has greatly complicated the ability of all employers to reach employees in a relatively efficient and effective manner. These competitive communicative technologies include such things as VCRs, fax transmissions, digital and cellular phones, electronic mail, conference calls, and computer-assisted communication. This phenomenon has produced a large number of communication vehicles, which have increased the demand on employees for message time and attention.

Increased Use of Video Technology

Another major development in the communication and awareness area is the increasing use of video media resources. This includes the use of video technology for information transfer, including the planned packaging of information for use in video productions. This process includes the packaging of information into short excerpts with a high degree of similarity to professionally developed television and entertainment media forms. This has had the effect of significantly "raising the bar" of expectation for communications on health and health promotion topics.

Tele- and Videoconferencing

The emergence of teleconferencing techniques and applications also has had a significant impact on how information is transmitted in work environments. The more sophisticated applications include uplinks and downlinks from satellite technology with voice and picture transmission. On the negative side, important elements of face-to-face relationships and communication are often lost due to the use of technology.

Personalization of Communication

A related historical development has been the personalization of communications. The use of computer technology, accessible and rewritable memory, and interactive capability have all contributed to the ability to personalize communication with individuals and to enhance its potential effectiveness if done carefully. The incorporation of personal names, personal statistics, tailored messages, and time-sensitive characteristics into communication exchanges are all elements in this historical development. As this expectation increases in employee populations, it may lessen the effectiveness and persuasiveness of health communications that are not tailored or personalized to a high degree.

Cultural Diversity of the Work Force

The growth of much more diversity in the composition of the American work force is another major development that has implications for how awareness and communications activities are conducted. The increasing diversity requires cultural and ethnic sensitivity in communications and requires more adaptation of the technology of awareness with employees and their family members.

Flexibility of Work Schedules

The increasing flexibility of work schedules through such techniques as the use of flex time, telecommuting, job sharing, and other developments, also influences how effective awareness programs can be with specific subgroups of employees. This increasing flexibility of work provides a very clear challenge to awareness program efforts. Also important are the very real, inherent behavioral change limitations in awareness programming. The bulk of the behavioral science and health education literature clearly identifies the inherent limitations in the effectiveness of awareness programming, by itself, in producing long-term behavioral change (Eyles, 1990; Bellicha & McGrath, 1990; Erickson, McKenna, & Romano, 1990; Farquhar, Fortman, Flora, Taylor, Haskell, & Williams, 1990). Hochbaum (1979) has cogently identified why results from awareness programming efforts can be expected to be somewhat modest. He contrasts awareness or health education with commercial marketing and arrives at the characterization contained in Table 6-5.

Table 6-5 Differences between Awareness and Commercial Marketing

Awareness/Health Education	Commercial Marketing
Decide what is good for people	Determine what people want and provide it
Try to convince people to change	Try to convince people that their need will be met through their product
Try to influence a complex, long-term decision	Try to influence a single purchase decision
Usually have very limited budgets	Usually have considerable resources
Usually lack skills and sophistication	Usually have considerable skills and sophistication

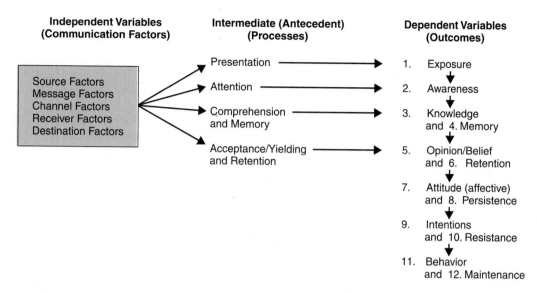

Figure 6-1 Flay's Model of Information Processing and Attitude and Behavior Change

The inherent limitations in awareness programming, as reflected in the writings of Hochbaum and others, are substantiated by relatively small increments of change in behavior over time. These sources usually highlight the fact that awareness activity needs to be linked to motivation and behavioral modification techniques in order to derive the greatest long-term behavioral impact.

ONE MODEL FOR AWARENESS INTERVENTIONS IN THE WORKSITE

There are a large number of theoretical models for awareness and communications activity presented in the behavioral, sociological, and communications literature (Macoby & Alexander, 1979; Fishbein & Ajzen, 1975; Nuttin, 1978). Each of these theoretical models have varying advantages and disadvantages. These include: comprehensiveness, fit with scientific evidence, degree of practical utility, understandability, breadth of usefulness of application, predictive ability, and flexibility in adaptation to unique settings. Based on these characteristics, the

awareness model that provides the most utility in the author's opinion is Flay's adaptation of McGuire's information-processing model (Flay, DiTecco, & Schliegel, 1990; McGuire, 1978). This information-processing model of the attitude and behavior change process includes an expanded twelve-level approach over McGuire's model and is much more useful for analysis of issues evolving from organized communication and mass media campaigns. The recommended model is illustrated in Figure 6-1.

The model uses a structure of independent variables, intermediate factors, and dependent variables to produce a framework that allows the structure, process, and outcome factors of awareness to be addressed in its component parts. The model also illustrates the complexity of communication. It has definite utility for the analysis and evaluation of organized institutional communication programs and mass media campaigns, as well as individual ideation and change processes. The model is useful for conceptualizing the various components and factors that affect the process of awareness and communication applied to health promotion issues.

SUGGESTIONS FOR EFFECTIVE AWARENESS STRATEGIES

There are some approaches that can help increase the effectiveness of awareness strategies. These strategies can be utilized in almost any setting or circumstance and are associated with the learning processes of adults (Chapman, 1996).

Strategy #1 SHOW-DISCUSS-APPLY

In the author's experience, one of the most important educational strategies with all learners is the SHOW-DISCUSS-APPLY principle of education. Simply put, when learners are shown something first in terms and ways they can understand, they will assimilate the information more readily. Next, the information should be discussed in order to let the learner assimilate the information more deeply through involvement with, and review of, its various facets. Finally, the information needs to be applied by the learner and adapted to the unique circumstances at hand. The SHOW-DISCUSS-APPLY model of learning is also important in developing a sense of ownership and involvement, which is critical to follow-through and cooperation. This model is useful for structuring brief presentations and for longer workshops as well. The SHOW-DISCUSS-APPLY activity can be repeated around desirable learning objectives, resulting in more effective educational intervention. This same strategy can also be used for health promotion and wellness presentations with senior management decision makers.

Strategy #2 REPETITIVE EXPOSURE

Another major educational strategy is based on repetitive exposure to information. It usually takes five to ten exposures to a new piece of information or a new concept before it is internalized comfortably by the learner (Wycoff, 1981). For this reason, a process of circulating key articles about worksite health promotion programs, including their cost-effectiveness, is a useful strategy to employ before having a group of decision makers consider funding a program. The multiple repetitions or exposures help the unfamiliar

become familiar. This also applies to new-to-the-learner concepts and principles concerning health behavior.

Strategy #3 EXPERIENTIAL LEARNING

A third major education strategy involves drawing the learner into an experiential learning situation (Davidson, 1989; Applebaum, 1974). This strategy has the learners actually experiencing the information or activity firsthand as much as possible. For example, have a senior management team undergo a wellness assessment as part of a management retreat to learn firsthand the value of what is or will be proposed for employees as part of an employee health promotion program. This is a very powerful learning strategy and should not be overlooked. This same kind of approach can be used with the members of an employee advisory group. It can help them gain a much more practical and insightful sense of what the likely reaction from participants will be for a proposed health promotion program activity. Experiential learning appears to be one of the most efficient and powerful ways of conveying information. One of its major disadvantages is the experiential exposure must be very well-tested and functioning before subjecting individuals to it, or the risk of rejection of the information is possible.

Strategy #4 SMALL INCREMENTS OF INFORMATION

A fourth educational strategy that is important to apply in awareness efforts is the need for small increments of information introduced over time (Wycoff, 1981). Overwhelming learners with too much information at one time may well result in less information being assimilated or fewer behavioral changes or results being implemented. By exceeding the learner's tolerance for information, it is possible to cause the learner to freeze up and not be willing to progress to the next step. Therefore, it is important to limit the informational exposure to a level that is within the learner's capability to respond. One practical application of this strategy is educational content that focuses on three points: a beginning point, a middle point, and a closing point. Each of these evidences a higher level of retention because it is easier to remember the beginning, middle, and last points in a presentation than a string of many points in one presentation. This issue becomes a careful process of selecting priorities in the educational content involved. Without clear priorities, very little information is likely to be retained.

Strategy #5 VALUE-ADDED APPROACH

Finally, the last key educational strategy recommended is based on the need to place the new information in a context in which the learner can see the direct benefit or value to his/her own interests (Reed, 1984). When presenting information, it is important to be able to demonstrate the value of the information to the individual involved in a way that can be clearly perceived by the learner. If the information is not seen as relevant by the learner, it will be very difficult for the learner to feel motivated to internalize the information or to assimilate it for future use.

CONCLUSION

The nature of the American worksite is undergoing far-reaching and significant change. The increasingly competitive nature of work and business is producing some profound changes for both public and private employers in terms of the increased economic pressures, need to increase productivity, relative scarcity of labor, and the cultural and educational diversification of the American work force. The report *Work Force 2000: The Revolution Reshaping American Business* (Boyett & Conn, 1991) highlights these changes and identifies for human resource professionals the breadth of issues that will shape employment for the decade ahead. Many of the changes will require adjustments and counterstrategies from health promotion professionals who function in workplace settings.

The major trends that are helping shape the future of the workplace include movement from production to information and service jobs; the increased cultural diversity of work groups; the increasing computerization of the work environment; the introduction of greater flexibility in work locations, job definitions, and role delineation; the increased pressure for greater productivity; the emphasis on business process improvement and its role in enhancing organizational effectiveness; the "re-engineering" of work; the changing expectations and capabilities of new labor entrants, such as Generation "X"ers into the work force; and the increased globalization of markets and productive capability (Boyett & Conn, 1991). These major trends will force changes in our work organizations, the process of work, and the way health promotion professionals deal with the objectives and purposes that reflect their organizational mandates.

A natural corollary of many of these major trends will be a greater need for health information to be segmented, tailored, and targeted to the unique needs of individual work groups and, ultimately, individuals. One of the primary implications of this increased segmentation will be the more highly refined targeting and packaging of services and products for defined market groups within an employer's work force. This will likely lead to higher degrees of specialization and focus within the health promotion vendor community and the specialization of health promotion professionals to an even greater degree.

Another implication of these major trends is that in order to successfully bring change to the worksite in the area of health promotion, it will require more creative approaches than what we have generally adopted in the past. The need for creative programming and nontraditional approaches to assisting employees and their family members in reaching higher levels of wellness will likely increase greatly in the decade ahead. Health care reform will also likely affect the conduct of health promotion in the worksite as it relates to the scope and conditions of health plan coverage.

An additional implication of the changing work environment for health promotion professionals is that health promotion and wellness-related concerns will become even more important because of the increasingly unstable nature of the work environment itself (Eyles, 1990). The major trends affecting the workplace will likely remove a significant portion of the stability that United States workers have enjoyed since the end of World War II. The age of acquisitions, mergers, and dislocations of organizational work cultures that follows, will make many of the areas of focus of health promotion even more important. A declining labor pool and expanded immigration will contribute to concerns such as stress, personal hardiness, self-esteem, spiritual health, relationship skills, sense of community and belonging, life-goal concerns, parenting and reparenting skills, and job satisfaction; other quality-of-life considerations will likely become more important dimensions for working populations in the years ahead. Awareness strategies, creatively applied, will help meet many of the challenges of the future inherent in these trends and implications.

References

Adams, R., & Victor, M. (1985). *Principles of neurology* (3rd ed.). Princeton, NJ: McGraw-Hill.

Applebaum, R. (1974). *The process of group communication.* Chicago: Science Research Associates, Inc.

Bandura, A. (1971). *Social learning theory.* Morristown, NJ: General Learning Press.

Bandura, A. (1978). The self system in reciprocal determinism. *American Psychologist, 33*, 344–58.

Becker, M. (Ed.). (1974). *The health belief model and personal health behavior.* Thorofare, NJ: C.B. Stack, Inc.

Bellicha, T,. & McGrath, J. (1990, May/June). Mass media approaches to reducing cardiovascular disease risk. *Public Health Reports*, pp. 245–53.

Boyett, I., & Conn, H. (1991). *Workforce 2000: The revolution reshaping American business.* Minneapolis, MN: E.F. Dutton.

Carlyon, W. (1984). Disease prevention/health promotion–Bridging the gap to wellness. *Health Values: Achieving High Level Wellness, 8*(3), 27–30.

Chapman, L. (1996). *Worksite wellness: Presenting the business case.* Seattle, WA: Summex Corporation.

Chapman, L. (1998a). *Planning wellness: Getting off to a good start.* Seattle, WA: Summex Corporation.

Chapman, L. (1998b). *Health management: Optimal approaches for managing the health of defined populations.* Seattle, WA: Summex Corporation.

Davidson, C. (1989). Employee benefits communication. *Employee Benefits Basics* (Fourth Quarter). Brookfield, WI: International Foundation of Employee Benefit Plans.

Erickson, A., McKenna, J., & Romano, R. (1990, May/June). Past lessons and new uses of mass media in reducing tobacco consumption. *Public Health Reports*, pp. 239–45.

Eyles, J. (1990, Winter). The problem of marketing health promotion strategies. *The Canadian Geographer*, pp. 341–48.

Farquhar, I., Fortman, S., Flora, J., Taylor, B., Haskell, W., & Williams, P. (1990). Effects of community-wide education on cardiovascular disease risk factors: The Stanford Five-City Project. *The Journal of the American Medical Association, 264,* 359–66.

Fishbein, M., & Ajzen, I. (1975). *Belief, attitude, intention and behavior.* Reading, MA: Addison-Wesley.

Flay, B., DiTecco, D., & Schlegel, R. (1990, Summer). Mass media in health promotion: An analysis using an extended information-processing model. *Health Education Quarterly,* 127–47.

Gooder, J., & Welberg-Ekvall, S. (1989). Extension of health and nutrition services via advanced telecommunications. *Journal of the American Diabetic Association, 11*(6), 821–26.

Graninger, R. (1990) Self-creation: Consciously changing patterns of behavior. *American Journal of Nursing, 17*(4), 15–16.

Hammad, A., & Mulholland, C. (1992, March) Functional literacy, health, and quality of life. *The Annuals of the American Academy of Political and Social Science, 520,* 103–2l.

Heller, M., & Krauss, H. (1991, June). Perceived self-efficacy as a predictor of aftercare treatment entry by the detoxification patient. *Psychological Reports, 85*(3), 1047–53.

Hochbaum, G. (1979, July/August) An alternative approach to health education. *Health Values, 3* (4), 197–201.

Lewin, K. (1951). Frontiers in group dynamics. In D. Cartwright (Ed.), *Field Theory in Social Sciences.* New York: Harper.

Lyons, P., & Burgard. (1990). *Great shape: The first fitness guide for large women.* Palo Alto, CA: Bull Publishing Co.

Macoby, N., & Alexander, J. (1979). Use of media in lifestyle programs. In P. Davidson (Ed.),

Behavioral Medicine; Changing Health Lifestyles. New York: Brunner/Mazel.

McGinnis, M. (1990, May/June). Communication for better health. *Public Health Reports, 105*(7), 217–19.

McGuire, W. (1978). An information-processing model of advertising effectiveness. In H. L. Davis & A. J. Silk (Eds.), *Behavioral and Management Science in Marketing.* New York: John Wiley & Sons.

Miller, K. et al. (1990, June). An integrated model of communication, stress and burnout in the workplace. *Communication Research, 17*(3), 300–27.

Nuttin, J. M. (1978). *The illusion of attitude change: Toward a response contagion theory of persuasion.* New York: Academic Press.

Ornstein, R., & Sobel, D. (1989). *Healthy Pleasures.* Reading, WA: Addison Wesley Publishing Company.

Pierce, J. (1990, May). Long-term effectiveness of mass media led anti-smoking campaigns in Australia. *The American Journal of Public Health, 80*(6), 565–69.

Prochaska, J., & DiClemente, C. (1989). *The transtheoretical approach.* Melbourne, FL: Krieger Publishing Company.

Reed, R. (1984, January). Is education the key to lower health care costs? *Personnel Journal,* 40–46.

Robison, J. (1997, January/February). Weight management: shifting the paradigm. *Journal of Health Education, 28*(1), 28–34.

Rudd, J., & Glantz, K. (1989, September). Influencing consumer health care choices with quality of care information. *Journal of Consumer Policy, 13*(6), 249–77.

Wycoff, E. (1981, March). Canons of communication. *Personnel Journal,* 208–12.

CHAPTER

7

Theoretically-Based Strategies for Health Behavior Change

Ken Wallston and Colin Armstrong

INTRODUCTION

How many times when you have been faced with clients who engaged in "unhealthy" behaviors (such as smoking cigarettes) or who refused to get involved in "healthy" behaviors (such as exercising on a regular basis) did you ask yourself, "Why do they do what they do?" or "What can I do to get them to change?" If these sound like familiar questions, this chapter may help you find some useful answers.

In their quest to understand human behavior, psychologists have long been interested in trying to understand why people do, or do not do, certain behaviors. This quest has led psychologists to speculate about a myriad of factors that influence behavior and to develop theories or models incorporating these factors. Social psychologists, in particular, have been in the forefront of such theorizing. Many of the theoretical frameworks developed by social psychologists have been applied to the understanding of health behavior. The purpose of this chapter is to describe

some of these psychological theories of health behavior and, more importantly, to show how strategies to change an individual's health behavior can be structured on the basis of the theories. As one of the founders of social psychology, Kurt Lewin, was fond of saying, "There is nothing quite as practical as a good theory" (Lewin, 1951).

In the first part of this chapter, we use two examples to illustrate the theories. The first example is that of an "addicted" cigarette smoker. The second example is someone who leads a very sedentary lifestyle with almost no exercise to speak of. It should be noted, however, that these theories are by no means restricted to these particular health behaviors. The examples could just as easily have been a person 20% above ideal weight, someone who sunbathes without using suntan lotion, or someone who never uses a seatbelt while riding in an automobile. These theories are applicable to a variety of health behaviors. Smoking is a highly addictive behavior and, as such, is very resistant to change. Not getting any exercise is also bad for our health, but it is sometimes easier to get somebody to adopt a new behavior (such as exercise) than to abandon an old one (such as smoking). In the second part of the chapter, we provide an introduction to some of the more well-accepted behavioral change strategies. If the theories and strategies presented below are helpful to understanding and working with committed smokers and "couch potatoes," they can be easily applied to other relevant situations.

THEORIES OF HEALTH BEHAVIOR

A number of theories have been developed to explain and understand health behavior. The following discussion explores some of them.

Health Belief Model

The first and, in many ways, most influential of these theories, the Health Belief Model, was, as the name implies, developed specifically to predict variations in health behavior as a function of certain beliefs about one's health. Four social psychologists–Godfrey

Hochbaum, Stephen Kegeles, Howard Leventhal, and Irwin Rosenstock–working in the 1950s for the U.S. Public Health Service, developed the Health Belief Model "in an effort to explain the widespread failure of people to participate in programs to prevent or to detect disease" (Rosenstock, 1990, p. 39). The Health Belief Model is portrayed in Figure 7-1.

Originally, the Health Belief Model had four major components: perceived susceptibility, perceived severity, perceived benefits, and perceived barriers. Perceived susceptibility refers to a person's subjective estimation of his or her own risk of developing a particular health condition (e.g., "I am not likely to develop lung cancer"), and perceived severity is a personal judgment of the seriousness of that condition (e.g., "Lung cancer is an awful condition"). Many users of the Health Belief Model have combined these two elements into a single dimension labeled "perceived threat" or "perceived vulnerability." In order for the person to feel threatened (or vulnerable), both perceived susceptibility and perceived severity must be high. According to this model, the

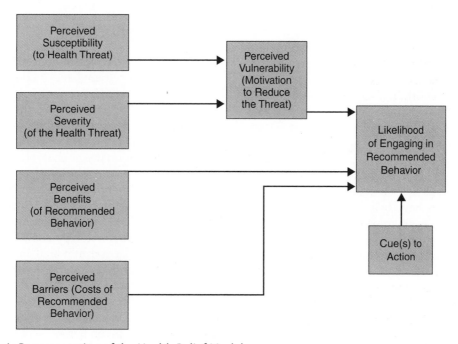

Figure 7-1   Classic Representation of the Health Belief Model

higher the perceived threat, the more motivated the person is to take action to reduce the threat.

Motivation to reduce the threat, however, is not enough of an explanation to understand why the threatened person chooses to engage (or fails to engage) in a particular health behavior. Many heavy smokers, for example, will readily admit that they are prime candidates for lung cancer and will say that lung cancer would be a terrible thing to have, and yet they continue to purchase and smoke pack after pack of cigarettes.

The other two dimensions in the Health Belief Model are in reference to a specific health recommendation (e.g., quit smoking cigarettes; exercise three times a week). Perceived benefits refers to a subjective estimation of the effectiveness of that recommendation in removing the threat (e.g., "Quitting smoking will greatly reduce my chances of getting heart disease"), and perceived barriers are any negative aspects or consequences of following the recommendation (e.g., "Exercise can be uncomfortable, plus it makes me sweat"). Perceived barriers are also sometimes referred to as perceived costs. A tenet of the theory is that people carry out a cost-benefit analysis whenever they contemplate following a particular recommendation. If the perceived threat is high enough *and* if the anticipated benefits outweigh the anticipated costs, the recommended action is likely to occur. As one of the originators of the Health Belief Model put it, "The combined levels of susceptibility and severity provided the energy or force to act and the perception of benefits ([minus] barriers) provided a preferred path of action" (Rosenstock, 1974, p. 332).

Although these four perceptual factors (i.e., beliefs) constitute the heart of the Health Belief Model, over the years other elements have been added. One of these, cues to action, refers to situational elements (including internal cues) that prompt the recommended health behavior. For example, any of the following—reading that the Surgeon General has come out with a new report linking cigarette smoking to premature death, viewing an anti-smoking commercial on television, seeing a poster announcing The Great American Smokeout, or waking up in the morning with a rasping two-hour coughing spell—might be the very thing that gets a smoker to take the first step toward quitting.

On its surface, the Health Belief Model looks as if it ought to be a very powerful tool for understanding all types of health behavior and for helping predict who will, and who will not, follow any conceivable recommendation. Because of its inherent appeal, literally hundreds of studies have been carried out testing the model's predictive validity. The results of these tests of the original Health Belief Model, however, have generally been disappointing. Although almost every published study has found some *statistically significant* findings, the amount of variability accounted for in the outcome measures (i.e., the actual health behaviors) has been so low as to be of little practical significance. (See Harrison, Mullen, & Green, 1992, for a meta-analysis backing up this assertion.)

A little later on in this chapter, we describe a revitalization of the Health Belief Model by Rosenstock and his colleagues that has a lot more promise than the earlier version. Before doing so, however, it is necessary to discuss two versions of social learning theory that have been very influential in understanding behavior in general and health behavior in particular.

Social Learning Theories

Rooted in learning theory concepts and principles (such as "reinforcement" and "acquired drives") that were first explicated in American psychology in the 1940s, modern social learning theories are highly cognitively oriented. That is, people's thoughts (e.g., their beliefs, attitudes, values, and expectancies) have a strong effect upon their behavior. This also works in the opposite direction: observing one's own behavior and its consequences influences one's thoughts. "Human behavior is explained in [social learning theory] in terms of a triadic, dynamic, and reciprocal model in which behavior, personal factors (including cognitions), and environmental influences all interact" (Perry, Baranowski, & Parcel, 1990, p. 161). Albert Bandura of Stanford University, a leading social learning theorist, includes the individual's capabilities to symbolize the meanings of behavior, to foresee the outcomes of given behavior patterns, to learn by observing others, to self-determine or self-regulate behavior, and to reflect and analyze experience among the critical personal factors that help determine whether or not a particular behavior will occur in a particular situation (Bandura, 1986).

One of the first social learning theories to be applied to health behavior evolved out of the work of Julian Rotter. Rotter, a clinical psychologist, developed the idea of "generalized expectancies of reinforcement." These are personality-like dispositions that the individual carries around from one situation to another. Rotter posited that a person's history of positive or negative reinforcement across a variety of situations shapes a belief as to whether or not the person's own actions lead to those reinforcements. He termed this belief orientation "internal vs. external locus of control of reinforcement" (Rotter, 1966). If a person thinks his own behavior determines his outcomes (or reinforcements), the person is said to have an internal locus-of-control orientation. Conversely, people who believe their outcomes are determined by chance, luck, fate, or powerful other persons are said to have an external locus-of-control orientation. Rotter's theory stated that a person's expectancies about reinforcements following behavior in a particular situation combined with the value (or importance) of that reinforcement in that situation to the person is predictive of whether or not the person performs the behavior in the situation (Rotter, 1954).

In the 1970s, Wallston and his colleagues at Vanderbilt began to apply Rotter's social learning theory to the prediction of health behavior. They developed measures of health locus-of-control beliefs and the value of health as a reinforcement. Then they began to explore whether these two constructs were sufficient to predict health behavior. Other investigators throughout the world have done similarly (see Wallston & Wallston, 1982, for reviews of this work), although often they failed to adequately measure or analyze differences in health value (Wallston, 1991).

Unfortunately, however, one's locus-of-control orientation (even moderated by the perceived value of the outcome) is insufficient, in and of itself, to predict much of the variability in health behavior. Rarely does health locus-of-control explain more than 10% of the variance in health behavior. Rotter's construct of locus-of-control goes only so far, but not far enough, when applied to health behavior (Wallston, 1992).

Having an "internal locus of control" belief about one's own health status is a necessary, but not a sufficient, determinant of health promotion behavior even if one places a high value on being healthy. If a smoker is to quit, believing his smoking affects his health is not enough; he also needs to believe he can do something about it. Similarly, very few people are going to begin an exercise program if they don't feel capable of exercising.

Bandura's version of social learning theory (which he now refers to as social cognitive theory; Bandura, 1986) has been shown to be far more useful to persons concerned with health behavior than has Rotter's version. This is principally due to Bandura's recognition that there is an important distinction to be made between outcome expectancies (such as locus-of-control beliefs) and behavioral expectancies (which Bandura termed "self-efficacy" beliefs). An internal locus-of-control belief merely signifies that the person thinks his behavior is responsible for his health status; for example, "I had a heart attack because I smoked two packs a day for 30 years and never got any exercise." Internality is only somewhat related to the person's belief that he can achieve good health outcomes. Self-efficacy, on the other hand, assesses the person's belief that he *can do* the behavior in order to achieve a desired outcome; for example, "I can quit smoking even if most of my friends smoke," or "I am confident that I can do whatever is necessary to beat this disease." This subtle difference, it turns out, makes all the difference in the world. If a smoker doesn't believe he can quit smoking, there is little likelihood he will attempt to quit, even if he believes that his smoking behavior is responsible for his poor health status.

Bandura's social cognitive theory is very highly thought of among academics and practitioners and is much richer than the constructs of outcome expectancies and self-efficacy. However, just as Rotter's social learning theory has become equated in most peoples' minds solely with the construct of locus of control, such is the case with social cognitive theory and self-efficacy. Readers are advised to read Bandura's (1986) book on social cognitive theory in order to fully appreciate the other constructs that make his theory attractive.

Ever since self-efficacy entered the public domain, every theoretician in the health behavior arena has scrambled to incorporate the construct into their own theoretical models. As hinted at above, Rosenstock (1990; Rosenstock, Strecher, & Becker, 1988) has added self-efficacy as a separate construct in the Health Belief Model, even though it can be argued that one potent "perceived barrier" to action is a lack of self-efficacy, thus negating the need to make it a separate dimension in the model. Additionally, Wallston modified Rotter's social learning theory for health by replacing health locus of control with health self-efficacy (or competence) as the major generalized expectancy belief and relegating internal health locus of control to the status of a moderator variable (Wallston, 1992). In this modified theory, health behavior is predicted mainly by one's self-efficacy beliefs (or perceived competence), but efficacy (or competence) only predicts behavior if an individual *both* values health as an outcome *and* believes that one's actions play a role in determining one's health status (i.e., one's locus of control is internal with respect to one's health).

The Theory of Planned Behavior

Another major theory that has been influenced by Bandura's work is Icek Ajzen's theory of planned behavior (see Figure 7-2). Ajzen's (1988) theory is an extension of the theory of reasoned action that Ajzen developed earlier with his mentor, Martin Fishbein. Fishbein and Ajzen did not set out to develop a theory of health behavior. Instead, they were interested in explaining virtually *any* behavior over which the individual has volitional control (i.e., any action that the person could choose to engage in, such as smoking or not smoking, exercising or not exercising).

A major assumption of the theory of reasoned action is that the *intention* to engage in a particular behavior is the principal determinant of whether or not the person will actually engage in the behavior (Fishbein, 1980). According to that earlier theory, there are only two factors that determine behavioral intention: one's own attitude toward the behavior itself, and one's impression of the social norms regarding the behavior. In the theory of planned behavior, Ajzen added "perceived behavioral control" as a third

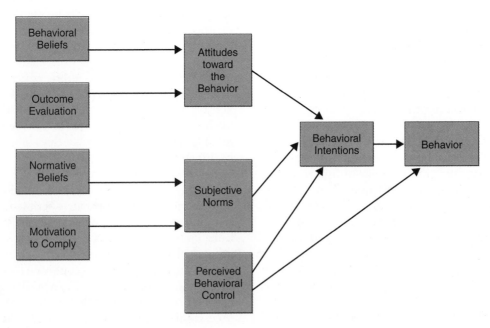

Figure 7-2 The Theory of Planned Behavior

determinant of behavioral intentions. As it turns out, Ajzen means pretty much the same thing by "perceived behavioral control" that Bandura means by self-efficacy: the belief that one has the resources necessary to perform the behavior.

In both the theory of reasoned action and the theory of planned behavior, the person's own attitude toward the behavior (i.e., whether or not one thinks the behavior is "good" or "bad") is determined by the person's belief that a given behavior will lead to a given outcome, weighted by how positively or negatively the person evaluates the outcome. "If I exercise every day, I will lose 10 pounds in the next month, and losing 10 pounds in a month would be fantastic." Similarly, subjective norms are determined by the person's belief about what salient other people might think the person should do, weighted by the extent to which she is motivated to comply with the wishes of those salient others. "My wife wants me to get more exercise, and I want to please my wife."

Perceived behavioral control (e.g., "I find it difficult to walk one mile in less than 20 minutes," or "I can easily build 30 minutes of exercise each day into my schedule") is also predictive of the intention to exercise. In addition, the theory of planned behavior states that perceived behavioral control predicts behavior independently (i.e., without going through intentions) in those instances in which there is no actual control possible over the behavior. This means that there is a direct link from perceived behavioral control to the behavior, a link that isn't necessarily mediated by intentions. The more we perceive control over a behavior, the more likely we are to engage in that behavior even if we don't intend to do so.

Although neither of Ajzen's two theories were specifically designed to be applied to health behavior, many investigators have attempted to do so, often with great success. In a review of 56 studies, Godin and Kok (1996) found that 41% of intentions and 34% of future behavior were explained by Ajzen's model, and perceived behavioral control explained an additional 11.5% of the variance in behavior above and beyond intentions.

Here is how the theory of planned behavior could be applied to understanding a person's intentions to quit smoking. The person's attitude toward quitting could either be assessed directly (by determining how positively or negatively the person felt about quitting smoking) or, as is more typical, indirectly by asking the person to respond to a number of belief statements. These statements would assess specific outcome expectancies (e.g., "Quitting smoking would enable me to breathe easier" and "Quitting smoking would make me more irritable") and also evaluations of the desirability of those outcomes (e.g., "Breathing easier would make my life much better" and "If I were more irritable, this would not be a good thing"). To determine a client's subjective norms, the client would be asked to indicate how much each "important" person in his life (from a short list of referent persons, such as spouse, child, parent, doctor) wants the client to quit smoking. He would also be asked to indicate how much he wants to go along with the others' wishes. As mentioned earlier, perceived behavioral control would typically be assessed by a series of statements about the ease or difficulty of carrying out the behavior (e.g., "It is easy for me to find time to exercise" or "I find it difficult to exercise by myself") or a set of self-efficacy beliefs (e.g., "I am confident that I can quit smoking any time I choose to" or "I can resist smoking in situations in which other people are smoking").

Typically, the theory of reasoned action does a better job of accounting for one's behavioral intentions than the Health Belief Model does of predicting behavior (see Schwarzer, 1992, or Wallston and Wallston, 1984, for reviews of this literature), and the theory of planned behavior does an even better job than the theory of reasoned action. However, even the theory of planned behavior fails to explain all of the variability in behavioral intentions and even less of the variability among individuals in their actual behavior. What this means, of course, is that there is room for improvement, and lots of theorists have jumped into the breach with their own models. Few are as parsimonious as the theories reviewed thus far in this chapter (i.e., most contain a relatively large number of explanatory factors), and none account for all of the variability that could be potentially explained.

The Health Action Process Approach

Ralf Schwarzer, a social psychologist at the Freie University of Berlin in Germany, developed what he calls a "Health Action Process Approach." Schwarzer (1992; 1999) contends that different factors are at work when a person is deciding which health action(s) to take—a period of time he calls the motivation (or decision-making) phase—than are operative during the action (or volition) phase. Thus, Schwarzer adds a time perspective to the previous models and also makes a more detailed analysis of the cognitions that guide ongoing behavior.

According to Schwarzer's theory (see Figure 7-3), during the motivation (or decision-making) phase, the individual forms an intention (or goal) to either adopt a health recommendation (e.g., begin exercising) or to change risk behaviors in favor of other behaviors (e.g., switch from non-filtered to filtered cigarettes). The model states that the most important predictors of intentions (or goals) are risk perceptions, outcome expectancies, and self-efficacy. As with Fishbein and Ajzen's theories, *social* outcome expectancies (e.g., "My family will think better of me if I start exercising") are explicitly given credence (along with other outcome expectancies) as determinants of intentions. Although Schwarzer's earlier (1992) portrayal of the Health Action Process Approach implied a causal ordering from risk perceptions to outcome expectancies to self-efficacy beliefs, his latest depiction of this model (Schwarzer, 1999) is less clear about the sequential pattern of these determinants of intentions.

Unlike the theory of reasoned action, Schwarzer does not assume that strong intentions necessarily guarantee corresponding actions. "In the motivation phase people choose which actions to take, whereas in the action or *volition phase* they plan the details, act, persist, possibly fail, and then recover" (Schwarzer, 1999, p. 118). Once a preference for a given behavior (e.g., quitting smoking cold turkey) has been shaped, it is necessary to transform that motivation into a detailed set of instructions on how to perform the desired action (e.g., set a quit date; throw away all cigarettes; don't buy or bum any more cigarettes; tell everyone you're quitting; stay away from people who smoke; carry low-calorie oral substitutes; begin exercise program; etc.). These action plans and their corresponding action control mechanisms are heavily influenced by the person's self-efficacy beliefs. During

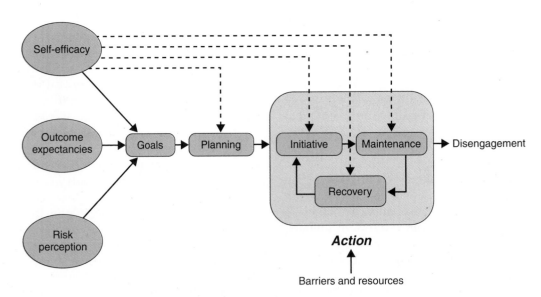

Figure 7-3 The Health Action Process Approach

the action phase, self-efficacy determines the amount of effort invested in the behavior and the amount of perseverance exhibited in the face of inevitable situational barriers.

In Schwarzer's model, actions are not only a function of intentions and cognitive control but are also influenced by the perceived and the actual environment. One's coworkers, for example, who ignore a person's attempts to quit by continuing to smoke in his presence, create a stressful situation which taxes the person's ability to achieve his goal. On the other hand, demonstrations of support for the person's quitting attempts by his family and coworkers can be extremely powerful means to help prevent relapses.

The Transtheoretical (or Stages of Change) Model

The Transtheoretical Model, also known as the Stages of Change Model, was developed by James Prochaska and Carlo DiClemente (Prochaska & DiClemente, 1982). Some of the earliest health issues to which the model was applied include smoking cessation (Prochaska & DiClemente, 1983), obesity (O'Connell & Velicer, 1988), ultraviolet light exposure (Rossi, 1989), alcohol use (DiClemente & Hughes, 1990), and participation in physical activity (Sonstroem, 1988; Marcus, Rakowski, & Rossi, 1992). This model has since been applied to numerous health problems and health behaviors, such as eating disorders, high fat diet, dietary intake of fruits and vegetables, mammography screening, condom use, medication compliance, radon testing, birth control practices, cocaine use, pain management, and the sterilization of needles among IV drug users (Prochaska & Velicer, 1997).

The Transtheoretical Model attempts to explain when and how individuals change their behavior, as well as which factors influence these changes (Prochaska, DiClemente, & Norcross, 1992). There are four major components to the model: stages of change, processes of change, self-efficacy, and decisional balance. Stages of change is the component that attempts to describe where individuals are in the change process (Prochaska et al., 1992). The processes of change focus on how individuals change (Prochaska et al., 1992). Decisional balance (Janis & Mann, 1977)

and self-efficacy (Bandura, 1977), two components adopted from other models of behavior change, are posited as factors that influence the change process.

The Stages of Change

The Transtheoretical Model postulates that individuals progress through five stages during the process of changing their behavior (Prochaska & DiClemente, 1983). These stages (see Figure 7-4) provide a dimension to the model that allows a better understanding of *when* changes occur in both an individual's intention for engaging in a particular behavior and in actual performance of that behavior (Prochaska et al., 1992). The earlier stages represent a set of tasks (i.e., changes in intentions and behaviors) necessary for progression to later stages (Prochaska & Velicer, 1997). Thus, like the Health Action Process Approach, the Transtheoretical Model is a dynamic model in which behavior change is viewed as a process, rather than as static states in which the person either engages or fails to engage in a particular behavior.

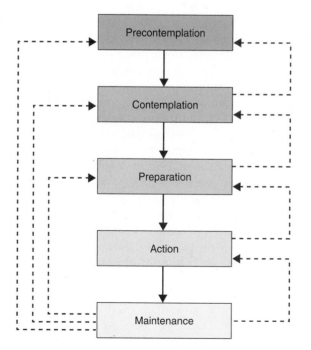

Figure 7-4 The Stages of Change

The five most widely recognized stages of change are precontemplation, contemplation, preparation, action, and maintenance (Prochaska & DiClemente, 1983). Although some researchers have identified a state of relapse, relapse is not considered a stage but is, instead, part of the process of progressing through the stages (Prochaska & Velicer, 1997). In addition, a stage of termination, reflecting zero temptation to return to an unhealthy state (e.g., smoking cigarettes), is included in some work on the stages of change but not in studies involving the adoption of a new behavior such as physical activity (Prochaska & Velicer, 1997). At this time, the vast majority of transtheoretical research is conducted employing the five-stage model described above.

Persons in the precontemplation stage are those who have no intention of changing their behavior in the near future, which is typically defined as within the next six months (Prochaska & Velicer, 1997). Precontemplators are often unaware that their current behavior poses a problem, although it may be very apparent to others, such as family members or employers (Prochaska et al., 1992). Persons in contemplation are aware of their problem behavior and are considering changing their behavior in the near future (e.g., within the next six months).

Persons in the preparation stage intend to change their behavior in the very near future (usually within the next month) and/or have been involved in recent sporadic behavior changes, such as decreasing their daily number of cigarettes or engaging in occasional bouts of physical activity (Prochaska & Marcus, 1994). Persons in the action stage are actively changing their behavior to a particular criterion level (such as exercising three times per week for 20 minutes or longer each time, or having stopped smoking within the past six months). To be considered to be in the maintenance stage, a person has to have sustained their behavior change for a period of time, usually operationally defined as six months or longer (Prochaska et al., 1992).

Although a linear progression through the five stages is possible and may even be normative, progress through the stages can best be conceptualized as occurring in a cyclical fashion (Prochaska et al., 1992; Prochaska & Velicer, 1997). Individuals cycle and recycle through the stages at different rates, often remaining in the earlier stages for prolonged periods of time. Also, often individuals progress to the later stages of action and maintenance only to relapse back to the earlier stages of precontemplation, contemplation, or preparation (Prochaska et al., 1992). Progression from some stages to other specific stages is more likely, such as from precontemplation to contemplation, and from contemplation to preparation (Prochaska et al., 1992). However, change from any one stage to almost any other stage is possible, although, by definition, one must pass through the stage of action to enter the stage of maintenance (Prochaska & Velicer, 1997).

The Processes of Change

The processes of change component of the transtheoretical model is aimed at describing and explaining *how* behavior change occurs (Prochaska et al., 1992). The processes are the experiences and activities that individuals engage in when they attempt to change their behavior (Prochaska & DiClemente, 1983). They represent categories of strategies and methods that individuals use and experiences that they report during the course of behavior change (Prochaska & DiClemente, 1983).

The Transtheoretical Model began as an attempt at integrating the important components of diverse systems of psychotherapy (Prochaska et al., 1992). Ten processes have been identified in diverse groups of psychotherapy patients and self-changers, and these processes have undergone many modifications and refinements (Prochaska & DiClemente, 1983; Prochaska & Velicer, 1997). One of the most important findings to emerge from these studies was the fact that self-changers generally use as many as ten different processes during the course of changing their behavior, while most leading systems of therapy theoretically include only two or three processes (Prochaska et al., 1992). According to Prochaska and his colleagues (e.g., Prochaska et al., 1992), the ten processes with the most theoretical and empirical support across different problem behaviors can be classified as either experiential (consciousness-raising, dramatic relief, self-reevaluation, environmental reevaluation, self-liberation, and social liberation) or behavioral (counterconditioning, reinforcement management, stimulus control, and helping relationships). Outside of Prochaska and his colleagues, not as much research has been done on the processes of change as has been done on the stages of change, particularly as applied to health behaviors.

Self-Efficacy

As mentioned above, Bandura proposed that self-efficacy reflects an individual's judgment of his or her capability to perform particular behaviors in specific situations (Bandura, 1977, 1986). Not only has self-efficacy been found to be a strong correlate and predictor of participation in many health behaviors, such as physical activity (e.g., Armstrong, Sallis, Hovell, & Hofstetter, 1993; Sallis, Hovell, Hofstetter, & Barrington, 1992) and smoking cessation (DiClemente, Prochaska, & Gibertini, 1985), it has also been shown to be related to the stages of change. Self-efficacy scores tend to increase in a linear fashion from precontemplation to maintenance (e.g., DiClemente et al., 1985; Marcus & Owen, 1992).

Decisional Balance

Based upon the research of Janis and Mann (1977), the notion of decisional balance has also been incorporated into the Transtheoretical Model (Prochaska et al., 1992). Studies based on this model have identified two important constructs that individuals balance when contemplating behavior change: the pros (i.e., benefits) and cons (i.e., barriers) associated with that behavior (Prochaska et al., 1992). The pros and cons have been shown to be related to stage of change (e.g., DiClemente, Prochaska, Fairhurst, Velicer, & Wayne, 1991; Marcus, et al., 1992). The perceived cons of making a healthy change (e.g., adopting physical activity, decreasing dietary fat intake, quitting smoking) tend to decrease in a linear fashion from precontemplation to maintenance, while the pros of making that same change tend to increase. The Transtheoretical Model postulates that perceived pros and cons of engaging in a particular behavior "crossover" either in contemplation or preparation, depending on the behavior in

question (Prochaska et al., 1994). That is, at some point in the change process, an individual's perceptions of the benefits of changing his or her behavior begins to outweigh the drawbacks of changing. At that point, the individual becomes ready for action. This part of the Transtheoretical Model is very congruent with the Health Belief Model.

Discussion

Although the concept of self-efficacy is the one piece of Bandura's social cognitive theory that has revolutionized our thinking about determinants of health behavior, Bandura (1986) and other social learning theorists (e.g., Walter Mischel) have put forth other constructs that are deserving of attention. One is the notion of vicarious learning. A person does not have to experience something directly in order to learn from that experience but can learn from hearing about and/or observing others' experiences and modeling their actions.

Another pertinent concept from Bandura is that of reciprocal determinism. This refers to the constant, dynamic interaction that takes place among a person, the person's behavior, and the environment in which the behavior takes place. As with any other system, change in any one of those three elements inevitably results in change in the others. This is particularly relevant when examining health behavior change in the workplace. Extrapolating from social learning theory, the workplace provides the social and physical situation within which the person must function. Thus, the workplace also provides the incentives and disincentives that influence workers' behavior. A change in the workplace (such as adopting a no-smoking policy) will have an effect on the people in the workplace and on their smoking behavior. Similarly, if a group of workers were to increase or decrease their smoking behavior, this would have a profound change on the workplace environment. "Reciprocal determinism may be used to advantage in developing programs that do not focus on behavior in isolation but focus instead on changes in the environment and in the individual as well" (Perry et al., 1990, p. 167).

There are additional theories that have been related to health behavior—Triandis' (1980) theory of social behavior, Rogers' protection motivation theory (Prentice-Dunn & Rogers, 1986), Pender's Health Promotion Model (Pender, Walker, Sechrist, & Frank-Stromborg, 1990), and O'Donnell's theory of health promotion behavior (O'Donnell, in press)–that are not covered here because of space considerations. All four of these approaches have much to offer practitioners concerned with changing health behaviors. In particular, Triandis introduces a number of "social factors" (including specific interpersonal agreements to perform the behavior) that are potentially highly predictive of whether or not a particular behavior will be performed. Unique to Rogers' model are the notions of fear arousal (which factors into "threat appraisal") and "coping appraisal" (which is partially determined by self-efficacy), both of which determine the extent to which the individual is motivated to protect him- or herself against real or imagined health threats. Pender's model adds the constructs "definition of health" and "health value," and O'Donnell's model makes explicit the point that one's prior experience with the behavior (such as the number of times one has tried to quit smoking or start exercising in the past) is an important determinant of both intentions and behavior.

This concludes the discussion of the theories of health behavior. The newest theories (e.g., Schwarzer's and O'Donnell's) hold a great deal of promise although, to date, neither has received sufficient empirical investigation. Probably neither will be the final word on the subject. In each of these theories, self-efficacy beliefs play a central role in predicting both intentions and behavior. This fact alone assures that the theories will "work." The newer theories also incorporate the construct of social support as an important determinant of whether one's intentions do, indeed, get translated into action. Other chapters in this book (Chapters 8 and 17) elaborate on the important role of social networks and social support in modifying health behaviors and should be read along with this one. Health promotion specialists looking for theoretical justification or assistance in developing programs to change individuals' health behaviors could turn to any of the theories described or mentioned above for a wealth of support. In addition, Irving Janis, formerly a social psychologist at Yale University, has done extensive work on developing short-term counseling strategies for effective behavior change that have been successfully applied to health behaviors such as smoking cessation and weight loss. Some of Janis' strategies will be described in the next section of this chapter. As will be apparent, Janis' approach is fully compatible with many of the existing models, especially those that have a social component.

STRATEGIES FOR HEALTH BEHAVIOR CHANGE

There exist a wide variety of strategies useful for promoting adoption of and adherence to healthy behavioral changes, and a complete overview of these strategies is well beyond the scope of this chapter. Instead, the following reflects only a basic introduction to some of the more well-accepted behavioral change strategies. The following behavior change strategies are frequently implemented by professionals who lack formal training in the use of psychotherapeutic techniques. This is appropriate, given that the majority of those requiring behavioral change will not have access to or will not seek out the assistance of an appropriately-trained therapist. However, the reader should remain aware that *all* behavior change strategies have the potential for misuse. Although it may seem unlikely that some of these techniques (e.g., self-monitoring, goal-setting) could actually cause harm to a client, harm could occur if such techniques are implemented while potentially important contributors to treatment nonadherence (e.g., marital conflict, depression) are overlooked. Readers should view the following as only the most basic introduction to behavioral change strategies. Readers unfamiliar with these strategies are urged to seek out additional readings and, whenever possible, training opportunities (e.g., training workshops). Strategies that by definition require advanced training (e.g., motivational interviewing) are not included below.

Assessing Readiness to Change

The most basic place to begin is with an assessment of the client's (or clients') need for and readiness to change. As mentioned above, a person in the precontemplation stage is not at all ready to change, despite "objective" evidence of the person's need to make a change. There are many ways to assess readiness; many, however, involve confronting the individual with an opportunity to act or to express a desire to act. For example, a worksite smoking cessation program is announced in the company newsletter, and all interested employees are invited to enroll. The act of enrolling in the program is taken as an indication of readiness to make a change.

There are numerous questionnaires designed to assess a client's readiness to change. Stages of change scales have been developed to assess a person's readiness to change various health behaviors (Prochaska & Velicer, 1997). For example, physical activity stages of change (hereafter referred to as "stage") instruments present subjects with an operational definition of physical activity or exercise in terms of frequency, duration, and, sometimes, intensity. After reading the definition, the subject answers a series of questions or selects a description of activity patterns that most closely describes his or her own pattern. Stage instruments vary in their response formats (e.g., multiple responses, as in a Likert scale vs. dichotomous responses, such as "yes/no") and in how the stages are operationally defined. However, numerous studies have supported the validity of various stages of change instruments (see Armstrong, 1998, for a review).

A related approach is to administer an instrument such as the Decisional Balance Scale developed by O'Connell and Velicer (1988). The client is asked to respond to a number of "pro" and "con" statements with respect to the new behavior. The relative number of pros and cons have been shown to be related to stage of change (e.g., 1991; Marcus et al., 1992). In individual or small group counseling sessions or workshops, clients can be asked to simply write out their "pros" and "cons." This strategy typically yields much information for discussion and identifies areas in which the client may require additional education.

Framing Messages

Most of the theories discussed above, from the Health Belief Model on up, clearly state that the more benefits a person believes will follow an action, the more likely the person will engage in that action. (This is the same as saying that motivation is directly a function of the number of "pro" statements the person makes about the behavior on some instrument like the Decisional Balance Scale.) Because of this, most health education messages are written in positive (or "gain frame") language, pointing out all of the benefits that will accrue to the person who follows a particular health recommendation.

In an interesting paradoxical twist, cognitive psychologists have pointed out that what is even more motivational than "gain frame" language is to make salient what the individual will lose if the individual fails to adopt the recommended action. According to this logic, a message framed in "loss" language (e.g., "If you fail to quit smoking, you'll lose the chance to know what it feels like to walk up a flight of stairs without wheezing") is more motivating than simply pointing out the "gains" to be had by quitting (e.g., "When you quit smoking, you will be able to walk up a flight of stairs without wheezing). (See Wilson, Purdon, & Wallston, 1988, for further details about gain frames vs. loss frames.)

A different type of message frame, incorporated into protection motivation theory, is designed to cut through a person's denial defenses and raise perceived threat or vulnerability. Such a message is called a "fear appeal." For example, a smoker might be told, "If you continue smoking, your lungs will become all black, and you'll suffer from emphysema or die of cancer or a heart attack." Fear arousal does, indeed, work some of the time, but only with people who have an ample supply of ego defenses, such as a high sense of self-esteem. All too often, threatening people, even short of scaring them to death, simply backfires and gets them to avoid both the recommendation and the recommender. (According to Gregg, Foote, Erfurt, & Heirich, 1990, this approach should only be used as a last resort.)

Building Up One's Referent Power

A number of the theories discussed in the first section of this chapter indicate that people will often be motivated to initiate specific health actions because they think some other person or persons wishes them to do the behavior and, for whatever reason, they choose to go along with the other person's wishes. When a "significant other" has the ability to influence another's actions, the person is said to possess "referent power." Helping "professionals are most likely to have referent power when their clients perceive them not only as useful and likeable but also as benevolent, admirable, and accepting" (Janis, 1983, p. 19).

Janis (1983) states there are three critical phases to the motivating power of helpers as change agents. During the first phase, the helper builds motivating power; in phase two, the helper uses the motivating power to effect the desired change; and, in the last phase, the helper promotes the client's internalization of the changes that were begun in phase two. (See Table 7-1 for a list of Janis' critical phases and key variables within each phase.)

Table 7-1 Critical Phases and Techniques in Janis's Short-Term Counseling Approach

Phase 1: Building up Motivating Power
    a. Encourage self-disclosures from clients.
    b. Give positive feedback to clients' disclosures.
    c. Use own self-disclosures to give insight and cognitive restructuring.

Phase 2: Using Motivating Power
    a. Make directive statements; endorse specific action recommendations.
    b. Elicit commitment to the recommended course of action.
    c. Attribute the norms being endorsed to a respected secondary group.
    d. Give selected positive feedback.
    e. Communicate a sense of client's personal responsibility for behavioral changes.

Phase 3: Maintaining Motivating Power While Promoting Internalization
    a. Give reassurances of continued maintenance of positive regard for client.
    b. Make arrangements for follow-up contact with client.
    c. Give reminders fostering client's sense of personal responsibility.
    d. Build client's self-confidence about succeeding without the aid of the counselor.

The initial phase is critical, according to Janis. It "involves overcoming the usual tendency toward reticence, suspiciousness, and defensiveness that prevents a person from trusting someone who purports to be trying to help change his or her behavior" (Janis, 1983, p. 26). Janis states there are three things a helper can do during this initial phase to maximize the acquisition of motivating power. The first is to encourage a *moderate* amount of self-disclosure from the client, enough so that the client senses you are interested in him as a person but not too heavy lest the client reveal all his or her weaknesses. The second strategy is to give *unconditional* positive acceptance and understanding to the client, regardless of the client's disclosures, and avoid giving neutral or negative feedback. The objective is to be perceived as someone whom the client can depend on to maintain or enhance the client's self-esteem, not to tear it down. Third, the client's self-disclosures are used as a way of giving insight and cognitive restructuring. For example, a client who reveals, "I'm such a weak-willed person because I can't seem to quit smoking," can be helped to realize how powerful an addictive drug nicotine really is (United States Department of Health and Human Services, 1988). In this manner, an external attribution for failure replaces an internal attribution, thus helping to bolster the individual's self-esteem.

Once the helper has acquired motivating power, the next step is to use that power to motivate the person to change. At the beginning of the second phase, according to Janis, the helper assumes the role of "norm-sender." In the role of norm-sender, the helper gives unambiguous recommendations or directives, making clear that the client is expected to carry out a stressful course of action. For example, it is important to say to a smoker: "I expect you to stop smoking cigarettes." Doing so, however, has a downside. "Any such demand creates a crisis in the newly formed relationship because of the threat that henceforth acceptance will be provided on a strictly conditional basis, which adversely affects the affiliative bond" (Janis, 1983, p. 33). However, if the helper refrains from making such demands, there is little likelihood that any behavior change will take place. The helper does not have to be the only referent person insisting on the behavior change. Attributing the norm being endorsed to other persons or groups the client respects is another strategy favored by Janis during this phase and one that is wholly consistent with Fishbein's, Ajzen's, and Triandis' theories.

Eliciting Commitment to Change

The next step in phase two is to elicit some degree of commitment from the client to try to make the behavior change. Getting the smoker to commit to a "quit date," for example, has been shown to be one of the most important aspects of all of the successful smoking cessation programs. At this point the helper needs to switch from being an unconditional source of positive feedback to being more selective. "Clients can come to realize that they will mostly receive spontaneous acceptance . . . *except* when they fail to make a sincere effort to live up to a *limited* set of norms" (Janis, 1983, p. 35). Eliciting a commitment on the part of the client to make a change is exactly equivalent to Triandis' construct of an interpersonal agreement to act. When a person says "I will do thus-and-so," the person forms a self-image consistent with doing the behavior. According to Triandis' (1980) theory of social behavior, having such a self-image increases the likelihood that the person will act appropriately.

Self-Monitoring

Self-monitoring is a technique in which clients are taught to carefully observe and monitor specific factors that influence their health. This often includes monitoring of a client's engagement in a specific health behavior (e.g., number of cigarettes smoked), physical symptoms (e.g., degree of muscular tension), environmental factors that might influence their behavior (e.g., stressors in the environment), cognitive factors (e.g., thoughts that precede their reaching for a cigarette), and the consequences of their behavior (e.g., do they feel relaxed or guilty?).

Self-monitoring is often used prior to treatment to establish a baseline for a particular behavior and to track progress during treatment. However, it can also be useful to motivate a person toward changing his or her behavior. For example, simply having an obese person monitor their caloric intake may help increase their motivation to make changes. Self-monitoring by itself can lead to substantial behavioral changes (reactivity), often in the desired direction. Self-monitoring occurs in many forms including electronic counters and paper-and-pencil monitoring charts and graphs. The results of self-monitoring are typically utilized by psychologists to perform a behavior (or functional) analysis, identifying the factors that strongly influence a person's behavior and the most appropriate targets of treatment.

Goal-Setting

As the name implies, goal-setting is the process of helping the client set appropriate goals for behavioral change. A goal can be a simple one-time event, such as setting a "quit date" in smoking cessation. Typically, however, the goal-setting process is more involved. During this process the client is taught to set goals that are clearly defined, measurable, and attainable, while at the same time challenging the client to make progress in the appropriate direction.

What defines an "appropriate" goal depends on numerous factors, including the consequences of the current behavior and the client's confidence (self-efficacy) in their ability to change. In general, goals for specific *behavioral changes* (e.g., reducing the number of fat grams consumed per day to 30 or less) are more useful than goals for specific *outcomes* (e.g., losing 20 pounds). In addition, proximal goals (e.g., "what I will do today") tend to be more useful than distal goals (e.g., "what I will be able to do in one year"), although the two are often used in combination. In general, individualized goals that are self-determined and/or negotiated between the client and health care professional are more likely to be accepted than are inflexible goals that are not tailored to the client.

Reinforcement/Incentive Strategies

A variety of reinforcement strategies can be utilized to promote healthy behavioral changes. These strategies either involve having a designated person (e.g., a clinician, program manager, or family member) reward the client for changes in behavior or having the client reward him- or herself (self-reward). Reinforcement strategies are highly congruent with social cognitive theory. They can be especially useful in the early stages of behavior change. For example, reinforcement can help a new exerciser get past the early drawbacks of adopting exercise (e.g., muscular soreness, added time burden) to get to the point where the intrinsic benefits of exercise (e.g., increased self-esteem) become more apparent.

Incentives can take many forms: symbolic rewards that provide public recognition for one's achievements; direct monetary payments given every time the behavior is emitted; small tangible "gifts"; tokens or credits that can be accumulated and cashed in for larger rewards; the return of a portion of the client's program fees; and, even, time for the client to interact one-on-one with the professional helper. Very often, a reinforcement program is set up so that external incentives (e.g., tokens) are gradually faded out over time while the client is taught to focus more on the intrinsic benefits of their behavioral change.

Reinforcement strategies require very clear definitions of the specific behavioral changes required of the client, the incentives to be utilized, the consequences (if any) of failing to make specific changes, and clear methods of documenting the changes. In general, the rewards must have incentive value to the client (although, as mentioned above, they do not have to be of monetary value), they must be received only if the desired behavioral change is achieved, and they should follow the behavior as soon as possible. A related set of strategies—referred to as "response-cost"—involve the client paying a price for not making or not adhering to a healthy change.

Behavioral Contracting

Often, important components of the behavioral change program (e.g., a client's goals and how they will be rewarded for reaching these goals) are incorporated into a written behavioral contract. As with goal-setting, it is important that both the client and professional agree to the specifics of this contract. Having the client participate actively in the contracting process fosters a higher sense of behavioral

control and commitment to the behavior change program. Often the contract is drafted and signed by both the client and the professional (health care provider, program manager, etc). Clients may be encouraged to post the contract in a place where they (and, sometimes, others) may see it. However, as noted above, it is important to remember that *all* behavior change techniques can be misused, and this is definitely the case with reinforcement strategies and contracts. For example, a contract may prompt some clients to adhere to their healthy change, but similar contracts may actually contribute to treatment dropout for others (such as when a client feels guilty about his or her performance and decides to avoid the treatment professional). Much has been written about the proper use and potential misuse of reinforcement strategies and contracts (e.g., Boehm, 1989; Kanfer & Schefft, 1988; Winett, King, & Altman, 1989), and readers are strongly encouraged to pursue additional reading and training before utilizing this strategy.

Stimulus Control Strategies

Stimulus control strategies are designed to intervene on the antecedents of a particular behavior, whether the antecedents are environmental (e.g., seeing another person smoke) or cognitive (e.g., thinking about how good a cigarette would taste). As described above, these antecedents are often identified via self-monitoring. *Cueing* strategies, suggested by the Health Belief Model, are often useful for promoting healthy changes. These involve introducing new "cues" to prompt a healthy behavior (e.g., putting up a reminder on the bathroom cabinet to take one's medications; placing one's walking shoes by the front door). They also include strategies for eliminating, or at least decreasing, the impact of cues that support unhealthy behaviors (e.g., putting unhealthy foods out of sight).

Modifying Self-Statements

Our health behaviors are often influenced by the statements we make to ourselves before, during, and after the behavior of interest. Statements that one makes to him/herself can have an impact on whether or not one initiates a specific activity (e.g., "I don't have time for exercise" vs. "I'll be more productive if I take this time to exercise"); one's degree of enjoyment of the activity (e.g., "This hurts" vs. "I'm doing my body good"); and how one feels after the activity (e.g., "That was a waste of time" vs. "I feel so much better now"). The topic of self-statements is sometimes discussed under the topics of stimulus control or self-reward strategies, depending upon how the self-statements are utilized (e.g., as when a positive self-statement is used as a form of self-reward). Very basically, clients are taught to identify and either alter or eliminate those self-statements that interfere with healthy behavior changes and to adopt self-statements that promote adoption and adherence. This is a very important part of cognitive-behavior therapy, a type of psychotherapy that definitely requires advanced training.

Enhancing Self-Efficacy Beliefs

Although being confident of one's ability to change can, indeed, motivate one's desire and intention to change, self-efficacy generally has its greatest impact during initial behavioral change (i.e., the stages of preparation and action in the Transtheoretical Model). Bandura (1977, 1986) says there are four principal ways to change a person's efficacy beliefs. The most effective way is to help the person have an *authentic mastery experience*. Nothing builds up a person's confidence better and faster than being successful. This is the basis for the behavioral strategy of setting small, attainable goals (e.g., quit smoking for one day) as opposed to large goals that are almost doomed to failure from the start (e.g., never smoke another cigarette for the rest of your life).

In those instances in which the individual clients themselves cannot easily have their own personal mastery experiences, Bandura suggests the use of *modeling* as a means of enhancing self-efficacy. Observing others similar to oneself persist at a task and succeed has a positive effect on one's own feelings of confidence. This type of vicarious learning has many potential benefits. Competent models can teach ob-

servers skills and effective strategies for dealing with challenging or threatening situations. One key point here is that the more similar the model is to the client, the more effective this strategy will be. Although professional helpers can and ought to be "role models," it is even more effective to have the client observe fellow clients successfully complete the behavior.

When neither direct nor vicarious mastery experiences are feasible, a third approach toward enhancing self-efficacy is through *social persuasion*. If the communicator is credible, there are many times when a person can be talked into believing that he or she is, in fact, capable. According to Bandura, realistic increases in efficacy beliefs that lead people to exert greater effort should increase their likelihood of success. However, raising unrealistic beliefs of personal efficacy might lead to failures, which, in turn, might discredit the credibility of the persuaders and undermine perceptions of personal efficacy.

A fourth means of enhancing self-efficacy beliefs, according to Bandura, is to modify peoples' physiological reactions and/or how they interpret signals from their body. For example, not only can a person quitting smoking be given nicotine replacement therapy as a means of eliminating withdrawal symptoms ("cravings"), which make the experience harder to endure, but they can also be helped to reframe a withdrawal symptom into a positive sign that they are conquering their habit.

Teaching/Coaching

A basic strategy for guiding behavior change is to teach or coach the client on how best to carry out the new behavior(s). In fact, with many behaviors, this teaching/coaching function is critical. It is unreasonable to expect someone to carry out a complex set of behaviors without knowing what to do and why it is being done. The teacher/coach must continuously guard against the tendency to do *too much* for the client. The truly supportive teacher/coach will simultaneously teach the client to monitor his/her own progress and will share the responsibility of supervising the client's progress with the client.

Promoting Social Support

Both Schwarzer's Health Action Process Approach and O'Donnell's theory of health promotion behavior assert that the provision of support from other people facilitates successful behavior change. There are undoubtedly a few self-motivated and self-directed people out there who can make and maintain health behavior changes without the support of a single other person; most people, however, need support from at least one other individual in order to change. This support can come from a variety of sources: family, friends, coworkers, other people "in the same boat," even professional helpers. As far as is known, the more support, the better, but only if it encourages and enables the individual to be as independent as possible, thus fostering a sense of self-responsibility. Support that "takes over" for the individual and induces a state of dependency on the support-giver is not helpful and can even be harmful in the long run.

Clients can be taught to actively increase the degree of social support that they receive from others, rather than merely hoping that others will be supportive. Clients can identify important persons (e.g., family members, friends, coworkers) who can provide support and identify specific ways each person could be supportive. For example, a client could ask a coworker to remind them of the importance of leaving work on time so he/she can exercise or ask a family member not to smoke or eat high-fat foods in their presence.

One means of seeing that the client receives support on an ongoing basis is to help the client locate one or more "buddies" who are attempting to make the very same behavioral changes and who can be supportive to one another. Buddy systems that are externally imposed do not often last, but those that are generated by the clients themselves can be very useful. Getting family members to be supportive buddies is especially desirable but often very difficult to carry out. In addition, although buddy systems can be useful, clients must be prepared for the possibility that their buddy may not adhere to their behavioral changes and should have contingency plans to continue on their own.

Fading Out Contact

The amount of direct contact required between helpers and clients can be greater in the early stages of behavior change and can be decreased in the later stages. All clients need to be prepared for the termination of the active phase of their behavior change program. Janis (1983) states that some form of continued contact, either real or symbolic, should be encouraged, perhaps by making arrangements for phone calls, exchange of letters, or some other form of ongoing communication. The helper needs to continue to build up the client's confidence in being able to succeed on his own, and the best way to do this is to reinforce the client's sense of personal responsibility (or internal locus of control) for the positive behavior changes that occurred during the action phase. The more the client can attribute success to his own actions, the better.

Relapse Prevention

In a real sense, relapse prevention strategies (Brownell, Marlatt, Lichtenstein, & Wilson, 1986) need to be incorporated throughout the change process. Bringing about a behavior change, such as getting a smoker to quit, is relatively easy compared with helping him never to resume smoking again. Many of the strategies described above serve double-duty as relapse prevention strategies, but there are others—such as "programmed lapses" and preparing the client for slips—that are uniquely relapse prevention strategies. In preparing people for the possibility (if not the inevitability) of a slip, it is important to recognize and to counter the "abstinence violation effect," which involves the loss of control that follows the violation of self-imposed rules. The ex-smoker who vows to himself that he will never smoke another cigarette will suffer from the abstinence violation effect even upon taking the very first puff. This psychological letdown, coupled with the reinforcing properties of the nicotine, make a full-blown relapse highly likely. One way to prevent such a relapse from occurring is to convince the person that the slip was due entirely to the situation rather than to some character weakness, such as lack of willpower.

A *programmed lapse* is a lapse in which the therapist/counselor directs the client who has made a change (such as quitting smoking) to deliberately go back to the previous behavior pattern. "This would be done only after the person has received extensive instruction in the cognitive and behavioral coping skills mentioned above. The purpose is to have the inevitable lapse occur under supervision and to demonstrate that self-management skills can be used to prevent the lapse from becoming a relapse. It may also be a useful paradoxical technique; because the therapist controls the lapse, perceptions about lack of control may change" (Brownell et al., 1986, p. 776). It must be pointed out, however, that programmed lapses have a high probability of backfiring and should only be used in a highly selective fashion.

CONCLUSION

This chapter introduced the reader to a number of psychological theories of why people do (or don't do) things that are good for their health. The most important single theoretical construct is undoubtedly self-efficacy: the belief than one can do (or cannot do) the health promoting behavior. But self-efficacy does not operate alone as an explanation of behavior. Other cognitions and situational influences work in combination with efficacy to influence behavioral intentions and behavior. Human behavior is multidetermined; there are no simple answers to why a person does or does not follow a particular recommendation. This is why many of the newer theories in this area contain a relatively large number of explanatory constructs. Although these newer theories, such as Schwarzer's Health Action Process Approach and O'Donnell's Model of Health Promotion Behavior, have great promise, the empirical support for their superiority over less complex theories, such as Ajzen's theory of planned behavior, is yet to be developed.

Similarly, this chapter points out a number of psychological strategies linked to these theories that can be used by health promotion specialists to motivate clients to adopt particular health recommendations and to guide client's actions while they make these changes. None of these strategies are "surefire"; some work better with some persons than with others, and all are more effective in some circumstances than in others. There is research to support the utility of each of these strategies, but there are limits to all of them. As with the theoretical constructs, no one single strategy is the magic answer, but some combination of these strategies will prove useful in almost any situation. Also, as pointed out in the introduction to the second section of the chapter, readers should remain cognizant of the potential for misuse and even abuse of all behavioral change strategies and are encouraged to seek out additional readings, appropriate training, and, if possible, consultation regarding their use.

One important caveat to the theories and strategies discussed in this chapter is that, for the most part, they focus on what is going on in an individual person's mind or in the interaction between an individual person and a limited number of other people. These person-focused theories and strategies provide only a limited worldview. "What has been omitted in the theories and strategies discussed in this chapter are structural features of the sociophysical environment that affect individual and collective well-being, either directly or interactively in conjunction with biopsychobehavioral factors. These *envirogenic* processes in health and illness subsume geographic, architectural, and technological features of the physical environment and sociogenic qualities of the social and cultural environment that influence the etiology of health and illness" (Stokols, 1992, p. 12).

Thus, this chapter can not and should not stand alone. It must be integrated with other chapters in this book, particularly others in this section of the book, in order to round out the picture.

References

Ajzen, I. (1988). *Attitudes, personality, and behavior.* Chicago, IL: Dorsey Press.

Armstrong, C. A., Sallis, J. F., Hovell, M. F., & Hofstetter, C. R. (1993). Stages of change, self-efficacy, and the adoption of vigorous exercise: A prospective analysis. *Journal of Sport and Exercise Psychology, 15,* 390–402.

Armstrong, C. A. (1998). *The stages of change in exercise adoption and adherence: Evaluation of measures with self-report and objective data.* Unpublished doctoral dissertation, University of California, San-Diego, and San Diego State University.

Bandura, A. (1977). Self-efficacy: Toward a unifying theory of behavior change. *Psychological Bulletin, 84,* 191–215.

Bandura, A. (1986). *Social foundations of thought and action: A social cognitive theory.* Englewood Cliffs, N.J.: Prentice-Hall.

Boehm, S. (1989). Patient contracting. *Annual Review of Nursing Research, 8,* 143–153.

Brownell, K. D., Marlatt, G. A., Lichtenstein, E., & Wilson, G. T. (1986). Understanding and preventing relapse. *American Psychologist, 41,* 765–782.

DiClemente, C. C., & Hughes, S. O. (1990). Stages of change profiles in outpatient alcoholism treatment. *Journal of Substance Abuse, 2,* 217–235.

DiClemente, C. C., Prochaska, J. O., & Gibertini, M. (1985). Self-efficacy and the stages of self-change of smoking. *Cognitive Therapy and Research, 9*(2), 181–200.

DiClemente, C. C., Prochaska, J. O., Fairhurst, S. K., Velicer, W. F. & Wayne (1991). The process of smoking cessation: An analysis of precontemplation, contemplation, and preparation stages of change. *Journal of Consulting and Clinical Psychology, 59*(2), 295–304.

Fishbein, M. (1980). A theory of reasoned action: Some applications and implications. In M. M. Page (Ed.), *Nebraska symposium on motivation, 1979.* Lincoln, NE: University of Nebraska Press.

Godin, G., & Kok, G. (1996). The Theory of Planned Behavior: A review of its applications to health-related behaviors. *American Journal of Health Promotion, 11*(2), 87–98.

Gregg, W., Foote, A., Erfurt, J. C., & Heirich, M. A. (1990). Worksite follow-up and engagement strategies for initiating health risk behavior changes. *Health Education Quarterly, 17,* 455–478.

Harrison, J. A., Mullen, P. D., & Green, L. W. (1992). A meta-analysis of studies of the health belief model with adults. *Health Education Research, Theory & Practice, 7,* 107–116.

Janis, I. L. (1983). *Short-term counseling: Guidelines based on recent research.* New Haven, CT: Yale University Press.

Janis, I. L., & Mann, L. (1977). *Decision making.* New York: Macmillan.

Kanfer, F. H., & Schefft, B. K. (1988). *Guiding the process of therapeutic change.* Champaign, IL: Research Press.

Lewin, K. (1951). The nature of field theory. In M. H. Marx (Ed.), *Psychological theory.* New York: Macmillan.

Marcus, B. H., & Owen, N. (1992). Motivational readiness, self-efficacy and decision-making for exercise. *Journal of Applied Social Psychology, 22,* 3–16.

Marcus, B. H., Rakowski, W., & Rossi, J. S. (1992). Assessing motivational readiness and decision-making for exercise. *Health Psychology, 11*(4), 257–261.

O'Connell, D., & Velicer, W. F. (1988). A decisional balance measure and the stages of change model. *The International Journal of the Addictions, 23,* 729–750.

O'Donnell, M. (in press). Predicting intentions and amount of future leisure time exercise in an employed population using the Model of Health Promotion Behavior.

Pender, N. J., Walker, S. N., Sechrist, K. R., & Frank-Stromborg, M. (1990). Predicting health-promoting lifestyles in the workplace. *Nursing Research, 39,* 326–332.

Perry, C. L., Baranowski, T., & Parcel, G. (1990). How individuals, environments, and health behavior interact: Social learning theory. In K. Glanz, F. M. Lewis, & B. K. Rimer (Eds.), *Health behavior and health education: Theory, research, and practice.* San Francisco: Jossey-Bass.

Prentice-Dunn, S., & Rogers, R. W. (1986). Protection motivation theory and preventive health: Beyond the health belief model. *Health Education Research, Theory and Practice, 1,* 153–161.

Prochaska, J. O., & DiClemente, C. C. (1982). Transtheoretical therapy: Toward a more integrative model of change. *Psychotherapy: Theory, Research, and Practice, 19,* 276–288.

Prochaska, J. O., & DiClemente, C. C. (1983). Stages and processes of self-change of smoking: Toward an integrative model of change. *Journal of Consulting and Clinical Psychology, 51*(3), 390–395.

Prochaska, J. O., DiClemente, C. C., & Norcross, J. C. (1992). In search of how people change: Applications to addictive behaviors. *American Psychologist, 47*(9), 1102–1114.

Prochaska, J. O., & Marcus, B. H. (1994). The transtheoretical model: Applications to exercise. In R. K. Dishman (Ed.), *Advances in exercise adherence* (pp. 1–9). Champaign, IL: Human Kinetics Books.

Prochaska, J. O., & Velicer, W. F. (1997). The transtheoretical model of health behavior change. *American Journal of Health Promotion, 12*(1), 38–48.

Prochaska, J. O., Velicer, W. F., Rossi, J. S., Goldstein, M. G., Marcus, B. H., Rakowski, W., Fiore, C., Harlow, L. L., Redding, C. A., Rosenbloom, D., & Rossi, S. R. (1994). Stages of change and decisional balance for 12 problem behaviors. *Health Psychology, 13*(1), 39–46.

Rosenstock, I. M. (1974). Historical origins of the health belief model. *Health Education Monographs, 2*, 328–335.

Rosenstock, I. M. (1990). The health belief model: Explaining health behavior through expectancies. In K. Glanz, F. M. Lewis, & B. K. Rimer (Eds.), *Health behavior and health education: Theory, research, and practice*. San Francisco: Jossey-Bass.

Rosenstock, I. M., Strecher, V. J., & Becker, M. H. (1988). Social learning theory and the health belief model. *Health Education Quarterly, 15*, 175–183.

Rossi, J. S. (1989). The hazards of sunlight: A report on the Consensus Development Conference on Sunlight, Ultraviolet Radiation, and the Skin. *The Health Psychologist, 11*(3), 4–6.

Rotter, J. B. (1954). *Social learning and clinical psychology*. Englewood Cliffs, NJ: Prentice-Hall.

Rotter, J. B. (1966). Generalized expectancies for internal versus external control of reinforcement. *Psychological Monographs, 80*, 1–28.

Sallis, J. F., Hovell, M. F., & Hofstetter, C. R. & Barrington (1992). Predictors of adoption and maintenance of vigorous physical activity in men and women. *Preventive Medicine, 21*, 237–251.

Schwarzer, R. (1992). Adaptation and maintenance of health behaviors: A critical review of theoretical approaches. In R. Schwarzer (Ed.), *Self-efficacy: Thought control of action*. New York: Hemisphere.

Schwarzer, R. (1999). Self-regulatory processes in the adoption and maintenance of health behaviors: The role of optimism, goals, and threats. *Journal of Health Psychology, 4*(2), 115–127.

Sonstroem, R. J. (1988). Psychological models. In R. K. Dishman (Ed.), *Exercise adherence: Its impact on public health* (pp. 125–154). Champaign, IL: Human Kinetics Books.

Stokols, D. (1992). Establishing and maintaining healthy environments: Toward a social ecology of health promotion. *American Psychologist, 47*, 6–22.

Triandis, H. C. (1980). Values, attitudes, and interpersonal behavior. In M. M. Page (Ed.), *Nebraska symposium on motivation, 1979*. Lincoln, NE: University of Nebraska Press.

United States Department of Health and Human Services (1988). *The health consequences of smoking: Nicotine addiction. A report to the Surgeon General* (DHHS Publication No. CDC 88-8406). Rockville, MD: U. S. Department of Health and Human Services, Public Health Service, Centers for Disease Control, Center for Chronic Disease Prevention and Health Promotion, Office on Smoking and Health.

Wallston, B. S., & Wallston, K. A. (1984). Social psychological models of health behavior: An examination and integration. In A. Baum, S. Taylor, & J. Singer (Eds.), *Handbook of psychology and health* (Vol. 4, pp. 23–53). Hillsdale, NJ: Erlbaum.

Wallston, K. A. (1991). The importance of placing measures of health locus of control in a theoretical context. *Health Education Research, Theory and Practice, 6*, 251–252.

Wallston, K. A. (1992). Hocus-pocus, the focus isn't strictly on locus: Rotter's social learning theory modified for health. *Cognitive Therapy and Research, 16*, 183–199.

Wallston, K. A., & Wallston, B. S. (1982). Who is responsible for your health? The construct of health locus of control. In G. S. Sanders, & J. Suls (Eds.), *Social psychology of health and illness* (pp. 65–95). Hillsdale, NJ: Erlbaum.

Wilson, D. K., Purdon, S. E., & Wallston, K. A. (1988). Compliance to health recommendations: A theoretical overview of message framing. *Health Education Research, Theory & Practice, 3*, 161–171.

Winett, R. A., King, A. C., & Altman, D. G. (1989). *Health psychology and public health: An integrative approach*. New York: Pergamon Press.

CHAPTER

Building Supportive Cultural Environments

Judd Robert Allen

INTRODUCTION

Imagine a workplace where most people live 10 to 20 years beyond today's usual life expectancy, where the people you meet have a spring in their step and a sense of joy in their lives, where people care about themselves and about one another, where people achieve their full productive and creative potential. Such a workplace is available to us today. It is not something we have to wait for. Our bodies and minds are more than ready for it. And what's more, it wouldn't cost more than a small fraction of dollars currently wasted on unhealthy lifestyles.

So what's the catch? How is it that most workforces achieve only a fraction of their health potential? There doesn't seem to be a lack of interest on the part of employees and employers. Many employers are pursuing policies and programs to promote employee health (Eikhoff-Shemek & Ryan, 1995). Furthermore, every year roughly 70 percent of the workforce attempts to adopt healthier lifestyle choices (Allen, 1998a). Most smokers have tried to quit smoking. Most overweight people have attempted to lose excess pounds. Most stressed-out employees want to

better balance work, rest, and play. However, less than 20 percent of change attempts result in lasting lifestyle change (Allen, 1998a).

Over the past 20 years, I have assisted over 500 businesses and community organizations to examine their cultures and the impact of the social environment on lifestyle practices. Although the empirical research necessary to show a causal relationship between health behaviors and culture has yet to be conducted, the following observations describe my general observational findings.

- Employees do not naturally gravitate toward unhealthy lifestyle practices. These practices are learned through the culture.
- When workers seek to alter their unhealthy practices without addressing the underlying cultural forces, the culture overwhelms or undermines the lifestyle improvement effort.
- With some notable exceptions–for example, new norms for not smoking and for buckling seatbelts–family, workplace, and broad community norms undermine efforts to adopt healthier and more productive lifestyles. In some areas–stress, exercise, and nutrition–the culture has become so toxic that few escape unscathed.

In my opinion, the impact of the culture on lifestyle has been largely overlooked. An exclusive focus on the individual in the pursuit of self-improvement is a central value in North American culture and dates back to the advent of participatory democracies about 4,000 years ago. At that point, self-concepts began to get redefined, so that individual preferences became important to decision-making and the functioning of the clan, family, or group. Migration to America, either as a pioneer or as a slave, broke traditional clan and family bonds. Individualism became a part of patriotic folklore, evident in tales of Davy Crockett, the *Autobiography of Benjamin Franklin* (Franklin, 1998), and the *Adventures of Huckleberry Finn* (Twain, 1993). Western psychology redefined mental health in terms of an individual's capacity for self-change. The very idea that someone was dependent on another person was diagnostic of any number of pathologies.

This chapter is based on the premise that an individual's effort to live a healthy lifestyle can be greatly enhanced by a supportive cultural environment. This premise breaks with common health promotion practices that focus almost exclusively on the individual. The learning objectives for this chapter are to be able to define key culture change concepts, develop strategies for measuring the culture, and work with processes for bringing about sustained cultural change. First, the theoretical and historical contexts of the culture change approach are discussed. Key concepts and their measurement are reviewed. Then an overview of the Normative Systems Culture Change Process is presented. Finally, suggestions are made for integrating culture change into established health promotion programs.

THEORETICAL CONTEXT: BORN OUT OF A QUEST FOR SUSTAINED RESULTS

The culture-based approach discussed herein was initially developed by the psychologist Robert F. Allen. In the early 1960s, a team of psychologists received a grant to help court-appointed delinquent youths (Allen, Dubin, Pilnick, & Youtz, 1981). The results seemed promising until the participants graduated from the program and returned to the street. One of the psychologists, Robert Allen, recognized that individual psychotherapeutic approaches to behavior change were ineffective in helping children break free of their illegal and frequently life-threatening lifestyle practices (e.g., drugs, robbery, vandalism, etc.). Allen found that the street culture was overwhelming young people's efforts to adopt healthy lifestyles. Allen's solution was to teach kids how to create non-delinquent subcultures.

Allen extended his work to hundreds of different organizational and social problems, ranging from litter reduction to corporate productivity and educational reform (Allen & Kraft, 1980). Allen's clients included government agencies, unions, schools, small businesses, and Fortune 500 companies. These programs are discussed in two books, *Beat the System: A Way to Create More Human Environments* (Allen & Kraft, 1980) and *The Organizational Unconscious* (Allen, Allen, Kraft, & Certner, 1987). Allen formed a behavioral science organization—the Human Resources Institute—to advance culture-based approaches to change. In the 1970s the Human Resources Institute developed the first culture-based health promotion programs at two pharmaceutical firms: Johnson & Johnson and Hoffman LaRoche. These projects led to the Lifegain model of culture-based health promotion (Allen & Linde, 1981).

Allen was strongly influenced by both anthropology and psychology. A discussion of the major theorists and how they influenced Allen's work is presented in Table 8-1.

PARALLEL THEORIES

Several social environmental approaches parallel the culture change methods developed by Allen. Among these strategies are conditioning (Skinner, 1953), social learning theory (Rotter, 1954; Bandura, 1977), theory of reasoned action (Ajzen & Fishbein, 1980), and social marketing (Novelli, 1984). While it is beyond the scope of this chapter to discuss each fully, a brief review of each approach is presented in Table 8-2.

Table 8-1 Contributors to Robert Allen's Culture Change Approach

- *Sigmund Freud (1900)*–recognized that much of human behavior is influenced by unconscious forces in the human psyche. Allen saw the culture as operating at an unconscious level to influence group behavior.
- *Solomon Asch (1955) and Stanley Milgram (1965)*–demonstrated that conformity to group expectations could lead people to highly destructive behavior. Allen recognized that skills in understanding and shaping cultural environments freed people from conformity.
- *Ashley Montagu (1986) and A.J. Bronowski (1974)*–recognized the importance of human contact in health and well-being. Allen saw that people's need for each other makes it virtually impossible to ignore culture in finding solutions to human problems.
- *Ruth Benedict (1934)*–recognized the importance of cultural norms in shaping perceptions of human nature. Allen saw that people could be taught to critically examine norms and choose norms that are more consistent with shared values.
- *Fritz Heider (1958)*–found that people tend to overestimate the role of personal choice and underestimate situational forces in decision-making. In keeping with Heider's attribution theory, Allen recognized that people use behavior rather than statements of personal belief to estimate individual values. Allen saw that people underestimate the power of culture in shaping behavior and, as a result, make false and negative judgments about individual values.
- *Kurt Lewin (1951)*–recognized the importance of a feedback loop in planning community and organizational change. Allen incorporated Lewin's concern for feedback in his four-phase change model (Normative Systems).

Table 8-2 Social Environmental Theories of Behavior

Theory	Definition
Operant conditioning	Holds that behavior is influenced by rewards. Healthy lifestyle practices are to be rewarded. At the very least, unhealthy behaviors should not be rewarded.
Social learning theory	Proposes that the probability of a given behavior is determined by the belief one can perform the necessary behavior, by the expectations of attaining a goal that follows that activity, and by the personal value of that goal. Role models can serve an important function by illustrating the positive outcome associated with health behavior.
Theory of reasoned action	Finds that behavior is most closely linked to individual intentions to act. Such intentions are in turn influenced by both an individual's attitudes toward a behavior and his or her perceptions about what is normal conduct. In accordance with this approach, practitioners determine the relative importance of attitudes versus norms in shaping a given intention, then a plan is devised to influence the most important factors.
Social marketing	Underscores the value of communicating the benefits of health behavior. Mass media can serve as advocates for healthy lifestyle practices.

THE BUILDING BLOCKS OF CULTURE

Five cultural factors work together to shape long-term behavior (see Figure 8-1 and Table 8-3). Assessing the impact of these cultural dimensions is the first step in empowering members of a workforce to choose healthy and productive cultures.

Discovering Wellness Values

A value is a heartfelt belief about the appropriate way to approach living. Values develop at all levels of the organization. The concept is most familiar on an individual level. For example, a friend might be seen as valuing honesty, frugality, and compassion. Organi-

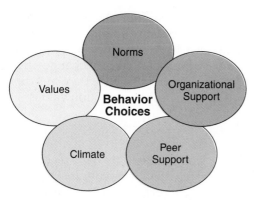

Figure 8-1 Cultural Factors that Shape Long-Term Behavior

Table 8-3 Elements of Culture

Values: Heartfelt beliefs about the appropriate way to approach living. Both individual and collective initiatives are driven by personal and shared cultural values.

Norms: Expected and accepted behavior. Norms are "the way we do things around here."

Organizational Support: The system of informal and formal structures, policies, and procedures that maintain the culture. Organizational support factors—such as modeling, rewards, and training—must be adjusted to provide ongoing support for desired behavior.

Peer Support: Assistance from family, friends, coworkers, and immediate supervisors. Support can take the form of emotional encouragement (such as kind words) and instrumental resources (such as help covering work responsibilities).

Climate: The cultural equivalent of yeast in bread making. Three social atmosphere factors—sense of community, shared vision, and positive outlook—enable constructive individual and collective change.

zations also adopt values. "Lean and mean" was a value theme for the 1980s. In the early 1990s, quality was the core value focus. In the later part of the 1990s, it turned to speed of innovation. Just as organizational development values such as innovation are gaining attention in the workplace, health promotion

values such as self-care need to become part of the way companies do business. For example, it would be possible to promote four wellness values—healthy fun, mutual respect, self-responsibility, and full potential—that are evident in companies listed in the book, *The 100 Best Companies to Work For in America* (Levering & Moskowitz, 1994); the companies in which these values prevail also tend to be more profitable than their peers.

Worksite health promotion professionals can identify health-enhancing values and translate them into the language of the corporate culture. For example:

- Describe past health promotion efforts and then ask people's opinions about these initiatives. Examine this input to identify desired values.
- Ask leaders how health promotion themes might fit with their vision for organizational growth.
- Ask members of the culture to list goals for the health promotion effort, then identify values that encompass those goals.
- Describe programs and activities that can be used to support employee wellness, then ask people to determine principles and values that will be important for delivering successful programs.
- Describe wellness and health promotion, then determine what aspects are the biggest motivators. Choose values to highlight those qualities.
- Once you have a preliminary list of four or five themes, ask people to translate the themes into the language of the culture.

Using these techniques, some organizations have adopted highly innovative value sets that match the organization's vision. Conoco, for example, organized its efforts around healthy pleasure and self-understanding. The YMCA strives to work with the whole person—mind, body, and spirit.

Core program values such as these provide needed direction for culture change. They enable employees to decide how health promotion matches their personal values. Such a match fosters commitment and enthusiasm. This positive attitude toward shared values is the cornerstone of a corporate culture that supports health.

Demystifying Cultural Norms

In a culture that emphasizes the individual, there is a tendency to believe that the behavior is guided by personal values. However, it is just as likely for the behavior of organizational members to be guided by cultural norms. A norm is an expected and accepted behavior: "It's the way we do things around here." For example, most people value eating healthful diets, but norms rarely support a balanced diet that is low in fat and sugar and high in grains, fresh fruits, and vegetables.

For better and for worse, norms guide most health behavior. There are social standards for everything, from when to seek help with an alcohol problem to whether or not to exercise during lunch breaks. Now that it is a norm to wear car safety belts, it has become much easier to buckle up. Changing norms for adult smoking have made it easier for adults to quit. In contrast, cultural norms for long work weeks, fast-paced lifestyles, and two-income households make it extremely difficult to manage stress (see Table 8-4).

Dissatisfaction and discomfort with current cultural norms reflect poor alignment between values and cultural norms. To close this gap, ask employees to rank whether a given norm exists among their peers on a scale of "strongly agree" to "strongly disagree." Then, to measure employee values, ask employees about what norms they would desire. One important purpose of a culture change effort is to modify cultural norms so that they are consistent with widely held health promotion values.

Organizational Support: The Backbone of Culture

Each workplace develops its own mechanisms for defining and perpetuating its culture. Formal personnel policies dictate such things as hours of work, employee benefits, and procedures. Informal structures, such as "the grapevine" and leadership modeling, are equally powerful. In order to bring about lasting changes in the culture, both informal and formal organizational support systems need to be brought into alignment with health promotion values.

There are a variety of ways to measure organizational support. Strategies include a review of job descriptions and performance evaluations. An evaluator might attend a company orientation for new employees or training sessions. Focus group interviews can reveal how friendships develop and determine rituals, symbols, celebrations, and company myths. Reading the company newsletters and e-mail bulletins can also reveal how the culture

Table 8-4 Sample Stress-Related Norm Gap Profile

Low				High	
1	2	3	4	5	
					Balance work, rest, and play
		Norm Gap			Adopt a stress management technique
					Resolve conflicts in positive ways
					Laugh and tell jokes
Existing Culture		Desired Culture			Take on only as much responsibility as you can handle

Table 8-5 Organizational Support: One Company's Findings

Support Mechanism	Strength	Opportunity for Improvement
Modeling	The CEO frequently jogs during lunch.	Middle managers tend to exercise at private health clubs instead of at the company facility. Their efforts are not visible to most employees.
Training	The company offers courses on job safety, exercise, and smoking cessation.	Too frequently, informal lessons in coping are also lessons in dishonesty (in other words, "tell the bosses what they want to hear").
Rewards and Recognition	The company recognizes work groups for achieving health goals around absenteeism and safety.	The company provides special breaks for smokers.
Confrontation	Employees confront those who violate no-smoking policies.	Employees make fun of lunchtime exercisers by calling them health nuts.
Orientation	New employees are immediately invited to join in company-sponsored exercise activities.	The orientation program does not describe the company's health promotion program as a primary benefit. Instead, there is a heavy emphasis on medical coverage and sick leave. This leaves employees with the unintended impression that they need to be sick to take advantage of company benefits.
Relationships and Interactions	Company-sponsored sport teams often provide opportunities for people to get to know each other better.	Many employees find their friendships in designated smoking areas.
Resource Allocation	The company will reimburse employees' fitness center membership fees.	Employees are not given release time to participate in health promotion activities and seminars.
Rituals, Myths, and Symbols	The Golden Carrot Award is given to people who exemplify balance in their lives.	The myth is that the founder always worked and never slept. Therefore, employees should always work late and not take breaks.

works. Observing how space is used and how employees interact is another strategy. Table 8-5 provides an illustration of organizational support findings drawn from an actual cultural analysis of small business.

A caution about organizational support: If only one factor is changed without attending to the others, unforeseen and frequently undesired consequences can result. For example, if the CEO is the only jogger, the CEO may become isolated from others. If smoking is confronted without providing smoking cessation programs, smokers may quit the company before quitting smoking.

Peer Support: Acts of Kindness that Work

People often think of peer support in terms of such special health promotion programs as Alcoholics Anonymous or Weight Watchers, but natural support systems provided by family, friends, and coworkers are also important sources of support. Ideally, such support systems provide both emotional support (in the form of kind words of encouragement) and instrumental support (such as money and time off).

Workplace wellness programs can offer training specifically designed to increase the effectiveness of support provided by coworkers and supervisors.

Table 8-6 Peer Support Skills

- **Goal Setting**–Helping to establish meaningful and specific goals using the Stages of Change framework (Prochaska, Norcross, & DiClemente, 1994).

- **Identifying Role Models**–Finding someone who has successfully achieved a similar goal.

- **Eliminating Barriers to Change**–Developing strategies for obtaining needed time, equipment, and other resources.

- **Locating Supportive Environments**–Helping to find people and places that support lifestyle improvement goals.

- **Working Through Relapse**–Helping to get back on track.

- **Celebrating Success**–Cheering someone on and acknowledging accomplishments.

For example, training can be organized around primary support skills (Allen, 1998b). Table 8-6 explains some of the peer support skills that have been included in health promotion programs.

Mentoring programs have proven successful in a variety of circumstances. For example, Union Pacific Railroad's Lifegain Health Culture Audit survey results revealed a need to increase support from coworkers and supervisors. In order to address these concerns, the railroad has begun an ambitious strategy of training Wellness Mentors (Allen, 1998b). The one-day training teaches skills for establishing trust and for goal setting using the "stages of change" approach (Prochaska, Norcross, & DiClemente, 1994). In addition to goalsetting, employees learn skills for identifying role models, eliminating barriers to change, locating supportive environments, working through relapse, and celebrating success. The mentoring program gives coworkers and supervisors opportunities to become partners in lifestyle change. Developing peer support resources has been particularly helpful in addressing the diverse needs of an employee population that is spread out along hundreds of miles of railroad track.

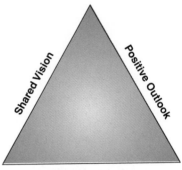

Climate in the Workplace

Figure 8-2 Climate in the Workplace

Climate: The Cultural Equivalent of Yeast in Bread Making

Three work climate factors—a sense of community, a shared vision, and a positive outlook—are the cultural equivalent of yeast in bread making (Allen & Allen, 1987). Where they are noticeably absent, individual and organizational growth grind to a halt. Where a sense of community, a shared vision, and a positive outlook are abundant, cooperative action and individual transformation proceed smoothly (see Figure 8-2).

A sense of community is present when people feel as if they belong and they trust one another. This sense of belonging includes an awareness that others "care" and that the individual, in turn, has a responsibility to care for others. Furthermore, when a sense of community exists, people tend to know one another beyond familiarity with job roles. What does this mean for health promotion? People are more receptive to advice about lifestyle if they believe it is given in a spirit of caring. In addition, community provides a level of comfort needed to try new behavior. Physiological addiction also appears less pronounced when people feel a sense of community (Horn, 1972).

It is possible to build a sense of community through multidimensional sharing. In our culture, informal conversation rarely gets beyond the weather and current events. Building community involves giving people a chance to get to know one another in multidimensional ways—beyond job responsibilities. Health promotion activities can challenge this norm for superficial conversation by giving people a chance to share their responses about the following aspects of their lives:

- Places you have lived in your life
- A major change you have made in your life
- One thing others would need to know in order to understand you better
- A childhood experience that has had a lasting effect on you
- A person who has had an important impact on you
- How you happened to choose your present work
- An experience you've had in the last year or two that has made a significant impression on you
- An obstacle you've had to overcome
- A personal achievement
- Your hobbies and/or special interests

A shared vision inspires peak individual and organizational performance. When people have a shared vision, they are enthusiastic about the organization's goals and have a common view about how to achieve them. When no shared vision exists, people end up working at cross-purposes. There is little common agreement about what the organization is trying to achieve, and it is hard to figure out why people should work together to achieve health promotion goals.

Shared vision emerges when people have a chance to integrate their own personal goals and approaches with those of the organization, program, or project. This is particularly important in health promotion because people are working with a variety of personal and organizational goals.

With **a positive outlook,** people look for opportunities rather than obstacles and for strengths rather than weaknesses in one another. In health promotion, it is our strengths rather than weaknesses that enable us to move forward. For example, with a positive outlook, the feedback from a health risk appraisal will be seen as recognizing many lifestyle strengths and a few opportunities for lifestyle enhancement. In a more negative culture, the same health risk appraisal feedback might leave employees feeling inadequate and many believing that survey results will be used to weed out unhealthy employees.

TOOLS FOR TAPPING INTO THE ORGANIZATIONAL UNCONSCIOUS

Most members of groups and organizations are blind to the influence of culture. For this reason, it is necessary to measure culture and its impact on behavior. Cultural anthropologists and other behavioral scientists have developed a variety of cultural analysis techniques. Strategies include focus group interviews, participant observation, examination of organizational documents, and conduction of field experiments and surveys. For example, a field experiment might have a new employee publicly practice a recommended stress management technique (or some other healthy lifestyle practice) then, after a few days, interviewing the employee and coworkers to determine how this behavior is treated in the culture.

One cultural analysis tool, the *Lifegain Health Culture Audit,* was designed specifically for health promotion program planning and evaluation. Versions of the survey have been used by hundreds of companies, schools, and government organizations. A one-page *Lifegain Health Culture Audit* is reprinted in Table 8-7 (online scoring is available at www.healthy-culture.com). Sample results are given in Table 8-8.

JUMP-STARTING A NEW HEALTH PROMOTION PROGRAM

Cultures are complex systems that respond best to a systematic change process that empowers organizational members to consciously choose their cultural environments. New health promotion programs can get off to a great start by organizing the program vision and processes to assure long-term success. The following four-phase Normative Systems Culture Change Process was developed specifically to change complex cultural environments (see Figure 8-3) (Allen & Silverzweig, 1977). The four-phase approach for changing culture should be part of the strategic planning process.

Table 8-7 Lifegain Health Culture Audit

Organizational culture plays an important role in supporting healthy lifestyles. The following confidential and anonymous survey measures how this works in your organization. Survey results will be used to help enhance existing health promotion services

Note: There are no right or wrong answers. We are asking for your opinion.

Please indicate your level of agreement with the statements below using the following scale:
1–Strongly Disagree, 2–Disagree, 3–Undecided/Don't Know, 4–Agree, or 5–Strongly Agree

1	2	3	4	5	
○	○	○	○	○	Living a healthy lifestyle is important to me.
○	○	○	○	○	My immediate supervisor models a healthy lifestyle.
○	○	○	○	○	My workplace demonstrates its commitment to supporting healthy lifestyles through its use of resources such as time, space, and money.
○	○	○	○	○	People in my work unit are taught skills needed to achieve a healthy lifestyle.
○	○	○	○	○	New employees at my work unit are made aware of the organization's support for healthy lifestyles.
○	○	○	○	○	In my work unit, people are rewarded and recognized for efforts to live a healthy lifestyle.
○	○	○	○	○	In my work unit, participation in healthy activities is a primary way to renew friendships and to meet new people.
○	○	○	○	○	In my work unit, unhealthy behavior (such as smoking and excess drinking) is discouraged and confronted.
○	○	○	○	○	My work unit has a sense of community (for example, people really get to know one another, feel as if they belong, and care for one another in times of need).
○	○	○	○	○	My work unit has a shared vision (for example, people feel that the organization's conduct is consistent with their personal values, and people are clear about how they fit in with the big picture).
○	○	○	○	○	My work unit has a positive outlook (for example, people enjoy their work, celebrate accomplishments, adopt a "we can do it" attitude, and bring out the best in each other).
○	○	○	○	○	My immediate supervisor supports employees' efforts to adopt healthier lifestyle practices.
○	○	○	○	○	My immediate coworkers support one another's efforts to adopt healthier lifestyle practices.
○	○	○	○	○	My family members and/or housemates support one another's efforts to adopt healthier lifestyle practices.

In my immediate work unit, it is normal for people to . . .

1	2	3	4	5	
○	○	○	○	○	Exercise regularly (at least 3 times a week).
○	○	○	○	○	Maintain a healthy weight.
○	○	○	○	○	Eat foods that are low in fat and refined sugar.
○	○	○	○	○	Drink alcohol moderately, if at all (that is, not more than 14 drinks per week or more than 5 drinks on a single day).
○	○	○	○	○	Use car safetybelts.
○	○	○	○	○	Follow safety precautions at work (including practicing good lifting techniques and organizing the work environment to avoid injury).
○	○	○	○	○	Not smoke.
○	○	○	○	○	Stay current on medical screenings.

Lifestyle Change Questions

In the past year have you attempted one or more health-supporting lifestyle changes, such as trying to lose weight, exercise, or manage stress?

    ○ Yes   ○ No

If you did attempt lifestyle change last year, how successful were you in maintaining your new desired lifestyle?

    ○ Very Successful   ○ Moderately Successful   ○ Not Successful

Table 8-8 Results of Union Pacific Railroad *Lifegain Health Culture Audit* Findings

- Each year 75% of Union Pacific employees attempt to adopt a new health practice. Just 16% of these efforts are seen as "very successful."
- Employees believe that health is important and that their quality of life is greatly influenced by personal lifestyle practices.
- Since 1992, when the survey was last conducted, progress has been made in norms associated with nutrition, substance abuse, safety, and work climate. Norms for taking on too much responsibility and for failing to balance work, rest, and play appear to be on the rise.
- Lack of time is the primary barrier to participation in health promotion activities.
- Family and friends are the primary sources of support for lifestyle improvements.
- Employees report moderate levels of organizational support in the dimensions of leadership modeling, rewards, training, resource commitment, and the orientation of new employees.

Phase I: Analysis, Objective Setting, and Leadership Commitment

The first phase involves analyzing the culture, setting objectives, and gaining leadership commitment. Leadership support is vital to successful culture change efforts (Allen, Hunnicutt, & Johnson, 1999). One strategy for working with leaders is to help define their role (see Table 8-9); leadership "ownership" is further achieved by acquainting leaders with health

Table 8-9 Developing Leadership Roles

Sharing the Wellness Program Vision
- Explaining how wellness contributes to the overall goals of the organization (such as improving morale, increasing productive capabilities, valuing employees, and reducing costs).
- Explaining the directions, purposes, structure, and philosophy of the wellness program.
- Asking questions that are useful for aligning the wellness program with overall organizational direction and mission.

Serving as a Role Model
- Sharing your enthusiasm for adopting a health and wellness philosophy in your own life.
- Telling about personal efforts to adopt healthier lifestyle practices.
- Participating in organizational health and wellness activities.

Gaining Resource Commitment
- Assisting with planning an adequate health promotion budget.
- Helping to modify institutional/organizational policies and procedures so that they better support wellness (such as assistance with smoking policies and release time for wellness activities).
- Working to reduce internal political barriers (such as ensuring that department heads support the program by providing appropriate resources in their areas).

Rewarding Success
- Recognizing employee progress in achieving healthier lifestyle practices.
- Tracking outcomes and celebrating positive results.
- Honoring those involved in the delivery of the health promotion program.

Normative Systems Culture Change Process

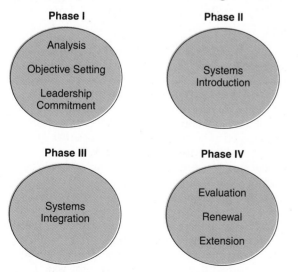

Figure 8-3 Normative Systems Culture Change Process

promotion goals and the culture change process that will be used for achieving them. Leaders are also encouraged to develop their own personal plans for modeling lifestyle improvement. As part of this first phase, baseline data are gathered from which later progress can be measured, and the program is tailored to meet the specific needs of the organization. Health risk appraisals, health screenings, focus group interviews, observational research, and employee surveys are frequently incorporated into this phase of project development.

Phase II: Systems Introduction

The second phase introduces the health promotion effort to the wider organizational community. One Phase II objective is to create an understanding of the value of health promotion and the role of the culture in supporting positive health practices. This can be accomplished by sharing findings generated during Phase I. Another Phase II objective is to help employees to assess their current situation and set meaningful individual and workteam goals. A third Phase II objective is to develop individual and group action plans. These action plans form the bulk of activities to be performed during the third phase of systems integration.

A letter from the president and articles in the company newsletter provide an overview of program goals and strategies. Company-sponsored games and contests have also been used to share the overall program vision with employees. For example, one university held a wellness contest. The contest manual introduced the philosophy of the wellness program, and individual participants and university departments won prizes for taking part in a variety of wellness activities.

It is often highly beneficial to kick off Phase II by inviting employees to attend a wellness workshop. Ideally such an introductory workshop would use group activities and discussions to provide its participants with an opportunity to experience the desired wellness culture during the workshop. The agenda should consist of at least three parts:

1. **Understanding**–To create an understanding of the value of health promotion and the role of culture in shaping health practices.

2. **Identifying**–To help participants identify their current situation and to set meaningful individual and workteam goals.
3. **Changing**–To develop a plan for personal and cultural change.

Phase III: Systems Integration

Support for healthy lifestyles needs to become a part of the fabric of organizational life. Phase III initiatives include many of the resources now being featured in traditional health promotion programs. For example, during this phase a health newsletter or Internet resource could be provided to employees. Support group programs such as Weight Watchers would be offered during Phase III. Increased access to fitness facilities and classes such as yoga would also be a part of Phase III. Activities should be provided in a varied format that matches the interests of the workforce (see Table 8-10 for a list of possible formats).

Day-to-day organizational functions should be adjusted to reflect a commitment to health. Phase III efforts address organizational supports such as communication systems, rewards, employee orientation, training, leadership modeling, policies, and procedures. Changing smoking policies is a highly visible example of such a policy change. Smaller changes in the way the organization conducts its business can also reinforce new health values and norms. For example, it

Table 8-10 Offer Culture Change Programming in a Variety of Formats

1. Provide self-help educational materials (such as educational brochures, books, videos, and access to health information on the Internet) that incorporate a discussion of finding or building supportive family, work, and community environments.
2. Offer support group programs or link employees with support group programs available in the community or on the Internet.
3. Foster periodic workgroup discussions of employee health promotion goals (at regular managers' meetings or in the monthly safety meeting).
4. Involve employees in health promotion task forces (for example, ask a group to help change the vending machines or to develop an incentive program).

may be possible to include healthier food choices in vending machines and the company cafeteria.

Phase IV: Evaluation, Renewal, and Extension

The final phase is ongoing evaluation, renewal, and extension. The evaluation should encompass three broad categories of assessment: performance, programmatic, and cultural.

- **Performance evaluation** examines the "bottom-line" results. Performance evaluation includes assessing the program's economic impact, illnesses avoided, productivity improvements, morale changes, and health behavior changes.
- **Programmatic evaluation** examines how well the initiative was implemented. For example, a determination can be made of participation rates, participant satisfaction, and the pace of changes in organizational policies and procedures.
- **Cultural evaluation** examines changes in values, norms, peer support, organizational support, and climate. Frequently the evaluation includes re-administering the cultural assessment survey (see *Lifegain Health Culture Audit*), as well as conducting focus interviews and field experiments.

Celebrate successes. Picnics, banquets, retreats, annual reports, award ceremonies, and shareholders' meetings are appropriate venues for celebrating health promotion outcomes. Celebrating is an important rite of passage to a new culture. During such activities, leaders can acknowledge how the culture has improved. Celebrating success provides participants with an opportunity to fully appreciate the value of their efforts. In addition, such celebrations further clarify the vision of a healthier and more productive culture. They enable participants to further commit to individual and organizational health. Such celebrations also reinforce project principles (such as approaching change systematically or being results-oriented).

Renew and extend the program. This may involve the commitment of additional resources to areas that are particularly resistant to change. One nice thing about culture change is that problems really do go away. For example, new norms for regular exercise reduce the need to offer special enticements for trying

out exercise. Fitness just becomes "the way we do things around here." For this reason, other health and productivity concerns would become the focus of renewal and extension efforts. Build on successes by approaching other areas, such as self-management, teamwork, quality, customer service, and speed of innovation. The same systematic culture-based approach can be applied to a broad range of organizational objectives.

Finally, people need to be encouraged to bring changes to new settings. Program extension is critical; employees who become the "teachers" are often the most successful in maintaining personal lifestyle changes.

ADDING CULTURE CHANGE COMPONENTS TO AN ESTABLISHED PROGRAM

Those involved in mature programs may find it difficult to restructure their overall program design around the four-phase Normative Systems Culture Change Process. For these programs, traditional health promotion elements can be adjusted to address cultural issues.

Conduct Periodic Cultural Assessments

Mature programs should conduct a periodic assessment of their cultures. Such assessments can either focus on a broad range of wellness goals (see *Lifegain Health Culture Audit*) or focus on those aspects of the culture that are the current focus of program interventions. For example, a program that is emphasizing medical self-care could look specifically at norms, values, peer support, and organizational support factors that influence self-care behavior. Is it a norm, for example, to consult a self-care book before seeking nonemergency medical care? In terms of organizational support, are people being rewarded and recognized for their medical self-care efforts?

It is recommended that a broad cultural assessment, such as the *Lifegain Health Culture Audit*, be conducted every three to five years. Broad cultural assessments keep programs on track. Program priorities can be set to address large gaps between the current and the desired culture. For example, in one hospital's audit it was determined that norms related to financial wellness and weight management had the largest gaps. As a result, health promotion managers are emphasizing these norms in their program design.

Periodic cultural assessments reveal shifts in employee needs. Many organizations are finding that mergers, downsizing, and changes in employee demographics require modifications in their program design. For example, work-family life balance issues may have become the priority for a workforce. As a result, health promotion programs must accommodate family members and housemates. Or maybe the cultural assessment will determine that the organization has a very unhealthy work climate. As a result, the first priority in the program design would be to foster a sense of community, a shared vision, and a positive outlook.

Develop Leadership Support

Culture is the link between traditional health promotion activities and leadership. CEOs, vice presidents, managers, and supervisors need to be able to define their roles in supporting wellness.

- Leaders can share a vision for a healthier and more productive workforce. Translating health promotion goals into business terms and philosophy is an important leadership function. Almost all management initiatives (such as customer service, learning organizations, or quality) are fertile ground for sharing about the importance of a healthy workforce. Leaders can articulate their vision in written and verbal statements about how business goals can best be achieved by supporting employee wellness.
- Leaders can serve as role models. Their healthy lifestyle choices and participation in health promotion activities inspire employees.
- Leaders can assist in setting budget and human resource priorities that reflect a commitment to employee health.
- Leaders can recognize individual and organizational progress. For example, leaders can acknowledge cost savings and overall reductions in employee illness achieved through the wellness program.

Develop Peer Support

The support of family, friends, coworkers, and supervisors can be a force for individual and cultural transformation. Mutual support for healthy lifestyles can be nurtured through work team discussions, mentoring programs, and support groups. At one university, for example, a "Well-Department Awards" program was introduced to foster department discussions of mutual support for health. Departments competed to achieve high scores on an anonymous survey designed to measure support for wellness. At an oil and gas company, work groups participated in the *Game of Lifestyle Change* (Allen, Jeagar, Torres, Leutzinger, & Baun, 1998). Work groups earned game points by participating in individual and group activities designed to enhance mutual support for healthy lifestyles.

Develop Organizational Support Systems

Traditional health promotion programs frequently offer new forms of organizational support, such as health newsletters and classroom experiences designed to promote employee health. These new health promotion programs are added to an existing array of organizational rewards, communication systems, and training (see Organizational Support: The Backbone of Culture). In order to cut organizational clutter, organizational policies, procedures, and programs (outside the health promotion program) should be examined to see if they can be adjusted to better support healthy lifestyle choices. For example, a system can be established for rewarding healthy lifestyle choices with reduced employee insurance premiums. In this way, health promotion can be more fully integrated into day-to-day operations without adding a new layer of programs and activities.

Develop a Healthier Work Climate

Without a sense of community, a shared vision, and a positive outlook, productivity, innovation, and morale suffer. Health promotion activities can be retooled to build a healthier work climate. For example, fitness classes can include "get-to-know-you" activities before and after the workout. Employees can utilize *Knowing Tree* software (Allen, 1999), an Internet and intranet application that builds a sense of community around shared health interests. To better nurture a shared vision, wellness mentoring programs can include a discussion of how personal goals fit with the overall direction of the company. To foster a more positive outlook, health newsletters can emphasize individual and organizational achievements.

THE FUTURE OF CULTURE CHANGE APPROACHES

We live in cultures of self-improvement. Thanks to abundant scientific evidence about the benefits of healthy lifestyles, every year most people attempt to enhance the quality and quantity of their lives through some sort of lifestyle change (Allen, 1998a). Dieting, adopting regular exercise practices, overcoming addictions to alcohol and nicotine, managing stress, advancing a career interest, and improving interpersonal relationships are just some of the many ways we attempt to improve our health. Sometimes we call these efforts New Year's Resolutions. Other times, we choose our goals to increase our sex appeal and attractiveness. Or, maybe we are responding to recommendations from a health professional.

A more systematic culture-based approach will enhance individual lifestyle improvement efforts. As O'Donnell (1989) notes, "Lifestyle change can be facilitated through a combination of efforts to enhance awareness, change behavior, and create environments that support good health practices. Of the three, supportive environments will probably have the greatest impact in producing lasting change." State-of-the-art individual change programs now embrace a process approach to change. For example, James Prochaska and his colleagues have identified six stages of individual change that are necessary to lasting self-improvement (Prochaska, Norcross, & DiClemente, 1994). Unfortunately, it is not a cultural norm to approach personal or organizational change as a process. It is normal to see change as a question of personal revelation or a function of picking the right goals. To improve success rates, health promotion practitioners will need to change this "quick fix" culture to one that embraces systematic, ongoing change.

The three primary points needed for culture-based health promotion are:

1. **Be Systematic.** Consider using the first couple of months of each year to analyze the culture, set goals, and develop leadership commitment. Then take a couple of months to introduce culture change goals and to involve people in the solution. Over the subsequent six to nine months, integrate the changes into the fabric of the culture. Use December to evaluate, celebrate success, and address those aspects of the culture that were resistant to change.
2. **Be Results Oriented.** Activities can be counterproductive if they do not lead to lasting and positive change. You are not trying to exhaust people and resources. Instead, try to change the conditions that are causing unhealthy behavior.
3. **Have Fun.** Work with others to create a unique and wondrous culture that is both healthy and enjoyable. We are all in this business for the long haul, so let's keep our senses of humor and have some fun.

CONCLUSION

As the field of health promotion matures, it is likely that companies will begin to adopt approaches that focus simultaneously on individual change processes and culture change processes. Improved health promotion research is increasing the likelihood that practitioners will move beyond random delivery of individual-focused health promotion activities. Benchmark studies are presenting compelling evidence concerning the need to create supportive cultural environments (O'Donnell, Bishop, & Kaplan, 1997). In addition, high failure rates of health promotion and other organizational development initiatives make leaders more receptive to alternative culture-based interventions. Furthermore, technologies such as the Internet, distance learning, and community building software applications are increasing access to culture change methodology.

The future and spirit of the culture-based approach is summarized in the words of the late Robert F. Allen: "We must transform our cultures so that our need for one another is not an obstacle to overcome, but rather a virtue to be celebrated" (Allen, 1981).

The editors gratefully acknowledge the contribution of Robert F. Allen for his chapter, The Importance of Cultural Variables in Program Design, which appeared in the first edition of Health Promotion in the Workplace. *The editors also acknowledge Rick Bellingham for his contribution to the chapter, Building Supportive Environments, which appeared in the second edition of* Health Promotion in the Workplace. *Joe Leutzinger of Union Pacific Railroad also made substantial contributions to this chapter.*

References

Ajzen, I., & Fishbein, M. (1980). *Understanding attitudes and predicting social behavior.* Englewood Cliffs, NJ: Prentice-Hall.

Allen, J. R. (1998a). *Lifestyle change attempt and success rate findings from Lifegain Health Culture Audit surveys conducted at over 50 companies.* Burlington, Vermont: Human Resources Institute.

Allen, J. R. (1998b, Summer). Wellness mentoring can help rebuild the corporate culture. *Worksite Health, 5*(3), 27–30.

Allen, J. R. (1999). *KnowingTree* [on-line]. Available: Healthyculture.com.

Allen, J. R., Hunnicutt, D., & Johnson, J. (1999). *Fostering wellness leadership: A new model* [Special Report]. Omaha, NE: Wellness Councils of America.

Allen, J. R., Jeager, M., Torres, M., Leutzinger, J., & Baun, W. (1998). *The game of lifestyle change* [On-line]. Available: http://healthyculture.com/Resource_Sheets/RSglc.asp.

Allen, R., Allen, J., Kraft, C., & Certner, B. (1987). The organizational unconscious. Burlington, VT: Human Resources Institute.

Allen, R. F. (1981). Quoted from address given in honor of receiving the Plattsburgh State University College Distinguished Alumnus Award.

Allen, R. F., & Allen, J. R. (1987). A sense of community, a shared vision, and a positive culture: Core enabling factors in culture-based health promotion efforts. *American Journal of Health Promotion, 1*(3), 40–47.

Allen, R. F., Dubin, H. N., Pilnick, S., & Youtz, A. C. (1981). *Collegefields: From delinquency to freedom.* New York: Irvington Publishers.

Allen, R. F., & Kraft, C. (1980). *Beat the system: A way to create more human environments.* Burlington, VT: Human Resources Institute Press.

Allen, R. F., & Linde, S. (1981). *Lifegain: The exciting new program that will change your health—and your life.* Burlington, VT: Human Resources Institute Press.

Allen, R. F. & Silver Zwelg, S. (1977). *Changing the Corporate Culture.* Sloan Management Review, *17*(3), 141–154.

Asch, S. E. (1955). Opinions and social pressure. *Scientific American, 193*(5), 31–35.

Bandura, A. (1977). *Social learning theory.* Englewood Cliffs, NJ: Prentice-Hall, Inc.

Benedict, R. (1934). *Patterns of culture.* Boston/New York: Houghton Mifflin.

Bronowski, J. (1976). *The ascent of man.* Boston: Little Brown.

Eikhoff-Shemek, J. M., & Ryan, K. F. (1995). A comparison of Omaha worksite health promotion activities to the 1992 National Survey with a special perspective on program intervention. *American Journal of Health Promotion, 10* (2), 132–139.

Franklin, B. (1998). *The Autobiography of Benjamin Franklin.* New York: Wordsworth Editions.

Freud, S. (1900). The interpretation of dreams. In J. Strachey (Ed. & Trans.), *The standard edition of the complete psychological works of Freud* (Vol. 5). London: Hogarth Press.

Heider, F. (1958). *The psychology of interpersonal relationships.* New York: Wiley.

Horn, D. (1972). Determinants of change. In J. C. Stone, F. Cohen, and N. E. Adler (Eds.), *The Second World Conference on Smoking and Health.* London: Pitman Medical.

Levering, R., & Moskowitz, M. (1994). *The 100 Best Companies to Work for in America.* New York: Plume.

Lewin, K. (1951). *Field theory in social science.* New York: Harper and Row.

Montague, A. (1986). *Touching: The human significance of skin.* New York: Harper and Row.

Milgram, S. (1974). Obedience to authority. New York: Harper and Row.

Novelli, W. D. (1984). Developing marketing programs. In I. Frederiksen, L. Solomon, &

K. Brehony (Eds.), *Marketing health behavior.* New York: Plenum.

O'Donnell, M. P. (1989). Definition of health promotion: Part III: Expanding the definition. *American Journal of Health Promotion, 3*(3), 5.

O'Donnell, M. P., Bishop, C. A., & Kaplan, K. L. (1997, March/April). Benchmarking best practices in workplace health promotion. *The Art and Science of Health Promotion, 1* (1) 1–8.

Prochaska, J. O, Norcross, J. C., & DiClemente, C. C. (1994). *Changing for good: A revolutionary six stage program for overcoming bad habits and moving your life positively forward.* New York: William Morrow and Company.

Rotter, J. B. (1954). *Social learning in clinical psychology.* Englewood Cliffs, NJ: Prentice-Hall.

Skinner, B. F. (1953). *Science and human behavior.* New York: Macmillan.

Twain, M. (1993). *The adventures of Huckleberry Finn.* New York: Modern Library.

CHAPTER

9

Health Assessment

David R. Anderson, Seth Serxner, and Paul Terry

INTRODUCTION

Health assessment, which may be broadly defined as any analysis of health-related data that evaluates health status or health risk at the individual or organizational level, is a key element of worksite health promotion programs (U.S. Department of Health and Human Services [USDHHS], 1993). At the organizational level, health assessment is an important planning and evaluation tool because it provides information on many aspects of employee and organizational health and well-being. These include health care utilization and costs, employee health behavior, and employee attitudes and beliefs. At the individual level, health assessment can play an important role in a worksite health promotion program by creating a "teachable moment" for the participating employee. In this teachable moment, the employee receives health information and relevant recommendations that may act as a catalyst for initiating behavioral change and health risk reduction.

As in the broader arena of health care, business and economics are clearly intertwined with science in decisions about worksite health promotion and, thus, health assessment. Indeed, many have named cost containment as the primary driver of worksite health promotion. A recent study suggested that improving employee health was only the fourth priority of employers implementing health promotion, coming after reducing health care costs, improving productivity, and retaining employees (William M. Mercer, Inc., 1996). This economic imperative introduces a fundamental difference between worksite health promotion programs and many other population health initiatives. While an axiom of population health programs is to provide "the greatest good for the greatest number," the economics of worksite health promotion programs factor cost-effectiveness or cost-benefit into their criteria for success.

The focus of worksite health promotion on economic outcomes changes many aspects of health assessment. Fundamental health assessment dimensions will vary depending on whether an employer's primary program goal is lowering costs or improving population health. That goal determines which risks are measured and how, which populations are targeted for measurement and ongoing surveillance, follow-up measurement intervals, and how the data are used.

This chapter explores how health assessment data can be used in planning, program development, motivating individuals, monitoring progress, and evaluating outcomes. **Health risk appraisal (HRA)** is a very popular approach to worksite health assessment, partly because it provides informative and action-oriented feedback both to the organization and to the individual employee. Because of its importance in worksite health promotion, HRA will be a focus of this chapter. **Biomedical screening**, which can be implemented independently or in conjunction with HRA, is another important health assessment approach that will be discussed in some detail. In addition to reviewing a range of health assessment approaches, this chapter discusses several HRA applications that are closely linked to the goal of reducing health-related costs.

PLANNING HEALTH ASSESSMENTS

The role and implementation of health assessments vary considerably across different worksite health promotion initiatives. In some worksite programs, gathering health assessment data occurs before planning, while in others the plans are developed first and health assessment serves as a baseline for measuring progress toward goals. Planning and evaluation overlap continuously in most cases, however, with health assessment serving both purposes. Ideally, both health assessment implementation and the overall program are driven by corporate health improvement goals. In turn, health assessment procedures and instruments can be used to support the mission and direction of the program. Additionally, developing a program evaluation strategy begins with an analysis of how program interventions can be monitored with measurable outcome data such as that provided by health assessments.

Value of Health Assessment

Health assessments are a fundamental element of worksite health promotion programs because of their value in planning, program development, motivating individuals, and monitoring progress. Additionally, health assessments provide a perceived benefit to the employee and tend to be viewed as a valuable employee benefit. Finally, health assessments in themselves serve as an intervention by creating a "teachable moment" and providing a context for follow-up interventions.

The value of the planning aspect of health assessments is found in the ability to link the findings of health assessments to prioritizing interventions that will have outcomes consistent with the strategic intent of the organization. As noted earlier in this chapter, much of the impetus for worksite health promotion programs comes from the intention to contain costs. Health assessment data can give a clear picture of which health risks are currently driving health and productivity-related costs and, even more importantly, which are likely to drive future costs. In turn, this information can be used to allocate limited resources to have the highest probability of a positive return on investment. Other chapters in this book provide more detail on targeted intervention strategies that can be used once a given at-risk population has been identified.

Health assessment data also serve as a key element in measuring individual progress and overall program impact. Initial health assessment data serves as the benchmark against which future measures can be compared. Individuals can monitor their progress and work with health professionals to improve their health. Program management staff can monitor the overall impact of their program on key health and behavioral outcomes to determine if they are meeting organizational objectives.

Finally, health assessments in themselves can be an important intervention. Effective feedback of individual health assessment results can create an opportunity to teach and motivate employees to make positive lifestyle changes. The health assessment data also provide program managers with information that can be used to target and tailor interventions to individual risks, readiness, and learning preferences. Various forms of health assessments will be discussed in the following sections.

Health Assessment Framework

No single health assessment measure captures all of the information needed to effectively plan a worksite health promotion program. Furthermore, the nonexperimental, uncontrolled nature of most evaluations of worksite health promotion programs casts doubt on the validity of results based on any single outcome measure. Accordingly, a worksite health assessment strategy that includes a variety of measurement tools is the most likely to provide an adequate understanding of both short-term and long-term program effects (Anderson & Jose, 1987; Hoover, Jensen, Murphy, & Anderson, 1994). A truly comprehensive health assessment approach includes four types of program evaluation measures, with multiple measures within each category: process measures, impact measures, outcome measures, and return-on-investment measures.

Conducting a meaningful evaluation of a worksite health promotion program usually requires developing an analytic database that links individual employees' medical charges to their program data. Because true experimental designs are not usually feasible, this type of database is necessary to correlate program participation and changes in health risks to changes in health care utilization and costs. Some employers have the unique resources required to link program data with medical charges. For most employers, however, such analysis is probably not a useful investment of limited health promotion resources. The process of linking claims data with HRA and program participation data also raises legal and ethical concerns about assuring the confidentiality and privacy of highly sensitive health and medical data. These concerns are serious enough that many employers conclude they outweigh the benefits such linkages could provide in documenting program outcomes.

In addition to the practical difficulties in getting access to data from employer-sponsored health promotion programs, ethical concerns about the need to maintain anonymity raise problems for researchers intent on understanding risk-cost relationships. These conflicts make it very challenging to build an evidence base for the economic benefits of worksite health promotion programs. The need to instill confidence among employees that their health assessment, HRA, and other program data are private, however, is inherently greater than the need to study a relationship that will explain only a fraction of the variation in medical resource use. If employees do not participate in a worksite health promotion program because they fear misuse of program data, the issue of outcome evaluation will be irrelevant.

General Health Screening Assessments

Setting worksite health program goals most often begins with an assessment of current health problems and needs. The specific health assessment requirements and recommended measurement approaches may vary considerably, depending on the size and type of an organization. Small employers with modest program goals may rely almost entirely on the findings of population-based health assessments already conducted by industries like theirs or by their local or state health agencies. Aside from using normative data available in the public domain, small employers often use relatively informal assessment options ranging from oral interviews to focus groups to self-developed surveys. Large employers, on the other hand, are more likely to plan and implement health promotion programs by using a subset of the following assessment resources:

1. **Health Risk Appraisal (HRA):** This popular health assessment tool uses computer software to analyze and report on individual health risks. Input data for the HRA software are obtained from a questionnaire that includes self-reported health behaviors, personal health history, family health history, and, depending on the HRA tool and feasibility, biomedical screening data that is either self-reported or obtained at a worksite health screening. Figure 9-1 provides a sample of typical HRA questions. A key advantage of using HRA as a health assessment tool is its dual role—in addition to providing the organization an aggregate employee health profile for program planning, HRA is particularly valuable when used at the individual level to target health education counseling and other behavioral and risk-reduction interventions.

Well Being

22. Stress can range from minor annoyances to fairly major pressures, problems or difficulties. How stressful is your life?
    a. Not at all stressful
    b. Only slightly stressful
    c. Somewhat stressful
    d. Quite stressful
    e. Extremely stressful

23. How effective are you at dealing with stress in your life?
    a. Not at all effective
    b. Only slightly effective
    c. Somewhat effective
    d. Quite effective
    e. Extremely effective

Activity and Exercise

58. How many **days** per week do you get 30 minutes or more of any **moderate-intensity** physical activity? Examples include walking (moderate pace), dancing, mowing (push mower), slow cycling, softball and golf (on foot).
    a. 7 days
    b. 5 or 6 days
    c. 3 or 4 days
    d. 2 days
    e. 1 day
    f. None

59. How many **days** per week do you participate in 20 minutes or more of **vigorous exercise**? (Examples: brisk walking, running, fast cycling, swimming, aerobics, racquetball, stair/ski/rowing machine).
    a. 5 or more days
    b. 4 days
    c. 3 days
    d. 2 days
    e. 1 day
    f. None

Figure 9-1 Sample HRA Questions

Source: HealthPath Health Risk Assessment, The StayWell Company. Reprinted with permission.

2. **Biomedical Screening:** Aggregate biomedical screening data can be used to assess organizational health risks. Many worksite health promotion programs offer biomedical health screening, sometimes on a stand-alone basis but most often in conjunction with an HRA. In the latter case, the biomedical measurements (such as weight, blood pressure, and blood chemistries) are combined with the HRA's self-reported behavioral, family, and personal health history data in scoring the individual results. Some worksite health promotion programs, particularly those with on-site fitness centers, also include fitness testing in their health assessment protocol. Fitness testing is sometimes implemented along with other biomedical measurements in the HRA screening protocol, in which case it is typically made available to all of those who participate in the HRA. If fitness testing is implemented specifically to support fitness center operation, however, it is most commonly offered on a stand-alone basis to fitness center members at the time of initial enrollment to establish a baseline for exercise program prescription and periodically thereafter to monitor progress. In this case, fitness testing is less useful for organizational health assessment because results are only reflective of fitness center members whose fitness levels are likely to be higher than the broader employee population. Other chapters in this book go into detailed discussion of the assessment of various risk factors.

3. **Employee Health Survey:** A census survey of health needs in an employee population or a random-sample survey, typically administered anonymously, is sometimes used to assess the health and safety needs of the population. These surveys may focus on a single issue (e.g., attitudes about a proposed corporate smoking policy) or encompass a broad range of issues, such as health habits and psychological well-being, worksite stress and job satisfaction, health history, health awareness, attitudes about organizational health policies, and individual health needs and preferences. If the cost of health screening and HRA is considered too high, an employee health survey can be a low-cost substitute that still provides some of the planning and evaluation features of an HRA. Unlike an HRA, however, the benefit to the respondent is minimal, and there is no opportunity for program delivery staff to follow up with individual participants to offer interventions or to link the data to objective measures such as health screening or claims data. When getting a representative profile of employee health is a concern, an employee health survey is sometimes recommended instead of a voluntary employee health screening or HRA. It should be kept in mind,

however, that a method for achieving a high response rate is still necessary to avoid the typical problem of more educated or health-oriented employees being overrepresented among survey respondents.

4. **Health Interest Survey:** While HRA is typically focused on health risks, interest surveys concentrate on gathering information on employee preferences among alternative opportunities for learning at the worksite. A challenge for program planners is to match assessment findings about health problems with the types of programs that would be widely used by employees. It is helpful in meeting this challenge to survey employees' readiness to change (Prochaska & DiClemente, 1992; Prochaska, Norcross, & DiClemente, 1994) in various health areas, as well as to survey their learning preferences. Interest surveys are a convenient and parsimonious means of keeping plans relevant and timely for employees. Fortunately for program planners, some HRAs have begun including interest measures, which offers them the advantage of obtaining individual targeting data as well as organization-level assessment.

HRA and biomedical screening are probably the most widely used health assessment approaches in worksite health promotion programs, with both offering the distinct advantage of informing and motivating the individual participant as well as providing aggregate data. Because of their widespread use, it is important to understand their limitations as well as their strengths. Although both can be important catalysts for employees considering lifestyle improvements, HRA and screening are both usually voluntary and may be particularly attractive to the more motivated or "worried well" employees. This type of systematic variation in participation rates can yield aggregate health risk profiles that do not accurately reflect the overall employee population, a problem statisticians call "selection bias." Despite this common limitation, HRA and screening data can play a valuable role in documenting the value of worksite health promotion, as illustrated in a recent study by the Health Enhancement Research Organization (see Figure 9-2).

Assessment resources in successful health promotion programs place an emphasis on program evaluation for the purposes of cost justification and continuous quality improvement. Health assessment resources need to be inextricably linked to program planning, goals, and objectives if worksite health promotion is to improve organizational health and save money for the employer.

HEALTH RISK APPRAISAL IN WORKSITE HEALTH PROMOTION

HRA has become a popular fixture in worksite health promotion programs. According to a national survey of worksite health promotion activities, the majority of large employers have used HRA in their health promotion programs. This 1992 study indicated that activities to measure employee health status/health risk were offered at 52% of worksites with fifty or more employees (USDHHS, 1993). As a further indicator of their proliferation, the Society of Prospective Medicine, a professional organization that supports the development of health assessment tools, listed 43 commercial HRA products available from 34 different companies in their most recent edition of the *SPM Handbook of Health Assessment Tools* (Hyner et al., 1999).

Disease Prediction versus Health Promotion

The genesis of HRA was in the clinical medicine and epidemiological thinking of 30 years ago (Robbins & Hall, 1970). Many HRAs continue to provide the participant with prescriptive and "medicalized" feedback, couched in clinical language and often reporting "health age" or similar complex statistical concepts developed in the earliest HRA instruments. This "mortality-based" approach is based on algorithms (i.e., logical and mathematical calculations) that predict an individual participant's risk of death from various diseases over some future period, most often the next ten years, as a statistical probability. These mortality calculations are compared to population averages to generate feedback that focuses on the participant's relative risk of dying from particular diseases, with supporting feedback that identifies risk factors (i.e., health-related behaviors and biomedical

One of the most promising new developments in building a scientifically credible economic case for worksite health promotion is the recent emergence of the Health Enhancement Research Organization (HERO). HERO is a consortium of industry and scientific experts committed to evaluating the cost-effectiveness and return on investment of health promotion and disease prevention (Whitmer & Dundon, 1997). HERO has taken a significant first step toward fulfilling this commitment by assembling a large multi-employer database containing health risk appraisal (HRA), biomedical screening, medical plan enrollment, and medical claims data on more than 46,000 employees over a six-year period. Findings of the first study using this database suggest a strong link between health risks and medical costs–key support for the idea that the return on investment in worksite health promotion can be increased by targeting high-risk employees (Goetzel et al., 1998). The figure below summarizes the results of the first HERO study, showing the impact of health risks on individual health care costs.

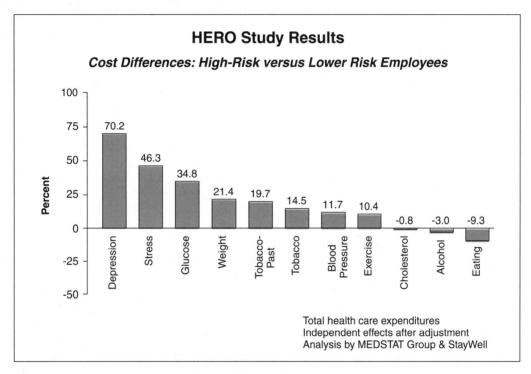

Figure 9-2 The HERO Database

measures) related to each cause of death. Additional calculations produce an "achievable health age" and achievable risk of death from the various causes, which represent the reduction in risk the participant could achieve by reducing their controllable risk factors to minimum levels. This type of feedback on current mortality risk and the potential impact of risk-factor modification on mortality risk was assumed by the developers of these mortality prediction tools to be an effective stimulus for healthy lifestyle change.

There is little scientific evidence, however, to support the notion that a mortality-based approach to HRA is likely to be effective in influencing future health risks. If an HRA is intended to shape future health behavior, it is not clear why a review of likely causes of death or the cost of illness would contribute to an understanding of how to change health habits. It is this conceptual gap that compelled proponents of innovation in HRA to support a change in the theoretical foundation of HRA from a mortality-based to a habit-based, or behavioral, approach that focuses on the individual's health behaviors (Terry, 1987). This shift is also consistent with the experience of most worksite health promotion practitioners, who favor a more positive approach to providing individual feedback with an emphasis on employee assets rather than illness.

The popular perception of HRA is that it reliably predicts an individual's mortality or other health-related risks even though the feedback is based on group probabilities (DeFriese, 1987). Since most practitioners view HRA as an appealing means of motivating employees to consider participating in health improvement programs, concern about the prescriptive capacity of the instrument is seldom expressed. Indeed, HRA feedback has significant educational and motivational value even when presented most accurately as the "average risk" for a person of the participant's age, sex, health history, and risk profile. Nevertheless, health promotion practitioners and other users of HRA tools should recognize that an individual's true risk is probably only marginally related to probabilities based on highly variable group risk distributions. Although there is good evidence supporting the "predictive validity" of HRA mortality projections at the group level (Smith, McKinlay, & Thorington, 1987), neither HRA nor any other current risk projection technology can predict an individual's future health status with a great degree of accuracy.

In addition to the ability of HRA to project group-level mortality, research has also documented the association between HRA results and other health-related outcomes. Studies have linked HRA-based health age or risk factor measurements to concurrent or prospective health care costs (Brink, 1987; Goetzel et al., 1998; Golaszewski, Lynch, Clearie, & Vickery, 1989; Vickery, Golaszewski, Wright, & McPhee, 1986) and to absenteeism (Bertera, 1991; Yen, Edington, & Witting, 1992). Such studies provide further support for the predictive validity of HRA at the group level. Their results also suggest that HRA may become a useful instrument for projecting the cost impact of health promotion programs, especially if changes in health care costs and absenteeism can be linked directly to corresponding changes in HRA results.

HRA as a Behavior Change Intervention

Research has documented little effectiveness of HRAs as a stand-alone behavior change intervention. This general lack of behavioral impact found in HRA research, however, may be because the tools used in published research (as well as most other existing HRA tools) were developed by biomedical experts rather than experts in behavior change theory and practice (Anderson & Staufacker, 1996). Victor Strecher of the University of Michigan and Matthew Kreuter of Saint Louis University acknowledge the lack of behavior-change expertise in most past HRA development but express optimism about the potential to develop HRAs that are effective behavior change tools (Strecher & Kreuter, 1999). Analyzing the role of HRA feedback using the Health Belief Model (Becker, 1974), which conceptualizes health behavior change as a function of perceived threat of a negative health outcome and perceived benefits (minus perceived barriers) of a preventive activity, Strecher and Kreuter make three recommendations for designing more behaviorally-focused HRAs.

Their first recommendation is to "provide feedback designed to correct users' inaccurate perceptions of their own risk." A substantial amount of research indicates that most people tend to underestimate their health risk (e.g., Avis, Smith, & McKinlay, 1989; Skinner, Kreuter, & Strecher, 1998; Weinstein, 1984). Others—called the "worried well" in the health promotion profession—overestimate their risk and, consequently, often seek health care unnecessarily. If it were designed to take advantage of what researchers have discovered about the causes of these inaccurate perceptions, Strecher and Kreuter believe HRA feedback could move users toward more accurate perceptions of their level of risk. Although acknowledging that changes in perceptions alone are not sufficient to elicit changes in behavior, they believe it is an essential step in the change process. After all, people who underestimate their risk are not likely to be motivated to change.

Strecher and Kreuter's second recommendation is to "provide feedback that establishes behavior change priorities when multiple risk factors exist." The importance of this prioritization becomes clear when one reviews typical HRA feedback to high-risk participants–faced with a seemingly impossible list of firmly entrenched behaviors and risk factors that the HRA recommends be changed, it is not surprising that many of these individuals would be overwhelmed and consequently less likely to act on recommendations. As well as focusing high-risk participants on changing a small number of habits at a time, it is also important that the right criteria be used in establishing this prioritization. Strecher and Kreuter identify five specific criteria they believe are important in prioritizing change recommendations: epidemiologic risk, readiness to make behavioral changes, self-efficacy for behavioral changes, quality-adjusted life years, and gateways to behavioral change.

With the exception of epidemiologic risk, which HRA feedback has traditionally relied on in the form of mortality risk or morbidity risk, all of these criteria are psychosocial factors. Readiness to change (see Table 9-1) refers to the importance of focusing behavioral recommendations on risks the employee is interested in changing (Prochaska & DiClemente, 1992; Prochaska et al., 1994), a seemingly obvious notion

that has often been ignored in the health promotion profession. Self-efficacy refers to the individual's confidence that he or she can succeed in modifying the unhealthy behavior or risk factor (Bandura, 1977). Quality-adjusted life years move beyond a simplistic measure of mortality risk to take into account the individual's experience of those additional years of life (Kaplan, 1985). Gateways to behavioral change refer to the idea that certain key health-related changes, such as engaging in physical activity or reducing stress, may "open the gate" to making other changes like quitting smoking, reducing depression, or losing weight (Landsbergis et al., 1998; USDHHS, 1996).

The final recommendation Strecher and Kreuter make is to "provide feedback that enhances the user's ability to make recommended health behavior changes." The feedback many HRAs provide on recommended changes is behaviorally very weak, often just telling the user what behaviors need to be changed to reduce their risk with no individually tailored information on how to go about making the changes. To become more effective as a behavior-change tool, an HRA questionnaire needs to assess

Table 9-1   Prochaska's "Stages of Change" Model of Behavior Change

Prochaska's Transtheoretical Model of behavior change, most commonly referred to as the "Stages of Change" Model, provides a very useful framework for discussing the role of the HRA in the behavior change process. Briefly, the model asserts that individuals move through six discrete stages in changing an unhealthy behavior or other problem behavior. (It should be noted that one should be able to apply the "stages of change" model equally well to describing changes in positive behaviors.) Each subsequent stage represents a heightened "readiness" to change, and successfully navigating each stage in the change process requires different cognitive, motivational, or behavioral processes. Individuals typically cycle through these stages multiple times before achieving the final stage (Prochaska & DiClemente, 1992; Prochaska, Norcross, & DiClemente, 1994).

Stage	Description
Precontemplation	The individual denies the problem or recognizes it but is not motivated to change.
Contemplation	The individual begins to think about change in the distant future and to consider the "pros" and "cons".
Preparation	Once the "pros" of change sufficiently outweigh the "cons," the individual commits to the change in the immediate future and makes specific plans.
Action	The individual initiates overt behavior changes.
Maintenance	Focus is on solidifying new behaviors to last a lifetime.
Termination	Individuals no longer think about the past, unhealthy behaviors or feel temptation to return to them.

The following is feedback to a currently sedentary HRA participant who is also overweight:

STEPS YOU CAN TAKE TODAY Imagine how your life would change if you lived an active lifestyle. The benefits of becoming more active include reducing your weight, developing stronger heart and lungs, improving your self-esteem, and feeling more energetic. Record these and other "pros" of living an active lifestyle and compare them to your list of "cons." Review this list frequently.

Figure 9-3 Sample HRA Feedback Tailored to Stage of Change

Source: HealthPath Health Risk Assessment, The StayWell Company. Reprinted with permission.

not only an individual's health risks, but also behavioral and psychosocial factors that affect their motivation and ability to change health behaviors, and HRA feedback needs to capitalize on this additional information. For example, collecting information on barriers to change and addressing these barriers in educational feedback has been shown to increase positive behavior change (Skinner, Strecher, & Hospers, 1994; Strecher et al., 1994). Figure 9-3 provides another example, in which the participant's HRA feedback has been tailored according to stage of change–see if you can identify the stage from the feedback.

The Optimal Role of HRA in the Change Process

With changes such as those recommended by Strecher and Kreuter, it is likely that HRAs can become more effective in stimulating a modest level of health-related behavior change, even without follow-up interventions. No matter how well behavioral science and individually tailored messaging are incorporated into HRA feedback design, however, many individuals will still require ongoing support and follow-up over an extended time period in order to successfully navigate the change process. For this reason, experienced health promotion practitioners consider HRA to be a potentially valuable educational and motivational tool for *initiating* the behavior-change process. They clearly recognize, however, that many high-risk individuals and others attempting to

change long-term unhealthy habits also need follow-up interventions focused on developing behavior change and maintenance skills.

Viewed from the conceptual framework of the stages of change model, HRAs are most useful in helping participants move through the early stages of change—from precontemplation to contemplation and from contemplation to preparation. HRAs can create positive movement through these stages by heightening participants' awareness about their susceptibility to poor health outcomes, consequences of their unhealthy behaviors, what they can do to reduce their risks, and the many benefits of change (Becker, 1974). As noted by Strecher and Kreuter (1999), HRAs can also support movement through the stages by suggesting strategies for overcoming barriers to change.

In addition to their direct role in the behavior-change process, HRAs can be designed to provide exactly the data needed to help steer participants to the follow-up interventions that will be most effective in helping them change. If the HRA includes behavioral and psychosocial data, these data can be used to fine-tune the intervention targeting process. For example, sedentary individuals who indicate on their HRA a high state of readiness to exercise in the near future and who also request support can be referred to a fitness program. Depending on their preferences, they could be offered a group program, one-on-one counseling, or serial self-help mailings. On the other hand, those not currently interested in exercise can be offered information about the health effects of a sedentary lifestyle or can be offered appropriate programs targeting other risks that this individual is currently ready to change. Figure 9-3 provides a sample of feedback targeted to stage of change.

Selecting the Right HRA

Since the development of HRA has evolved more because of the needs of practitioners than of the findings of systematic research, it behooves worksite health promotion practitioners to be vigilant in choosing an HRA that meets the needs unique to their organization. Admittedly, evaluating the effectiveness of alternative HRA tools in influencing health practices is difficult given the sparse data currently available. Still, the worksite practitioner is ultimately responsible for choosing an HRA that supports the vision and mission of the organization's health promotion program. Practitioners should examine each aspect of a proposed HRA tool and ask the designers why their tool is desirable. The Society of Prospective Medicine's recently published handbook on health assessment tools provides a great deal of information on how to select the right HRA for a particular application, as well as extensive information on commercially available tools (Hyner et al., 1999). Evaluating potential HRA tools requires getting answers to an extensive set of questions about each tool being considered. Table 9-2 provides examples of some of the kinds of questions that should be asked when selecting an HRA tool. The discussion of behavioral issues in HRA design earlier in this chapter provides additional ideas for important questions to ask in evaluating various HRA tools.

BIOMEDICAL SCREENING IN WORKSITE HEALTH PROMOTION

Many HRA tools, particularly the first-generation HRAs that evolved from the mortality-based tradition of prospective medicine, are designed to provide mortality projections that depend substantially on biomedical screening data. As well as being used in the HRA scoring algorithms, the results of screening tests are typically included in the HRA participant's report along with feedback based on self-reported data. Today's most advanced HRAs fully integrate the biomedical screening results into the participant's report and further personalize the report by tailoring messages throughout based on health risks, psychosocial/behavioral data, and other relevant information.

Early worksite health promotion programs often consisted solely of a health assessment process that combined a limited HRA with a very extensive biomedical screening battery. This narrow approach was based on the assumption that screening results

Table 9-2 Sample Questions in Selecting an HRA

1. Services Needed
   - Can "instant HRA feedback" be provided at a worksite screening or health fair?
   - Is the HRA available online via the internet/intranet?
2. Adequacy of the Science Base
   - Is information available about the science on which the HRA is based?
   - What elements are included from the Health Belief Model, the Stages of Change Model, or another scientifically validated behavior-change model?
3. Ease of Participation
   - How long does it take to complete the HRA questionnaire and read the report?
   - What is the reading level of the HRA material?
4. Use of Questionnaires
   - Are the health areas covered appropriate for the intended audience?
   - Are instructions clear for completing and returning the questionnaire?

5. Use of Individual Reports
   - Will participants be able to understand the statistics, terminology, and graphics?
   - What percent of the text is standard, and what percent is individualized? How much can it be tailored to the participant or client organization?
6. Availability of Aggregate and Group Data
   - To whom does the data in the database belong?
   - What aggregate reports can be created without custom programming?
7. Systems Considerations
   - What are the vendor's plans for updating software and systems requirements?
   - How are data backed up, stored, and retained for future access?
8. Customer Service
   - What staff is available to support my program?
   - How am I charged for the products and services I receive?

Source: G. Hyner et al., *SPM Handbook of Health Assessment Tools*, 1999. Adapted with permission.

providing "objective medical evidence" of a significant health risk would be sufficiently threatening to motivate participants to take prescribed actions to reduce their risk. This "common-sense" notion that awareness of risk alone is sufficient to motivate widespread, long-term behavior change, whether based on self-reported HRA or biomedical screening results, has largely disappeared from the health promotion landscape. Research has established what experienced practitioners already recognized—health information can play an important role in reducing health risks but only if it is integrated into a comprehensive health promotion process that includes behavior change skill-building and maintenance components (Anderson & Staufacker, 1996).

Decisions about which biomedical measures to include in worksite health promotion have been influenced markedly in the past decade by the recommendations of the U.S. Preventive Services Task Force (1996). With its evidence-based approach to decisions about preventive screening and its advocacy for more counseling and less population-wide testing, the Task Force called for the virtual abandonment of the "annual physical exam" and other screening tests with unproven effectiveness. The shift to more conservative and targeted use of biomedical screening tests is consistent with the focus of managed care organizations and other capitated health care systems on demand-side management and evidence of return on investment. Biomedical screening tests and other assessment measures that are now being sought for most worksite-based health promotion initiatives, are most useful for generating the individual data needed to manage targeted follow-up interventions, assess aggregate employee health risk, and evaluate program impact (Anderson & Staufacker, 1996).

In addition to science-based recommendations about conducting specific biomedical screening tests, there are very practical considerations for the program planner in deciding whether to implement biomedical screening and in selecting tests to include in the screening protocol. Screening opportunities such as blood pressure or cholesterol tests are extremely popular employee benefits. Employees al-most universally find it much more interesting to get feedback on their vital measures than solely to get feedback on self-reported HRA data. For that reason, many health promotion program planners try to increase HRA participation by administering it as part of an annual or biannual screening event or health fair. Because some biomedical measures are recommended less often than this for most people (e.g., lipid measurement is recommended every five years for low risk individuals) and some screening tests can be relatively costly, program planners often stagger the screening components from year to year. For example, low-cost screening measures like height, weight, and blood pressure may be done with every HRA, while blood chemistries and fitness testing are done in alternate years. Although most contemporary HRAs produce valid risk feedback with or without clinical values, program planners should insure that the HRA they use can accommodate variation in the screening protocol and that recommended screening intervals and risk criteria are consistent with the organization's health care philosophy and policies.

In some instances, the scientific evidence for performing clinical tests is equivocal and the recommended intervals for conducting the exams are controversial. In these cases, employee preferences should be considered in determining the health screening protocol. For example, the American Cancer Society recommends mammograms every 1–2 years for all women beginning at age 40 and annually beginning at age 50, while the U.S. Preventive Services Task Force recommends screening every 1–2 years only for women aged 50–69 or those aged 40–49 or 70+ who are at high risk. Similar contradictions based on a review of the same scientific evidence exist for stool occult blood tests, prostate specific antigen (PSA) tests, and digital rectal exams. Given the absence of clear evidence for or against a particular clinical recommendation, it behooves the health promotion planner to make allowances for the values of the employee in determining the best approach. It is also important that program planners responsible for health screening distinguish between science-based recommendations and values-based personal choices.

Blood Pressure Screening

Given the prevalence and serious complications of hypertension, its ease of detection, and the effectiveness of treatment, periodic blood pressure screening is recommended for all persons aged 21 or above (U.S. Preventive Services Task Force, 1996). Furthermore, the workplace has been identified as a useful setting for hypertension detection and follow-up programs (Alderman and Lamport, 1988).

While blood pressure measurement can be highly accurate, potential sources of error must be considered. Sphygmomanometry (i.e., blood pressure measurement) errors can occur from machine or cuff malfunction. All blood pressure measuring equipment requires periodic calibration for proper functioning. Table 9-3 includes guidelines for blood pressure measurement offered by the U.S. Preventive Services Task Force (1996).

Normal blood pressure, which is an "average" level for good health, is considered by medical experts to be 120/80 mm Hg. Anyone with blood pressure consistently at or above 140/90 (i.e., systolic reading of 140+ or diastolic 90+) is considered to have hypertension and be "at risk" for related medical complications like cardiovascular and kidney disease. Those consistently at or above 160/100 are considered to be "at high risk." Table 9-4 provides standards for use in worksite blood pressure screenings (National High Blood Pressure Education Program, 1992).

Combining blood pressure screening with ongoing hypertension monitoring is a key component of disease management programming. A study of the hypertension management program at HealthSystem Minnesota shows the value of standardized approaches to measurement in detecting hypertension. Out of 275 participants referred for screening, 78% had normal blood pressure. This data suggests that screening techniques using multiple measures insure that participants will not be unnecessarily treated. The study also indicates the value of educational interventions in helping participants control their blood pressure. At entry into the management phase of the program, only 17% of participants had blood pressure within controlled limits. By the 12-month follow-up, this proportion had increased to 44% versus 27% in the comparison group. The 6 mm Hg average decrease in systolic blood pressure found in this study is associated with a 34% reduction in strokes and a 24% reduction in heart disease (Pheley, Terry, Pietz, Fowles, McCoy, & Smith, 1995).

Weight and Body Composition Screening

Despite the widely publicized health consequences of obesity and billions of dollars spent annually on weight loss efforts, the prevalence of overweight has increased steadily in the United States in recent decades (Kuczmarski, Flegal, Campbell, & Johnson, 1994; Galuska, Serdula, Pamuk, Siegel, & Byers, 1996). Most health complications of obesity are actually attributable to body fatness, with "male-pattern" fat distribution (i.e., excess abdominal fat) predicting the highest coronary heart disease risks (Pollock & Wilmore, 1990). Since body fatness can be more difficult to measure reliably than weight, however, many practitioners and researchers use body mass index (BMI) as a proxy for body composition. BMI is

Table 9-3 Guidelines for Sphygmomanometry

- Clients should be seated with bare arm at heart level.
- Clients should have had no recent smoking, caffeine, or exertion and should rest quietly for five minutes before measuring.
- An appropriate cuff size with the bladder encircling at least two-thirds of the arm should be used.
- Measurement should be taken preferably with a mercury sphygmomanometer (a recently calibrated aneroid sphygmomanometer or a validated device can also be used).
- Both systolic and diastolic pressures, using the disappearance of sound as the diastolic, should be recorded.
- Two or more readings, separated by 2 minutes, should be averaged. If the first two readings differ by more than 5mm Hg, additional readings should be obtained and averaged.

Source: Joint National Committee on Prevention, Detection, Evaluation and Treatment of High Blood Pressure, *Archives of Internal Medicine*, 1997.

Table 9-4 Worksite Blood Pressure Screening Standards and Follow-up Criteria

A. Initial Screening–Standards for Blood Pressure

Blood Pressure		
Low Risk	Moderate Risk	High Risk
>140/90	140/90–159/99	160/100+

B. Follow-up Recommendations for Initial Blood Pressure Measurements in Adults 18 Years or Older

Initial Screening Blood Pressure (mm Hg)*		Follow-up Criteria[†]
Systolic	Diastolic	
<130	<85	Recheck in 2 years
130–139	85–89	Recheck in 1 year**
140–159	90–99	Confirm within 2 months
160–179	100–109	Evaluate or refer to source of care within 1 month.
180–209	110–119	Evaluate or refer to source of care within 1 week.
≥210	≥120	Evaluate or refer to source of care immediately.

Note. *If the systolic and diastolic categories are different, follow recommendation for the shorter time follow-up (e.g., 160/85 mm Hg should be evaluated or referred to source of care within 1 month). Blood pressure measurement and follow-up criteria are based on the average of two or more readings.
†The scheduling of follow-up should be modified by reliable information about past blood pressure measurements, other cardiovascular risk factors, or target-organ disease.
**Consider providing advice about lifestyle modifications.
Source: Adapted from the National High Blood Pressure Education Program, *The Fifth Report of the Joint National Committee on Detection, Evaluation, and Treatment of High Blood Pressure*, 1992.

defined as weight in kilograms divided by the square of the individual's height in meters and is highly correlated with total body fat.

In response to the increasing problem of obesity, the National Institutes of Health recently issued the first federal guidelines on the identification, evaluation, and treatment of overweight and obesity in adults (National Heart, Lung and Blood Institute, 1999). According to the guidelines, assessment of overweight involves the evaluation of three key measures–BMI, waist circumference, and risk factors for diseases and conditions associated with obesity. Periodic assessment was recommended every two years. The guidelines identify **overweight** for both men and women as a BMI of 25 to 29.9 and **obesity** as a BMI of 30 and above. A BMI of 30, which is approximately 30 pounds overweight through the middle of the height range, equals 221 pounds for a 6-foot person and 186 pounds for a 5-foot 6-inch person. The panel recognized that very muscular people could have a high BMI without health risk, which is partially addressed by adding waist circumference to the risk assessment process. A waist circumference of over 40 inches in men and over 35 inches in women is associated with increased risk in those who have a BMI of 25 to 34.9. The presence of associated risk factors (see Table 9-5) further increases the risk level of overweight or obese individuals.

Table 9-5 Risk Factors Affecting Risk Level of Overweight and Obese Persons

Risk Factor	Examples
Disease conditions	established coronary heart disease (CHD), other atherosclerotic diseases, type II diabetes, and sleep apnea (Patients with these conditions are classified as being at very high risk for disease complications and mortality.)
Other obesity-associated diseases	gynecological abnormalities, osteoarthritis, gallstones and their complications, and stress incontinence.
Cardiovascular risk factors	cigarette smoking, hypertension (systolic blood pressure $\geq$ 140 mm Hg or diastolic blood pressure $\geq$ 90 mm Hg, or the patient is taking antihypertensive agents), high-risk LDL (low-density lipoprotein) cholesterol ($\geq$ 160 mg/dL), low HDL (high-density lipoprotein) cholesterol (>35 mg/dL), impaired fasting glucose (fasting plasma glucose of 110 to 125 mg/dL), family history of premature CHD (definite myocardial infarction or sudden death at or before 55 years of age in father or other male first-degree relative, or at or before 65 years of age in mother or other female first-degree relative), and age (men $\geq$ 45 years and women $\geq$ 55 years or postmenopausal). (Patients can be classified as being at high absolute risk if they have three of these risk factors.)
Other risk factors	physical inactivity and high serum triglycerides (> 200 mg/dL). (When these factors are present, patients can be considered to have incremental absolute risk above that estimated from the preceding risk factors. Quantitative risk contribution is not available for these risk factors, but their presence heightens the need for weight reduction in obese persons.)

Source: National Heart, Lung and Blood Institute, *Clinical guidelines on the identification, evaluation, and treatment of overweight and obesity in adults*, 1999.

Obesity can also be defined based on body fatness as an excessive percentage of body fat relative to total body mass, with suggested cutoff points of 35% in women and 30% in men (Wadden & Bell, 1990). Body fat can be estimated using electrical impedance testing, skin-fold caliper readings, body circumference measures, and, more recently, infrared reflected-light technology.

Skin-fold measures have assumed common practice in estimating body fat because they are relatively easy to administer, inexpensive calipers are widely available, and various equations have been developed to convert body density to percent body fat. Sites generally tested include some combination of chest, axilla, triceps, subscapula, abdominal, suprailium, and thigh (Pollock & Wilmore, 1990). Tester technique, site selection, skin-fold size, leanness, age, and sex are all determinants of adipose density and predicted body-fat percentage. Based on their observations, Martin, Ross, Drinkwater, and Clarys (1985) concluded that skin-fold thickness alone, without being transformed by a mathematical formula into percent fat, is a reasonable indicator of body structure that can be measured serially for change. These authors called for skilled technicians making repeated measures on a number of sites, including arm, anterior and posterior torso, and leg. The skin-fold measure is quite consistent over brief measurement intervals.

Bioelectrical impedance is another method for estimating body composition that has the advantage of largely eliminating tester error. However, the reliability of this body fat measure requires standardization and control of a number of variables, including body position, hydration status, consumption of food and beverages, ambient air and skin temperature, recent physical activity, and conductance of the examining table (National Institutes of Health, 1994). Although bioelectrical impedance is popular with participants because of its "high-tech" nature, which makes it an attractive tool for increasing participation in worksite screenings, it should probably not be used in an uncontrolled setting like the worksite if precise measurement is required. Newer techniques that rely on reflected light appear to eliminate some of these control problems but must await further validation studies.

Obesity has been associated with a wide range of health problems, and weight control remains one of the most popular worksite health promotion programs. Unfortunately, those who participate in weight loss programs are often those who need them the least (i.e., they are participating for "cosmetic" purposes). Health promotion program planners should also take into consideration the effectiveness of the weight loss options available to employees. A stark but reasonable conclusion is that no interventions have been proven to be highly effective in population-based weight management (Brownell, 1993). Nevertheless, obesity is such an insidious and costly problem, both medically and personally, that planners may decide it deserves continued intervention efforts and compassionate and creative attempts at implementing effective programs. Because weight "recycling" is the most common result of weight loss attempts and can have a variety of unhealthy consequences (Brownell & Rodin, 1994), screening and intervention for obesity must be considered within the context of an ongoing plan for targeted interventions and relapse prevention (Brownell & Wadden, 1992).

Because of the well-documented foibles of weight management programs, many have concluded that decreased health risks and increased well-being and self-esteem, rather than a focus on weight per se, should be the goal of treatment (Foreyt & Goodrick, 1994). With this approach, some planners may even conclude that screening for weight is superfluous. Companies that have offered worksite health promotion programs for many years may find the notion of discontinuing screening for weight counterintuitive. It is incumbent on the health promotion advocate, however, either to be prepared to refute the value of weight as an independent risk factor or to be prepared to offer a workable solution to the obesity epidemic. Given weight loss intervention results to date, neither position will be easy or comfortable to defend.

Blood Chemistry Screening

A large and growing number of parameters of health and organ function can be assayed with a small specimen of blood. With the ability to collect so much information at minimal incremental cost per parameter tested, far-ranging blood chemistry analysis is difficult for many health assessment planners to resist. They ask themselves, "why just do a few tests when, for very little additional cost, I can do a full battery of tests of metabolic function (glucose, uric acid, cholesterol, triglycerides, LDL and HDL cholesterols), liver function (transaminases, bilirubin, alkaline phosphatase), muscle function (LDH, CPK), and proteins (albumin, total protein)?"

In asking this question, however, they must understand that the "normal" range for each test is based on the statistical distribution of a measure with less than perfect reliability. There is a very real probability of two types of erroneous results on each test administered—a **false positive** when the test result is abnormal but the underlying condition is not present, or a **false negative** when the test result is normal but the underlying condition is present. The more tests administered to an individual, the greater the probability of one or more erroneous abnormal results. Further, administering a test to an asymptomatic person for a condition with a low prevalence rate means that the abnormal result will most commonly be a false positive. In these cases, the test is positive (i.e., abnormal), but the disease is not present. A false abnormal result on even one test (a high probability event when a SMAC-20 or similar comprehensive blood panel is done) results in needless anxiety for the employee and needless costs associated with referring the employee to a physician for follow-up evaluation and even more testing.

For this reason, experienced worksite health promotion planners include in periodic population-wide screenings only tests for conditions that are prevalent, potentially serious, and for which the test is reasonably specific and sensitive. (A "specific" test is one with a low rate of false positives; a sensitive test is one with a low rate of false negatives.) Follow-up testing is targeted to the subset of individuals determined to be at high risk for a specific condition. Based on these criteria, the blood chemistry tests recommended for population-wide use at the worksite include blood cholesterol (total and HDL) to screen for the very prevalent heart disease risk, and blood glucose to screen for the very serious problem of diabetes (U.S. Preventive Services Task Force, 1996).

Blood Cholesterol Screening

Although the coronary heart disease (CHD) mortality rate has decreased in recent decades, CHD remains by far the leading cause of death in the United States (Hunink et al., 1997). Along with smoking and hypertension, high total blood cholesterol is a major risk factor for CHD (Kannel, Castelli & Gordon, 1979), and lowering blood cholesterol has been shown to significantly reduce CHD risk (Frick et al., 1987).

The most recent recommendations of the expert panel for cholesterol management convened by the National Cholesterol Education Program established three categories for total blood cholesterol. Less than 200 mg/dL of total blood cholesterol is "desirable" to lower one's risk of heart disease; 200–239 mg/dL is "borderline-high" and increases one's risk; 240 mg/dL or above is "high" risk (Expert Panel on Detection, Evaluation, and Treatment of High Blood Cholesterol in Adults, 1993). Based on growing evidence that low HDL cholesterol (i.e., high-density lipoprotein) increases risk of CHD, the expert panel also classified low HDL (< 35 mg/dL) as a major risk factor for CHD and recommended including HDL with total blood cholesterol in initial screening. The expert panel further indicated that testing should only be done if accuracy of measurement, appropriate counseling, and follow-up could be assured.

Follow-up lipoprotein analysis and therapeutic prescription by a physician was recommended by the expert panel for all those initially screened who fell into the "high-risk" group due to total blood cholesterol of 240 or above or due to HDL less than 35. Those in the 200–239 borderline-high range were classified as high-risk and referred for follow-up testing if they had two or more CHD risk factors. The expert panel guidelines and follow-up lipid analysis criteria are presented in more detail in Table 9-6.

Blood Glucose Screening

Diabetes is one of the most serious and costly health problems in the United States. It is the seventh leading cause of death and is estimated to cost $44.1 billion annually in direct medical costs and $54 billion in indirect costs (disability, lost productivity, mortality). Unfortunately, many people first become aware that they have diabetes when they develop one of its complications, including heart disease and stroke, blindness, kidney disease, nerve disease and amputations, and impotence. In fact, of the estimated 15.7 million people in the United States who have diabetes, fully 5.4 million (34%) are not aware they have the disease (American Diabetes Association, 1997).

With the high costs of diabetes, both economically and personally, it is critical to identify the large undiagnosed population and triage them to appropriate interventions. Fortunately, diabetes screening can be accomplished with a simple blood glucose test. Testing can either be non-fasting or fasting (for 8 hours prior to testing), with the latter recommended if practical. A fasting glucose level of less than 110 mg/dL is considered normal, and a result of greater than 125 mg/dL yields a provisional diagnosis of diabetes that must be medically confirmed. Those whose values fall in the 110–125 range are classified as having impaired glucose tolerance, which is a risk factor for both diabetes and heart disease (American Diabetes Association, 1999a).

Although diabetes can be extremely destructive, many of its complications can be avoided or ameliorated for a majority of diabetics solely through weight loss, improved nutrition, exercise and, possibly, other lifestyle modifications. A minority of those with diabetes may also require insulin and/or other medications to manage the disease (American Diabetes Association, 1999b).

Fitness Testing

It is important to conduct fitness testing prior to exercise participation in order to screen for those at higher risk of a cardiac event during exercise, to prescribe safe and effective exercise, and to determine baseline functional capacity for ongoing monitoring and program evaluation. Fitness testing is particularly important for

Table 9-6 Blood Cholesterol Screening Standards and Follow-up Criteria

Cholesterol (mg/dL)		
Desirable	**Borderline-High**	**High**
< 200	200–239	240+

Cholesterol (mg/dL)		
High Rank	**Normal**	**Protective**
< 35	35–59	60+

Follow-up Recommendations for Adults with No Personal History of CHD*

Cholesterol Value	HDL Value	Follow-up Recommendation
Desirable blood cholesterol < 200 mg/dL	HDL ≥ 35 mg/dL	Repeat total cholesterol and HDL measurements within 5 years or with physical exam
	HDL < 35 mg/dL	Refer for lipoprotein analysis
Borderline-high blood cholesterol 200–239 mg/dL	HDL ≥ 60 mg/dL *and* < 3 nonlipid CHD risk factors** or HDL 35 – 59 mg/dL *and* < 2 nonlipid CHD risk factors	Reevaluate in 1 to 2 years by repeating total cholesterol and HDL measurements
	HDL ≥ 60 mg/dL *and* ≥ 3 nonlipid CHD risk factors or HDL 35 – 59 mg/dL *and* ≥ 2 nonlipid CHD risk factors or HDL < 35 mg/dL	Refer for lipoprotein analysis
High blood cholesterol ≥ 240 mg/dL	Any Value	Refer for lipoprotein analysis

Note. *All individuals with CHD should be referred to their physician for follow-up.
**Nonlipid CHD risk factors: age (men 45+; women 55+), family history of premature CHD, smoking, hypertension, diabetes.
Source: Expert Panel on Detection, Evaluation, and Treatment of High Blood Cholesterol in Adults, *Journal of the American Medical Association*, 1993.

employers with on-site fitness facilities to manage the liability risk associated with exercise supervision. The components of a fitness test include the following:

- Functional test of cardiovascular endurance to measure or estimate aerobic capacity

- Body composition and circumference measurements to determine body fatness and lean body mass (see earlier section)
- Measurements of flexibility, strength, and muscular endurance to assess the function of joints and muscles

Functional Capacity Test of Cardiovascular Endurance

Functional capacity tests are used to measure or estimate maximal oxygen uptake or aerobic capacity (VO_2max), the largest amount of oxygen one can use under the most strenuous conditions (Pollock & Wilmore, 1990). Normative information on aerobic capacity, which is useful in providing feedback on test results, has been developed by the Institute for Aerobics Research (1989). There are four principles for testing functional capacity (McKiman & Froelicher, 1987):

1. The work must involve large muscle groups.
2. The work must be measurable and reproducible.
3. Test conditions must be such that the results are comparable and repeatable.
4. Testing must be well-tolerated and must not require unusual skill.

Fitness-testing labs affiliated with medical facilities typically conduct a maximal graded exercise test on a motor-driven treadmill or bicycle ergometer, combined with electrocardiographic (EKG) blood pressure monitoring and physician attendance to detect signs of subclinical heart disease. The American College of Sports Medicine (1986) and the American College of Cardiology (Subcommittee on Exercise Testing, 1986) recommend such EKG-monitored, maximal graded exercise tests on those over age 40 or on those with two or more coronary risk factors prior to their participating in a strenuous exercise program. The U.S. Preventive Services Task Force (1996), however, concluded that there was good evidence to recommend *not* using an exercise EKG for screening purposes in clinically healthy persons due to its expense and the low probability that disease would be detected.

Submaximal tests using a treadmill, bicycle ergometer, steps, or timed run or walk are much less useful for the diagnosis of asymptomatic coronary artery disease, but these tests can be used to reliably estimate functional capacity. Submaximal tests rely on attaining a steady state heart rate for a given work load, and then using the heart rate and work load data to project maximum heart rate and VO_2max from nomograms (Pollock & Wilmore, 1990). Distinct advantages of submaximal tests are that they are relatively inexpensive, do not require the presence of a physician, and may or may not use EKG monitoring. They are used most often and appropriately in young healthy populations or in mass testing outside of the lab environment. Bicycle ergometer testing uses a mechanically braked bicycle pedaled at a constant rate over increasing resistance. It has the key advantages of being portable and producing less upper body movement than the treadmill, which makes heart rate and blood pressure measurements easier to obtain.

The easiest and least expensive submaximal tests are the field tests described by Balke (1963) and Cooper (1968) and more recently reviewed and modified by Kline et al. (1987). Kline and his coworkers used a repeated, fast one-mile track walk and treadmill-measured VO_2 to develop a predictive equation for estimating VO_2max in 30- to 69-year-old adults. The advantages over previous studies were use of a larger and older sample size, the high correlation of the prediction equation, and the simplicity of the test, which requires only a measured one-mile flat surface, a stop watch, and accurate pulse measurements (Kline et al., 1987).

Field tests like the timed one-mile walk can be administered safely to most employees at a worksite and repeated whenever necessary to document changes in fitness. However, employees who are committed to a program of vigorous physical activity and who are at high risk of heart disease because of their age and the presence of other coronary risk factors should be referred to their physician for evaluation before beginning their program.

Flexibility, Muscle Strength, and Endurance Testing

Much of the public equates the benefits of exercise with aerobic exercise. However, exercises that improve strength and flexibility may enhance the performance and decrease the risks of vigorous aerobic exercise, while providing additional health benefits of their own. For example, back injury prevention programs, arthritis treatment programs, and the prevention of falls in the elderly typically include exercises that promote strength and flexibility. For this reason, tests of strength and flexibility can be useful as part of an overall fitness assessment. Testing standards and normative information are less established for strength and flexibility testing than for aerobic fitness testing, but helpful information is available from the Institute for Aerobics Research (1989) and the President's Council on Physical Fitness and Sports in Washington, DC. Similarly, there is considerably less scientific documentation of the benefits of exercises to improve strength or flexibility than there is for aerobic exercise.

As with aerobic exercise, strength and flexibility development will occur only with sustained participation in enjoyable and safe activities. Whether sophisticated laboratory or simple field fitness tests help accomplish this goal has not been conclusively proven. It would seem reasonable to conduct baseline fitness testing where doubt exists regarding an employee's underlying health or his or her attention to safety issues during exercise. Additionally, periodic fitness test results can motivate employees by showing them the results of their exercise program. Too great a focus on test results rather than the broader health benefits of exercise, however, can be counterproductive. Overall, exercise specialists might be best advised to emphasize compliance, motivation, and enjoyment issues in exercise counseling and support rather than focusing on testing.

KEY APPLICATIONS OF HEALTH RISK ASSESSMENT IN WORKSITE HEALTH PROMOTION

Periodic population-wide HRA (with or without biomedical screening), as well as more frequent, ongoing monitoring of high-risk employees identified in the population-wide assessment process, can be very helpful in planning worksite health promotion programs and targeting intervention components to employees who will benefit the most from them. Research has clearly established that targeting educational interventions is much more effective in attracting participation than less focused approaches, as well as being more effective in improving health outcomes (Erfurt, Foote, & Heirich, 1991; Erfurt, Foote, Heirich, & Gregg, 1990; Heaney & Goetzel, 1997).

Key issues in maximizing the effectiveness of worksite health promotion programs include targeting the right employees for the right interventions, as well as maximizing levels of participation and risk reduction. HRA and biomedical screening can play a key role in segmenting the population but only if participation in these assessment activities is consistently high. To achieve acceptable levels of participation, an increasing number of employers are offering financial incentives. Many are also attempting to encourage risk reduction through the use of incentives. This section explores the role of HRA and biomedical screening in targeting interventions, administering incentives, and monitoring program impact.

Targeting High-Risk Populations

Now that computer-based HRA technology has made targeting specific segments of large employee populations practical, comparing the value of short-term versus long-term health improvement strategies is more important than ever. Given the limited resources currently available for health promotion programming, it is likely that targeting the highest-risk employees for intensive intervention will come at the expense of programming for the general population. This strategy is usually justified by the argument that a small proportion of employees uses a disproportionately large portion of total health care resources. Herein lies a serious question regarding the logic of a growing number of health promotion practitioners. While it may be true that a small number of employees with chronic conditions use the preponderance of medical services today, it is also true that an even larger number with poor health habits will suffer from these same conditions in the future. Will more money be saved by reducing the current high costs of a small number of people or by preventing unnecessary increased future costs for a far greater number? It is reasonable to speculate that even minimally improving the health practices of a large population, moving many individuals to just a slightly lower risk level, may be more cost-effective than targeting only a small number of currently high-cost employees in order to achieve cost savings. (Edington, Yen, & Witting, 1997). Research that carefully explores the balancing point between these two alternatives, and how this point varies depending on population characteristics (e.g., compensation patterns, turnover rate), is very important to both the health promotion and disease management fields.

Another compelling reason to question the logic of exclusively targeting the highest-risk employees relates to the assumption that disease management will inherently save money. While this is often true, the opposite can also occur. For example, if clinical guidelines representing "best practices" for chronic conditions were fully implemented, many believe the total costs of care in the U.S. would increase dramatically (Terry, 1994). The unfortunate reality of "usual care" for most chronic conditions is that patients do not receive the amount of care they need. Effective disease management often means more doctor visits, more expensive medication, more employee education, and more programming aimed at employee compliance with treatment regimens. In some cases, interventions may yield immediate or long-term net savings; in other cases the intervention, while improving health, may add substantially to total costs in the short term. Again, research is sorely needed to determine which areas of disease management will yield optimal economic and health returns and over what time periods these returns will occur.

Despite these caveats, targeting the right high-risk employees can be a compassionate and cost-effective strategy for organizations with enough resources to implement programs that encompass both prevention and high-risk management. Although HRA technology makes targeting the right high-risk employees easy, resistance has centered on concerns that the programs can be viewed as coercive rather than supportive. The national fervor over managed care and the trend to vilify HMOs is a clear signal that this concern needs to be taken seriously. Targeting high-risk employees, however, does have historical precedence in the worksite health promotion field. Back awareness education for physically demanding jobs, prenatal education for young female employees, and on-site cardiac rehabilitation programs are examples of very successful and welcome high-risk reduction initiatives.

Today's most successful worksite health promotion programs use an exemplary approach to targeting interventions that preserve employees' privacy while offering the support they are seeking. To accomplish this result, several attributes need to be present in an HRA tool. Of paramount importance is a mechanism for employee "informed consent." The HRA questionnaire should clearly indicate that follow-up on the results of the assessment is an option in the program. The HRA tool or screening process should also offer participants a clear choice about whether or not they want to be contacted about programs related to their specific risks. Fortunately, in addition to addressing the privacy issue, today's more sophisticated HRA instruments allow targeting based on participants' risks, readiness to change, and other health-related psychosocial and behavioral measures. This enables the program planner to target follow-up interventions, not only according to willingness to be contacted but also in terms of tailoring the specific intervention to the participant's stage in the change process and other individual factors.

HRA and the Use and Misuse of Incentives

One of the most controversial uses of HRA and biomedical screening at the worksite has been that of linking results to financial incentives. Often referred to as "risk rating," benefit managers adjusted employee health care premium payments according to measured or self-reported risk factors. The greater the number of risks, the higher the monthly premium payments. Published programs averaged premium differentials of $200 between low-risk and high-risk employees, with differentials of as much as $700 more per year being paid by employees at highest risk in some programs (Frierson, 1992). The ethical issues related to this practice have been discussed elsewhere (Terry, 1994), as has the cost-shifting principle behind the practice (Terry, Fowler, & Fowles, 1998). Although some experts advised that risk rating could be challenged under the Americans with Disabilities Act (Kaelin, Barr, Golaszewski, & Warshaw, 1992), a significant number of employers continued to adopt risk-rating schemes until recently. In 1996, Congress enacted the Health Insurance Portability and

Accountability Act (HIPAA). Many employers have discontinued risk rating since the enactment of HIPAA.

The HIPAA law was intended, in part, to prevent health insurance discrimination by prohibiting premium penalties based on "health status-related" factors (HIPAA, 1996). The law, which also applies to self-insured companies, states that "a group health plan . . . may not require any individual (as a condition of enrollment or continued enrollment under the plan) to pay a premium or contribution which is greater than such premium or contribution for a similarly situated individual enrolled in the plan on the basis of any health status-related factor in relation to the individual." All but the most emboldened benefit designers would define habits like smoking or conditions like hypertension as "health status-related factors." Still, in the same year that Congress approved HIPAA, a survey found that 66% of corporate benefit managers supported "charging higher premiums to individuals engaging in unhealthy behavior, such as smoking" (Hewitt Associates, 1996).

In spite of the restrictions established by HIPAA, some continue to advocate behavioral incentives and point out that the law explicitly allows their use in worksite health promotion programs (Chapman, 1998). The referent section of the law includes the statement: "Nothing in paragraph (1) should be construed . . . to prevent a group health plan . . . from establishing premium discounts or rebates or modifying otherwise applicable co-payments or deductibles in return for adherence to programs of health promotion and disease prevention." A reasonable interpretation of this clause would be that employers can reward participation in programs but need to stay away from premium incentives related solely to risk-related outcomes. As an example, an employer can offer a financial incentive to an employee for attending a weight loss class, but it cannot penalize the employee with higher insurance premiums if they stay overweight despite this effort to change.

Those committed to using incentives will no longer be able to simply pay for results but will need to reinforce effort, a decidedly more complex undertaking. For example, while the use of incentives may increase short-term compliance, research also indicates that externally motivated short-term behavioral commitments generally lead to relapse. Employees return to their usual lifestyle after the reinforcement has been paid. Regarding weight control in particular, such weight recycling appears to lead to higher rates of disability and death than would occur for those who remain at high-risk but have stable weights (Brownell & Rodin, 1994). A more effective approach to incentives, if behavior change were the objective, would be to use a "variable interval schedule" of reinforcement. That is, employee participation in programs would be monitored at frequent and unpredictable times, and they would need to demonstrate sustained program involvement to earn the reward or avoid the penalty. While HIPAA appears to allow reward for participation, this more sophisticated approach to reinforcing progress toward goals will be much more administratively difficult.

Despite the demise of risk rating, the use of health assessment to qualify for incentives continues in other, less controversial forms. For example, a very effective approach is to provide incentives for participating in the HRA process. One of the authors recently completed a study with a large employer that increased participation in a mail-delivered HRA program from the typical 20–25% range without incentives to approximately 50% using a $10 incentive and nearly 70% using a $25 incentive. This high rate of participation in the assessment component of a comprehensive health promotion program is very important, since it yields much greater penetration into the at-risk segments of the employee population, who can then be targeted for stage-appropriate follow-up interventions.

Monitoring and Follow-up

The most valuable HRAs are those with the built-in capability to provide comparisons over time. An HRA can serve as a catalyst for behavior change when employees benefit from seeing how their risks have improved or worsened since a previous assessment. Similarly, HRA technology that has programmed memory and retention of time-over-time data in a database allows employers to monitor on an aggregate level the progress of employees participating in

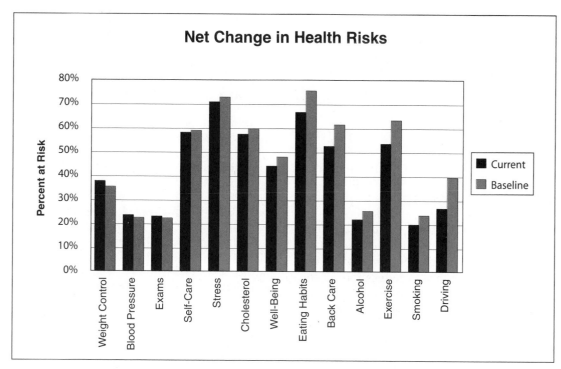

Figure 9-4 Example of Aggregate Time-Over-Time HRA Results
Source: HealthPath Health Risk Assessment, The StayWell Company. Reprinted with permission.

specific programs and the change in the overall health of their population. Figure 9-4 provides a graphical example of time-over-time aggregate health risk changes based on HRA data. Based on changes in health risks, some HRA tools also include estimates of the financial impact of risk reduction in their standard aggregate reports.

Unfortunately, time-over-time aggregate HRA results often give visibility to the progressive decline in the health of an employee population. Too often employers, lured by the false promise of being able to manage health-related costs through health assessment alone, invest heavily in the assessment phase of their program while remaining overly frugal in implementing a comprehensive range of follow-up health promotion interventions for employees. Subsequent HRAs reveal the all-too-obvious fact that no amount of assessment will meaningfully slow the decline in the health of an aging workforce. Only effective interventions can do that.

CONCLUSION

For worksite health promotion programs to be successful, it is critical that HRA, biomedical screening, and other health assessment approaches be combined with behavioral interventions and used for monitoring and follow-up. It is also critical that health assessments be positioned positively within the organization to gain the greatest level of participation. The contribution of health assessment in worksite health promotion can be summarized as follows:

1. Health assessment is a fundamental element of worksite health promotion programs because it provides a basis for program planning and development, serves as an intervention platform, and allows monitoring of both individual and organizational progress.
2. When planning worksite health promotion programs, appropriately selected health assessments

offer the most comprehensive and cost-effective information available for developing educational content for employee decision support, medical self-care, disease management, and lifestyle improvement, as well as providing an organization's senior management with the economic justification for funding interventions.

3. Ongoing administration of health assessments to measure time-over-time trends is a key component in evaluating worksite health promotion programs by providing information to support quality improvement, program redesign, and outcomes measurement.

4. Health risk appraisal (HRA) and biomedical screening are the most economical assessment approaches currently available for determining employees' health risks, health education needs, health interests, and readiness to change.

5. Results from biomedical screenings and HRAs can be operationally linked to behavioral interventions such as telephonic counseling, materials-based fulfillment campaigns, on-site group programs, or individual instruction in health improvement and disease management.

References

Alderman, M. H., & Lamport, B. (1988). Treatment of hypertension at the workplace: An opportunity to link service and research. *Health Psychology, 7,* 283–295.

American College of Sports Medicine. (1986). *Guidelines for graded exercise testing and exercise prescription* (3rd ed). Philadelphia, PA: Lea and Febiger.

American Diabetes Association. (1997). *Diabetes facts and figures* [Brochure]. Alexandria, VA: American Diabetes Association.

American Diabetes Association. (1999a). Report of the expert committee on the diagnosis and classification of diabetes mellitus. *Diabetes Care* 22(1).

American Diabetes Association. (1999b). Position statement: Standards of medical care for patients with diabetes mellitus. *Diabetes Care* 22(1).

Anderson, D. R., & Jose, W. S. (1987). Comprehensive evaluation of a worksite health promotion program: The StayWell program at Control Data. In S. H. Klarreich (Ed.), *Health and fitness in the workplace* 284–298. New York: Praeger.

Anderson, D. R., & Staufacker, M. J. (1996). The impact of worksite-based health risk appraisal on health-related outcomes: A review of the literature. *American Journal of Health Promotion, 10*(6), 499–508.

Avis, N., Smith, K., & McKinlay, J. (1989). Accuracy of perceptions of heart attack risk: What influences perceptions and can they be changed? *American Journal of Public Health, 79,* 1608–1612.

Balke, B. (1963). A simple field test for the assessment of physical fitness. *CARI Report 63-6.* Oklahoma City, OK: Civil Aeromedical Research Institute, Federal Aviation Agency.

Bandura, A. (1977). Toward a unifying theory of behavior change. *Psychological Review, 84,* 191–215.

Becker, M. H. (1974). The Health Belief Model and personal health behavior. *Health Education Monograph, 2,* 324–472.

Bertera, R. L. (1991). The effects of behavioral risks on absenteeism and health-care costs in the workplace. *Journal of Occupational Medicine, 33,* 1119–1124.

Brink, S. D. (1987). *Health risks and behavior: The impact on medical costs.* Brookfield, WI: Milliman & Robertson.

Brownell, K. D. (1993). Whether obesity should be treated. *Health Psychology, 12,* 339–341.

Brownell, K. D., & Rodin, J. (1994). Medical, metabolic and psychological effects of weight cycling. *Archives of Internal Medicine, 154,* 1325–1330.

Brownell, K. D., & Wadden, T. A. (1992). Etiology and treatment of obesity: Understanding a serious, prevalent, and refractory disorder. *Journal of Consulting and Clinical Psychology, 60,* 505–517.

Chapman, L. (1998). The use of incentives: The Health Insurance Portability and Accountability Act of 1996. *Art and Science of Health Promotion, 1*(3), 4–7.

Cooper, K. H. (1968). A means of assessing maximal oxygen uptake. Correlation between field and treadmill testing. *Journal of the American Medical Association, 203,* 135–138.

DeFriese, G. (1987). A research agenda for personal health risk assessment. *Health Services Research, 22,* 581–594.

Erfurt, J. C., Foote, A., & Heirich, M. A. (1991). Worksite wellness programs: Incremental comparison of screening and referral alone, health education, follow-up counseling, and plant organization. *American Journal of Health Promotion, 5,* 438–448.

Erfurt, J. C., Foote, A., Heirich, M. A., & Gregg, W. (1990). Improving participation in worksite wellness programs: Comparing health education classes, a menu approach, and follow-up counseling. *American Journal of Health Promotion, 4,* 270–278.

Expert Panel on Detection, Evaluation, and Treatment of High Blood Cholesterol in Adults. (1993). Summary of the second report of the National Cholesterol Education Program (NCEP) expert panel on detection, evaluation, and treatment of high blood cholesterol in adults (Adult Treatment Panel II). *Journal of the American Medical Association, 269,* 3015–3023.

Foreyt, J. P., & Goodrick, G. K. (1994). *Living without dieting.* New York: Warner.

Frick, M. H., Elo, O., Haapa, K., Heinonen, O. P., Heinsalmi, P., Helo, P., Huttunen, J. K., Kaitaniemi, P., Koskinen, P., Manninen, V., Maenpaa, H., Malkonen, M., Manttari, M., Norola, S., Pasternack, A., Pikkarainen, J., Romo, M., Sjoblom, T., & Nikkila, E. A. (1987). Helsinki heart study: Primary-prevention trial with gemfibrozil in middle-aged men with dyslipidemia. *New England Journal of Medicine, 317,* 1237–1245.

Frierson, J. G. (1992, May/June). New laws may make employee health incentive plans illegal. *Journal of Compensation and Benefits, 7*(6), 5–9.

Galuska, D. A., Serdula, M., Pamuk, E., Siegel, P. Z., & Byers, T. (1996). Trends in overweight among US adults from 1987 to 1993: A multistate telephone survey. *American Journal of Public Health, 86,* 1729–1735.

Goetzel, R. Z., Anderson, D. R., Whitmer, R. W., Ozminkowski, R. J., Dunn, R. L., & Wasserman, J. (1998). The relationship between modifiable health risks and health care expenditures: An analysis of the multi-employer HERO health risk and cost database. *Journal of Occupational and Environmental Medicine, 40,* 843–854.

Golaszewski, T., Lynch, W., Clearie, A., & Vickery, D. M. (1989). The relationship between retrospective health insurance claims and a health risk appraisal-generated measure of health status. *Journal of Occupational Medicine, 31,* 262–264.

Health Insurance Portability and Accountability Act, H. R. Bill 3103, Title 27 (1996).

Heaney, C. A., & Goetzel, R. Z. (1997). A review of health-related outcomes of multi-component worksite health promotion programs. *American Journal of Health Promotion, 11,* 290–307.

Hewitt Associates. (1996). Who is responsible for health care costs? *Corporate communications survey of benefits administrators.* Chicago, IL: Author.

Hoover, S., Jensen, M., Murphy, R., & Anderson, D. (1994). Evaluation: Guidelines for the accountable health promotion professional. In J. P. Opatz (Ed.), *Economic impact of worksite health promotion* (pp. 99–120). Champaign, IL: Human Kinetics.

Hunink, M. G. M., Goldman, L., Tosteson, A. N. A., Mittleman, M. A., Goldman, P. A., Williams, L. W., Tsevat, J., & Weinstein, M. C. (1997). The recent decline in mortality from coronary heart disease, 1980–1990. *Journal of the American Medical Association, 277,* 535–542.

Hyner, G., Peterson, K., Travis, J., Dewey, J., Foerster, J., & Framer, E. (Eds.). (1999). *The SPM handbook of health assessment tools.* Pittsburgh, PA: The Society of Preventive Medicine & The Institute for Health and Productivity Management.

Institute for Aerobics Research. (1989). *Physical fitness specialist course.* Dallas, TX: Institute for Aerobics Research.

Joint National Committee on Prevention, Detection, Evaluation and Treatment of High Blood Pressure. (1997, November 24). The sixth report of the Joint National Committee on Prevention, Detection, Evaluation and Treatment of High Blood Pressure. *Archives of Internal Medicine, 157,* 2413–2446.

Kaelin, M. A., Barr, J. K., Golaszewski, T., & Warshaw, L. J. (1992). Risk-rated health insurance programs: A review of designs and important issues. *American Journal of Health Promotion, 7,* 118–128.

Kannel, W. B., Castelli, W. P., Gordon, T. (1979). Cholesterol in the prediction of atherosclerotic disease: New perspectives based on the

Framingham study. *Annals of Internal Medicine, 90*, 85–91.

Kaplan, R. (1985). Quantification of health outcomes for policy studies in behavioral epidemiology. In R. Kaplan, & M. Criqui (Eds.), *Behavioral epidemiology and disease prevention* (31–54). New York, NY: Plenum.

Kline, G. M., Porcari, J. P., Hintermeister, R., Freedson, P. S., Ward, A., McCarron, R. F., Ross, J., & Rippe, J. M. (1987). Estimation of VO_2 max from a one-mile track walk, gender, age, and body weight. *Medicine and Science in Sports and Exercise, 19*, 253–259.

Kuczmarski, R. J., Flegal, K. M., Campbell, S. M., & Johnson, C. L. (1994). Increasing prevalence of overweight among US adults: The National Health and Nutrition Examination Survey, 1960 to 1991. *Journal of the American Medical Association, 272*, 205–211.

Landsbergis, P., Schnall, P., Deitz, D., Warren, K., Pickering, T., & Schwartz, J. (1998). Job strain and health behaviors: Results of a prospective study. *American Journal of Health Promotion, 12*, 237–245.

Martin, A. D., Ross, W. D., Drinkwater, D. T., & Clarys, J. P. (1985). Prediction of body fat by skinfold caliper: Assumptions and cadaver evidence. *International Journal of Obesity, 9*, 31–39.

McKiman, M. D., & Froelicher, V. F. (1987). General principles of exercise testing. In J. S. Skinner (Ed.), *Exercise testing and exercise prescription for special casts. Theoretical basis and clinical application* (3–19). Philadelphia, PA: Lea and Febiger.

National Heart, Lung and Blood Institute. (1999). *Clinical guidelines on the identification, evaluation, and treatment of overweight and obesity in adults.* Bethesda, MD: NHLBI Information Center.

National High Blood Pressure Education Program. (1992). *The fifth report of the Joint National Committee on Detection, Evaluation, and Treatment of High Blood Pressure (JNC V).* Bethesda, MD: National Heart, Lung, and Blood Institute, NHLBI Information Center.

National Institutes of Health. (1994). *Bioelectrical impedance analysis of body composition measurement. Technology assessment conference statement.* Bethesda, MD: National Institutes of Health Technology Assessment Program.

Pheley, A. M., Terry, P., Pietz, L., Fowles, J., McCoy, C. E., & Smith, H. (1995). The effectiveness of a nurse-based hypertension management program. *Journal of Cardiovascular Nursing, 23*, 133–138.

Pollock, M. L., & Wilmore, J. H. (1990). *Exercise in health and disease: Evaluation and prescription for prevention and rehabilitation* (2nd ed.). Philadelphia: Saunders.

Prochaska, J. O., & DiClemente, C. C. (1992). Stages of change in the modification of problem behaviors. In M. Hersen, R. M. Eisler, & P. M. Miller (Eds.), *Progress in behavior modification: Vol. 28* (pp. 183–213). New York: Sycamore.

Prochaska, J. O., Norcross, J. C., & DiClemente, C. C. (1994). *Changing for good.* New York: William Morrow.

Robbins, L. C., & Hall, J. H. (1970). *How to practice prospective medicine.* Indianapolis, IN: Methodist Hospital of Indiana.

Skinner, C., Kreuter, M., & Strecher, V. (1998). Perceived and actual breast cancer risk. *Journal of Health Psychology, 3*, 181–193.

Skinner, C., Strecher, V., & Hospers, H. (1994). Physicians' recommendations for mammography: Do tailored messages make a difference? *American Journal of Public Health, 84*, 43–49.

Smith, K. W., McKinlay, S. M., & Thorington, B. D. (1987). The validity of health risk appraisal instruments for assessing coronary heart disease risk. *American Journal of Public Health, 77*(4), 419–424.

Strecher, V. J., & Kreuter, M. W. (1999). Health risk appraisal from a behavioral perspective: Present and future. In G. C. Hyner, K. W. Peterson, J. W. Travis, J. E. Dewey, J. J. Foerster, & E. M. Framer (Eds.), *The SPM handbook of health assessment tools* (75–82. Pittsburgh, PA: The Society of Preventive Medicine & The Institute for Health and Productivity Management.

Strecher, V., Kreuter, M., DenBoer, D., Kobrin, S., Hospers, H., & Skinner, C. (1994). The effects of computer-tailored smoking cessation messages in family practice settings. *Journal of Family Practice, 39*, 262–270.

Subcommittee on Exercise Testing. (1986). Guidelines for exercise testing. A report on the American College of Cardiology/American Heart Association task force on assessment of cardiovascular procedures. *Journal of the American College of Cardiology, 8*, 725–738.

Terry, P. (1987). The role of health risk appraisal in the workplace: assessment versus behavior change. *American Journal of Health Promotion, 2,* 18–22, 36.

Terry, P. (1994). A case for no-fault insurance: From the "worried well" to the "guilty ill." *American Journal of Health Promotion, 8,* 165–168.

Terry, P., Fowler, E., & Fowles, J. (1998). Are health risks related to medical care charges in the short-term? Challenging traditional assumptions. *American Journal of Health Promotion, 12,* 340–347.

U.S. Department of Health and Human Services. (1996). *A Report of the Surgeon General: Physical Activity and Health.* Atlanta, GA: Centers for Disease Control and Prevention; Washington, DC: President's Council on Physical Fitness and Sports.

U.S. Department of Health and Human Services, Public Health Service. (1993). 1992 National survey of worksite health promotion activities: summary. *American Journal of Health Promotion, 7,* 452–464.

U.S. Preventive Services Task Force. (1996). *Guide to Clinical Preventive Services* (2nd ed.). Baltimore, MD: Williams & Wilkins.

Vickery, D., Golaszewski, T., Wright, E., & McPhee, L. (1986). Life-style and organizational health insurance costs. *Journal of Occupational Medicine, 28,* 1165–1168.

Wadden, T. A., & Bell, S. T. (1990). Obesity. In A. S. Bellack, M. Hersen, & A. E. Kazdin (Eds.), *International handbook of behavior modification and therapy* (448–473). New York: Plenum.

Weinstein, N. (1984). Why it won't happen to me: Perceptions of risk factors and illness susceptibility. *Health Psychology, 2,* 11–20.

Whitmer, R. W., & Dundon, M. W. (1997). The Health Enhancement Research Organization (HERO). *American Journal of Health Promotion, 11,* 388–393.

William M. Mercer, Inc. (1996). *Why Health Promotion in the Worksite?* [Monograph]. New York, NY: William M. Mercer, Incorporated.

Yen, L., Edington, D., & Witting, P. (1992). Predictions of prospective medical claims and absenteeism costs for 1284 hourly workers from a manufacturing company. *Journal of Occupational Medicine, 34,* 428–435.

CHAPTER

10

Physical Activity in the Workplace

Mark G. Wilson, C. Shannon Griffin-Blake, and David M. DeJoy

INTRODUCTION

Physical activity has been an integral part of health promotion and disease prevention efforts at the worksite for three decades. Many early health promotion and disease prevention efforts were related to increasing physical activity (Wilson, 1999). Although many of these first programs were perks primarily offered to company executives, they did open the door for programs that were more inclusive and provided the foundation for current physical activity efforts. As the evidence for the health-related benefits of physical activity grows, so does the need for well-developed programs targeted to ensure their maximum effectiveness.

This chapter will first review the relationship of physical activity and health, highlight physical activity trends, discuss organizational benefits, and reflect upon the many opportunities that lie ahead for increasing physical activity in worksite populations. The primary focus of the chapter will be a review of physical activity and behavior change, highlighting specific strategies that may be used throughout the

change process. The chapter will conclude by hypothesizing about the future direction of physical activity and the role worksites play in that future.

PHYSICAL ACTIVITY AND HEALTH

The body's physiologic response to physical activity is well documented. The cardiovascular, respiratory, musculoskeletal, endocrine, and immune systems are all positively impacted by aerobic and/or resistance exercise (Bouchard, Shephard, & Stephens, 1994; Plowman & Smith, 1997; Robergs & Roberts, 1997; Wilmore & Costill, 1994). Exercise has been shown in controlled clinical studies to increase cardiac output, blood flow, oxygen uptake, energy levels, metabolic rate, and hormone levels and to decrease blood pressure (systolic and diastolic), cholesterol (triglycerides), and blood glucose levels (Bouchard et al., 1994; Fletcher et al., 1996; Plowman & Smith, 1997; Robergs & Roberts, 1997; Wilmore & Costill, 1994). These changes are largely constant from adolescence to adulthood but slowly deteriorate as a function of the aging process (Bouchard et al., 1994; Hasberg, 1994; Malina, 1994; Plowman & Smith, 1997; Robergs & Roberts, 1997; Wilmore & Costill, 1994). Generally speaking, men and women have similar physiologic responses to physical activity, assuming equal size and activity level (U.S. Department of Health and Human Services [USDHHS], 1996; Wilmore & Costill, 1994). Although the research is limited, persons with disabilities appear to respond to physical activity in a similar manner to persons without disabilities (USDHHS, 1996).

Hundreds of studies have examined the impact of physical activity on the health and well-being of the individual. These were recently summarized in the first Report of the Surgeon General on Physical Activity and Health (USDHHS, 1996), the most comprehensive review of the physical activity research literature conducted to date. According to Donna Shalala, Secretary of the Department of Health and Human Services, this report is a "work of real significance, on par with the Surgeon General's historic first report on smoking and health published in 1964" (USDHHS, 1996, p. i). The report's key finding was that people of all ages can improve their quality of life through a lifelong practice of regular physical activity. In addition, there appears to be a dose-response relationship between physical activity and disease prevention, with higher levels of activity being most beneficial but lower levels also demonstrating significant benefits. According to the Surgeon General's report, regular physical activity:

- is associated with lower overall mortality rates in both older and younger adults (higher and moderate levels of activity compared to inactive individuals)
- decreases the risk of cardiovascular disease and coronary heart disease mortality (the level of decreased risk is similar to that for not smoking cigarettes)
- prevents or delays the development of hypertension
- is associated with a decreased risk of colon cancer
- lowers the risk of developing non-insulin-dependent diabetes mellitus
- probably reduces the risk of developing obesity
- may reduce the risk of developing depression (it does seem to relieve symptoms of depression and anxiety)
- appears to improve health-related quality of life

Although recent studies have indicated that the benefits of physical activity may be derived from several short activity sessions (3 times for 10 minutes) as opposed to one long session (30 minutes) (Fletcher et al., 1996), individuals who maintain a regular regimen of physical activity that is of longer duration or more vigorous intensity are likely to derive greater benefits (Haskell, 1994; USDHHS, 1996). The problem is that the majority of the United States population is not regularly active at either level.

PHYSICAL ACTIVITY TRENDS

Physical activity during leisure time has been one of the most frequently measured health risk variables over the last decade. Many nationwide surveys of health risk (Behavioral Risk Factor Surveillance System, National Health and Nutrition Examination Survey, National Health Interview Survey, and Youth Risk Behavior Survey) include measures of physical activity (or inactivity) (USDHHS, 1996). Although the various surveys differ slightly on the wording of the questions, sampling frames, time of year, and definitions of physical activity, the data collected from the various surveys are consistent in illustrating trends of self-reported physical activity (USDHHS, 1996).

The proportion of U. S. adults 18 years of age or older who report engaging in regular vigorous physical activity had increased gradually to its highest level (14.1%) in 1996, the last year data were available (see Figure 10-1) (Centers for Disease Control and Prevention, 1997a; USDHHS, 1996). For this same period of time, the percentage of respondents reporting regular sustained activity remained relatively constant (range: 18.8% to 21.0%), and those indicating they engaged in no physical activity during the previous two to four weeks declined significantly (from 32.8% to 27.8%). Overall, men report lower levels of inactivity than women (see Figure 10-2); however, women consistently report higher levels of vigorous activity than men. Physical activity also varies by ethnic status with white, nonhispanic women reporting the highest levels of vigorous physical activity and black, nonhispanic women reporting the lowest levels

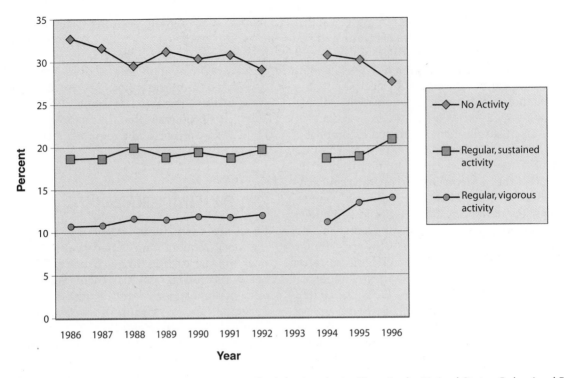

Figure 10-1 Trends in Leisure-Time Physical Activity of Adults Aged 18+ Years in the United States, Behavioral Risk Factor Surveillance System* [BRFSS].

Sources: U.S. Department of Health and Human Services, *Physical activity and health: A report of the Surgeon General*, 1996; Centers for Disease Control and Prevention, National Center for Chronic Disease Prevention and Health Promotion, BRFSS, 1995 & 1996.

*Physical activity data not collected in the 1993 survey.

(see Table 10-1). Other studies have demonstrated that physical activity levels are lowest during the winter months (November–February) and highest during summer months (May–August) (Centers for Disease Control and Prevention, 1997b) and are higher among persons living in urban areas than those in rural areas (Centers for Disease Control and Prevention, 1998).

The most widely cited surveys documenting the prevalence of physical activity programs in worksites were conducted by the Office of Disease Prevention and Health Promotion in 1985 and 1992 (USDHHS, 1987, 1992). The surveys showed that the percent of worksites that offered physical activity programs to their employees almost doubled between 1985 and 1992 (see Figure 10-3). Large worksites were significantly more likely to offer physical activity programs,

and there was also significant variation in prevalence by industry classification (USDHHS, 1987, 1992). A recent survey conducted by the Centers for Disease Control and Prevention tended to corroborate these findings, albeit at slightly lower levels (Wilson, DeJoy, Jorgensen, & Crump, 1999). This trend clearly indicates that organizations see some benefit of regular physical activity for their employees.

ORGANIZATIONAL BENEFITS

A growing body of literature has examined the benefits of physical activity programs to the organization, much of which has been summarized in a series of reviews (Dishman, Oldenburg, O'Neal, & Shephard, 1998; Gebhardt & Crump, 1990; Kaman & Patton, 1994; Shephard, 1989, 1996). The majority of this lit-

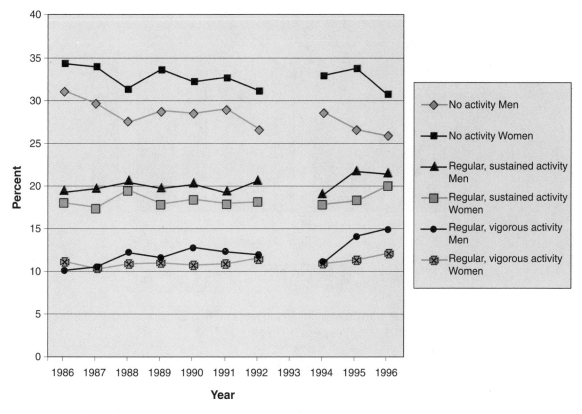

Figure 10-2 Trends in Leisure-Time Physical Activity by Gender of Adults Aged 18+ Years in the United States, Behavioral Risk Factor Surveillance System* [BRFSS].

Sources: U.S. Department of Health and Human Services, *Physical activity and health: A report of the Surgeon General*, 1996; Centers for Disease Control and Prevention, National Center for Chronic Disease Prevention and Health Promotion, BRFSS, 1995 & 1996.

*Physical activity data was not collected in 1993 survey.

erature has as its foundation the health-related benefits of physical activity to the individual. For example, worksite studies have documented positive changes in participants' body mass, blood pressure, cholesterol, and smoking status (Gebhardt & Crump, 1990; Shephard, 1996) as a result of a physical activity program.

At the same time, the expectation on the part of many organizations is that reduced health risks result in increased overall health, which can positively impact the organization. In the physical activity area, the organizational impact has usually been measured as a reduction of medical care claims and/or absenteeism. The evidence supporting the impact of physi-

cal activity programs on these variables is positive and continuing to grow but only suggestive at this time. Some studies have been successful in demonstrating a link between physical activity and absenteeism (Baun, Bernacki, & Tsai, 1986; Blair et al., 1986; Cox, Shephard, & Corey, 1981; Lechner, de Vries, Adriaansen, & Drabbels, 1997; Lynch, Golaszewski, Clearie, Snow, & Vickery, 1990; Steinhardt, Greenhow, & Stewart, 1991; Tucker, Aldana, & Friedman, 1990; Wood, 1997). However, many of these studies suffered from methodological weaknesses that limit the conclusions that may be drawn. In addition, any absenteeism study is confounded by the facts that it is extremely difficult to separate sick leave from

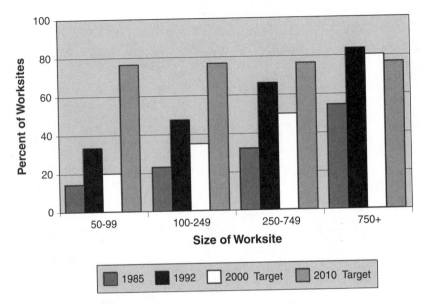

Figure 10-3 Percent of Private Worksites with 50 or More Employees Offering Exercise or Fitness Program by Size, 1985, 1992, Healthy People 2000 target, Healthy People 2010 target.

Source: U.S. Department of Health and Human Services, *National Survey of Worksite Health Promotion Activities*, 1985; U.S. Department of Health and Human Services, *1992 National Survey of Worksite Health Promotion Activities*, 1992; U.S. Department of Health and Human Services, *Healthy People 2000. National Health Promotion and Disease Prevention Objectives*, 1991; U.S. Department of Health and Human Services, *Healthy People 2010*, 2000.

Table 10-1 Percentage of Adults Aged 18+ Years Participating in Regular, Vigorous Physical Activity, by Various Demographic Characteristics, Behavioral Risk Factor Surveillance System (1992)

Race/Ethnicity	Participation in Physical Activity	
White, nonhispanic	15.3%	(14.9, 15.7)*
Males	13.3	(12.7, 13.9)
Females	17.1	(16.5, 17.7)
Black, nonhispanic	9.4	(8.6, 10.2)
Males	9.5	(8.1, 10.9)
Females	9.4	(8.4, 10.4)
Hispanic	11.9	(10.5, 13.3)
Males	12.4	(10.2, 14.6)
Females	11.4	(9.8, 13.0)
Other	11.8	(10.0, 13.6)
Males	11.5	(9.0, 14.0)
Females	12.2	(10.0, 14.4)

Source: U.S. Department of Health and Human Services, *Physical activity and health: A report of the Surgeon General*, 1996.
*95% Confidence intervals.

personal leave and that organizational absenteeism records are notoriously unreliable. Clearly, additional research is needed to establish a conclusive link between physical activity and absenteeism.

The evidence linking physical activity programs with a decrease in health care costs is promising (Baun, et al., 1986; Bell & Blanke, 1992; Bowne, Russell, Morgan, Optenberg, & Clarke, 1984; Shephard, Corey, Renzland, & Cox, 1982) but suffers from many of the same methodological limitations as the absenteeism studies. This is true of many other worksite health promotion programs and is largely related to the difficulty in documenting the link between the behavior and medical claims. Physical activity programs also yield higher overhead costs, which significantly impact the cost savings demonstrated by the programs. For example, annual costs typically range from $150 to $550 per worker or $700 to $2800 per participant to cover the costs of facilities, maintenance and cleaning, depreciation of equipment, and accident insurance. Even for programs that collect employee contributions or user fees, these overhead costs have a significant effect on the program's ability to demonstrate cost-effectiveness or favorable cost-benefit ratios.

Additional studies have examined the effects of physical activity programs on productivity (Cox, et al., 1981; Shephard, Cox, & Corey, 1981), turnover (Leatt, Hattin, West, & Shephard, 1988; Tsai, Baun, & Bernacki, 1987), work culture (Rudman & Steinhardt, 1988), and job performance (Bernacki & Baun, 1984) with some positive but limited effects. Clearly, drawing the link between physical activity programs and organizational benefits is difficult to demonstrate directly. The exception may be increased employee morale. A number of studies have reported the positive effect of physical activity programs on employee morale, and 26% of organizations surveyed indicated that employee morale was one of the main benefits of offering health promotion programs for their employees (USDHHS, 1992).

OPPORTUNITIES AHEAD

Healthy People 2000, the National Health Promotion and Disease Prevention Objectives for the 1990s, contained a number of objectives for increasing the proportion of health promotion programs being offered at the worksite (USDHHS, 1991). Only one of those objectives was directly related to physical fitness programs:

Objective 1.10 Increase the proportion of worksites offering employer-sponsored physical activity and fitness programs as follows:

worksite size	1985 baseline	2000 target	2001 target
50–99 employees	14%	20%	75%
100–249 employees	23%	35%	75%
250–749 employees	32%	50%	75%
750+ employees	54%	80%	75%

When comparing the Healthy People 2000 target levels for physical activity programming with results reported in the 1992 National Survey of Worksite Health Promotion Activities (USDHHS, 1992), it is evident that worksites have achieved the objective well before the end of the decade (see Figure 10-3). Although this does not provide insights into the efficiency or efficacy of those programs, it does reflect a growing interest on the part of worksites to provide these type of activities to their employees. So where do we go from here?

The Healthy People 2010 Objectives strive to top the best proportion by increasing the proportion of worksites offering employer-sponsored physical activity and fitness programs to 75% (USDHHS, 2000). This appears to be very achievable for large worksites but becomes increasingly more difficult to achieve as the size of the worksite decreases.

In order to continue the growth of worksite physical activity programs over the next decade, practitioners must work toward increasing the number of medium and small worksites that offer physical activity and fitness programs for their employees. This may be a considerable challenge for small worksites that are constrained by limited manpower and resources and may require a collaborative effort between private and public health organizations to overcome the barriers. At the same time, for large organizations and/or those organizations already offering physical activity and fitness programs to their employees, practitioners should strive to increase the sophistication of their programmatic efforts to demonstrate greater benefits. Emphasis should be placed on offering programs that are conceptually sound, grounded in behavioral theory, and utilize proven strategies for achieving behavior change. The remainder of the chapter will provide a framework for this approach.

PHYSICAL ACTIVITY BEHAVIOR CHANGE

Traditional Approach

Most physical activity behavior change programs conducted at the worksite have taken a similar approach. Typically, individuals sign up for the program and attend an orientation session. The orientation session usually includes some combination of the following: a) risk assessment, which may be specific to physical activity or more broad-based like a health risk appraisal, b) an education and/or information period that will talk about the health-related benefits of exercise, potential barriers and how to overcome them, and types of activities and benefits of each, c) an introduction to the layout, rules and regulations, and equipment of the fitness facility, if applicable, d) a fitness test for those that qualify, and e) completion of the necessary paperwork to register participants in the organization's system and meet insurance and/or liability requirements. Next, participants meet with a trained facilitator, who sets up a physical activity program or exercise prescription. Usually this is conducted one-on-one but may be performed in small groups if necessary. The facilitator then meets with each individual at the first exercise session to help them start their program. Finally, a facilitator may periodically contact the participant over the following few weeks to monitor progress and make modifications in their physical activity program as needed.

This "one size fits all" approach to worksite physical activity has some inherent limitations that may affect the overall impact of the program. First, the approach initially rests on the assumption that all individuals are at the same level of readiness for becoming physically active. Practitioners tend to believe that everyone who signs up for a physical activity program is ready to take action to be regularly physically active. Many are subsequently surprised and disappointed when 50% of participants drop out of the program in the first six weeks, even though research shows that approximately one-third (32–39%) of individuals initially beginning an exercise program are in precontemplation or contemplation stages (Marcus, Banspach et al., 1992; Marcus, Emmons et al., 1998) and approximately another one-quarter to one-third (14–37%) are in preparation (Marcus, Emmons et al., 1998; Marcus, Banspach et al., 1992).

Second, the one-size-fits-all approach assumes that the same behavior change strategies work for everyone, regardless of background or interests. Third, the approach allows little personalized or one-on-one contact between the participant and the exercise specialist. Research has clearly demonstrated that intensive, multiple-contact programs are more effective (Marcus, Owen, Forsyth, Cavill, & Fridinger, 1998). Finally, the approach does not readily support the use of relapse prevention strategies or long-term monitoring of participant progress that have been shown to reduce program dropout.

Stage-Based Approach

In contrast to the traditional approach to health behavior change, the stage-based approach assumes that behavior change occurs through a series of qualitatively distinct phases or stages. These different stages of behavior can be thought of as representing different levels of motivational readiness. Although the general idea of stage-based models of behavior change have been discussed by a number of different authors (e.g., Horn, 1976; Janis & Mann, 1977; Weinstein, 1988), the Transtheoretical Model developed by Prochaska and colleagues (e.g., Prochaska & DiClemente, 1983; Prochaska, DiClemente, & Norcross, 1992; Prochaska & Velicer, 1997) has been the most widely studied and applied. The Transtheoretical Model postulates that health behavior change progresses through at least five stages: *precontemplation* (not intending to make a change in the foreseeable future); *contemplation* (seriously considering making a change but not yet committed to changing); *preparation* (intending to change in the near future [i.e., the next month] and having taken some small or preliminary steps toward action); *action* (engaging in overt behavior change for a period of six months or less); and *maintenance* (sustaining behavior change for six months or more) (Cardinal & Sachs, 1996; Prochaska & DiClemente, 1983; Prochaska & Velicer, 1997).

The most important implication of adopting a stage-based approach is the recognition that people at the different stages of the change process are receptive to different types of information and intervention strategies. In other words, the stage-based approach to physical activity requires that we abandon the traditional, or one-size-fits-all, approach to programming. Secondly, it is important to recognize that change is quite often gradual and occurs only after repeated attempts. Third, the stages of the Transtheoretical Model are often depicted as a spiral shaped diagram to show that advancement through the stages occurs at varying rates, and relapse may cause an individual to leave and reenter the change process at the same or an earlier stage. For example, a person who relapses during the action stage may recycle back to the preparation or to the contemplation stage. In thinking about how people change problem behaviors, relapse is integral to the process and should be considered directly in developing behavior change programs.

The processes of change are a second major aspect of the Transtheoretical Model. The processes of change refer to the techniques used by people as they progress through the various stages in the change process. Each process of change can be viewed as a broad category encompassing multiple techniques, methods, and programming concepts associated with distinct theoretical orientations (Perz, DiClemente, & Carbonari, 1996; Prochaska, DiClemente, & Norcross, 1992). The processes of change can also be organized in a hierarchical manner and divided into experiential and behavioral categories. Table 10-2 shows these two categories as Marcus and colleagues have applied them to exercise (Marcus, Simkin, Rossi, & Pinto, 1996).

Research suggests that certain processes are more useful at particular stages and can lead to effective programming and progression towards behavioral change (DiClemente, Prochaska, et al., 1991; Marcus, et al., 1996; Marcus, Rossi, Selby, Niaura, & Abrams, 1992; Perz et al., 1996; Prochaska & DiClemente, 1983, 1984; Prochaska, Norcross, Fowler, Follick, & Abrams, 1992; Samuelson, 1998). According to Prochaska and colleagues, individuals in the precontemplation stage are more likely to respond to consciousness raising, dramatic relief, and environmental reevaluation strategies; contemplators will benefit most from self-reevaluation approaches; individuals in preparation will be more receptive to self-liberation approaches; and individuals in the action stage will respond more to reinforcement management, helping relationships, counterconditioning, stimulus control, and social liberation strategies (Prochaska, DiClemente, & Norcross, 1992).

Stage-matched interventions that integrate the stages and processes of change can accelerate individuals to

Table 10-2 The Processes of Exercise Behavior Change

Process	Definition
Experiential	
Consciousness raising	Efforts by the individual to recall and seek new information related to exercise and adoption of activity (e.g., the benefits of exercise)
Dramatic relief	Affective or intense emotional experiences related to sedentary lifestyle (e.g., thinking about the negative health consequences in inactivity)
Environmental reevaluation	Consideration and self-assessment of how exercise impacts others in the physical and social environment
Social liberation	Awareness, availability, and acceptance by the individual of societal and social influences on encouraging and promoting exercise
Self-reevaluation	Emotional and cognitive reappraisal by the individual with respect to exercise activity
Behavioral	
Counterconditioning	Use of exercise to cope with unpleasant emotions (e.g., stress, fatigue)
Helping relationships	Trusting, accepting, and using the support of others to enhance and assist with the individual's exercise activity
Reinforcement management	Changing the contingencies that control or maintain sedentary behavior (e.g., use of positive reinforcement and goal setting to increase exercise)
Stimulus control	Control of situations and other causes which trigger inactivity
Self-liberation	The individual's choice and commitment to maintain exercise

Source: B. H. Marcus, L. R. Simkin, J. S. Rossi, & B. M. Pinto. *American Journal of Health Promotion*, 1996.

higher levels of readiness to change and possibly result in the initiation and adoption of a health behavior (Laforge, Velicer, Richmond, & Owen, 1999; Prochaska & DiClemente, 1983; Prochaska & Velicer, 1997; Prochaska, Velicer, DiClemente, & Fava, 1988). Stage-matched (also called motivationally tailored) interventions have successfully demonstrated the utility of the Transtheoretical Model in studies on smoking (Prochaska, DiClemente, Velicer, & Rossi, 1993), exercise (LaForge et al., 1999; Marcus, Emmons, et al., 1998), condom use (Centers for Disease Control and Prevention, 1996), dietary fat reduction (Campbell et al., 1994), sun exposure (Rossi, Blais, Redding, & Weinstock, 1995; Rossi, Weinstock, Redding, Cottrill, & Maddock, 1997), mammography (Rakowski et al., 1997; Rakowski et al., 1998; Skinner, Strecher, & Hospers, 1994), and alcohol (Heather, Rollnick, Bell, & Richmond, 1996).

General Guidelines for Stage-Based Programming

Adoption of the stage-based approach to worksite physical activity programming requires embracing two key concepts. First, applying the stage-based approach means tailoring intervention strategies to the individual's particular stage of behavior change or level of motivational readiness. This means that different strategies will be required to affect those in the precontemplation stage than those who are in the maintenance stage. For example, getting employees to begin to think seriously about engaging in regular, health-enhancing exercise (i.e., helping a person move from precontemplation to contemplation) is quite different from trying to help people avoid relapse and to maintain an already established pattern of physical activity. Second, stage-based programming needs to be multi-faceted and continuous. In any given population of employees at any given point in time, people can be expected to be at different stages in the change process; and, over time, some of these people will move forward, some will move backward, and others will not move at all. Traditional one shot fitness initiatives or programs relying on a single intervention approach conducted over a specific period of time are not consistent with stage-based programming.

A multifaceted, stage-based exercise program at the worksite involves attention to three interactive domains or programming dimensions: a) the stages of motivational readiness, b) the social-organizational context, and c) the admixture of specific educational and behavior change strategies. Simply acknowledging that people are at different stages of motivational readiness does not provide a very rich or detailed blueprint for program development. The multilevel model of workplace health behavior change presented in Figure 10-4 combines these three dimensions (DeJoy, Wilson, & Huddy, 1995). The interactive nature of these dimensions and relative merits of multilevel programming at the worksite have been discussed by a number of authors (e.g., Abrams, Elder, Carleton, Lasater, & Artz, 1986; DeJoy & Southern, 1993; Winett, King, & Altman, 1989). The three aspects of this cube-shaped model are labeled stages of change, levels of intervention, and strategies, respectively. The stages of change are similar to those discussed above and embrace the notion that behavior change is not an all-or-none phenomenon.

The levels of intervention dimension consists of three levels: individual, group, and organizational. One of the unique aspects of the workplace as a setting for health promotion is that there are potentially powerful incentives and social factors that can be used to support and reinforce health behavior change. Abrams and associates (Abrams et al., 1986) refer to the three levels portrayed in Figure 10-4 as the three qualitatively different but interactive systems that comprise the organizational social structure. At the individual level, primary interest is with the individual's knowledge, attitudes, and skills. The individual level is typically emphasized in most worksite health promotion activities (DeJoy & Southern, 1993). The group level focuses on the individual's immediate social environment at work but can also include family and other important nonwork social networks. The organization level emphasizes the organization's formal and informal rules, standards, expectations, and norms. These factors contribute to the organization's climate or culture (e.g., Ribisl & Reischl, 1993), as does the overall environment of the workplace and the available resources and assets.

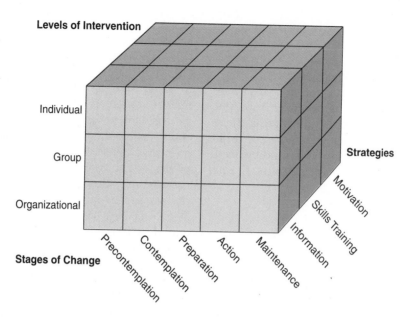

Figure 10-4 A Multilevel Model of Workplace Behavior Change.

Source: D. M. DeJoy, M. G. Wilson, & D. C. Huddy. Health behavior change in the workplace. In D. DeJoy and M. Wilson (Eds.), *Critical Issues in Worksite Health Promotion*, 1995.

The strategies dimension involves activities related to informing employees, providing them with the behavioral skills necessary to initiate and maintain positive health-related changes in their health behaviors, and creating an emotional environment or climate that motivates and supports positive change. These three sets of strategies have been viewed as critical to comprehensive workplace health promotion programming (O'Donnell & Ainsworth, 1984). The three dimensions should not be construed as being mutually exclusive or exhaustive; however, they do underscore the fact that information-based programs alone are seldom sufficient to produce and maintain behavior change in the long term.

This three-dimensional model is fundamentally an ecological or contextual model (e.g., McLeroy, Bibeau, Steckler, and Glanz, 1988) in that it recognizes that group- and organization-level efforts can contribute in positive (or negative) ways to individual behavior change. Indeed, most current definitions of health promotion are ecological and emphasize the interaction of behavioral and environmental factors (e.g., Green, Richard, & Potvin, 1996; Green & Kreuter,

1990; O'Donnell, 1989). In developing a stage-based physical activity program at the workplace, the primary goal is individual behavior change; however, this can be best accomplished through a combination of individual, group, and organizational level strategies. Group and organizational strategies play particularly important roles in supporting and reinforcing desired behaviors. To a considerable extent, if we ignore the complex interrelationships that exist between behavioral and environmental influences, we lose much of the richness of the workplace as a setting for health promotion efforts.

Using the multidimensional model to develop workplace physical activity programs involves developing strategies that a) impart information, build necessary skills, provide motivation, and energize action, b) are specifically tailored to each of the five stages of behavior change, and c) include group and organizational strategies and actions to augment the individual behavior change process. For example, it is easy to see how various financial incentives, such as company-subsidized health club memberships, could be used to provide important motivation for employees who are in the contemplation stage. In this regard, subsidized memberships would be a stage-specific strategy that is organizational in terms of level and motivational in terms of focus. This sounds complex but is really quite simple. The challenge lies in developing and tailoring the multiple strategies to the individual and administering them at the correct time. This is where interactive computer-mediated or web-based formats could be used for program delivery and tracking (Marcus, Owen et al., 1998).

Stage-Specific Programming

Before any stage-based programming may begin, individuals must be categorized into their appropriate stage of motivational readiness. This is commonly accomplished through a self-administered questionnaire using a specific staging question. One commonly used question was developed by Marcus and colleagues (Marcus & Simpkin, 1993) and asks respondents to circle the correct response(s):

1. I currently do not exercise.   a. True   b. False
2. I intend to exercise in the
   next 6 months.   a. True   b. False
3. I currently exercise *regularly*. a. True   b. False
4. I have exercised *regularly* for
   the past 6 months.   a. True   b. False

The scoring instructions for each stage:
  If Item 1 = true and Item 2 = false,
     then stage = Precontemplation
  If Item 1 = true and Item 2 = true,
     then stage = Contemplation
  If Item 1 = false and Item 3 = false,
     then stage = Preparation
  If Item 3 = true and Item 4 = false,
     then stage = Action
  If Item 3 = true and Item 4 = true,
     then stage = Maintenance

To increase the reliability, the staging questions should be preceded by a definition of exercise such as: "Exercise includes activities such as brisk walking, jogging, swimming, aerobic dancing, biking, rowing,

etc. Activities that are primarily sedentary, such as bowling or playing golf with a cart, would not be considered exercise. REGULAR EXERCISE = 3 TIMES OR MORE PER WEEK" (Reed, Velicer, Prochaska, Rossi, & Marcus, 1997, p. 59). The staging question may be combined with a health risk or physical activity assessment or other questionnaire designed to elicit participation or programmatic data. Additional questions determining the individual's level of the processes of change (where they stand on each process) may be added to help guide programmatic decisions (see Marcus, Rakowski, & Rossi, 1992; Marcus, Rossi et al., 1992). For example, questions may be added to determine if the individual has low or high physical activity self-efficacy.

In the sections that follow, overviews are provided for worksite physical activity programming in each of the five stages of behavior change. Table 10-3 contains a summary of various strategies that might be used and the stage in which they should be initiated. These are arranged by level: individual, group, and organizational.

Precontemplation

Precontemplation is the stage in which the individual has no real intention to change his or her behavior in the foreseeable future (at least not within the next six months). The challenge here is reaching people who are not really interested in or motivated to change their behavior. These individuals are not thinking about change and typically process less information about their problems and behaviors, dedicate less time and energy to reevaluating themselves, undergo fewer emotional reactions to the negative aspects of their behavior, and are not as candid with significant others about their problems (Marcus, Rossi et al., 1992; Prochaska, Norcross et al., 1992). Because these individuals do not perceive physical inactivity as a problem, physical activity becomes unimportant in their lives. For progression to occur, precontemplators need to take ownership of their behaviors, increase their awareness of the benefits of changing and consequences of not changing their behavior, and accurately evaluate self-regulation capacities (Allan, 1997; DiClemente & Prochaska, 1985).

Table 10-3 Suggested Strategies for Stage-Specific Physical Activity Programs

	Precontemplation	Contemplation	Preparation	Action	Maintenance
Individual	Information/Awareness Health Communication ("why")		Information/ Knowledge ("how to")	Information/Knowledge ("staying motivated/ avoiding obstacles")	
		Skill-Building Activities (decision-making/goal-setting/ self-efficacy/self-reinforcement)			
Group		Peer Group Support Informal/Peer Leaders Team-based Activities		Peer Group Support Feedback/Recognition Competitions/Incentives	
Organizational	Endorsement/Sponsorship Management/Leadership Visibility Position Statements/Policies Environmental Supports		Supportive/Enabling Policies Facilities/Equipment/Resources Incentives/Reinforcers Management/Leadership Participation Environmental Supports		

Information and awareness activities directed at consciousness-raising, such as health communication strategies, decisional balance scales, and health risk appraisals and/or fitness testing, can be used with this group of individuals to assist them in recalling and seeking new information related to adoption of physical activity. The emphasis at this stage is on strategies that provide information and impart knowledge about *why* people should be physically active. Health communication strategies may encompass mass media methods, fliers, brochures, bulletin boards, and face-to-face communication. These types of educational materials can be used at any stage (Table 10-3), but are particularly important in precontemplation, by making physical activity information more accessible to employees and increasing the awareness of the benefit of regular physical activity. Having a variety of written materials on the consequences of remaining sedentary can provide a person with answers to the questions of the "whys" and "why nots" surrounding their exercise behaviors. These written materials should foster the importance of physical activity as an integral part of one's lifestyle.

The pros and cons of behavior change or decisional balance (Janis & Mann, 1977; Velicer, DiClemente, Prochaska, & Brandenburg, 1985) can be measured by "a balance sheet of the comparative gains and losses" concerning one's exercise behavior (Janis & Mann, 1977; Marcus, Rakowski et al., 1992). The transition to each stage of motivational readiness is based on the individual weighing and comparing the benefits (pros) and costs (cons) of initiating and maintaining the new behavior (Prochaska & DiClemente, 1983; Prochaska & Velicer, 1997). Reviewing the five stages, the cons appear to significantly decrease as one moves from precontemplation to a later stage; and, in contrast, the pros significantly increase from precontemplation to maintenance (Hellman, 1997; Lechner & de Vries, 1995; Marcus, Banspaugh et al., 1992). Considerable evidence shows that perceived barriers to exercise impact both intention and actual behavior (Clarke & Eves, 1997; Godwin & Shephard, 1986; Prochaska & Velicer, 1997; Tappe, Duda, Menges-Erhnwald, 1989); thus, an individual's attitudes must be modified before they can be expected to take action. Interventions that have been found to be successful in progressing precontemplators toward higher stages employed decisional balance sheets as activities for this stage (Cardinal & Sachs, 1996, Marcus, Emmons et al., 1998). The key to the success of the decisional balance strategies is to integrate them with the health communication strategies discussed earlier.

Health risk appraisals and/or fitness testing can serve to raise an individual's awareness of various personal risk factors and/or poor physical conditioning and the potential impact these factors have on their health. Precontemplators, some of whom were probably active as youths or work in physically demanding jobs, may be unaware of the extent of deterioration of their physical conditioning that has occurred over time. Demonstration of this in a perceived scientific, unbiased fashion may counter the denial that this "doesn't affect me".

At the group level, many organizations have regular meetings that can be used as conduits to provide information and create awareness about a sedentary lifestyle. For example, many manufacturing organizations have monthly safety meetings for which attendance is mandatory. Individuals who organize and conduct these meetings are usually open to sharing information about a variety of health- and safety-related issues. Organization-level strategies can also be important for precontemplators and can include company sponsorship/endorsement of information/ awareness campaigns, management participation in information forums and other information-oriented events, and the development and dissemination of position statements or policies related to physical activity and employee health and well-being.

Contemplation

Contemplation is the stage in which the individual is aware of the problem or needed change but has not made a firm commitment to take action. According to the definition used in the Transtheoretical Model, persons in contemplation are seriously considering changing their behavior in the next six months. However, the amount of time individuals remain within this stage (or any given stage) can vary widely. Some individuals have been found to remain in the contemplation stage for two years without any progress

(Prochaska & DiClemente, 1984; DiClemente & Prochaska, 1985). Similar to precontemplators, contemplators have been found to be responsive to consciousness-raising techniques, such as feedback, educational messages, and face-to-face communication (Table 10-3) (Prochaska & DiClemente, 1984; Prochaska, DiClemente et al., 1992; Prochaska & Velicer, 1997). In addition, dramatic relief experiences (such as role playing, media campaigns, or personal testimonies), which may raise emotions and reduce negative affects if the person changes his or her behavior, have been found effective with contemplators (Prochaska & DiClemente, 1992; Prochaska, DiClemente et al., 1992; Prochaska, Norcross et al., 1992; Prochaska & Velicer, 1997). Personal testimonies from individuals who have overcome the barriers of incorporating exercise into their busy schedules or starting an exercise program after years of remaining sedentary may empower other individuals to consider their own health choices and begin evaluating their priorities. Dramatic relief strategies may be considered a success if employees' thinking about physical activity advances to improved motivational readiness.

Reevaluating one's values, problems, and ultimately themselves, both affectively and cognitively, provides an opportunity for an individual to gain greater understanding of how the presence or absence of personal behaviors impact their physical and social environment (Marcus et al., 1996; Prochaska, Norcross et al., 1992; Prochaska & Velicer, 1997). Ultimately, an individual's behavior or motivation to exercise is based on the meaning of the physical activity or what value is procured through action (Maehr & Braskamp, 1986). A need or reason for change must be felt before intention may develop. Consequently, during contemplation, the strategies utilized should emphasize the plethora of benefits of exercise while debunking barriers or reasons for not exercising (Marcus, Emmons et al., 1998; Marcus, Banspaugh, et al., 1992) and provide an opportunity to assess current behaviors through a behavioral assessment activity (Cardinal & Sachs, 1996). A physical activity index or health risk appraisal would be a useful tool for a contemplator to evaluate his or her health status and current activity level.

Self-efficacy enhancement becomes important during contemplation (Prochaska & DiClemente, 1992) in that the individual must feel capable of increasing his or her activity level before strong behavioral intention can occur. No one wants to begin a new behavior if failure is the likely outcome. Thus, an activity pyramid (see Figure 10-5), which helps to educate and encourage small lifestyle activity changes, could be an effective approach to empower someone to consider these small changes (Cardinal & Sachs, 1996; King, Marcus, Pinto, Emmons, & Abrams, 1995; Jakicic, Wing, Butler, & Robertson, 1995; Norstrom & Conray, 1995; Robison & Rogers, 1995). The activity pyramid promotes making exercise a part of every

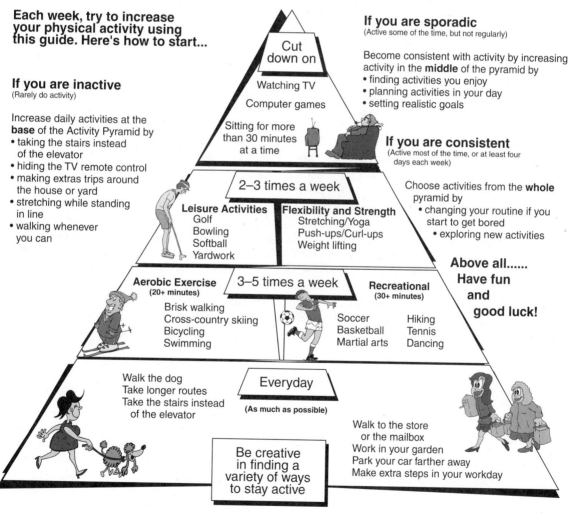

Figure 10-5 The Activity Pyramid.

Source: Copyright © 1997 Park Nicollet *HealthSource*® Institute for Research and Education. Reprinted by permission.

day activities, such as taking the stairs, walking to perform errands, and gardening, and can be considered as an entry point for reaching American College of Sports Medicine guidelines (American College of Sports Medicine [ACSM] 1998) for physical activity. As people become more able to visualize themselves as being more physically active, it becomes easier to set a date for making this change and making other related preparations.

As shown in Table 10-3, group level strategies become increasingly important during contemplation. Activities that involve the immediate work group, and sometimes family members, can be used to help contemplators to emphasize the benefits of exercise, minimize associated barriers, and enhance self-efficacy expectations. Group level activities typically provide a) opportunities to receive emotional support and encouragement, b) exposure to role models, c) opportunities to participate in structured or semi-structured team-based activities, and d) various reinforcers or incentives. For example, physical activity interventions using a team-based approach have demonstrated success in facilitating stage progression (Cole, Leonard, Hammond, & Fridinger, 1998). Basically, the same organizational strategies that were discussed for precontemplation are also useful for those in contemplation; but as individuals make the transition from contemplation to preparation, workplace policies and incentives (for example, flextime and activity fee waivers or reimbursement), facilities and equipment, and other types of environmental supports become increasingly important in fostering motivational readiness.

Preparation

Preparation is the stage that combines intention and behavioral criteria. Individuals at this stage have formed a specific intention to change their behavior in the near-term (i.e., within the next month) and/or may have taken some preliminary or tentative steps toward acting on their newly formed behavioral intention. It is important to recognize that some people reaching the preparation stage will have been there before. For these individuals, it is useful to examine what went wrong in earlier attempts and what has been learned from these experiences. Within the stage change perspective, it is important to view relapse as part of the change process and as an opportunity to learn and improve. Use of experiential, or cognitive, processes continues during preparation, but behavioral adjustments begin to prepare the individual for change (Perz et al., 1996). Self-liberation, a central process utilized during this stage, requires the individual to make a choice of and commitment to the specific physical activity regimen (Marcus et al., 1996; Prochaska & DiClemente, 1992; Prochaska & Velicer, 1997). One means for doing so would be to ask individuals to specify (in writing) what activity they are going to perform, when they will perform it, where it will be performed, and for how long it will be performed, thus publicly demonstrating their choice and commitment.

Individual strategies important during preparation can be grouped into two categories: information/knowledge and skill-building activities. During preparation, information/knowledge strategies focus less on *why* people should be physically active and more on *how to* become more physically active. Although there should be continued emphasis on the benefits of physical activity, other more action-oriented information and knowledge is required. This may include specific suggestions for starting an exercise program, selecting activities, training and safety tips, and equipment, facility, and resource options and considerations.

Decision-making, goalsetting, self-efficacy strategies, and self-management/self-reinforcement techniques are examples of skill development activities (Table 10-3) that are applicable for enhancing the progression from preparation toward action (Allan, 1997; Cardinal & Sachs, 1996; Marcus, Emmons et al., 1998; Marcus, Selby, Niavra, & Rossi, 1992). Goalsetting should involve goals that strike a balance among being realistic, difficult enough to elicit significant effort, while not exceeding the individual's perception of their ability to accomplish the goal (self-efficacy) (Strecher et al., 1995). Short- and long-term goals should be developed and written down in order for a strategic action plan to be delineated. As discussed earlier, the activity pyramid provides a means of making small but gradual exercise changes that can lead to reaching a certain activity criterion (i.e., 3 times per week) and increase levels of self-efficacy. Thus, a progressive plan could be developed from the pyramid, which meets the personal goals, exercise knowledge, and self-efficacy levels of the individual.

Self-management strategies typically emphasize personal responsibility for behavior change and the development of skills for solving problems and managing the change process. Self-management skills are important because, ultimately, each person must take responsibility for maintaining his or her own level of physical activity and for dealing with various problems and obstacles. Kanfer and colleagues (e.g., Kanfer & Gaelick-Buys, 1991) describe the self-management process in terms of three stages: self-monitoring, self-evaluation, and self-reinforcement. In this instance, self-monitoring would involve direct observation of one's own physical activity over time. This may simply involve keeping a record of one's level of physical activity on a daily basis. Notations might also be made with respect to various internal and/or external stimuli or conditions that appear to influence the pattern of activity. Self-monitoring helps the individual to understand the dimensions of the target behavior and gets them involved in the change process. At its most basic level, self-evaluation involves comparing the information obtained from self-monitoring with some standard of recommended behavior (e.g., exercise guidelines).

Self-monitoring and self-evaluation set the stage for goalsetting and for developing action plans for meeting these goals. Self-reinforcement refers to how people react cognitively and emotionally to the results of the self-evaluation. To the extent that exercise goals are met, self-efficacy is enhanced and expectations for future behavior become more positive. Even negative feedback is useful in helping participants to revise their goals, make needed changes in their plans, and identify and remove barriers. In most instances, people who succeed with long-term behavior change efforts do develop some type of self-reinforcement system and self-administer rewards based on meeting personal goals (Green, Wilson, & Lovato, 1986). With the behavioral science literature, considerable evidence suggests that self-administered incentives can be just as effective, or even more effective, in maintaining behavior change than external rewards or incentives (Thoresen & Mahoney, 1974).

At the group and organizational levels, those in preparation will benefit from many of the same strategies as those who are in precontemplation and contemplation. However, at the group level, opportunities exist for somewhat more direct peer group support through the use of planned activities such as buddy systems, teams, and even more formal strategies such as contests/competitions or behavioral contracting (Wilson & DeJoy, 1995). A similar transition occurs at the organizational level with official exercise-friendly policies and programs becoming increasingly more relevant as people move through preparation into action.

Action

Action is the stage in which commitment is translated into overt behavior change. On average, the action stage extends for approximately six months from the initiation of change (when an individual starts exercising). Greater levels of self-liberation, counterconditioning, and stimulus control are found among action-oriented individuals (Marcus et al, 1996; Prochaska, DiClemente et al., 1992). Individual strategies during the action stage focus on helping the individual to sustain his or her motivation and to minimize and cope with obstacles that may prompt relapse. For example, counterconditioning involves learning of healthier alternatives for problem behaviors and using relaxation, assertion, and positive self-statements as methods to encourage behavioral change. Encouraging individuals to cross-train (Marcus, Banspaugh et al., 1992) or attempt different exercises within their routines may decrease boredom, prevent injury, and improve motivation and self-confidence. When an individual gets discouraged, cognitive restructuring (also called cognitive reappraisal) may help an individual reframe or favorably alter a negative self-defeating perception into a positive one. The individual should think positively about becoming physically active and use positive self-talk to encourage exercise adherence.

Stimulus control (avoiding stimuli or situations that elicit the problem behavior and adding prompts for healthier alternatives) promotes relapse prevention by restructuring one's environment and avoiding high-risk cues. For example, individuals may place reminders around the office (e.g., on their datebook or calendar) or at home (e.g., on the refrigerator) to remind them to exercise. In the action stage, individuals have been found to rely on support networks and understanding from helping relationships. The influence of others affects attitudes and behaviors and molds the choices a person makes. Lewthwaite (1990) stated that actions and beliefs of family and friends can either undermine or reinforce exercise behaviors. Interaction and support from exercise partners, peers, fitness program staff, and family have been shown to have a positive impact on exercise adherence (Dishman, Sallis, & Orenstein, 1985; Horne, 1994; Siegel, Johnson, & Newhof, 1988; Wankel, 1984). As an example, Horne (1994) found that women, especially mothers, use their peers as emotional sounding boards to discuss exercise barriers that may affect the amount of time they spend exercising. Allan (1997) recommends letting others know about one's exercise goals and finding support groups, such as family members, co-workers, or a mentor, who will foster the physical activity routine. As such, significant opportunities exist to use the work group or peer network at the workplace to foster and sustain physical activity. Buddy systems and organized group or team activities can be beneficial, especially when they feature opportunities for feedback and recognition that acknowledge and reinforce the newly established pattern of behavior and altered attitudes about exercise.

Competitions or contests between departments or other work groups can be a useful way to take advantage of group loyalties and natural intergroup rivalries in the workplace. Competitions have been used with success in facilitating behavior change in workplace weight loss (Abrams & Follick, 1983; Brownell & Felix, 1987; Brownell, Stunkard, McKeon, & Felix, 1983; Cohen, Stunkard, & Felix, 1987; Stunkard, Cohen, & Felix, 1989) and smoking cessation programs (Cummings, Hellmann, & Emont, 1988; Jason, Jayaraj, Blitz, Michaels, & Klett, 1990; Klesges, Glasgow, Klesges, Morray, & Quale, 1987). This basic approach could be readily adapted to exercise. The workgroup would monitor its physical activity per-

formance, perhaps using some type of points system to quantify individual levels of physical activity across different types of activities and to calculate a mean score for the workgroup. These performance data would then be posted and compared across groups. The workgroup with the best performance for the week or month would receive some type of monetary award or other incentive. Practitioners should be careful that the value of the prizes reflect the amount of effort expected in the program, the competition increases camaraderie among participants rather than malice, the competition minimizes overzealous participation, and all participants are made to feel like winners, even though only one of them won the competition (Wilson & DeJoy, 1995). Group level contingencies can be powerful motivators in the workplace (Brownell & Felix, 1987). Competitions provide opportunities for peer group support and public recognition, but they also provide opportunities to employ performance feedback, goal setting, and self-management processes at the group level.

Organizational level strategies can be very important during the action stage. DeJoy, Wilson, and Huddy (1995) argue that organizational level actions are important in three respects. First, they help establish a sense of shared responsibility for employee health within the organization (Jaffe-Sandroff, Bradford, & Gilligan, 1990). If the organization wishes its members to practice healthy lifestyle behaviors, then the organization should take an active role in supporting these behaviors and accept a share of responsibility for fostering and enabling them. This is crucial, if only for the fact that employees spend almost half of their waking hours at work. Second, organizational level actions are frequently needed to remove some of the very real barriers that stand in the way of healthy behavior change. Various organizational level incentives can be used to alter the benefits/barriers ratio for various healthy behaviors, including exercise. Companies can use financial incentives, such as prizes, rebates, vouchers, or reduced insurance premiums, to recognize and reinforce desired lifestyle behaviors. Organizations can simplify the logistics of participation by providing convenient onsite facilities and equipment, allowing employees to participate on company time, offering flexible scheduling of work hours, and maintaining adequate staffing, support, and visibility for the health promotion effort.

Third, organizational level actions are essential to creating a corporate culture that encourages and supports physical activity and comprehensive health promotion efforts. According to DeJoy and associates (DeJoy et al., 1995, p. 115), "a strong health promotion culture exists where top management actively supports health promotion through resource allocation, supportive policy development, and it is hoped, participation." At the same time, it is important to realize that culture change is a long-term process that often involves fundamental changes in the organization's values, assumptions, and beliefs about human resources and the value of a healthy and productive workforce (Jaffe, 1995; Shein, 1985). The creation of supportive cultures can sometimes be speeded up through systematic and deliberate program planning, by involving managers and employees in the planning process, and by systematically evaluating programming efforts (Baun, 1995; Allen, Allen, Kraft, & Certner, 1987). This is essentially an evidence-based approach, in which the organizational benefits of physical activity programming are systematically assessed and analyzed.

Maintenance

Maintenance is the stage in which individuals strive to prevent relapse and consolidate the gains attained during action. The maintenance stage is generally thought to begin about six months after the initial behavior change and may be indeterminate in duration for many lifestyle changes. In practical terms, the time period from six months to five years is often used to set boundaries for the maintenance stage (Prochaska and Velicer, 1997). Stabilization of the changed behavior and avoidance of relapse are the hallmarks of the maintenance stage. However, as suggested by the spiral model used to portray the Transtheoretical Model, progression toward action and maintenance often does not take a linear path. The spiral model suggests that individuals have the potential to learn from their attempts and failures and can learn to try a new alternative or technique on the next attempt

(DiClemente et al., 1991; Evers, Harlow, Redding, & LaForge, 1998; Prochaska & DiClemente, 1992). Fortunately for exercise behaviors, only fifteen percent of people regress from action or maintenance stages completely back to precontemplation. In fact, the majority of individuals who relapse return either to contemplation or preparation for another attempt at behavioral change (Prochaska & Velicer, 1997). The processes utilized during the action stage help build a foundation for success during maintenance. Other processes, such as helping relationships (social support) and reinforcement management, can be used to advance long-term adherence (Prochaska, DiClemente et al., 1992).

The group and organizational strategies discussed for the action stage remain relevant and important throughout maintenance. The principal goals during the maintenance stage are to help people remain motivated and assist them in recognizing and negotiating the inevitable obstacles and competing demands that can get in the way of their newly established exercise habit. Most activities and programs that help people become active can also be used to help them stay active. For example, workgroup social relationships provide an opportunity to be open about one's problems with others who care, and continual support can be provided through social networks, buddy systems, and self-help groups (Marcus, Banspaugh et al., 1992; Marcus et al., 1996; Prochaska, Norcross et al., 1992). Having a group of co-workers who walk during lunchtime is a prime example of such a network. These individuals not only serve as role models for continued exercise behavior but also provide a supportive environment in which to discuss issues affecting workouts or temptations to return to a sedentary lifestyle.

In addition, reinforcement strategies reward the person for making behavioral changes and may be furnished through incentives, recognition, self-rewards, or contingency contracts. Reinforcement strategies can employ either individual or group level contingencies. Marcus and colleagues (1998) incorporated rewards into their exercise intervention at both action and maintenance stages. The rewards may be provided when an individual or group reaches a specific goal or remains consistent with established goals or benchmarks for a set amount of time. These rewards or incentives are techniques to prevent temporary relapses and provide a certain amount of motivation to remain consistent with the exercise behavior. It is important to make sure the rewards are reflective of the effort and time put into to achieving them (Wilson & DeJoy, 1995).

Finally, relapse may occur at any stage; however, relapse prevention is especially important as individuals make exercise a regular part of their everyday lives. Thus, the reasons for first starting an exercise program should be revisited. The benefits of exercise are numerous and remain potent as exercise continues as part of one's lifestyle; therefore, the pros of long-term physical activity should be highlighted, and future exercise goals should be set in order to plan ahead to remain active (Allan, 1997; Marcus, Owen et al., 1998).

Relapse Prevention

Although relapse is a construct of the Transtheoretical Model that dovetails with many of the stages, there has been enough research into the causes of relapse and relapse prevention strategies that a separate discussion is warranted. Realistically speaking, relapse is probably the most common outcome of health behavior change programs. With respect to exercise programs, relapse rates average 50% in the first six months (Dishman, 1988). It should be noted that there is a distinct difference between **lapse** and **relapse.** A lapse is a single event, the reemergence of the previous behavior that may or may not result in relapse (Brownell, Marlatt, Lichtenstein, & Wilson, 1986). An individual who is too busy to exercise one particular week or an ex-smoker who has one cigarette are examples of lapses. If the individual returns to their previous inactivity pattern or smoking behavior as a result of the lapse, then relapse has occurred. In other words, the individual's response to the lapse determines whether or not relapse will occur (Brownell et al., 1986). Individuals need to understand that an occasional slip-up or mistake does not automatically trigger relapse and that they are still able to correct themselves and continue the positive behavior.

Although the causes of relapse are varied, there seem to be similarities across different health behaviors. The most commonly cited antecedents for relapse include: negative emotional states or stress events, inadequate motivation, inadequate coping skills to deal with the event, lack of social support, withdrawal effects associated with an addictive behavior (e.g., smoking, alcohol), and environmental cues (finding oneself in a situation that was previously associated with the behavior) (Brownell et al., 1986; DeJoy et al., 1995; Taylor, 1991). Most relapse prevention strategies are designed to prevent or control these antecedents.

Since the majority of relapse (50–60%) occurs in the first three months (Lovato and Green, 1990; Marlatt and Gordon, 1985), relapse prevention strategies should be incorporated into the physical activity program from the very beginning. Brownell and colleagues suggest a three-pronged approach designed to affect: motivation and commitment, initial behavior change, and maintenance (Brownell et al., 1986). First, enhancing motivation and commitment before individuals formally begin the change process (preparation) will pay dividends down the road. Strategies used in this approach may include increasing motivation through education (touting the benefits of the action) or incentives, goalsetting, and screening to determine those most likely to succeed and, consequently, those requiring additional attention. Second, during initial behavior change (action), three areas should be emphasized: decision-making, cognitive restructuring, and coping skills. Decision-making prepares an individual for analyzing the determinants of relapse and selecting the appropriate coping skills to counter the event. Cognitive restructuring teaches an individual to interpret events in a rational way and respond constructively to crises or stressful events. Coping skills are the specific skills used to handle the event, such as scheduling a specific time for exercise after being away for a week or walking away from a social event at which a number of people are smoking. Finally, during maintenance, recommended strategies include: continued monitoring, social support, and general lifestyle change or lifestyle rebalancing. Strategies designed to maintain long-term contact with the individual, increase social support, and promote other positive health changes in their lifestyle will reduce the likelihood of relapse during maintenance. Ironically, exercise is increasingly being cited as a positive health change to reduce the likelihood of relapse for other behaviors, particularly addictive behaviors (Brownell et al., 1986).

Finally, one of the strongest predictors of behavior change is previous attempts at change (King et al., 1992). Consequently, relapse should not be considered a failure, just another step toward permanent change. Individuals may learn from the relapse experience to acquire additional information about their weaknesses and test means for coping with them. As infants, we learned to walk through trial and error, so it seems natural that we would use the same process to modify our current behaviors. Individuals need to perceive the relapse as a learning experience rather than a failure that can not be corrected. Incorporating these "lessons learned" into the next change effort may be the boost they need to attain permanent change.

Implementing Physical Activity Program Components

The previous section detailed various stage-based strategies that could be used for tailoring worksite physical activity change efforts. Table 10-4 takes that one step further by summarizing various program components that are commonly used in worksite physical activity programs and recommending the stage during which the component would be most effectively implemented. It should be noted that this list is not all inclusive and that worksite programs should

Table 10-4 Programmatic Options and Suggested Stage of Implementation

Programs	Precontemplation	Contemplation	Preparation	Action	Maintenance
Health fair	X	X			
Health risk appraisal	X	X			
Health screening (blood pressure, blood sugar, etc.)	X	X	X		
Bulletin boards	X	X			
Lunch and learn programs	X	X	X		
Fitness assessment	X	X	X	X	
Incentive programs		X	X	X	X
Exercise prescription		X	X	X	
Health library		X	X		
Fitness web page		X	X	X	X
Fitness centers (in-house)			X	X	X
Health club memberships				X	X
Recreation clubs (bowling, softball, etc.)			X	X	
Aerobics classes				X	X
Spin classes				X	X
Circuit weight training				X	X
Computerized exercise logs				X	X
Competitions			X	X	X
Running/walking clubs				X	X
"Fun run" sponsorship		X	X	X	X
Support groups			X	X	X

not be judged by how many of these components they offer. Offering these components without incorporating the tailoring concepts discussed previously greatly reduces their effectiveness. Worksite practitioners should strive to incorporate stage-based constructs into the program component where appropriate with the understanding that not all constructs will necessarily work in all the components. For example, such constructs as social support, walking/running clubs, and computerized exercise logs are suggested components for the maintenance stage (see Table 10-4). However, walking/running clubs obviously lend themselves to incorporating social support strategies much more readily than do exercise logs, which do not necessarily require social support.

FITNESS PRINCIPLES

While using a stage-based approach it is still important to incorporate basic fitness principles into the physical activity program. These principles have been extensively discussed in most exercise physiology textbooks (readers interested in a more detailed discussion of these principles are referred to the following: Bouchard et al., 1994; Plowman & Smith, 1997; Robergs & Roberts, 1997; Wilmore & Costill, 1994). This section will summarize the key elements and suggest guidelines for prescribing physical activity regimens. The following suggestions are intended for apparently healthy individuals.

Components of Fitness

Health-related fitness consists of the following components (Bouchard et al., 1994; Collingwood, 1994; Robergs & Roberts, 1997; Wilmore & Costill, 1994): a) **flexibility,** the ability to have range of motion, b) **body composition,** the relationship between fat and fat-free tissue and the comparison between the two, c) **muscular strength and endurance,** the absolute strength or muscles' capability to generate force and muscular endurance in terms of muscles' capability to make repeated contractions, and d) **cardiorespiratory endurance** (aerobic power), the ability of the body to transport oxygen and perform work on a sustained basis. These components, in addition to the dimensions of intensity, frequency, duration, and

mode provide a foundation for all physical activity programs.

Fitness Prescription Dimensions

The foundations of any fitness program are intensity, frequency, duration, and mode. These factors should be considered and incorporated into all physical activity prescriptions.

Intensity

Exercise intensity refers to the level of stress achieved during the exercise period (Robergs & Roberts, 1997). Three specific methods may be used to examine intensity: metabolic equivalents (METs), heart rate, and perceived exertion.

A graded exercise stress test may be used to determine an individual's functional aerobic capacity. Exercise prescription, defined by METs, is the most sophisticated and detailed type of prescription commonly used. A MET quantifies intensity in terms of oxygen required to perform a certain level of work. One MET is assumed to be equal to an oxygen uptake of 3.5 milliliters per kilogram of body weight per minute (mL/kg) or a caloric expenditure of 50 kilocalories per square meter of body surface per hour. For example, if a person's VO_2 max of 35 mL/kg/min is equal to 10 METs then, according to American College of Sports Medicine guidelines, this individual should exercise within 50% to 85% of maximum oxygen uptake (VO_2 max) or between 5 to 8.5 METs.

The heart rate method assumes there is a relationship between heart rate and oxygen consumption. For the majority of aerobic enthusiasts, this form of monitoring exercise intensity provides a safe, effective, and quick way of ensuring that they are reaping the health benefits of their exercise program through adequate effort levels. To determine what heart rate range is best for any individual, the four-step Karvonen process can be used.

1. Determine your predicted maximal heart rate by subtracting the age of the individual from 220 (for women), or subtracting half the age from 205 (for men). [For example for a 40-year-old woman: $220 - 40 = 180$]

2. Subtract the resting heart rate in beats per minute from the predicted maximal heart rate. The best time to estimate the resting heart rate is in the morning. [Continuing our example: $180 - 60 = 120$]
3. For most healthy adults, 65% to 90% of predicted maximal heart rate is the optimal range. So, multiply the predicted maximal heart rate by 65% to determine the lower end of the range and by 90% to determine the upper end of the range. [$120 \times 0.65 = 78$ and $120 \times 0.90 = 108$]
4. Finally, add the resting heart rate back into the heart rate range at the lower and upper ends of the range to estimate the aerobic training zone. [$78 + 60 = 138$ and $108 + 60 = 168$]

The rate of perceived exertion method is performed by asking the individual to rate the feelings of exertion caused by an aerobic activity (Borg, 1982). Using a scale for rate of perceived exertion, the intensity may be assessed by having the individual describe the sensations of energy or effort exerted during a particular bout of exercise using a scale ranging from 6 to 20. On this scale a rating of 6–7 would be considered "very, very light," 12–13 "somewhat hard," 15–16 "hard," and 19–20 "very, very hard." To exercise at 60% to 80% of maximal heart rate, the individual should be the range of 12–15.

Frequency

The frequency refers to the number of sessions per week. The amount of improvement in oxygen uptake increases with the frequency of aerobic training and has been found to result in less meaningful increases when below 2 days per week and a plateau when frequency rises above 3 days per week. Importantly, it takes about two weeks for a significant amount of detraining to occur. Thus, if the individual misses a training session, it is best to try to get back into the workout regimen very soon.

Duration

Duration refers to the length of time of the physical activity session. The intensity and duration of exercise may be considered inversely related: the higher the exercise intensity, the shorter the duration of the

exercise (Robergs & Roberts, 1997). Thus, the duration of the activity should be increased when the activity is performed at lower intensities, as is usually the case with beginning exercisers. One hour following a workout, an individual should feel rested. Performing too much too soon may lead to overtraining and reduced adherence rates.

Mode

Mode refers to the type of activity performed during the physical activity session. The mode is dependent upon the individual's physical activity goals. For example, to improve muscular strength and endurance, weight training will be the focus of activity, while goals centered on weight reduction and improving aerobic metabolism will include activities such as running, biking, and swimming. A variety of activities, such as running, cycling, swimming, hiking, cross-country skiing, and dancing, should be prescribed to allow a person to cross-train (perform both aerobic and strength training) in order to benefit from a well-rounded training effect (ACSM, 1998).

Physical Activity Program Guidelines

Table 10-5, which was updated from Collingwood (1994), outlines exercise prescription guidelines established by the American College of Sports Medicine (1998). These guidelines are the minimum threshold values for cardiorespiratory endurance, muscular strength and endurance, and flexibility. The remainder of this section will discuss additional suggestions for programs in these three areas.

Cardiorespiratory Endurance (Aerobic Training)

Aerobic exercise is defined as any activity that rhythmically utilizes large muscle groups for a continuous period. The selection of the mode of exercise should be dependent on the individual's goals, past exercise experiences, budget, current fitness level, and preferences (Robergs & Roberts, 1997). The most common forms of aerobic exercise include walking, running, swimming, and biking. Cardiorespiratory endurance may be the most important health-related component of physical activity due to its impact on coronary

Table 10-5 Exercise Prescription Guidelines

Aerobic Power–Cardiorespiratory Endurance

Intensity	65–90% maximum HR; 50–85% VO$_2$max
Frequency	3–5 days/week
Duration	20–60 minutes (dependent on intensity)
Mode	large muscle movement

Flexibility

Intensity	stretch to easy point of tension
Frequency	minimum of 2+ times/week
Duration	hold 10–30 seconds for static stretch
Mode	stretching, active and passive

Strength

Frequency	2–3 days/week (every other day)
Duration	1 set initially, work toward 3 sets
Intensity	*endurance* (dynamic strength) = low resistance, high repetitions
	strength (absolute strength) = high resistance, low repetitions
Mode	isometrics, isotonic, isokinetic
	1 set of 8–12 repetitions of 8–10 exercises

Source: American College of Sports Medicine, *Medicine and Science in Sports and Exercise*, 1998.

heart disease risk factors and other chronic diseases (Bishop & Aldana, 1999).

Muscular Strength and Endurance (Strength Training)

Muscular performance involves the effectiveness of how our muscles use energy and entails both muscular strength (the maximal level at which a muscle can exert a force) and endurance (the muscle's ability to make repeated contractions against resistance). For strength, a key concept behind muscular performance is the resistance, or overload, principle. Resistance may come in the form of an external force, such as a barbell, or one's own body weight. The goal is to increase the load a muscle can bear in order for that area of the body to become larger, stronger, and more efficient at working against such force. Through progressive resistance training, increasing the force (or "overloading" the muscle) will in turn improve strength. For endurance, interval training, which involves short times of exertion that are followed by recovery periods, can be used. Endurance is built

through an individual increasing the number of times they can perform the repetitions. Training for the healthy adult includes performing contractions at moderate-to-slow speed, through the full range of motion, and using a normal breathing pattern during lifting movements.

Flexibility

Flexibility may be defined as the body's ability to move freely over a wide range of motion while being void of stiffness and resistance. Flexible muscles are less prone to soreness and injury and can help to improve overall muscular performance due to ability to lengthen and stretch. Stretching may be performed as often as an individual desires and should focus on the area(s) of the body that needs improvement in range of motion. For a period of five to ten minutes, preexercise stretching can help reduce one's risk of injury during vigorous exercise bouts, and for a similar length of time, stretching at the end of a workout can prevent muscle soreness. The optimal way of working on the flexibility of a muscle is through slow, gentle stretching, without bouncing. Keeping a stretch slow and controlled throughout the range of motion is important in avoiding hyperextension or pushing a joint beyond its limits. The "sitting toe-touch" is an example of a flexibility stretch that examines the limberness of the lower back and hamstrings. This test can be used to assess an individual's lower body flexibility and as a means of developing an exercise program that can help improve the stiffness of these muscles and prevent future injury or lower back pain.

PROGRAM MANAGEMENT

In order for worksite health promotion to be successful, the encompassing activities and events must be well-planned, -organized, and -implemented. Program management provides a blueprint for certain policies and procedures that can ensure that employee needs are being met and programs are functioning efficiently. Program management includes the areas of program planning, maintenance, and marketing. This discussion serves to highlight program management issues specific to exercise programs. An in depth discussion of all program management issues may be found in Chapter 4.

First, program planning starts with the development of a mission statement and goals for the health promotion program. Program activities can be developed and prioritized based on a needs assessment performed within the workforce. This needs assessment helps to identify the health risk behaviors of the employees and provides a focus to the programs' events based on the needs of the population. Needs assessments could include: an employee survey of health/program interests, a climate survey (observer examines the work environment for physical and mental factors that may impact employee health), a fitness assessment and/or health risk appraisal (a survey which helps to identify specific health risks based on individual lifestyle choices), and an examination of company records (i.e., employee health insurance claims).

Second, maintenance of the program involves carrying out the tasks of a program in the proper manner and other implementation issues, such as those involving personnel and evaluation. For example, the staff of a worksite health promotion program must not only exhibit fidelity in providing services and completing certain tasks (such as cleaning equipment, familiarizing employees with exercise machines, and documenting participation) but must also have adequate education and proper experience. Besides formal education within a university/college setting, national certifications are available for fitness instructors, personal trainers, and program directors (e.g., American College of Sports Medicine, National Academy of Sports Medicine, American Council on Exercise, Aerobics and Fitness Association of America). Having an educated and well-informed staff is an essential step in providing safe and effective services. Evaluation within an exercise program should include assessing an employee's health status to determine the most effective physical activity program, assessing program implementation, and determining program effectiveness.

Finally, marketing entails a variety of strategies designed to increase program awareness and participation. Payroll stuffers, workteam meeting announcements, posters in the lunchroom, and program incentives (e.g., raffle for television, participant T-shirt) are all methods that may attract employee attention and enhance participation rates. The key to the success of the marketing effort will be to incorporate a customer-centered philosophy throughout the program. This philosophy must permeate all planning and implementation efforts.

CONCLUSION

Physical activity programs have served as the cornerstone for many worksite health promotion programs for the past three decades. During this time, the interest in and support for physical activity programs at the worksite has increased significantly. At the same time, practitioners face a number of challenges to sustain the viability of these programs in the future. The major challenges facing all practitioners, but particularly those in worksite settings, include: a) making physical activity attractive to the masses, b) increasing the sophistication of physical activity interventions, and c) increasing environmental and organizational support for physical activity.

Probably the biggest challenge facing practitioners over the next decade is to get the 50–66% of the population that is not regularly active or is inactive to embrace physical activity as a part of their normal routine. This may require a radical departure from the current approach to physical activity programming, necessitate adopting principles or strategies originally developed for other types of behavior change interventions (e.g., smoking, hypertension), involve a coordinated effort conducted at the national, regional, state, and local (worksite) level, be focused entirely on yet unreached subgroups, and/or utilize modern technology to encourage rather than discourage physical activity. All this will need to be accomplished during a time of rapid change. Telecommuting, decentralized work structures, global operations, and an increasingly aging and multicultural workforce will magnify the complexity of this challenge.

The second challenge is not unique to fitness practitioners but is one faced by all health promotion professionals attempting to facilitate behavior change. There is growing awareness of the need to build all health promotion programs on a sound theoretical foundation, one supported by the best available evidence at that point in time. However, the key to the success of those programs, and the real challenge, is to link specific intervention strategies to the underlying theoretical construct and then demonstrate the impact of those strategies on the construct. The typical health promotion intervention is like making soup. Practitioners throw in a bunch of ingredients and determine whether or not it is pleasing to the taste without really knowing which specific ingredients are pleasing and which are not. So the next time they make soup, they are not really sure which ingredients to add or remove to make it more pleasing. Furthermore, if the soup was not pleasing, they throw out the entire recipe and start over, even though only a fraction of ingredients might have been the cause for the bad taste. We need to start developing and testing the individual ingredients (strategies) of our interventions to better understand which impact the targeted behavior and which can be "thrown out."

The final challenge is one of developing a support structure for physical activity. This support structure goes beyond an individual social support-type of approach to include the organization's environment and culture and the community in which it resides. This support can take a variety of forms from the provision of space and equipment, to providing flex time, to reducing health insurance deductibles and/or copayments. Many companies have provided beautiful facilities for employee use, but how many have provided time "on the clock" to exercise? A variety of companies have covered part or all of the cost of using the exercise facility or joining another, but how many have lowered health insurance premiums or deductibles for those who are regularly active? Organizations need to model the behavior they wish the employees to adopt and get away from a "do what I say, not what I do" mentality. Practitioners are challenged to build a healthy organization, one that values its employees, integrates it through its philosophy, and demonstrates it through its actions.

These are considerable challenges that can not be easily addressed or overcome. However, they *must* be confronted if worksite physical activity programs are going to significantly impact the health and well-being of the employees, and in turn the organization, in the future. This will require a coordinated effort on the part of practitioners, researchers, administrators, and policy makers to ensure that a majority, rather than a minority, are physically active.

References

Abrams, D. B., Elder, J. P., Carleton, R. A., Lasater, T. M., & Artz, L. M. (1986). Social learning principles for organizational health promotion: An integrated approach. In M. F. Cataldo & T. J. Coates (Eds.), *Health & industry: A behavioral medicine perspective* (pp. 28–51). New York: John Wiley & Sons.

Abrams, D. B., & Follick, M. J. (1983). Behavioral weight loss intervention at the worksite: Feasibility and maintenance. *Journal of Consulting and Clinical Psychology, 51*, 226–233.

Allan, J. (1997). Lifestyle change success rates: Our greatest challenge. *American Worksite Health Promotion, 4*, 29–31.

Allen, R. F., Allen, J. R., Kraft, C., & Certner, B. (1987). *The organizational unconscious: How to create the corporate culture you want and need.* Morristown, NJ: Human Resource Institute.

American College of Sports Medicine. (1998). The recommended quality and quantity of exercise for developing and maintaining cardiorespiratory and muscular fitness, and flexibility in healthy adults. *Medicine and Science in Sports and Exercise, 30*, 975–991.

Baun, W. B. (1995). Culture change in worksite health promotion. In D. M. DeJoy and M.G. Wilson (Eds.), *Critical issues in worksite health promotion* (pp. 29–49). Boston: Allyn & Bacon.

Baun, W. B., Bernacki, E. J., & Tsai, S. P. (1986). A preliminary investigation: Effect of a corporate fitness program on absenteeism and health care cost. *Journal of Occupational Medicine, 28*(1), 18–22.

Bell, B. C., & Blanke, D. J. (1992). The effects of an employee fitness program on health care costs and utilization. *Health Values, 16*(3), 3–13.

Bernacki, E. J. & Baun, W. B. (1984). The relationship of job performance to exercise adherence in a corporate fitness program. *Journal of Occupational Medicine, 26*, 529–531.

Bishop, J. G., & Aldana, S. G. (1999). *Step up to wellness. A stage based approach.* Boston: Allyn & Bacon.

Blair, S. N., Smith, M., Collingwood, T. R., Reynolds, R., Prentice, M. C., & Sterling, C. L. (1986). Health promotion for educators: Impact on absenteeism. *Preventive Medicine, 15,* 166–175.

Borg, G. A. V. (1982). Psychophysical bases of physical exertion. *Medicine and Science in Sports and Exercise, 14,* 377–87.

Bouchard, C., Shephard, R. J., & Stephens, T. (Eds.). (1994). *Physical activity, fitness and health. International proceedings and consensus statement.* Champaign, IL: Human Kinetics.

Bowne, D. W., Russell, M. L., Morgan, J. L., Optenberg, S. A., & Clarke, A. E. (1984). Reduced disability and health care costs in an industrial fitness program. *Journal of Occupational Medicine, 26,* 809–816.

Brownell, K. D., & Felix, M. R. (1987). Competitions to facilitate health promotion: Review and conceptual analysis. *American Journal of Health Promotion, 2,* 28–36.

Brownell, K. D., Marlatt, G. A., Lichtenstein, E., & Wilson, G. T. (1986). Understanding and preventing relapse. *American Psychologist, 41,* 765–782.

Brownell, K. D., Stunkard, M., McKeon, P., & Felix, M. R. (1983). *Cooperation competition: Four studies in department stores and banks.* Paper presented at the American Psychological Association Annual Convention, Anaheim, CA.

Campbell, M. K., DeVellis, B. M., Stretcher, V. J., Ammerman, A. S., DeVellis, R. F., & Sandler, R. S. (1994). Improving dietary behavior: The effectiveness of tailored messages in primary care settings. *American Journal of Public Health, 4,* 783–787.

Cardinal, B. J., & Sachs, M. L. (1996). Effects of mail-mediated, stage-matched exercise strategies on female adults' leisure-time exercise behavior. *Journal of Sports Medicine and Physical Fitness, 36,* 100–107.

Centers for Disease Control and Prevention. (1995). *Behavioral risk factor surveillance system* [On-line]. Available: http://www.cdc.gov/nccdphp/brfss.

Centers for Disease Control and Prevention. (1996). *Behavioral risk factor surveillance system* [On-line]. Available: http://www.cdc.gov/nccdphp/brfss.

Centers for Disease Control and Prevention. (1998). Self-reported physical inactivity by degree of urbanization–United States, 1996. *Morbidity Mortality Weekly Report, 47,* 1097–1100.

Centers for Disease Control and Prevention. (1997a). Monthly estimates of leisure-time physical inactivity–United States, 1994. *Morbidity Mortality Weekly Report, 46,* 393–397.

Centers for Disease Control and Prevention. (1997b). *1997 Summary report.* Atlanta, GA: National Center for Chronic Disease Prevention and Health Promotion, Behavioral Risk Factor Surveillance System.

Centers for Disease Control and Prevention. (1996). Community-level prevention of human immunodeficiency virus infection among high-risk populations: The AIDS community demonstration projects. *Morbidity Mortality Weekly Report, 45,* 1–24.

Clarke, P., & Eves, F. (1997). Applying the Transtheoretical Model to the study of exercise on prescription. *Journal of Health Psychology, 2,* 195–207.

Cohen, R. Y., Stunkard, A. J., & Felix, M. R. J. (1987). Comparison of three worksite weight-loss competitions. *Journal of Behavioral Medicine, 10,* 467–479.

Cole, G., Leonard, B., Hammond, S., & Fridinger, F. (1998). Using "stages of behavioral change" constructs to measure the short-term effects of a worksite-based intervention to increase moderate physical activity. *Psychological Reports, 82,* 615–618.

Collingwood, T. R. (1994). Fitness programs. In M. P. O'Donnell & J. S. Harris (Eds.), *Health promotion in the workplace* (2nd ed., pp. 240–270). Albany, NY: Delmar.

Cox, M., Shephard, R. J., & Corey, P. (1981). Influence of an employee fitness programme upon fitness, productivity, and absenteeism. *Ergonomics, 24,* 795–806.

Cummings, K. M., Hellmann, R., & Emont, S. L. (1988). Correlates of participation in a worksite stop-smoking contest. *Journal of Behavioral Medicine, 11,* 267–277.

DeJoy, D. M., Wilson, M. G., & Huddy, D. C. (1995). Health behavior change in the workplace. In D. M. DeJoy & M. G. Wilson (Eds.), *Critical issues in worksite health promotion* (pp. 97–122). Boston: Allyn & Bacon.

DeJoy, D. M., & Southern, D. J. (1993). An integrative perspective on worksite health promotion. *Journal of Occupational Medicine, 35,* 1221–1230.

DiClemente, C. C., & Prochaska, J. O. (1985). Processes and stages of self-change: Coping and competence in smoking behavior change. In S. Schiffman & T. A. Wills (Eds.), *Coping and substance use* (pp. 319–343). San Diego, CA: Academic Press.

DiClemente, C. C., Prochaska, J. O., Fairhurst, S. K., Velicer, W. F., Velasquez, M. M., & Rossi, J. S. (1991). The process of smoking cessation: An analysis of precontemplation, contemplation, and preparation stages of change. *Journal of Consulting and Clinical Psychology, 59,* 295–304.

Dishman, R. K. (1988). *Exercise adherence: Its impact on public health.* Champaign, IL: Human Kinetics.

Dishman, R. K., Oldenburg, B., O'Neal, H., & Shephard, R. J. (1998). Worksite physical activity interventions. *American Journal of Preventive Medicine, 15*(4), 344–361.

Dishman, R. K., Sallis, J. F., & Orenstein, D. R. (1985). The determinants of physical activity and exercise. *Public Health Reports, 100,* 158–171.

Evers, K. E., Harlow, L. L., Redding, C. A., & LaForge, R. G. (1998). Longitudinal changes in stages of change for condom use in women. *American Journal of Health Promotion, 13,* 19–25.

Fletcher, G. F., Balady, G., Blair, S. N., Blumenthal, J., Casperson, C., Chaitman, B., Epstein, S., Froelicher, E. S., Froelicher, V. F., Pina, I. L., & Pollock, M. L. (1996). Statement on exercise: Benefits and recommendations for physical activity programs for all Americans. *Circulation, 94,* 857–862.

Gebhardt, D. L., & Crump, C. E. (1990). Employee fitness and wellness programs in the workplace. *American Psychologist, 45*(2), 262–272.

Godwin, G., & Shephard, R. J. (1986). Importance of type of attitude to the study of behavior. *Psychological Reports, 58,* 991–1000.

Green, L. W., & Kreuter, M. S. (1990). *Health promotion planning: An educational and environmental approach.* Toronto: Mayfield.

Green, L. W., Richard, L., & Potvin, L. (1996). Ecological foundations of health promotion. *American Journal of Health Promotion, 10,* 270–281.

Green, L. W., Wilson, A. L., & Lovato, C. Y. (1986). What changes can health promotion achieve and how long do these changes last? The trade-offs between expediency and durability. *Preventive Medicine, 15,* 508–521.

Hasberg, J. M. (1994). Fitness, health and aging. In C. Bouchard, R. J. Shephard, & T. Stephens (Eds.), *Physical activity, fitness and health. International proceedings and consensus statement* (pp. 993–1005). Champaign, IL: Human Kinetics.

Haskell, W. L. (1994). Dose-response issues from a biological perspective. In C. Bouchard, R. J. Shephard, & T. Stephens (Eds.), *Physical activity, fitness and health. International proceedings and consensus statement* (pp. 1030–39). Champaign, IL: Human Kinetics.

Heather, N., Rollnick, S., Bell, A., & Richmond, R. (1996). Effects of brief counseling among male heavy drinkers identified on general hospital wards. *Drug and Alcohol Review, 15,* 29–38.

Hellman, E. A. (1997). Use of the stage of change in exercise adherence model among older adults with cardiac diagnosis. *Journal of Cardiopulmonary Rehabilitation, 17,* 145–155.

Horn, D. A. (1976). A model for the study of personal choice health behavior. *International Journal of Health Education, 19,* 89–98.

Horne, T. E. (1994). Predictors of physical activity intentions and behavior for rural homemakers. *Revue Canadienne de Sante Publique, 85,* 132–135.

Jaffe, D. T. (1995). The healthy company: Research paradigms for personal and organizational health. In S. L. Sauter & L. R. Murphy (Eds.), *Organizational risk factors for job stress* (pp. 13–39). Washington, DC: American Psychological Association.

Jaffe-Sandroff, D., Bradford, S., & Gilligan, V. F. (1990). Meeting the health promotion challenge through a model of shared responsibility. In M. E. Scofield (Ed.), *Occupational medicine: State of the art reviews: Worksite health promotion, 5,* 677–690.

Jakicic, J. M., Wing, R. R., Butler, B. A., & Robertson, R. J. (1995). Prescribing exercise in multiple short bouts versus one continuous bout; Effects on adherence, cardiorespiratory fitness, and weight loss in overweight women. *International Journal of Obesity, 19,* 893–901.

Janis, I. L., & Mann, L. A. (1977). *Decision making: A psychological analysis of conflict, choice, and commitment.* New York: Collier MacMillan.

Jason, L. A., Jayaraj, S., Blitz, C. C., Michaels, M. H., & Klett, L. E. (1990). Incentives and competition in a worksite smoking cessation intervention. *American Journal of Public Health, 80,* 205–206.

Kaman, R. L., & Patton, R. W. (1994). Costs and benefits of an active versus an inactive society. In C. Bruchard, R. J. Shephard, & T. Stephens (Eds.), *Physical activity, fitness and health: International proceedings and consensus statement* (pp. 134–144). Champaign, IL: Human Kinetics.

Kanfer, F. & Gaelick-Buys, L. (1991). Self-management methods. In F. Kanfer &

A. Goldstein (Eds.), *Helping people change: A textbook of methods* (pp. 305–360). New York: Pergamon Press.

King, A. C., Blair, S. N., Bild, D. E., Dishman, R. K., Dubbert, P. M, & Marcus, B. H. (1992). Determinants of physical activity and interventions in adults. *Medicine and Science in Sports and Exercise, 24* (Suppl.), S221–S236.

King, T. K., Marcus, B. H., Pinto, B. M., Emmons, K. M., & Abrams, D. B. (1995). Cognitive-behavioral mediators of changing multiple behaviors: Smoking and a sedentary lifestyle. *Preventive Medicine, 25,* 684–691.

Klesges, R. C., Glasgow, R. E., Klesges, L. M., Morray, K., & Quale, R. (1987). Competition and relapse prevention training in worksite smoking modification. *Health Education Research, 2,* 5–14.

Laforge, R. G., Velicer, W. F., Richmond, R. L., & Owen, N. (1999). Stage distribution for five health behaviors in the United States and Austria. *Preventive Medicine, 28,* 61–74.

Leatt, P., Hattin, H., West, C., & Shephard, R. J. (1988). Seven year follow-up of employee fitness program. *Canadian Journal of Public Health, 79,* 20–25.

Lechner, L., & de Vries, H. D. (1995). Participation in an employee fitness program: Determinants of high adherence, low adherence, and dropout. *Journal of Occupational and Environmental Medicine, 37,* 429–436.

Lechner, L., de Vries, H., Adriaansen, S., & Drabbels, L. (1997). Effects of an employee fitness program on reduced absenteeism. *Journal of Occupational and Environmental Medicine, 39,* 827–831.

Lewthwaite, R. (1990). Motivational considerations in physical activity involvement. *Physical Therapy, 70,* 808–819.

Lovato, C. Y., & Green, L. W. (1990). Maintaining employee participation in workplace health promotion programs. *Health Education Quarterly, 17,* 73–88.

Lynch, W. D., Golaszewski, T. J., Clearie, A. F., Snow, D., & Vickery, D. M. (1990). Impact of a facility-based corporate fitness program on the number of absences from work due to illnesses. *Journal of Occupational Medicine, 32,* 9–12.

Maehr, M. L., & Braskamp, L. A. (1986). *The motivational factor.* Lexington, MA: Lexington Press.

Malina, R. M. (1994). Physical activity: Relationship to growth, maturation, and physical fitness. In

C. Bouchard, R. J. Shephard, & T. Stephens (Eds.), *Physical activity, fitness and health. International proceedings and consensus statement* (pp. 918–930). Champaign, IL: Human Kinetics.

Marcus, B. H., Banspach, S. W., Lefebvre, R. C., Rossi, J. S., Carleton, R. A., & Abrams, D. B. (1992). Using stages of change model to increase the adoption of physical activity among community participants. *American Journal of Health Promotion, 6,* 424–429.

Marcus, B. H., Emmons, K. M., Simkin-Silverman, L. R., Linnan, L. A., Taylor, E.R., Bock, B.C., Roberts, M. B., Rossi, J. S., & Abrams, D. B. (1998). Evaluation of motivationally tailored vs. standard self-help physical activity interventions at the workplace. *American Journal of Health Promotion, 12,* 246–253.

Marcus, B. H., Owen, N., Forsyth, L. H., Cavill, N. A., & Fridinger, F. (1998). Physical activity interventions using mass media, print media, and information technology. *American Journal of Preventive Medicine, 15,* 362–378.

Marcus, B. H., Rakowski, W., & Rossi, J. S. (1992). Assessing motivational readiness and decision making for exercise. *Health Psychology, 11,* 257–261.

Marcus, B., Rossi, J., Selby, V., Niaura, R., & Abrams, D. (1992). The stages and processes of exercise adoption and maintenance in a worksite sample. *Health Psychology, 11,* 386–395.

Marcus, B. H., & Simkin, L. R. (1993). The stages of exercise behavior. *Journal of Sports Medicine and Physical Fitness, 33,* 83–88.

Marcus, B. H., Simkin, L. R., Rossi, J. S., & Pinto, B. M. (1996). Longitudinal shifts in employees' stages and processes of exercise behavior change. *American Journal of Health Promotion, 10,* 195–200.

Marcus, B., Selby, V. L., Niavra, R. S., & Rossi, J. S. (1997). Self-efficacy and the stages of exercise behavior change. *Research Quarterly for Exercise and Sport, 63,* 60–66.

Marlatt, G. A., & Gordon, J. R. (1985). *Relapse prevention: Maintenance strategies in addictive behavior change.* New York: Guilford Press.

McLeroy, K. R., Bibeau, D., Steckler, A., & Glanz, K. (1988). An ecological perspective on health promotion programs. *Health Education Quarterly, 15,* 351–377.

Norstrom, J. A., & Conray, W. E. (1995). The activity pyramid and the new physical activity recommendations. *The Bulletin, 2,* 107–111.

O'Donnell, M. P. (1989). Definition of health promotion: Part III: Expanding the definition. *American Journal of Health Promotion, 3,* 5.

O'Donnell, M. P., and Ainsworth, T. A. (1984). *Health promotion in the workplace.* New York: John Wiley & Sons.

Perz, C. A., DiClemente, C. C., & Carbonari, J. P. (1996). Doing the right thing at the right time? The interaction of stages and processes of change in successful smoking cessation. *Health Psychology, 15,* 462–468.

Plowman, S. A., & Smith, D. L. (1997). *Exercise physiology for health, fitness and performance.* Needham Heights, MA: Allyn & Bacon.

Prochaska, J. O., & DiClemente, C. C. (1983). Stages and processes of self-change in smoking: Towards an integrative model of change. *Journal of Consulting and Clinical Psychology, 51,* 390–395.

Prochaska, J. O., & DiClemente, C. C. (1984). *The transtheoretical approach: Crossing traditional boundaries of change.* Homewood, IL: Dorsey Press.

Prochaska, J. O., & DiClemente, C. C. (1992). Stages of change in the modification of problem behaviors. In M. Hersen, R. M. Eisler, & P. M. Miller (Eds.), *Progress in behavior modification* (pp. 184–214). Sycamore, IL: Sycamore Press.

Prochaska, J. O., DiClemente, C. C., & Norcross, J. C. (1992). In search of how people change: Applications to addictive behaviors. *American Psychologist, 47,* 1102–1114.

Prochaska, J. O., DiClemente, C. C, Velicer, W. F., & Rossi, J. S. (1993). Standardized, individualized, interactive, and personalized self-help programs for smoking cessation. *Health Psychology, 12,* 399–405.

Prochaska, J. O., Norcross, J. C., Fowler, M. J., Follick, M. J., & Abrams, D. B. (1992). Attendance and outcome in a worksite weight control program: Processes and stages of change as process and predictor variables. *Addictive Behaviors, 17,* 35–45.

Prochaska, J. O., & Velicer, W. F. (1997). The transtheoretical model of health behavior change. *American Journal of Health Promotion, 12,* 38–48.

Prochaska, J. O., Velicer, W. F., DiClemente, C. C., & Fava, J. (1988). Measuring processes of change: Applications to the cessation of smoking. *Journal of Consulting and Clinical Psychology, 56,* 520–528.

Rakowski, W., Ehrich, B. E., Goldstein, M. G., Dube, C. E., Clark, M. A., & Pearlman, D. N. (1997). *A stage-matched intervention for screening mammography.* Paper presented at the annual meeting of The Society of Behavioral Medicine, San Francisco, CA.

Rakowski, W., Ehrich, B. E., Goldstein, M. G., Dube, C. E., Clark, M. A., & Peterson, K. K. (1998). *Encouraging repeat screening mammography with a stage-matched, tailored intervention.* Paper presented at the annual meeting of The Society for Behavioral Medicine, New Orleans, LA.

Reed, G. R., Velicer, W. F., Prochaska, J. O., Rossi, J. S., & Marcus, B. H. (1997). What makes a good staging algorithm: Examples from regular exercise. *American Journal of Health Promotion, 12,* 57–66.

Ribisl, K. M., & Reischl, T. M. (1993). Measuring the climate for health at organizations: Development of the worksite health climate scales. *Journal of Occupational Medicine, 35,* 812–824.

Robergs, R. A., & Roberts, S. O. (1997). *Exercise physiology. Exercise, performance, and clinical applications.* St. Louis, MO: Mosby.

Robison, J. I., & Rogers, M. A. (1995). Impact of behavioral management programs on exercise adherence. *American Journal of Health Promotion, 9,* 379–382.

Rossi, J. S., Blais, L. M., Redding, C. A., & Weinstock, M. A. (1995). Behavior change for reducing sun and ultraviolet light exposure: Implications for interventions. *Dermatology Clinics, 13,* 613–622.

Rossi, J. S., Weinstock, M. A., Redding, C. A., Cottrill, S. D., & Maddock, J. E. (1997). *Effectiveness of stage-matched interventions for skin cancer prevention: A randomized clinical trial of high-risk beach bathers.* Paper presented at the annual meeting of The Society of Behavioral Medicine, San Francisco, CA.

Rudman, W. J., & Steinhardt, M. (1988). Fitness in the workplace: The effects of a corporate health and fitness program on work culture. *Health Values, 12,* 4–17.

Samuelson, M. (1998). Stages of change: From theory to practice. *The Art of Health Promotion, 2,* 1–7.

Shein, E. H. (1985). *Organizational culture and leadership.* San Francisco: Jossey-Bass.

Shephard, R. J. (1989). Current perspectives on the economics of fitness and sport with particular reference to worksite programmes. *Sports Medicine, 7,* 286–309.

Shephard, R. J. (1996). Worksite fitness and exercise programs: A review of methodology and health impact. *American Journal of Health Promotion, 10,* 436–452.

Shephard, R. J., Corey, P., Renzland, P., & Cox, M. (1982). The influence of an employee fitness and lifestyle modification program upon medical care costs. *Canadian Journal of Public Health, 73*, 259–263.

Shephard, R. J., Cox, M., & Corey, P. (1981). Fitness program participation: Its effect on worker performance. *Journal of Occupational Medicine, 23*, 359–363.

Siegel, D., Johnson, J., & Newhof, C. (1988). Adherence to exercise and sports classes by college women. *Journal of Sports Medicine and Physical Fitness, 28*, 181–188.

Skinner, C. S., Strecher, V. J., & Hospers, H. (1994). Physicians' recommendations for mammography: Do tailored messages make a difference? *American Journal of Public Health, 84*, 40–49.

Steinhardt, M., Greenhow, L., & Stewart, J. (1991). The relationship of physical activity and cardiovascular fitness to absenteeism and medical care claims among law enforcement officers. *American Journal of Health Promotion, 5*, 455–460.

Strecher, V. J., Seijts, G. H., Kok, G. J., Glasgow, R., DeVellis, B., & Meertens, R. M. (1995). Goal-setting as a strategy for health behavior-change. *Health Education Quarterly, 22*, 190–200.

Stunkard, A. J., Cohen, R. Y., & Felix, M. R. (1989). Weight loss competitions at the worksite: How they work and how well. *Preventive Medicine, 18*, 460–474.

Tappe, M. L., Duda, J. L., & Menges-Ehrnwald, P. (1989). Perceived barriers to exercise among adolescents. *Journal of Scholastic Health, 59*, 153–155.

Taylor, S. E. (1991). *Health psychology.* New York: McGraw-Hill.

Thoresen, C. E., & Mahoney, M. J. (1974). *Behavioral self-control.* New York: Holt.

Tsai, S. P., Baun, W. B., & Bernacki, E. J. (1987). Relationship of employee turnover to exercise adherence in a corporate fitness program. *Journal of Occupational Medicine, 29*, 572–575.

Tucker, L. A., Aldana, S. G., & Friedman, G. M. (1990). Cardiovascular fitness and absenteeism in 8,301 employed adults. *American Journal of Health Promotion, 5*, 140–145.

U. S. Department of Health and Human Services. (1987). *National survey of worksite health promotion activities. A summary.* National Technical Information Service (Publications No. PB88-129390). Washington, DC: Author.

U.S. Department of Health and Human Services. (2000). *Healthy people 2010.* U.S. Government Printing Office (Conference Edition). Washington DC: Author.

U. S. Department of Health and Human Services. (1991). *Healthy people 2000. National health promotion and disease prevention objectives.* U.S. Government Printing Office (Publication No. PHS 91-50212). Washington, DC: Author.

U. S. Department of Health and Human Services. (1992). *1992 national survey of worksite health promotion activities.* National Technical Information Service (Publications No. PB93-100204). Washington, DC: Author.

U. S. Department of Health and Human Services. (1996). *Physical activity and health. A report of the Surgeon General* (Publication No. PA 15250-7954). Atlanta, GA: Author.

Velicer, W. F., DiClemente, C. C., Prochaska, J. O., & Brandenburg, N. (1985). A decisional balance measure for assessing and predicting smoking status. *Journal of Personality and Social Psychology, 48*, 1279–1289.

Wankel, L. M. (1984). Decision-making and social support strategies for increasing exercise involvement. *Journal of Cardiac Rehabilitation, 4*, 124–135.

Weinstein, N. D. (1988). The precaution adoption process. *Health Psychology, 7*, 355–386.

Wilmore, J. H., & Costill, D. L. (1994). *Physiology of sport and exercise.* Champaign, IL: Human Kinetics.

Wilson, M. G. (1999). Health promotion in the workplace. In J. R. Rippe (Ed.), *Lifestyle Medicine.* Cambridge: Blackwell.

Wilson, M. G., & DeJoy, D. M. (1995). Maximizing participation and adherence in health promotion programs. In D. M. DeJoy & M. G. Wilson (Eds.), *Critical issues in worksite health promotion.* Boston: Allyn & Bacon.

Wilson, M. G., DeJoy, D. M., Jorgensen, C. J., & Crump, C. J. (1999). Health promotion in small worksites: Results of a national survey. *American Journal of Health Promotion, 13*, 358–365.

Winett, R. A., King, A. C., & Altman, D. G. (1989). *Health psychology and public health: An integrative approach.* New York: Pergamon Press.

Wood, E. A. (1997). Lifestyle risk factors and absenteeism trends: A six-year corporate study. *Worksite Health, 4*, 32–35.

C H A P T E R

11

Worksite Nutrition Programs

Karen Glanz and Alan R. Kristal

INTRODUCTION

Eating patterns have a substantial impact on health and quality of life. Worksite nutrition programs provide important opportunities to reach employees and their families with information, motivation, skills, and supportive environments to enhance health through good nutrition. Worksite nutrition programs have several advantages: convenience for workers; availability of daily eating situations; the potential to harness social support and social influence among coworkers and management; and the possibility of follow-up, monitoring, and reinforcement (Glanz & Seewald-Klein, 1986). They also can incorporate environmental supports for healthy eating through cafeterias, vending machines, and catering policies and can be less expensive than nutrition improvement programs offered elsewhere (Glanz, Sorensen, & Farmer, 1996).

National surveys of health promotion activities conducted in 1985 and 1992 in worksites with more than 50 employees suggest that the prevalence of employee nutrition and cholesterol-control programs has nearly doubled in the past decade (Office of Dis-

ease Prevention and Health Promotion & U.S. Public Health Service, 1987, 1993). More recently, the 1999 National Worksite Health Promotion Survey found that about 17% of small worksites (50–99 employees) and two-thirds of large worksites (with $\geq$ 750 employees) offer on-site nutrition education and cholesterol screenings (William M. Mercer, Inc., 1999). The 1999 survey also found that, overall, 43% of companies offer nutrition education and 59% provide cholesterol screening, either on-site or through employee health plans. Clearly, nutrition programs are integral to comprehensive worksite health promotion. They supplement and converge with activities in the areas of physical fitness, stress management, tobacco control, substance abuse reduction, and health screening.

This chapter addresses the rationale for and potential of worksite nutrition programs, the components and range of worksite nutrition strategies, and the results that have been found in previous program evaluations. (Weight control programs are discussed in depth in Chapter 12.) This chapter has five principal goals:

1. To describe the nature and magnitude of health, economic, and quality-of-life problems due to poor nutrition;

274

2. To familiarize readers with current guidelines for healthy eating patterns and key barriers to and supports for good nutrition;

3. To present the theoretical bases and range of options for effective worksite nutrition interventions;

4. To review recent and current strategies for worksite nutrition programs, the evidence regarding their impact, and contemporary "best strategies"; and

5. To introduce readers to the design and conduct of worksite nutrition program evaluations.

To accomplish these goals, this chapter summarizes what is currently known in practice and research on nutrition programs at the worksite, serves as a resource for readers, and aims to stimulate creative applications and advances in practice and research. Improved nutrition in working populations requires building on and extending past efforts in worksite nutrition.

NUTRITION AND HEALTH: OVERVIEW AND CURRENT GUIDELINES

There is a large and compelling body of evidence linking dietary patterns to health and disease (National Research Council & National Academy of Sciences, 1989). Most obviously, good nutrition contributes to our overall well-being. For many Americans, however, overconsumption of some dietary components contributes to obesity and to high risks of such chronic diseases as heart disease, cancers, and diabetes. Because eating patterns with too much of some foods tend to contain too little of other protective foods (e.g., fruits and vegetables), underconsumption is a related concern. These nutritionally-related diseases have high personal and social costs; they reduce quality of life and work productivity and increase health care costs, premature disability, and death.

In the United States and most other industrially developed countries, programs to promote healthful dietary patterns are public health priorities. This is because five of the ten leading causes of death (coronary heart disease, kidney diseases, cancer, stroke, and adult-onset diabetes) are nutrition related (see Table 11-1). If we also consider alcohol consumption as a dietary behavior, then accidents, suicide, and cirrhosis should also be counted among the leading causes of death that could be prevented by dietary change.

Below we review the major conclusions from laboratory, clinical, and epidemiological research linking diet to major chronic diseases. It is important to keep in mind that this research is evolving rapidly, with great media and public interest. Advances in molecular biology and an expansion in the number of very

Table 11-1 Leading Causes of Death in the United States in 1997

Rank	Diet Related?	Cause of Death	Numbers of Deaths	Rate (per 100,000)	Years of Potential Life Lost Before Age 75 (per 100,000)
1.	YES	Heart diseases	726,974	271.6	1,396
2.	YES	Cancers	539,577	201.6	1,755
3.	YES	Stroke	159,942	59.7	240
4.	NO	Chronic pulmonary diseases	109,029	40.7	189
5.	Alcohol	Accidents	95,644	35.7	1,079
6.	NO	Pneumonia and influenza	86,449	32.3	126
7.	YES	Diabetes mellitus	62,636	23.4	175
8.	Alcohol	Suicide	30,535	11.4	381
9.	YES	Kidney disease	35,331	9.5	281
10.	Alcohol	Chronic liver disease and cirrhosis	25,175	9.4	164

Source: *U.S. National Vital Statistics Reports*, 1999, U.S. Department of Health and Human Services.

large epidemiological studies of diet and disease are producing a steady stream of new (and often unexpected) findings in the scientific literature. The media tend to give new findings undue attention, even though it generally takes several years of additional research to confirm their importance. Thus, we focus below on associations between diet and disease for which there is substantial agreement among nutritional scientists.

Diet and Cardiovascular Disease

Cardiovascular diseases include coronary heart disease, other vascular diseases, and stroke. The relationships between diet and cardiovascular disease are complex (Knapp, 1996; Lichtenstein, 1996). Diet is directly associated with three of the major cardiovascular disease risk factors: high blood cholesterol, high blood pressure, and diabetes mellitus. These risk factors are also strongly affected by obesity. Finally, there are components in foods that directly affect cardiovascular disease risk, for example by reducing the likelihood of blood clots. The nutrients that contribute to high serum cholesterol are saturated fat and cholesterol, typically obtained from high-fat meats, full-fat dairy products, and egg yolk. In addition, high sodium intake predisposes some persons to high blood pressure. In contrast, some foods or food components decrease risk. Polyunsaturated fats, derived from vegetable oils, lower serum cholesterol. Fish and other seafoods, because they are a source of omega-3 fatty acids, reduce clot formation and thus decrease the risk of myocardial infarction (i.e., heart attack). Diets high in fruits and vegetables also reduce cardiovascular disease risk, probably because they are sources of folate and antioxidants. Finally, some whole-grain products (for example, oatmeal) reduce cholesterol absorption and can modestly lower serum cholesterol (Knapp, 1996; Lichtenstein, 1996).

Cancers

Cancers are a diverse group of diseases, and their relationships with diet vary (World Cancer Research Fund, 1997). The most consistent findings for many cancers are of protective effects of vegetables and, to a lesser extent, fruits. High intakes of vegetables and fruits decrease the risks of lung, stomach, colon, esophageal, and oral cavity cancers. Recent evidence also suggests protective effects for breast and prostate cancers. High fat intakes increase risk for prostate cancer, while high intakes of meat and/or saturated fat increase the risk of colon cancer. Alcohol, even in modest quantities, increases the risk of breast cancer, and high alcohol consumption increases risks of colon, liver, esophageal, and oral cavity cancers. Much progress is being made in understanding the associations of diet with cancer, with a focus on identifying the components of fruits and vegetables that reduce risk.

Obesity

Obesity is a complex disease but is ultimately the result of chronic excess energy intake. Maintaining a balance between energy intake and expenditure can be difficult for persons leading sedentary lifestyles, especially given the ready availability of low-price, tasty, high-calorie foods. Even a small positive energy balance can, over a number of years, lead to obesity. While controversial, most nutritionists believe that high-fat foods, because they are high in calories, contribute to obesity (Bray & Popkin, 1998). Many short-term feeding studies show that people tend to consume more energy when presented with high-fat compared to lower-fat foods, and dietary interventions to lower fat intake consistently lead to substantial weight loss. As for most other associations between diet and disease, there is considerable variability across individuals in their susceptibility to obesity. It is also clear that once a person becomes obese, it is very difficult to lose weight and maintain significant weight loss. Thus, prevention of obesity is a diet-related goal appropriate for everyone.

Osteoporosis

Osteoporosis, a condition that affects primarily post-menopausal women, is a weakening of bone caused by calcium loss. While the causes of osteoporosis are complex, inadequate calcium intake probably contributes to risk (Sowers, 1996).

Other Diet-Related Concerns for Working Adults

For working adults and their families, diet is a general concern for reasons other than major causes of chronic disease. For example, for women of child-bearing age, optimal nutrition plays a role in both fertility and pregnancy outcome. Dental health, child growth and development, and even surgical outcomes can be affected by diet and nutritional status. Food safety, whereby some infectious diseases may be avoided, can also contribute to overall health. Finally, dietary patterns are an integral part of one's culture, shared meals are a source of social cohesion, and food provides great pleasure.

Economic Consequences of Nutrition-Related Disease

There are substantial economic consequences, both to individuals and to society at large, from poor dietary practices. For individuals, these are primarily in lost income and high health care costs. For employers, consequences of poor dietary practices include absenteeism, reduced productivity, disability, and high health care utilization. While it is difficult to calculate the exact proportion of diet-related disease that is attributable to poor dietary practices, the total economic costs of diet-related diseases are enormous (see Table 11-2). Heart diseases, stroke, cancer, and diabetes cost society over $200 billion per year in medical costs and lost productivity (Frazao, 1996). And osteo-porosis affects 25 million women, with a cost of $13 to $18 billion annually for hip fractures alone (Barefield, 1996).

GUIDELINES FOR HEALTHY EATING PATTERNS

Developing dietary guidelines can be very controversial. This is especially true when scientific data are inconclusive or when significant economic interests are at stake. Further, guidelines specifically targeted to reduce the risk of one disease may increase the risk of other diseases. Governmental agencies, professional and scientific organizations, and voluntary health organizations have all developed recommendations and guidelines for healthful diets. Guidelines differ in their disease or risk factor emphasis, but there is surprising commonality in overall recommendations (Bal and Foerster, 1991). This is especially true when guidelines for specific nutrients (e.g., eat less than 10% of energy from saturated fat) are translated into recommendations for dietary patterns (e.g., choose low- or non-fat milk; trim fat off meat).

To develop general dietary guidelines for the U.S. population, expert panels convened by the U.S. Departments of Agriculture and of Health and Human Services achieved consensus around seven overarching recommendations in "Nutrition and Your Health: Dietary Guidelines for Americans." First developed in 1990 and revised every 5 years, these guidelines provide consistent and comprehensible messages to educate the public about nutrition and health (U.S.

Table 11-2 Costs of Diet-Related Diseases

Disease	Total Cost ($ Million)	Medical Cost ($ Million)	Lost Productivity ($ Million)
Heart diseases	56,300	48,300	8,000
Cancers	104,000	35,000	69,000
Stroke	19,700	16,900	2,800
Diabetes	40,000	-	-
Obesity	2,400	-	-
Hypertension	17,400	14,900	2,500
Osteoporosis	10,000	-	-

Source: E. Frazao, *Food Review*, 1999; Economic Research Service, U.S. Department of Agriculture.

Table 11-3 Dietary Guidelines for Americans

1. Aim for a healthy weight.
   - Evaluate your weight. Avoid weight gain or lose weight to improve you health.
   - Get regular physical activity to balance calories from food.
2. Be physically active each day.
   - Engage in at least 30 minutes of moderate physical activity each day.
   - Stay active throughout your life.
3. Let the pyramid guide your food choices.
   - Build your eating pattern on a variety of plant foods, including whole grains, fruits and vegetables.
4. Eat a variety of grains daily, especially whole grains.
   - Make a variety of grain products a foundation of your diet.
   - Eat six or more servings of grain products daily.
5. Choose a variety of fruits and vegetables daily.
   - Enjoy 5 a day.
   - Choose fresh, frozen or canned forms and a variety of colors and kinds.
6. Keep foods safe to eat.
   - Keep clean. Wash hands and surfaces often.
   - Cook foods to a safe temperature. Refrigerate perishable foods.
7. Choose a diet that is low in saturated fat and cholesterol and moderate in fat.
   - Limit use of solid fats, such a butter, hard margarines and hydrogenated shortnings.
   - Choose fat-free or low-fat dairy products, fish, lean meats and poultry.
8. Choose beverages and foods to moderate your intake of sugars.
   - Limit intake of beverages and foods that are high in added sugars.
   - Drink water often.
9. Choose and prepare foods with less salt.
   - Read the Nutrition Facts Label to identify foods lower in sodium.
   - Use herbs, spices and fruits to flavor food, and cut the amout of salt by half.
10. IF YOU DRINK ALCOHOLIC BEVERAGES, DO SO IN MODERATION.
    - Limit alcoholic beverages to 1 per day for women and 2 per day for men.
    - Some persons should not drink: women who are pregnant or trying to become pregnant; persons who cannot moderate their alcohol intake; persons using certain prescription and over-the-counter medications.

Source: U.S. Department of Agriculture and U.S. Department of Health and Human Services, *Nutrition and Your Health: Dietary Guidelines for Americans,* 2000.

Department of Agriculture [USDA] & U.S. Department of Health and Human Services [USDHHS], 2000). The ten guidelines, and details about each recommendation, are given in Table 11-3.

In 1992, to help consumers plan meals that fit into the dietary guidelines, the U.S. Department of Agriculture developed the Food Guide Pyramid (see Figure 11-1). The purpose to this graphic is to emphasize that grain products, fruits, and vegetables should be the foundation of a healthful diet, with modest amounts of dairy and meat products and little use of fats, oils, and sweets. Lastly, in 1994, the U.S. Food and Drug Administration introduced a new standardized food label format for giving nutrition information on packaged foods (see Figure 11-2). These "Nutrition Facts" labels are a significant improvement over previous labels for several reasons. Most importantly, foods now have standardized portion sizes, making it possible to compare across brands to select food more consistent with healthful dietary recommendations. Labels also introduced a measure, "% DV" or percent daily value, as an attempt to help people judge the contribution of that food to their daily requirement (or limit) for a particular nutrient.

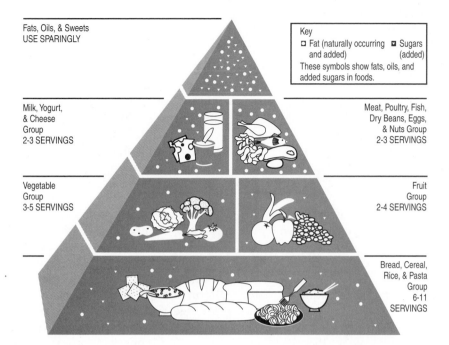

Figure 11-1 The Food Guide Pyramid
Source: U.S. Department of Agriculture and U.S.
Department of Health and Human Services

SERVING SIZE
gives usual
amount eaten.
Allows easy
comparison
among brands

NUTRIENTS
are those most
important for
dietary
guidelines

DAILY VALUE
shows the
contribution of the
food to the daily
goal (or limit) for
many nutrients

Nutrition Facts

Serving Size 3 cookies (34g/1.2oz.)
Servings Per Container About 5

Amount Per Serving

Calories 180   Calories from Fat 90

	% Daily Value
Total Fat 10g	15%
Saturated Fat 3.5g	18%
Polyunsaturated Fat 1g	
Monounsaturated Fat 5g	
Cholesterol 10mg	3%
Sodium 80mg	3%
Total Carbohydrate 21g	7%
Dietary Fiber 1g	4%
Sugars 11g	
Protein 2g	

Vitamin A 0%	•	Vitamin C 0%
Calcium 0%	•	Iron 4%
Thiamin 6%	•	Riboflavin 4%
Niacin 4%		

*Percent Daily Values are based on a 2,000
calorie diet. Your daily values may be higher
or lower depending on your calorie needs.

	Calories	2,000	2,500
Total Fat	Less than	85g	80g
Sat Fat	Less than	20g	25g
Cholesterol	Less than	300mg	300mg
Sodium	Less than	2,400mg	2,400mg
Total Carbohydrates		300g	375g
Dietary Fiber		25g	30g

Figure 11-2 Standardized food label for
packaged food in the United States
Source: U.S. Food and Drug Administration

The "Dietary Guidelines for Americans" and the Food Pyramid are starting points for any worksite healthy nutrition promotion program. However, in practice these guidelines are too broad to be all targeted in any single program. For worksite health promotion, goals should fit the following criteria:

- Address important and well-established dietary risk factors for major diseases
- Be generally applicable to healthy adults
- Be consistent with cultural norms of employee population(s)
- Avoid popular fads and extreme scientific viewpoints
- Be feasible for worksite implementation

From the perspective of disease prevention in the general adult population, we believe that the following areas are the most important for worksite health promotion:

- Weight management
- Reduction in total and saturated fat
- Increased consumption of vegetables and fruits
- Moderation of alcohol consumption

CURRENT TRENDS IN DIET AFFECTING WORKSITE NUTRITION PROGRAMS

Some progress has been made in the past few decades toward improving the quality of the U.S. diet, yet change has been modest (USDHHS, 1998). Total fat intake has decreased somewhat (Anand & Basiotis, 1998), with a marked shift toward more unsaturated and less saturated fats (Center for Nutrition Policy and Promotion, USDA, 1990–1994). This change in type of fat being consumed, which began as early as 1970, may explain some of the steep drop in cardiovascular disease rates that has occurred. However, starting in about 1990, both total energy and alcohol intakes increased in both men and women. There have also been recent trends for increased intakes of fruits and vegetables, and sodium intake remains unchanged. Still, only about 35% of the U.S. population meet the dietary goals for either total fat or fruits and vegetables.

Certainly the most disconcerting nutrition-related change in the health of the U.S. population has been the profound increase in obesity. Between 1980 and 1994, the rates of obesity increased from 25% to 35% of the adult population (Pamuk, Makuc, Heck, Reuben, & Lochner, 1998); and, based on a recently revised definition, about half of all Americans are now considered overweight (National Heart, Lung, and Blood Institute, 1998). The reasons for this marked rise are the subject of controversy, but they most certainly involve both increased total energy intake and decreased physical activity.

During the past decade, much more progress has been made in developing the programs and infrastructure required to promote healthful dietary change. Examples include the "5 A Day for Better Health" program, a large, national effort to promote increased consumption of fruits and vegetables (Havas, et al., 1994), and the development and dissemination of such nutrition education materials as the Dietary Guidelines for Americans and the Nutrition Facts food labels. As part of a broad program to improve public health overall, the Healthy People 2010 Objectives give specific goals for nutrition related concerns. In addition to the health status and dietary intake goals that match those of the Dietary Guidelines for Americans, the Healthy People Objectives include goals for health services delivery. For example, one goal for the proposed 2010 Objectives is that 85% of worksites with 50 or more employees offer nutrition education and/ or weight management programs for their employees (DHHS, 2000). Several federal- and state-led health programs offer guidelines, materials, and program components that are well-suited for worksite nutrition programs.

Worksite nutrition intervention programs should follow established health guidelines and reflect an accurate and timely understanding of social and economic trends that affect employees' food choices and other diet-related behavior. Perhaps foremost of these trends is the large proportion of women in the workforce and the resulting changes in types of meals served at home. Thus, in addition to taste and health, convenience has become one of the more important determinants of food choice (Glanz, Basil, Maibach,

Goldberg, & Snyder, 1998). Supermarkets now focus on providing convenience foods, either as "take-out" meals, frozen entrée's, or other types of foods requiring little or no preparation. The selection of convenience foods now includes more choices designed to conform to healthful dietary guidelines, especially in terms of containing less fat and less saturated fat. In addition, the new Nutrition Facts food labels make it easier for consumers to compare across brands and types of convenience foods to choose those with superior nutritional characteristics. Thus, this shift away from raw food preparation toward convenience meals is not necessarily a significant barrier to eating healthful foods at home. What is a significant challenge, however, is the increasing consumption of commercially-prepared foods eaten away from home, from restaurants in general and from fast-food restaurants in particular. On average in the U.S., about 30% of meals are from foods prepared away from home (Lin & Frazao, 1997). Among those of working age (18–59), almost half of all away-from-home meals are from fast-food restaurants. Restaurant-prepared meals are typically higher in total calories, fat, saturated fat, and sodium and lower in fruits and vegetables than meals made at home. This is one area in which worksite nutrition programs can directly affect the quality of their employees' diets: by making available tasty and convenient meals and snacks that are consistent with healthful dietary guidelines in employee cafeterias and vending machines.

THEORETICAL FOUNDATIONS FOR WORKSITE NUTRITION PROGRAMS

Successful nutrition programs for employees take many forms. Interventions to yield desirable changes in eating patterns can be best designed with an understanding of relevant theories of dietary behavior change and the ability to use them skillfully (Glanz, Lewis, & Rimer, 1997). While many early reports of worksite nutrition interventions did not cite a particular theory or model as the basis for the strategies they employ (Glanz & Seewald-Klein, 1986), the application of sound behavioral science theory in worksite nutrition programs is becoming increasingly common (Glanz & Eriksen, 1993). In fact, intervention

research conducted in occupational settings has been a major force in advancing our understanding of the theoretical foundations for dietary behavior (Abrams et al., 1994; Glanz, Kristal, Tilley, & Hirst, 1998; Glanz, Patterson et al., 1994; Kristal, Glanz et al. 1999; Kristal, Patterson et al., 1995; Sorensen, Stoddard, & Macario, 1998; Terborg, Hibbard, & Glasgow, 1995) and of ways to measure relevant theoretical constructs (Glanz, Kristal, Sorensen et al., 1993; Kristal, Glanz, Curry, & Patterson, 1999).

Common wisdom holds that worksite nutrition programs are most likely to be effective if they embrace an ecological perspective for health promotion (McLeroy, Bibeau, Steckler, & Glanz, 1988; Sallis & Owen, 1997). That is, they should not only be targeted at individuals but should also affect interpersonal, organizational, and environmental factors influencing dietary behavior (Glanz, Lankenau et al., 1995). We have identified four theoretical models that are particularly useful for understanding the processes of changing eating patterns in worksite settings: social cognitive theory, the stages of change construct from the Transtheoretical Model, consumer information processing, and diffusion of innovations (Glanz & Eriksen, 1993). The central elements of each theory and how they can be used to help formulate worksite nutrition programs are described next. (These and other theoretical models are discussed in greater detail in Chapter 7.)

Social Cognitive Theory

The principles of social cognitive theory, Bandura's contemporary version of social learning theory, postulate that there are dynamic relationships among personal factors, the social and physical environment, and behavior (Bandura, 1986). The key social cognitive theory construct of reciprocal determinism means that a person can be both an agent for change and a respondent to change. Thus, changes in the environment, the examples of role models, and reinforcements can be manipulated to promote healthier behavior. Also, self-efficacy, or a person's self-confidence about the ability to successfully carry out a behavior even when faced with challenges (Bandura, 1997), can be improved through program activities that incorporate goalsetting, feedback, external rewards, and self-reward (Glanz & Eriksen, 1993). Activities such as cooking demonstrations, problem-solving discussions, and self-monitoring are rooted in social cognitive theory and can be readily incorporated in worksite nutrition programs. Several recent large worksite nutrition programs have applied constructs from social cognitive theory (Brug, Steenhuis, Van Assema, Glanz, & De Vries, 1999; Sorensen, Hunt et al., 1998; Tilley et al., 1997).

Stages of Change

The stages of change construct from the Transtheoretical Model can be helpful in designing, delivering, and evaluating interventions to help employed persons adopt more healthful diets (Kristal, Glanz, Curry, & Patterson, 1999). Stages of change is a heuristic model that describes a sequence of steps in successful behavior change: precontemplation (no recognition of need for or interest in change); contemplation (thinking about changing); preparation (planning for change); action (adopting new habits); and maintenance (ongoing practice of new, healthier behavior) (Prochaska, DiClemente, & Norcross, 1992). The stages of change construct (or "model") suggests that interventions should be designed to match employees' stage of readiness to change. This can be done on a group or worksite level (Glanz, Patterson et al., 1998) or at the individual level within worksites (Tilley, Vernon et al., 1997). Multicomponent worksite nutrition programs might include strategies to increase awareness, develop new skills, and maintain new healthful eating skills and deliver those strategies based on participants' or workgroups' stage of readiness.

Over the past five years, there has been a substantial increase in research applying the stages of change model to dietary behavior (Campbell et al., 1999; Glanz et al., 1994; Kristal, Glanz, Curry, & Patterson, 1999). Several intervention trials have explicitly used this model to help shape their nutrition promotion programs (Sorensen et al., 1996; Sorensen, Stoddard, & Macario, 1998; Tilley et al., 1997). Prospective intervention research examining employees' readiness to change their eating patterns has revealed "forward movement" across the stage continuum in worksite nutrition studies and shown that changes in stage of change for healthy eating is significantly associated with dietary improvements (Glanz, Patterson et al., 1998; Kristal, Glanz, Tilley, & Li, 1999).

Consumer Information Processing

People require information about how to choose nutritious foods in order to follow guidelines for healthy eating. A central premise of consumer information processing theory is that individuals can process only a limited amount of information at one time (Glanz & Rimer, 1995; Rudd & Glanz, 1990). People tend to seek only enough information to make a satisfactory choice. They develop heuristics or rules of thumb to help them make choices quickly within their limited information-processing capacity (Rudd & Glanz, 1990). The nutrition information environment is often complex and confusing, especially when programs rely heavily on printed nutrition-education materials that may be written at too sophisticated a level in terms of wording and concepts (Glanz & Rudd, 1990). Recently, introduction of the new "Nutrition Facts" food labels (see Figure 11-2) have simplified generally available nutrition information somewhat and contributed to an increase in usual label use and satisfaction with their content (Kristal, Levy, Patterson, Li, & White, 1998).

There are several implications of consumer information processing theory for worksite nutrition education. Information that is provided should be made easily accessible, not confusing, and processable with limited effort. Messages that are food-focused rather than nutrient-focused may be particularly helpful (Hunt et al., 1997). Nutrition information should be tailored to the comprehension level of the audience, matched to their lifestyles and experience, and either be portable or available at or near the point of food selection (Rudd & Glanz, 1990).

Diffusion of Innovations

The last conceptual model is the diffusion of innovations, which provides guidance both for developing successful programs and assuring that they are optimally communicated through the social environment of the workplace. Diffusion concepts emphasize the macrolevel of social and dietary change (Rogers, 1983). A key implication of diffusion theory is that mediated information sources—that is, sources that rely on media rather than interpersonal communication (including brochures, mass media, etc.)—are most important in the early stages of adoption, such as awareness and interest-building. Interpersonal communication grows more important during active evaluation, trial, and adoption of new habits (Rogers, 1983). Diffusion principles are consistent with social cognitive theory concepts that suggest initially creating an environment conducive to change and disseminating the program and new ideas through successful examples (Bandura, 1986). However, it also appears that special efforts are required to sustain worksite nutrition interventions after an initial active period. An investigation of the durability and diffusion of the nutrition intervention in the Working Well Trial found that two years after the main intervention ended, the treatment sites did not have significantly more nutrition activity than control sites (Patterson, Kristal, Varnes et al., 1998). There is a need for further research on diffusion of effective intervention models, as few studies have addressed how best to disseminate tested interventions (Sorensen, Emmons, Hunt, & Johnston, 1998).

The challenge of successfully applying theoretical frameworks in worksite nutrition programs involves evaluating the frameworks and their key concepts in terms of both conceptual relevance and practical value (Glanz, Lewis, & Rimer, 1997). Also the integration of multiple theories into a comprehensive model tailored for a given worksite and its employees requires careful analysis of the audience and frequent reexamination during program design and implementation.

TYPES OF WORKSITE NUTRITION PROGRAMS

Theory and research suggest that the most effective worksite health promotion programs are those that use multiple strategies and aim to achieve multiple goals of awareness, information transmission, skill development, and supportive environments and policies (Glanz, Sorensen, & Farmer, 1996). However, the range of nutrition programs suitable for worksites is extensive and varied. Programs will differ based on their goals and objectives of the organization and the available resources, staff, and expertise. Nutrition programs can stand alone or be part of a broader, multicomponent and multiple-focus worksite health promotion program (Heaney & Goetzel, 1997).

The majority of published evaluations of worksite nutrition programs report on four types of interventions: group education, group education with individual counseling, cafeteria-based programs, and group education combined with cafeteria-based programs (Glanz, Sorensen, & Farmer, 1996). Across these types of, or formats for, programs, there are some emerging issues and trends that warrant consideration. These issues relate to choices on how to approach worksite nutrition interventions and contrast "traditional" ways of thinking with more innovative models. They are: clinical versus public health approaches; professional versus lay or self-help programs; direct instruction versus media methods; and individual versus environmental/organizational changes.

Clinical versus Public Health Approaches

Clinical approaches to worksite nutrition programs are among the most common and were some of the first nutrition interventions introduced in workplaces. They focus primarily on individuals at high risk for nutrition-related health problems or on self-selected groups of motivated and interested people. Clinical approaches tend to employ relatively intensive interventions, including screening, individual counseling, and classes; and they often involve medical personnel. Consequently, they have high costs per participant and often reach relatively small audiences.

Examples of the clinical approach applied to worksite nutrition programs include cholesterol screening and education/counseling efforts, some of which have been shown to effectively influence eating behavior and cholesterol levels (Glanz & Rogers 1994; Glanz, Sorensen, & Farmer, 1996). However they have attracted relatively small proportions of employee populations, usually between five and fifteen percent of the workforce. In contrast to the clinical model, public health approaches are of more recent vintage. They aim to improve the health and well-being of all employees at a worksite, not just the highly motivated and high-risk workers. Less intensive but broader-reaching programs can achieve small changes in a wide audience and thus result in broader population impact.

In recent years, the results of some population-oriented, or public health model, interventions have yielded significant but very small positive changes compared to no-treatment control worksites (Sorensen, Thompson et al., 1996). Yet a third alternative is to use population-based approaches on entire groups identified to be at some level of excessive risk. The Next Step Trial, a colorectal cancer screening and nutrition intervention in high-risk employees, used this type of approach and achieved favorable success in promoting diets low in fat, high in fiber, and high in fruits and vegetables (Tilley, Glanz et al., 1999).

Professional versus Lay or Self-Help Programs

Most worksite nutrition programs have been conducted by health professionals, such as dietitians, nutrition educators, and psychologists, who serve in direct program-delivery roles. This approach is often chosen because providers can assume responsibility for fine-tuning programs and answering questions that arise. Professionally delivered programs are consistent with a clinical approach, particularly those that use counseling, small groups, classes, and seminars. While this type of staffing provides a measure of quality assurance, it adds to the cost of programs and can be an inefficient use of professional time if attendance is low or attrition is high. Some programs have used non-professional, or lay, leaders successfully. While this began in the area of weight control (addressed in Chapter 12), it has grown with the expansion of employee planning or advisory groups who help design *and* deliver worksite health activities. Some low-intensity programs, including displays, competitions and contests, and self-help materials can be conducted with a minimum of professional time during their active delivery. The emphasis on personal responsibility in addition to the reduced cost

are benefits of this way of conducting programs. Professionals can then assume the roles of technical advisors and direct program planners to credible resources, but the employees' involvement can make the program more efficient and potentially more effective as well.

Direct Instruction versus Media Methods

Historically, the majority of worksite nutrition programs have relied on direct, face-to-face intervention methods, such as group sessions, classes, and counseling. Self-help programs using print and audiovisual media can extend a program's reach, reduce attrition rates, and, if well planned and implemented, may be as effective as traditional, direct approaches (Glanz, 1999). The use of videotapes, slide-tape shows, and "video magazines" are just a few of the types of media that may be more interesting than brochures, yet can be delivered at a much lower cost than live professional presentations.

Computerized assessments and Internet- and Web-based interventions have expanded the available options still further. However, it is important that program planners assure the scientific accuracy of information if they encourage workers to search out information on the Internet without supervision. Further innovations are available by designing programs to take advantage of the ever-increasing availability of worksite computer networks and desktop e-mail. In using these novel opportunities, careful planning is very important. Some workers (e.g., factory or field workers) may lack routine access to e-mail, and health promotion programs must be careful to avoid being intrusive on the daily work activities of employees.

Individual versus Environmental/Organizational Changes

Most of the discussion of worksite nutrition up to this point has focused on how to improve dietary practices of employees with strategies that require individuals to learn, modify their attitudes, and change their behavior. While these are important, the environmental and organizational context also plays an important role in shaping and maintaining individual change. Modification of cafeterias, dining facilities, and vending services, along with other supportive policies and incentives, are increasingly the focus of programs to encourage healthy eating patterns (Glanz, Lankenau et al., 1995; Glanz & Mullis, 1988).

Three general types of nutrition policy and environmental interventions can be implemented in the workplace: food access strategies (improving the healthfulness of available foods, establishing healthy catering policies), nutrition information policy and strategies (food labeling, point-of-choice nutrition information programs), and economic strategies (incentives, pricing to encourage healthy choices) (Glanz, Lankenau et al., 1995). One of the key features of these interventions is that they can reach all employees—not just those at high-risk or the more highly motivated workers.

Food access strategies can increase the availability of nutritious foods in cafeterias and vending machines, use recipe modifications to improve the composition of foods that are already available, or establish policy guidelines for foods served at company functions (i.e., catering policies). Point-of-choice programs provide nutrition information to individuals at the point of food selection or purchase, thereby increasing awareness and prompting people to select more healthful foods (Glanz, Hewitt, & Rudd, 1992; Mayer, Dubbert, & Elder, 1989). Economic strategies can reduce the prices of healthier choices. Incentive programs can be used to bolster participation on an organized worksite nutrition program or to draw attention to point-of-choice programs, awareness events, games, and competitions. While few evaluations have reported the results of programs trying to modify the worksite eating environment, the Working Well Trial intervention trial involving 111 workplaces found that, at the follow-up surveys, the intervention sites showed improved access to healthful food, more nutrition information at work, and more favorable social norms regarding dietary choices (Biener, Glanz et al., 1999).

THE IMPACT OF WORKSITE NUTRITION PROGRAMS

Information about the impact of worksite nutrition programs is increasingly available from large field trials that address nutrition only or nutrition along with other risk factors. During the mid 1990s, there were several new trials of worksite nutrition programs to reduce the risks of cardiovascular disease and cancer and to lower employees' elevated cholesterol levels. (As noted earlier, weight control interventions are described in Chapter 12). A rigorous literature review of worksite nutrition programs available in 1995 found 10 worksite nutrition studies and 16 worksite cholesterol intervention studies that reported nutrition and health outcomes (Glanz, Sorensen, & Farmer, 1996).

Worksite Nutrition Programs

The studies of worksite nutrition programs evaluated four types of interventions: group education, group education with individual counseling, cafeteria-based studies, and group education plus cafeteria-based programs. The evaluations used a variety of measures and designs and varied as to whether individuals or worksites were the unit of randomization and analysis (Glanz, Sorensen, & Farmer, 1996). Most of the studies used nonrandomized designs; while all of the nonrandomized studies reported some positive outcomes in employee knowledge, behaviors, or food purchasing, it was not possible to clearly attribute those results to the interventions. The randomized studies also reported generally positive results, including increased consumption of fruits and vegetables, consumption of higher-fiber foods, and lower-fat eating (Sorensen et al., 1990; Jeffery, French, Raether, & Baxter, 1994).

Results are now available from some more recent worksite nutrition intervention trials. The Working Well Trial used multiple strategies, including awareness activities, education, cafeteria changes, and participatory strategies to improve diet and reduce tobacco use. One hundred fourteen worksites were randomized to treatment or control conditions. After two years of intervention, there was a significant net decrease in energy from fat (-0.9% energy from fat), increase in fiber density ($+0.13$ g/1,000 kcal), increase in fruit and vegetable intake ($+0.18$ servings/day) (Sorensen et al., 1996), and improvements in the healthy eating environment (Biener et al., 1999). Post hoc analyses indicated that longer, interactive intervention efforts, such as contests and classes, resulted in more positive outcomes than one-time activities (such as kick-off events) or more passive efforts (such as use of printed materials) (Patterson, Kristal et al., 1997). However, it is difficult to determine the specific effective and/or ineffective components of the Working Well Trial intervention because the evaluation was designed to compare a multi-method program with a control condition. The changes were modest but significant because of the large sample (114 worksites, more than 30,000 workers); and the practical significance of the dietary changes found in the Working Well Trial, while considered encouraging, remains a matter of debate.

The Next Step Trial tested interventions that encouraged prevention and early detection practices in automotive-industry employees at increased colorectal risk. The nutrition intervention, provided at half of the 28 worksites that were randomly assigned to the experimental arm, included nutrition classes, self-help materials, and computer-generated personalized feedback (Tilley, Vernon et al., 1997). At one year, there were modest but significant intervention effects for fat (-0.9% energy from fat), fiber ($\pm.5$ g/1,000 kcal), and fruits/vegetables ($+0.2$ servings/day), all $p<0.007$. At two years, intervention effects were smaller and remained significant for fiber only. Intervention effects were larger in younger, active employees and those who attended classes (Tilley, Glanz et al., 1999).

The Take Heart Project sought to reduce dietary fat intake and serum cholesterol and to improve healthy eating environments in 26 moderate size worksites in Oregon. A variety of motivational, educational, policy/environmental, and employee steering committee strategies were used (Glasgow, Terborg et al., 1994). At the conclusion of the intervention, early and delayed intervention conditions did not differ on changes in dietary intake or cholesterol levels, and there was considerable variability in outcomes among worksites (Glasgow, Terborg, Hollis, Severson, & Boles, 1995). A revised intervention called Take Heart II used a steering committee/menu approach and evaluated it with a quasi-experimental matched-pairs design. Take Heart II produced modest effects favoring worksite intervention on eating patterns but showed no beneficial effect on cholesterol levels (Glasgow, Terborg, Strycker, Boles, & Hollis, 1997).

The Treatwell 5-A-Day study compared a minimal intervention control group, a worksite intervention, and a worksite-plus-family intervention for increasing fruit and vegetable intake in 22 community health center worksites. The intervention used a community-organizing strategy and was structured to target multiple levels of influence (Sorensen, Hunt et al., 1998). The control group showed no change, the worksite intervention group increased their fruit and vegetable intake by 7%, and the worksite-plus-family group increased total fruit and vegetable intake by 19%; the group with the largest increases improved by about one-half serving per day (Sorensen, Stoddard, Peterson et al., 1999).

The Seattle 5-A-Day Worksite Program evaluated an intervention based on the stage of change model and used 28 worksites randomly assigned to intervention or control arms. The intervention included an Employee Advisory Board, a study interventionist, and materials targeting transition points between stages of change and addressed both individual and worksite environments. There was a significant net intervention effect of 0.3 daily servings, favoring the intervention worksites (Beresford et al., 1999).

In a multiple risk factor intervention study that included nutrition among the outcomes, the Working Healthy Project, participants from half of the 26 manufacturing worksites studied completed a comprehensive risk assessment. They reported increased intake of fruits, vegetables, and fiber but no changes in percent energy from fat (Emmons, Linnan, Shadel, Marcus, & Abrams, 1999).

Another report describes a randomized evaluation of computer-tailored nutrition education interventions in employee populations in the Netherlands. The study recruited 315 participants from the worksites, but sent the materials to employees at their homes and were randomized as individuals. Computer-tailored materials provided either feedback about their diets only (control group) or about both their diet and psychosocial status, including attitudes, self-efficacy expectations, and perceived social support (Brug et al., 1999). After the intervention, both groups reported decreased fat consumption and increased consumption of fruits and vegetables, but no differences in consumption were found between the two groups (Brug et al., 1999).

What Strategies or Programs Work Best?

It is difficult to draw definitive conclusions about the strategies that work best in promoting dietary change as part of worksite nutrition programs. We cautiously conclude that group education programs produced some dietary changes. Cafeteria programs appear to hold promise, as do computer-tailored messages and worksite interventions enhanced with family outreach. Comprehensive programs addressing both individual and environmental changes deserve particular further attention, and it would be useful for future multiple-strategy studies to enable readers to discern the impact of various contributing strategies.

Cholesterol Intervention Programs

Most published worksite cholesterol intervention studies have used nonrandomized designs and report substantial attrition during the course of the studies. About half the studies showed changes in dietary behavior, and about half reported cholesterol reduction in intervention groups, irrespective of study design. Individual counseling appeared to be successful across studies when enhanced by follow-up and printed materials. Generally speaking, more intensive strategies appear to have achieved the largest effects (Glanz, Sorensen, & Farmer, 1996).

Quality of the Evidence for Worksite Nutrition and Cholesterol Programs

Because of limitations imposed by study designs used in many program evaluations, Glanz, Sorensen, and Farmer concluded in 1996 that the quality of evidence in the intervention literature on worksite nutrition and cholesterol programs lies between *suggestive* and *indicative*. It is clear that worksite nutrition and cholesterol programs are feasible and that participants do benefit in the short-term. More recent publications point to the promising strategies of family outreach, stage-based interventions, and group programs for large groups of high-risk workers. The designs have improved markedly in the past few years. However, it is still often difficult to determine which *strategies*

within a program account for observed effects; the effects are generally modest even where they are significant; and no single study can be taken as conclusive regarding a particular type of strategy. Important opportunities remain to evaluate innovative nutrition programs for employees and their worksite environments.

PROGRAM EVALUATION

One key to a successful worksite nutrition program is a clear plan for its evaluation. An evaluation plan requires the program to have clearly defined and realistic objectives. Well-planned and conducted evaluation can also give timely feedback at each stage of program implementation, allowing modifications to improve program effectiveness. The four types of evaluation that are most suitable for worksite nutrition programs are: (a) formative evaluation, focusing on program design; (b) process evaluation, emphasizing program implementation and employee reaction; (c) quality assurance monitoring, to confirm that the program is being delivered as planned; and (d) outcome evaluation, measuring the achievement of program objectives. Principles of program evaluation are given in Chapter 5, and we focus here on those aspects of evaluation that are specific to dietary intervention programs.

Formative Evaluation

One challenge for nutrition education programs is matching the content of the interventions to the interests and needs of the intended audience. Nutrition information is inherently complex, and it must balance between being scientifically correct and still comprehensible and useful to the intended audience. Information should be free of jargon and unnecessary scientific complexity. Intervention activities should also be reasonable in a worksite context. A series of weekly, hour-long nutrition intervention sessions may benefit the persons attending; however, if only small numbers of employees are willing to participate, other intervention modalities are more appropriate. Thus, at the stage of formative evaluation, it is most critical to make sure materials and programs are not too intensive, demanding, scientifically complex, inconvenient, or otherwise inconsistent with their intended use.

Process Evaluation

Once in place, it is important to know if the nutrition program is reaching its audience and how it is being received. Although not necessarily unique to nutrition programs, one problem here is that there is a tendency for persons who are already interested in nutrition, and are motivated to change, to participate. Historically, these have been predominantly women. Thus, at the stage of process evaluation, it is important to assure that program components successfully reach men, younger people, and other groups less likely to be drawn to programs in nutrition. This is also the stage at which to evaluate whether the audiences' reactions to the program are favorable or whether changes are needed to have a broader impact. For example, one may wish to monitor whether employees like new foods offered in the cafeteria and whether food service employees are comfortable with—and adhering to—changes in food preparation and signage.

Outcome Evaluation

There are four types of outcome evaluations that are useful in worksite nutrition programs. These are focused on: (a) environmental-level change, (b) changes in diet-related mediating factors, (c) changes in dietary behavior, and (d) evaluations of health improvements (e.g., cholesterol, blood pressure, weight change) (Glanz, Sorensen, & Farmer, 1996). It is important to recognize that the latter, reflecting changes in health risk factors, may reflect behaviors other than just nutritional practices, such as physical activity and medication adherence.

A comprehensive and scientifically rigorous evaluation of a worksite nutrition program is generally beyond the scope of any but a well-funded research study. However, there are a number of simplified approaches that can provide helpful information to interventionists and management to measure program success. For example, environmental assess-

ments might include a food service "food frequency questionnaire" to measure changes resulting from a cafeteria intervention program (Sorensen et al., 1990) or surveys of food service managers about changes in food availability and catering policies (Biener et al., 1999). Questionnaires using measures of stage of change, or "readiness to change," can be completed as part of a program to provide workers with personalized feedback and also be built into an evaluation design (Campbell et al., 1994; Glanz, Patterson, Kristal et al., 1998). And creative approaches to tracking food consumption, such as a "fruit and vegetable scoreboard," can serve as both motivational interventions and assessment tools over a period of time.

What Can be Expected? Program Design and Expectations of Results

Evaluation and worksite nutrition program design and delivery go hand in hand. Generally speaking, minimally intensive intervention efforts can reach large audiences but seldom lead to behavior changes. More intensive programs typically appeal to at-risk or motivated groups, cost more to offer, and can achieve relatively greater changes in knowledge, attitudes, and eating patterns (Glanz & Rogers, 1994). Key points to keep in mind are:

1. The method of delivery and/or use of a particular program determines the resources it will require, the participant burden, and the predicted impact.
2. More intensive methods usually cost more in staff time and resources and attract more motivated employees.
3. More intensive programs usually produce greater behavior change.
4. Not all worksites are suited to, or can afford, the "most effective" approach. The number of workers reached and the amount of impact per worker may be inversely related. What is important is to establish realistic expectations and goals.

The most effective program for a given workforce is one that matches the needs, interests, and resources available for the effort.

CONCLUSION

This chapter has shown that nutrition-related health problems are among the most significant and challenging public health issues today. To address these problems, a wide range of worksite programs have been developed and tested with varying degrees of success. The chapter also discussed some of the dilemmas that have challenged health promotion professionals as they work in this field. Clearly, much experience has been gained in the 1980s and 1990s in conducting and evaluating the worksite nutrition programs cited in this chapter. However, there is no universally acceptable, feasible, and effective worksite nutrition enhancement program that is suitable for every worksite. Nevertheless, one can extract a few kernels of wisdom from the experiences to date.

First, nutrition interventions must be sensitive to audience and contextual factors. Food selection decisions are made for many reasons other than just nutrition: taste, cost, convenience, and cultural factors all play significant roles (Glanz, Basil et al., 1998). The design and implementation of worksite nutrition programs must take these issues into consideration. The health promotion motto "know your audience" has a true and valuable meaning.

Second, change is incremental. Many people have practiced a lifetime of less-than-optimal nutrition behaviors. It is unreasonable to expect that significant and lasting changes will occur during the course of a program that lasts only a few months. Programs need to pull the work force along the continuum of change, being sure to be just in front of those most ready to change with attractive, innovative offerings. It may seem like an easy, comprehensive strategy to ban all junk food from worksite vending machines, for example. However, if employees are not prepared for and do not support such a radical change, the effort will not be well-received.

Third, the underlying program philosophy should not blame the victim. For many employees, access to fresh, wholesome, nutritious foods is quite restricted. In some worksites, for example, low-fat dairy products cannot be found in the cafeteria. In such cases, it is of limited value to adopt a program solely oriented toward modifying individual choice (e.g., teaching and persuading employees to choose low-fat dairy products). A more productive strategy would also include environmental change efforts, such as expanding the availability of more nutritious food choices. When this is done in conjunction with individual skill training, long-lasting and meaningful changes can be expected.

Finally, program designers ought to lighten up. Worksite health promotion may be the chosen profession of the program designer, and low-fat eating may be his or her avocation, but not everyone will share this passion. Nutrition interventions should be as entertaining and engaging as the other nonwork activities with which they are competing. Employees will want to participate if they can have fun with the nutrition programs. Emerging communication technologies are opening up new channels for engaging the interest of workers in better nutrition. Worksite e-mail support and motivation systems, "Internet buddies," and interactive Web-based approaches can be used creatively to promote healthful eating. The communication of nutrition information, no matter how important it is to good health, is secondary to attracting and retaining the interest and enthusiasm of the audience.

References

Abrams, D., Boutwell, W. B., Grizzle, J., Heimendinger, J., Sorensen, G., & Varnes, J. (1994). Cancer control at the workplace: The Working Well Trial. *Preventive Medicine, 23,* 15–27.

Anand, R., & Basiotis, P. (1998). Is total fat consumption really decreasing? *Nutrition Insights, 5.* [On-line]. Available: http://www.usda.gov/fcs/cnpp.htm.

Bal, D. G., & Foerster, S. B. (1991). Changing the American diet: Impact on cancer prevention policy recommendations and policy implications for the American Cancer Society. *Cancer, 67,* 2671–2680.

Bandura, A. (1986). *Social foundations of thought and action: A social cognitive theory.* Englewood Cliffs, NJ: Prentice-Hall.

Bandura, A. (1997). *Self-efficacy: The exercise of control.* New York: W. H. Freeman.

Barefield, E. (1996). Osterporosis-related hip fractures cost $13 billion to $18 billion yearly. *Food Review, 19,* 31–36.

Beresford, S. A., Thompson, B., Feng, Z., Christianson, A., McLerran, D., & Patrick, D. L. (1999). *Seattle 5 A Day worksite program to increase fruit and vegetable consumption.* Unpublished manuscript.

Biener, L., Glanz, K., McLerran, D., Sorensen, G., Thompson, B., Basen-Engquist, K., Linnan, L., & Varnes, J. (1999). Impact of the Working Well Trial on the worksite smoking and nutrition environment. *Health Education and Behavior, 16,* 478–494.

Bray, G. A., & Popkin, B. M. (1998). Dietary fat intake does affect obesity! *American Journal of Clinical Nutrition, 68,* 1157–1173.

Brug, J., Steenhuis, I., Van Assema, P., Glanz, K., & De Vries, H. (1999). Computer-tailored nutrition education: Differences between two interventions. *Health Education Research, 14,* 249–256.

Campbell, M. K., DeVellis, B. M., Strecher, V. J., Ammerman, A. S., DeVellis, R. F., & Sandler, R. S. (1994). Improving dietary behavior: The effectiveness of tailored messages in primary care settings. *American Journal of Public Health, 84,* 783–787.

Campbell, M. K., Reynolds, K. D., Havas, S., Curry, S., Bishop, D., Nicklas, T., Palombo, R., Buller, D., Feldman, R., Topor, M., Johnson, C., Beresford, S., Motsinger, B., Morrill, C., & Heimendinger, J. (1999). Stages of change for increasing fruit and vegetable consumption among adults and young adults participating in the National 5 A Day for Better Health Community Studies. *Health Education and Behavior, 26,* 513–534.

Frazao, E. (1996). The American diet: A costly problem. *Food Review, 19,* 2–6.

Gerrior, S., & Bente, L. (1999). *The nutrient content of the U.S. food supply 1990–94.* U.S. Department of Agriculture, Center for Nutrition Policy and Promotion, Home Economics Research Report No. 53.

Glanz, K. (1999). *Nutrition intervention in managed care settings.* Washington, D.C.: Center for the Advancement of Health.

Glanz, K., Basil, M., Maibach, E., Goldberg, J., & Snyder, D. (1998). Why Americans eat what they do: Taste, nutrition, cost, convenience, and weight control as influences on food consumption. *Journal of the American Dietetic Association, 98* (10), 1118–1126.

Glanz, K., & Eriksen, M. P. (1993). Individual and community models for dietary change. *Journal of Nutrition Education, 25,* 80–86.

Glanz, K., Hewitt, A. M., & Rudd, J. (1992). Consumer behavior and nutrition education: An integrative review. *Journal of Nutrition Education, 24,* 267–277.

Glanz, K., Kristal, A., Sorensen, G., Palombo, R., Heimendinger, J., & Probart, C. (1993). Development and validation of measures of psychosocial factors influencing fat- and fiber-related dietary behavior. *Preventive Medicine, 23,* 373–387.

Glanz, K., Kristal, A., Tilley, B., & Hirst, K. (1998). Psychosocial correlates of healthful diets among male auto workers. *Cancer, Epidemiology, Biomarkers, and Prevention, 7* (2), 119–126.

Glanz, K., Kristal, A. R., Tilley, B. C., & Li, S. (2000). Mediating factors in dietary change: Understanding the impact of a worksite nutrition information, *Health Education and Behavior, 27,* 112–125.

Glanz, K., Lankenau, B., Foerster, S., Temple, S., Mullis, R., & Schmid, T. (1995). Environmental and policy approaches to cardiovascular disease prevention through nutrition: Opportunities for state and local action. *Health Education Quarterly, 22* (4), 512–527.

Glanz, K., Lewis, F. M., & Rimer, B. K. (1997). *Health behavior and health education: Theory, research, and practice* (2nd ed.). San Francisco, CA: Jossey-Bass.

Glanz, K., & Mullis, R. M. (1988). Environmental interventions to promote healthy eating: A review of models, programs, and evidence. *Health Education Quarterly, 15* (4), 395–415.

Glanz, K., Patterson, R., Kristal, A., DiClemente, C., Heimendinger, J., Linnan, L., & McLerran, D. (1994). Stages of change in adopting healthy diets: Fat, fiber and correlates of nutrient intake. *Health Education Quarterly, 21* (4), 499–519.

Glanz, K., Patterson, R., Kristal, A., Feng, Z., Linnan, L., Heimendinger, J., & Hebert, J. R. (1998). Impact of worksite health promotion on stages of dietary change: The Working Well Trial. *Health Education and Behavior* (formerly *Health Education Quarterly*), 25, 448–463.

Glanz, K., & Rimer, B. K. (1995). Theory at a glance: A guide for health promotion practice [Monograph]. National Cancer Institute, NIH, Public Health Service. *U.S. Government Printing Office,* Publication No. 95-3896.

Glanz, K., & Rogers, T. (1994). Worksite nutrition programs. In M. P. O'Donnell, & J. S. Harris (Eds.), *Health promotion in the workplace* (2nd Ed., pp. 271–299). Albany, NY: Delmar.

Glanz, K., & Rudd, J. (1990). Readability and content analysis of written cholesterol education materials. *Patient Education and Counseling, 16,* 109–118.

Glanz, K., & Seewald-Klein, T. (1986). Nutrition at the worksite: An overview. *Journal of Nutrition Education, 18* (1, Suppl.), S1–S12.

Glanz, K., Sorensen, G., & Farmer, A. (1996). The health impact of worksite nutrition and cholesterol programs. *American Journal of Health Promotion, 10,* 453–470.

Glasgow, R. E., Terborg, J. R., & Hibbard, J. (1995). Behavior change at the worksite: does social support make a difference? *American Journal of Health Promotion, 10*(2), 125–31.

Glasgow, R. E., Terborg, J. R., Hollis, J. F., Severson, H. H., & Boles, S. M. (1995). Take heart: Results from the initial phase of a worksite wellness program. *American Journal of Public Health, 85,* 209–216.

Glasgow, R. E., Terborg, J. R., Hollis, J. F., Severson, H. H., Fisher, K. J., Boles, S., Pettigrew, E., Foster, L., Strycker, L., & Bischoff, S. (1994). Modifying dietary and tobacco use patterns in the worksite: The Take Heart Project. *Health Education Quarterly, 21,* 69–82.

Glasgow, R. E., Terborg, J. R., Strycker, L. A., Boles, S. M., & Hollis, J. F. (1997). Take Heart II: Replication of a worksite health promotion trial. *Journal of Behavioral Medicine, 20,* 143–161.

Havas, S., Heimendinger, J., Reynolds, K., Baranowski, T., Nicklas, T. A., Bishop, D., Buller, D., Sorensen, G., Beresford, S. A., & Owan, A. (1994). 5 A Day for better health: A new research initiative. *Journal of the American Dietetic Association, 94,* 32–36.

Heaney, C. A, & Goetzel, R. Z. (1997). A review of health-related outcomes of multi-component worksite health promotion programs. *American Journal of Health Promotion, 11,* 290–308.

Hunt, M. K, Stoddard, A. M., Glanz, K., Hebert, J. R., Probart, C., Sorensen, G., Thomson, S., Hixson, M. L., Linnan, L., & Palombo, R. (1997). Measures of food choice behavior related to intervention messages. *Journal of Nutrition Education, 29,* 3–11.

Jeffery, R. W., French, S. A., Raether, C., & Baxter, J. E. (1994). An environmental intervention to increase fruit and salad purchases in a cafeteria. *Preventive Medicine, 23,* 788–792.

Knapp, H. R. (1996). Nutritional aspects of hypertension. In E. E. Ziegler & L. J. Filer (Eds.), *Present knowledge in nutrition* (pp. 438–444). Washington, DC: International Life Sciences Institute.

Krebs-Smith, S. M., Cook, A., Subar, A. F., Cleveland, L., Friday, J. (1995). U.S. adults' fruit and vegetable intakes, 1989 to 1991: A revised baseline for the Healthy, People 2000 objective. *American Journal of Public Health, 85,* 1623–1629.

Kristal, A. R., Glanz, K., Curry, S. J., & Patterson, R. E. (1999). How can stages of change be best used in dietary interventions? *Journal of the American Dietetic Association, 99,* 679–684.

Kristal, A. R, Glanz, K., Tilley, B. C., & Li, S. (2000). Mediating factors in dietary change: Understanding the impact of a worksite nutrition intervention. *Health Education and Behavior, 27,* 112–125.

Kristal, A. R., Levy, L., Patterson, R. E., Li, S., & White, E. (1998). Trends in food label use associated with new nutrition labeling regulations. *American Journal of Public Health, 88,* 1212–1215.

Kristal, A., Patterson, R., Glanz, K., Heimendinger, J., Hebert, J., Feng, Z., & Probart, C. (1995). Psychosocial correlates of healthful diets: Baseline results from the Working Well Study. *Preventive Medicine, 24,* 221–228.

Lichtenstein, A. H. (1996). Atherosclerosis. In E. E. Ziegler & L. J. Filer (Eds.), *Present knowledge in nutrition* (pp. 430–437). Washington, DC: International Life Sciences Institute.

Lin, B., & Frazao, E. (1997). Nutritional quality of foods at and away from home. *Food Review, 20,* 33–40.

Mayer, J., Dubbert, P., & Elder, J. (1989). Promoting nutrition at the point-of-choice: A review. *Health Education Quarterly, 16,* 31–43.

Mayer, J. A., Brow, T. P., Heins, J. A., & Bishop, D. B. (1987). A multi-componat intervention for modifying food selections in a worksite cafeteria. *Journal of Nutrition Education, 19,* 277–280.

McLeroy, K., Bibeau, D., Steckler, A., & Glanz, K. (1988). An ecological perspective on health promotion programs. *Health Education Quarterly, 15* (4), 351–377.

National Heart, Lung, and Blood Institute. (1998). *Clinical Guidelines on the Identification, Evaluation, and Treatment of Overweight and Obesity in Adults. The Evidence Report.* Bethesda, MD: National Institutes of Health.

National Research Council, & National Academy of Sciences. (1989). *Diet and health: Implications for reducing chronic disease risk.* Washington, DC: National Academy Press.

Office of Disease Prevention and Health Promotion, & U.S. Public Health Service. (1987). *National survey of worksite health promotion activities. Summary Report.*

Office of Disease Prevention and Health Promotion, & U.S. Public Health Service. (1993). *National survey of worksite health promotion activities. Summary Report.*

Pamuk, E., Makuc, D., Heck, K., Reuben, C., & Lochner, K. (1998). *Socioeconomic status and health chartbook.* Health, United States. Hyattsville, MD: National Center for Health Statistics.

Patterson, R. E., Kristal, A., Glanz, K., McLerran, D., Hebert, J. R., Heimendinger, J., Linnan, L., Probart, C., & Chamberlain, R. M. (1997). Components of the Working Well Trial intervention associated with the adoption of healthful diets. *American Journal of Preventive Medicine, 13,* 271–276.

Patterson, R., Kristal, A., Varnes, J., Biener, L., Feng, Z., Glanz, K., Stables, G., Probart, C., & Chamberlain, R. (1998). Durability and dissemination of the nutrition intervention in the Working Well Trial. *Preventive Medicine, 27,* 668–673.

Prochaska, J. O., DiClemente, C. C., & Norcross, J. (1992). In search of how people change: Applications to addictive behaviors. *American Psychology, 47,* 1102–1114.

Rogers, E. M. (1983). *Diffusion of innovations* (3rd Ed.). New York: The Free Press.

Rudd, J., & Glanz, K. (1990). How individuals use information for health action: Consumer information processing. In K. Glanz, Lewis, & Rimer (Eds.), Health Behavior and Health Education: Theory, Research, and Practice (pp. 115–139). San Francisco, Jossey-Bass, Inc.

Sallis, J., & Owen, N. Ecological models. (1997). In K. Glanz, F. M. Lewis, & B. K. Rimer (Eds.), *Health behavior and health education: Theory, research, and practice* (2nd Ed., pp. 403–424). San Francisco, Jossey-Bass, Inc.

Sorensen, G., Hunt, M. K., Morris, D. H., Donnelly, G., Freeman, L., Ratcliffe, B. J., HSieh, J., Larson, K., Ockene, J. K. (1990). Promoting healthy eating patterns in the worksite: The treatwell intervention model. *Health Education Research,* 5(4), 505–515.

Sorensen, G., Emmons, K., Hunt, M. K., & Johnston, D. (1998). Implications of the results of community intervention trials. *Annual Review of Public Health, 19,* 379–416.

Sorensen, G., Hunt, M. K., Cohen, N., Stoddard, A., Stein, E., Phillips, J., Baker, F., Combe, C., Hebert, J., & Palombo, R. (1998). Worksite and family education for dietary change: The Treatwell 5-A-Day Program. *Health Education Research, 13,* 577–591.

Sorensen, G., Stoddard, A., & Macario, E. (1998). Social support and readiness to make dietary changes. *Health Education and Behavior, 25,* 586–598.

Sorensen, G., Stoddard, A., Peterson, K., Cohen, N., Hunt, M. K., Stein, E., Palombo, R., & Lederman, R. (1999). Increasing fruit and vegetable consumption through worksites and families in the Treatwell 5-a-Day study. *American Journal of Public Health, 89,* 54–60.

Sorensen, G., Thompson, B., Glanz, K., Feng, Z., Kinne, S., DiClemente, C., Emmons, K., Heimendinger, J., Probart, C., & Lichtenstein, E. (1996). Working well: Results from a worksite-based cancer prevention trial. *American Journal of Public Health, 86,* 939–947.

Sowers, M. F. (1996). Nutritional advances in osteoporosis. In E. E. Ziegler & L. J. Filer (Eds.), *Present knowledge in nutrition* (pp. 456–463). Washington, DC: International Life Sciences Institute.

Tilley, B., Glanz, K., Kristal, A., Hirst, K., Li, S., Vernon, S., & Myers, R. (1999). Nutrition intervention for high-risk auto workers: Results of the Next Step Trial. *Preventive Medicine, 28,* 284–292.

Tilley, B., Vernon, S., Glanz, K., Myers, R., Sanders, K., Lu, M., Hirst, K., Kristal, A., Smereka, C., & Sowers, M. F. (1997). Worksite cancer screening and nutrition intervention for high-risk auto workers: Design and baseline findings of the Next Step Trial. *Preventive Medicine, 26,* 227–235.

U. S. Department of Agriculture, & U.S. Department of Health and Human Services. (1995). *Nutrition and your health: Dietary guidelines for Americans* (Home and Garden Bulletin No. 232.) Washington, DC: U.S. Government Printing Office.

U.S. Department of Health and Human Services. (1998). *Nutrition. Healthy people 2010 objectives: Draft for public comment.* Washington, DC: U.S. Government Printing Office.

William M. Mercer, Inc. (1999). *National Worksite Health Promotion Survey, 1999.* New York: Author.

World Cancer Research Fund. (1997). *Food, nutrition and the prevention of cancer: A global perspective.* Washington, DC: American Institute for Cancer Research.

CHAPTER

12

Worksite Weight Management

Gordon D. Kaplan, Valerie Brinkman-Kaplan, and Edward M. Framer

INTRODUCTION

Most medical authorities recognize obesity as one of the most significant world health problems (Popkin & Doak, 1998). Over the past 30 years it has reached epidemic proportions in the United States (Kuczmarski, Flegal, Campbell, & Johnson, 1994). Obesity is associated with a wide variety of medical risk factors and serious health consequences. It results in both personal costs, in terms of quality and length of life for the individual, and a significant economic burden to the health care system. In the U.S., a large percent of this economic burden is borne by the private sector (Faltermayer, 1992); therefore, it is not surprising that worksite weight management programs have ranked relatively high in health promotion opportunities provided by employers (Office of Disease Prevention and Health Promotion, 1987), particularly in companies with over 750 employees (Fielding & Piserchia, 1989).

This chapter is divided into five sections. The first presents a brief background on the health problems and economic costs associated with obesity. Current population data and national health promotion goals are also reviewed. Section two describes treatment options for obesity, including a critique of their general effectiveness. The third section examines the application of these treatment options at the worksite and presents an analysis of their success. Section four describes a comprehensive model for obesity treatment at the worksite, and section five concludes with a discussion of major issues of program implementation.

BACKGROUND OF OBESITY AS A HEALTH AND ECONOMIC PROBLEM

The Definition and Measurement of Obesity

Obesity is a medical condition characterized by an excess of body fat and usually, but not necessarily always, by excess body weight. Researchers (e.g., Ditschuneit, 1991) have pointed out that it is possible for individuals, such as football players or bodybuilders who have excess lean body mass (muscle tissue), to be classified by height/weight charts as being overweight. However, they might not be obese. Likewise, an individual could be of normal body weight according to charts but carry an excess of body fat.

A body fat percent greater than 22% is considered obese for young men and over 25% is considered obese for older men; for women these figures are 32% and 35%, respectively (Gray, 1989).

The location of the excess body fat also has been shown to be an important factor in the relationship of obesity to health problems (Kissebah, Freedman, & Peiris, 1989). Centrally-located fat (distributed in the upper body around the waist) tends to be associated with a greater degree of medical risks than peripherally-located fat (distributed in the lower body around the hips). The waist-to-hip ratio is one of several measures of fat distribution that has been consistent in its relationships with medical risk factors independent of degree of overweight. Waist-to-hip ratios greater than 0.95 for men and 0.80 for women are associated with increased health risk (Keenan, Strogatz, James, Ammerman, & Rice, 1992).

Actual measurement of body fat is problematic for the standard outpatient medical practitioner. The most accurate methods (e.g., computed tomography, neutron activation, and nuclear magnetic resonance) also tend to be more difficult to perform and are more costly (Gray, 1989). Therefore, indices of body weight that correlate reasonably well with obesity and its health consequences are used most frequently.

The most common index is the Metropolitan Relative Weight. This is the percent over the midpoint of a desirable body weight range based on height/weight tables generated by the Metropolitan Life Insurance Company in 1959. Recently, however, a Consensus Panel convened by the National Institutes of Health National Heart, Lung, and Blood Institute (NHLBI) issued new guidelines based on the Body Mass Index (NHLBI Obesity Education Initiative Expert Panel, 1998). This index is derived by dividing an individual's weight (expressed in kilograms) by the square of his/her height (expressed in meters). For the health professional, the Body Mass Index (BMI) has the advantage of a large research base relating it to negative health consequences. It also allows a single set of recommendations to be used with both males and females. BMIs between 18.5 and 24.9 are within recommended limits. A BMI between 25 and 29.9 is considered overweight, and a BMI of 30 or greater is considered obese. From a nonprofessional

perspective, BMIs have the disadvantage of being more difficult to understand compared with scale weight. However, recommended BMI ranges may be translated easily back into weight ranges for the purposes of setting healthy weight goals with individuals. It should be noted that while BMI values are highly correlated with percent body fat ($r = 0.70$; Revicki & Israel, 1986), they can be inaccurate in populations with excess lean body mass (such as bodybuilders). This can lead to a false positive classification. In such specialized populations, a measurement of percent body fat would be desirable. However, the NHLBI Expert Panel has concluded that this issue does not "markedly influence the validity of BMI cutoffs either for classifying individuals into broad categories of overweight and obesity or for monitoring weight status of people in clinical settings" (NHLBI Obesity Education Initiative Expert Panel, 1998, p. 104S).

Worksites have a range of possibilities available for the assessment of body composition among employees. For those interested, a full description of methods is available in Heyward and Stolarczyk (1996). Of the available methods, measuring height and weight to calculate BMI is still the easiest, the least expensive, and the least prone to measurement error. Skinfold measurements may be used to supplement BMI calculations and may offer a way to cross-validate a questionable BMI in an individual who may have excess lean body mass. However, skinfold measurement requires a trained technician to assure accuracy. In some populations (e.g., the obese), the prediction equations for converting skinfold measures to percent body fat may be inaccurate, but such populations are not likely to be in question with regard to the need for weight management. Bioelectrical impedence or near-infrared measurements are also relatively inexpensive but require more training and are subject to larger and more frequent errors in misclassification. Hydrostatic (underwater) weighing has been the gold standard for body composition but requires a fairly expensive setup and a trained technician. This places it outside the scope of most worksite wellness facilities. Other methods, such as dual photon absorptiometry, are too expensive for most worksites to consider. For the purposes of this chapter, unless otherwise stated, we will use the NHLBI Consensus panel BMI definitions when referring to overweight and obese employees.

The Prevalence of Obesity

There is no doubt that obesity has risen to epidemic proportions in the United States. Today more than half of all adult Americans are overweight. Data from the NHANES III survey conducted in 1988–1991 indicated that the percentage of overweight men and women increased by 39% and 36% in men and women, respectively, over the past quarter century (Kuczmarski et al., 1994). Based on the new NHLBI definitions, 32.6% of men and 25.7% of women over age 20 qualify as being overweight (BMI between 25 and 24.9). An additional 22.3% of men and 25.0% of women are obese (BMI ≥ 30) (Kuczmarski, Carroll, Flegal, & Troiano, 1997). Data from the Centers for Disease Control indicate that both the prevalence of overweight and incidence of obesity are greatest among women (Williamson, Kahn, Remington, & Anda, 1990). Women were twice as likely as men to have experienced a major weight gain—approximately 35 or more pounds—over a ten-year period, and young women 25–34 years old were at greatest risk.

The Etiology of Obesity

Genetic Influence

Research has shown obesity to be a condition with a multifactorial etiology in which genetic, physiological, environmental, and behavioral factors all interact. Bouchard's (1994) analysis of recent studies places the genetic contribution to obesity between 25 and 40%. Adoption study data also indicate that obesity has a strong genetic component (Stunkard, Harris, & McClearn, 1990; Stunkard, Harris, Pederson, & McClearn 1990; & Stunkard, 1986). Allison, Faith, & Nathan (1996) compute that one's risk of being obese increases by a factor of 2–3 if one has a first-degree relative (for example, father, mother, or sibling) who is overweight, moderately obese, or severely obese. Stunkard concluded that the value of determining the genetic contribution to obesity lies in being able to better identify that segment of the population for

whom lifelong efforts at weight management may be necessary to prevent the development of the condition (Stunkard, 1986).

Influence of Energy Expenditure

Obesity results from an imbalance between energy intake and energy expenditure. Factors affecting energy expenditure include metabolic rate, diet-induced thermogenesis (energy expenditure associated with metabolizing food), and voluntary physical activity. Metabolic rate accounts for approximately 75% of daily energy expenditure. Shah & Jeffery (1991) have reviewed the literature on the influence of metabolic rate on obesity. It has been suggested that obese individuals may suffer from a reduced metabolic rate, greater metabolic efficiency, or both. However, studies consistently demonstrate that obese individuals have higher absolute metabolic rates (kcal/day) than their lean counterparts. This is due in part to the fact that obese individuals tend to have increased lean body mass in addition to their increased fat mass (Forbes & Welle, 1983). Additionally, metabolic rate is directly correlated both with total body mass in general and with lean body mass in particular (Nelson et al., 1992). Bruce et al. (1990) report no evidence of increased metabolic efficiency among grossly obese individuals compared to lean controls. Obese individuals do not need fewer calories to maintain their body weight. In fact, Forbes (1990) concluded that obese individuals actually require a greater energy intake to gain a given amount of weight than do leaner counterparts, implying metabolic inefficiency.

It also has been suggested that losing weight may result in a reduced metabolic rate and that this reduction in metabolic rate may be responsible for the difficulty in obese individuals maintaining weight loss. However, data are not consistent on this issue. For example, Foster et al. (1990) found decreases in metabolic rate that were proportional to the severity of caloric restriction. However, the overall decreases in metabolic rate were consistent with the degree of weight loss, particularly with fat-free mass loss. They concluded that no long-term reduction in metabolic rate occurred with either moderate or severe calorie restriction combined with physical activity (Wadden,

Foster, Letizia, & Mullen, 1990). DeGroot, van Es, van Raaij, Vogt, & Hautvast (1989, 1990) also noted no changes in metabolic efficiency following weight loss in follow-ups of one month and one year when metabolic rate was standardized to change in total body mass. A recent meta-analysis by Astrup et al. (1999) concluded that there was a 3–5% lower metabolic rate when adjusted for fat-free mass among formerly obese individuals when compared with never-obese individuals. However, it should be noted that this difference, while statistically significant, amounts only to 40–60 kcal/day. This would predict only a 4–6 pound difference in weight loss maintenance ability among formerly obese individuals.

Approximately 10% of daily calorie expenditure is estimated to come from thermogenesis, the metabolic cost of digesting and metabolizing food. It has been suggested that obese individuals may have a blunted thermogenic response to feeding, but studies have shown mixed results, possibly due to differing methodologies (D'Alessio, et al., 1988). In studies of obese subjects before and after weight loss and again after substantial weight regain, Jequier (1990) reported that, compared with lean controls, the obese subjects had an initially lower glucose-induced thermogenesis (6.8% vs. 8.3%), which was further reduced to an average of 3.8% after weight loss and returned to baseline following weight regain. Nelson et al. (1992) also found a reduced diet-induced thermogenesis among moderately obese women compared to never-obese controls who did not improve with weight normalization. While such a contribution may seem small, over a year's time even small but consistent decreases in energy requirements can contribute to weight gain. In addition, there are data to suggest that the location of the excess body fat may interact with the thermogenic response. Vansant, Van Gaal, & De Leeuw (1989) found that women with lower body obesity (waist-to-hip ratio < 0.80) had a three-hour glucose-induced thermogenic response, which was half that of women with upper body obesity (waist-to-hip ratio > 0.80).

Voluntary physical activity accounts for approximately 15% of daily energy expenditure under normal conditions. The rise in obesity in the United States has been associated with significant reductions in physical activity and increases in the nutrient density of our diets. Whereas pre-modern, pre-twentieth century lifestyles required substantial amounts of daily physical activity, today we engage in only a fraction of the energy expenditure of our great-grandparents (Blair, 1991). Particularly for those who have lost weight, substantial increases in physical activity may be critical to prevent regain of weight (Schoeller, Shay, & Kushner, 1997; Wing, 1999).

Influence of Energy Intake

Factors affecting energy intake include behavioral eating patterns and macronutrient composition of the diet. A complete exposition of the dramatic changes that have taken place in the American diet is beyond the scope of this chapter. Interested readers should refer to excellent reviews by Senauer, Asp, & Kinsey (1991) and by the Committee on Diet and Health of the Food and Nutrition Board, National Research Council Commission on Life Sciences (1989). Comments here are confined to a few examples of dietary changes that have affected the development of obesity in this country since 1900.

Both the macronutrient composition of the average American diet and the eating patterns of the average American have changed significantly during this period. In particular, the percentage of fat available in the food supply has increased from 32% in 1910 to 43% in 1985 (Senauer, Asp, & Kinsey, 1991). Data from the NHANES I survey indicated that by 1978 Americans were consuming about 41% of their daily calories as fat. Following major public health efforts since then, it is now estimated that adults consume an average of 36% of their daily calories in fat (Norris et al., 1997). However, this level is still considerably higher than dietary levels on which we evolved and under which we lived for millions of years (Eaton & Konner, 1985). In addition, as shown in Figure 12-1, while intake of saturated fat has declined since 1910, total per capita consumption of fat has actually increased due to a rise in vegetable fats.

From a weight management perspective, vegetable fat and animal fat are equivalent in calorie content. Hidden fat in animal products is a major contributor to the total fat content of the American diet. The con-

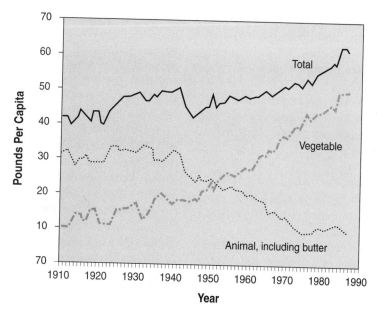

Figure 12-1 Since 1910, total per capita consumption of fat has increased due to increased intake of vegetable fats.
Source: B. Senauer, E. Asp, and J. Kinsey, *Food Trends and the Changing Consumer*, 1991. Reprinted with permission.

sumption of red meat rose significantly from 59 pounds per capita in 1900 to 95 pounds in 1976. Although there has been a dramatic decline to just over 70 pounds per capita in 1989, levels are still substantially higher than 1900 levels. While poultry consumption has risen in recent years, this has been due mainly to increased sales of fast foods in which fat is added during poultry preparation.

Survey data show that a greater percentage of individuals are eating meals away from home (National Research Council Commission on Life Sciences, 1986). Fast food establishments account for much of the eating done away from home, and the likelihood of obtaining a high-fat meal in these settings is perhaps greater. Data suggest that increased frequency of meals away from home is associated with a strikingly higher percentage of calories from fat (National Research Council Commission on Life Sciences, 1986). While some studies (Heitmann, Lissner, Sørenson, & Bengtsson, 1995) suggest that dietary fat intake may have an obesity-promoting effect, others (Golay et al., 1996) show that, under isocaloric conditions (i.e., with low-calorie intake kept constant), the percentage of

fat in the diet does not relate either to obesity or to weight loss success. However, under free-living conditions, the isocaloric requirement imposed by Golay et al. (1996) is rarely met. The primary result of the change in dietary fat consumption and increased food availability has been an increase in the ease with which individuals can consume total calories in excess of their daily energy requirements. Surveys confirm that men and women have increased calorie intake over the past 20 years (Koplan & Dietz, 1999). Thus, when methods of managing weight are considered, the reduction of dietary fat remains important, if not essential, for most individuals.

Summary

Regardless of issues of heredity, metabolic rate, and thermogenesis, voluntary control of body weight rests on factors that can be manipulated by the individual. These include physical activity, macronutrient composition of the diet, volume of energy intake, and various modifiable environmental determinants of intake. Our bodies evolved in a physically demanding environment, with limited access to food and very limited access to calorically high-dense foods. Therefore, weight regulation at non-obese levels was more likely even among those who might have been predisposed to the condition genetically. It should not be surprising that decreased energy expenditure combined with increased fat intake and greater availability of food should have produced a substantial rise in obesity prevalence.

The Health Risks of Obesity

In 1985 the National Institutes of Health Consensus Panel on the Health Implications of Obesity (1985) concluded that obesity constituted a clear public health risk. This conclusion was reaffirmed by the NIH NHLBI Consensus Panel on the Identification, Evaluation, and Treatment of Obesity (1998). Obesity increases risk for all-cause mortality (mortality from all causes), Figure 12-2 (Gray, 1989). It is the second leading cause of preventable death, contributing to over 300,000 deaths per year (Allison, Fontaine, Manson, Stevens, & VanItallie, 1999).

Obesity increases risk for coronary heart disease, diabetes, breast and colon cancers, hypertension, elevated total and LDL-cholesterol, stroke, osteoarthritis, gallbladder disease, and pregnancy complications (Cnattingius, Bergström, Lipworth, & Kramer, 1998; Colditz et al., 1990; Huang et al., 1998; Källén, 1998; Maclure et al., 1989; Manninen, Riihimäki, Heliövaara, & Mäkelä, 1996; Manson et al., 1990; Must et al., 1999; Rexrode et al., 1997; Shaw, Velie, & Schaffer, 1996; Siervogel et al., 1998; Trentham-Dietz et al., 1997; Witteman et al., 1989; Ziegler et al., 1996). A recent 12-year study of more than 9400 patients with coronary heart disease showed that the obese individuals were diagnosed at an earlier age, had 3–4 more years of illness, and died at a significantly earlier age (Eisenstein, Nelson, Shaw, Hakim, & Mark, 1999).

The health risks of obesity show remarkably consistent curvilinear relationships with respect to body mass, with risks beginning to escalate dramatically at BMIs beyond 27.8 (or 20% over desirable body weight as defined by the 1959 Metropolitan Life Insurance Tables). However, even lower BMI levels are associ-

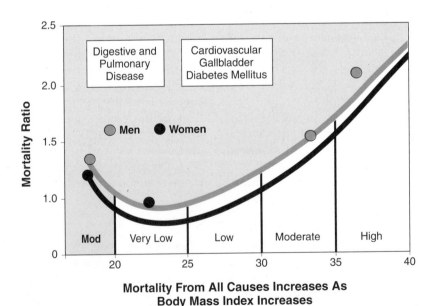

Figure 12-2 All-cause mortality as BMI increases.

Source: D. S. Gray, *Medical Clinics of North America* 73:1–13. Reprinted with permission from W. B. Saunders Company.

ated with health risks. For example, data from the Nurse's Health Study on coronary heart disease, hypertension, diabetes, and gallbladder disease show significant increases in risk for BMI levels above 25 (Colditz et al., 1990; Maclure et al., 1989; Manson et al., 1990; Witteman et al., 1989). New guidelines (NHLBI Obesity Education Initiative Expert Panel, 1998) recommend that health professionals be concerned either when BMIs exceed 24.9 and there are two or more comorbid risk factors or when BMIs exceed 29.9. Research from the U.S., Japan, and Finland indicate that the optimal BMI for adults to minimize morbidity and mortality is 22 (Castelli, 1989; Rissanen, Heliovaara, Knekt, Reunanen, & Aromaa, 1990; Tokunaga et al., 1990).

Quality of life is also impaired (Fontaine, Cheskin, & Barofsky, 1996; Rippe et al., 1998). For example, the obese are more likely to report pain (Barofsky, Fontaine, & Cheskin, 1997), fatigue (Chen, 1986), daytime sleepiness (Vgontzas et al., 1998), employment problems (van Gemert, Adang, Greve, & Soeters, 1998; Wolf & Colditz, 1996), and significant psychological consequences (Brownell, 1982).

Factors Modifying the Relationship between Overweight/Obesity and Health

It should be remembered that overweight/obesity is only one of a number of medical and lifestyle-related risk factors that influence longitudinal health status. Obesity does not usually occur in isolation. Most often other medical risk factors, such as high blood pressure, elevated total cholesterol:HDL cholesterol ratios, elevated triglycerides, and elevated blood glucose, are also present. In addition, the obese are less likely to be physically active (or fit). This chapter does not attempt to evaluate the independent health risks posed by obesity, nor does it attempt to rank in order the importance of obesity as a risk factor relative to other risk factors. However, there has been recent discussion about whether it might be possible to reduce the health risks of obesity by modifying other aspects of lifestyle. Specifically, Blair and colleagues (1989) have suggested that fitness may be far more important than weight (BMI). Data from the Cooper Institute for Aerobics Research, first presented by Blair et

al. (1989), do suggest that individuals with elevated BMI but also in the top two-fifths of fitness actually had lower all-cause mortality than those whose BMIs were in the lowest third but who were also in the bottom fifth of fitness. These data suggest that it may be possible to protect against the health risks of obesity by maintaining fitness. However, two issues must be considered. First, the cutpoints used by Blair et al. for BMI were: < 20.0; 20.0–25.0; and > 25.0. Thus, the lowest BMI category may have included individuals who were underweight and whose health risks would have been due in part to that condition. Second, no data were presented on individuals with greater BMIs, for example, over 30 or over 40. In such populations—if fitness were found—the protective effects might not be present. Prudence suggests that the Cooper data might be taken as evidence that, under conditions of overweight (BMI between 25 and 29.9), exercise and the resulting improvements in fitness may mitigate the health risks of obesity. However, individuals with excessive weight (BMI > 29.9) would still be well-advised to reduce weight while pursuing increases in physical activity.

Health Benefits of Weight Loss

Weight loss results in improvement in most medical risk factors, particularly among individuals with initially elevated levels. It also has become evident from a number of studies that the degree of weight loss needed to obtain significant medical benefits may be less than originally assumed (Blackburn & Kanders 1987; Goldstein, 1992; Van Gaal, Wauters, & De Leeuw, 1997). For example, weight loss is a recommended treatment for hypertension and is a cornerstone for the treatment of non-insulin-dependent (Type II) diabetes. Significant improvements in blood pressure among individuals with obese hypertension can be accomplished with weight losses averaging as little as 3.9 kg (Corrigan, Raczynski, Swencionis, & Jennings, 1991; Hypertension Prevention Trial Research Group, 1990). Weight losses of 22–41 lbs (9–18% of initial body weight) have been associated with significant improvements in fasting blood glucose, glycosylated hemoglobin levels, total cholesterol:HDL cholesterol ratios, and triglycerides among obese non-insulin-dependent diabetics (Anderson, Brinkman, & Hamilton, 1991; Wing et al., 1991). These improvements may be maintained despite some weight regain (Wing et al., 1991). Markovic et al. (1998) showed significant improvement in lipid profiles following weight loss, particularly associated with abdominal fat loss, among obese nondiabetic individuals. Finally, quality of life and self-esteem indices also have been shown to improve with weight loss (Rippe et al., 1998).

Health Risks of Weight Loss

There is also concern that voluntary weight loss may be associated with an increase in health risk if a pattern of weight cycling is present (Brownell, Greenwood, Stellar, & Shrager, 1986). Original data from animal studies suggested that cycles of weight fluctuation might result in a lowered metabolic rate and increased storage of body fat following each weight loss cycle. These effects would result in an increased percentage of body fat and decreased ability to maintain weight loss. Such concerns are consistent with the observation that most individuals who lose weight are not successful in maintaining weight loss.

Few human studies exist that relate weight cycling from voluntary dieting to metabolic rate and body composition. Steen, Oppliger, & Brownell (1988) reported decreased resting metabolic rate among weight-cycling wrestlers. However, Melby, Schmidt, and Corrigan (1990) have not found this to be the case among the wrestlers they studied. Blackburn et al. (1989) reported lower weight losses among patients restarting a protein-sparing modified fast, but compliance with the diet was not verified. Kaplan, Miller, & Anderson (1992) reported data on 22 patients who restarted a very-low-calorie diet after significant weight regain; there was no significant reduction in rate of weight loss but patients experienced more difficulty maintaining the diet during their second attempts. Beeson, Ray, Coxon, & Kreitzman (1989) also found no evidence of impaired ability to lose weight following weight loss and regain on a very-low-calorie diet, and Wadden, Foster, et al. (1990) have demonstrated that the decline in metabolic rate with weight loss is consistent with the amount of weight lost. Even the animal studies have not been

consistent in finding a negative effect of weight cycling on metabolic rate or body composition (Gray, Fisler, & Bray, 1988).

It has been suggested that weight fluctuation may increase coronary heart disease mortality (Lissner et al., 1991). Data from Framingham (Framington, Brownett, Lissner, & D'Agostano, 1991) showed a two-fold increase in risk among weight fluctuators; this risk was equivalent to that of remaining overweight. However, numerous studies have not supported this finding (Field et al., 1999; Hammer & Fisher, 1990; Jeffery, Wing, & French 1992; Schotte, Cohen, & Singh, 1990; Taylor, Jatulis, Fortmann, & Kraemer, 1995). There has also been concern that the repeated failures represented by weight cycling might lead to adverse psychological effects. However, the research has not found this to be the case (Bartlett, Wadden, & Vogt, 1996; Foster, Wadden, Kendall, Stunkard, & Vogt, 1996; Klem, Wing, McGuire, Seagle, & Hill, 1998; Simkin-Silverman, Wing, Plantinga, Matthews, & Kuller, 1998; Venditti, Wing, Jakicic, Butler, & Marcus, 1996).

Given the clear health risks associated with obesity, the benefits of weight loss currently outweigh potential hazards. However, the data emphasize the importance of maintaining weight loss and of potential dieters being committed to long-term lifestyle change. They also emphasize the need for providers of obesity programs to offer extended treatment following weight loss to help clients integrate lifestyle changes needed to maintain weight loss.

Economic Costs of Obesity

The successful prevention and treatment of obesity is important, considering its potential economic benefit. Thompson, Edelsberg, Colditz, Bird, & Oster (1999) estimated total lifetime costs associated with treating just five of the comorbid conditions associated with obesity (hypertension, hypercholesterolemia, diabetes, coronary heart disease, and stroke). They found that costs are $10,000 higher for obese individuals. The costs associated with obesity have been escalating dramatically. Colditz (1992) reported that $39.3 billion dollars (5.5% of the total costs of illness in the United States in 1986) could be attributed to obesity.

A more recent reanalysis showed that the total costs attributable to obesity in 1995 increased significantly to $99.2 billion, of which $51.64 billion were direct medical costs. These costs included 63% of the costs associated with diabetes, 17% of the costs for coronary heart disease, 8% of the costs for osteoarthritis, 6% of the costs due to hypertension, 5% of the costs due to gallbladder disease, and 4% of the costs for all cancers (Wolf & Colditz, 1998). These costs continue to escalate at a rapid pace. Estimates for 1999 suggest that healthcare costs for obese adults (BMI ≥ 30) will be $238 billion, of which $102 billion are in direct medical costs associated with 15 comorbid conditions (Rubin, 1999). Quesenberry, Caan, & Jacobson (1998) examined health care utilization and costs attributable to obesity within a large health maintenance organization and found similar results. Their analysis of over 17,000 members showed that, compared with non-obese individuals (BMI between 20 and 24.9), health care costs were 25% higher for those with a BMI from 30–34.9 and 44% higher for those with a BMI ≥ 35. Again, these costs were attributable to treatment for comorbid conditions, including heart disease, diabetes, and hypertension. Other countries also report that obesity contributes significantly to national health care expenditures. For example, in Canada and New Zealand, obesity accounted for 2.4% and 2.5% of total healthcare expenditures respectively (Birmingham, Muller, Palepu, Spinelli, & Anis, 1999; Swinburn et al., 1997).

Industry bears a large percentage of these costs. In the Wolf and Colditz (1998) analysis, productivity losses attributable to obesity (defined as BMI ≥ 30) were $3.9 billion. According to a report published jointly by the U.S. Office of Disease Prevention and Health Promotion, The American Dietetic Association, and the Society for Nutrition Education, "employees who are 40 percent overweight visit their physicians and miss work twice as often as average workers, costing employers an additional $1000 per year per overweight employee" (Armstrong, 1986, p. 53). Evaluating Control Data's StayWell® program, Jose and Anderson (1986) found that overweight employees' annual health care claims were nearly 25% higher ($1100 vs. $850). A subsequent analysis conducted by Milliman and Robertson, Inc. (1987) found

a similar relationship with monthly claims (excluding maternity) 11% higher for the high-risk overweight group than the low-risk group. In addition, high-risk overweight employees had 45% more hospital days per thousand (595 vs. 409) and were more likely to have claims over $5000 (4.0% vs. 2.7%). These high-risk overweight employees also were significantly more likely to have been absent from work more than 5 days during the year (18% vs. 14% of employees). Finally, an analysis of data on 10,825 employed men and women who had participated in a wellness screening program demonstrated that obese employees had significantly more absenteeism compared with non-obese employees (Tucker & Friedman, 1998). Obesity was defined by percent body fat (≥ 25% for men; ≥ 30% for women). There was a 74% increase in high-level absenteeism (7 or more absences over the past 6 months) and a 61% increase in moderate absenteeism (3–6 absences over the past 6 months). Such data demonstrate why it would be advantageous for industry to support effective treatment options for their obese employees. Such programs can be offered efficiently at the worksite, but concern must be given to long-term weight management if economic benefits are to be maintained.

Other costs of weight loss include personal costs associated with time, effort, and money. Of course, such costs are subjective in nature, and it is clear that as individuals become increasingly obese, the psychological and social consequences become more severe. In a survey of post-gastric-bypass patients, Rand and Macgregor (1991) found that, given the choice, these formerly morbidly obese individuals would choose any other disability (e.g., blindness, deafness, paralysis) rather than be morbidly obese. To put the personal costs of weight loss into a financial perspective, these same individuals would rather be normal weight than be morbidly obese multimillionaires.

Dieting Prevalence

Intentional dieting may well have surpassed baseball as the great American pastime. Jeffery, Adlis, & Forster (1991) found dieting to be so pervasive that it may be considered to be normative. Estimates range as high as 50% of the U.S. population being on a diet at any given time. The dieting industry has grown exponentially over the past two decades. According to a recent Federal Trade Commission report, total spending for weight loss products and services is $33 billion annually (Cleland et al., 1998). Forman, Trowbridge, Gentry, Marks, & Hogelin (1986) have reported data from the Behavioral Risk Factors Survey, a random sample of over 16,000 people from 49 states, which indicated that up to 37% of men and 52% of women are currently dieting. Data from the 1996 Behavioral Risk Factor Surveillance System estimate that 28.8% of men and 43.6% of women are attempting weight loss, and an additional 35.1% of men and 34.4% of women are working on weight maintenance (Serdula et al., 1999). As part of their Healthy Worker Project, Jeffery, Adlis, and Forster (1991) conducted a survey of dieting prevalence among workers randomly selected from 32 worksites ranging in size from 235 to 915 employees. They found that 47% of men and 75% of women reported dieting for weight loss at some point in their lives. Moreover, 13% of men and 26% of women were currently dieting, 1% and 6%, respectively, in an organized weight loss program.

Given these data, the potential need in industry for weight management programs is great. It is also clear that there is a demand for such programs. In a survey conducted by Reid and Dunkley (1989) of 611 employees from two high-tech companies in Canada in 1985, 75% of the men and 92% of the women with a BMI greater than 25 (44% and 21% of the sample, respectively) were interested in participating in a worksite weight management program. In 1989 Fielding and Piserchia (1989) reported that 48% of worksites with 750 or more employees offered health promotion activities in the area of weight management. Weisbrod, Pirie, Bracht, and Elstun (1991) surveyed worksites with over 100 employees in four Midwest communities and found that weight loss programs were offered by 33%. In the 1992 National Survey of Worksite Health Promotion Activities, only 24% of worksites surveyed offered weight control interventions (U.S. Department of Health and Human Services, 1993). However, Wilson, DeJoy, Jorgenson, and Crump (1999) surveyed 3628 randomly selected worksites from the American Business Lists in 1995 and found that 31% of small (15–99 employees) and 46% of larger (100+ employees) worksites reported offering weight management programs during the previous 12 months. The most recent survey of worksite health promotion, conducted by William M. Mercer, Inc. (1999), indicated that 38% of worksites sampled offered weight management programs for their employees, the majority being services offered offsite. Only 15% of worksites offered weight management onsite. Of interest is the finding that 30% of worksites reported weight management services being offered through one or more of their health plans.

National Health Promotion Goals

The U.S. Surgeon General (U.S. Public Health Service, 1999) has established a goal for the year 2010 that the prevalence of obesity (BMI $\geq$ 30) be reduced to no more than 15% of the adult population. For industry another goal was recommended to increase to at least 50% the proportion of worksites with 50 or more employees that offer nutrition education and/or weight management programs for their employees. In 1985 these levels were 17% (nutrition education) and 15% (weight management), respectively. Therefore, the worksite is seen as an integral part of the eventual solution to the obesity epidemic in the United States. However, it is also clear that achieving these goals will require coordinated efforts from public, private, and professional sectors.

TREATMENT OPTIONS FOR OBESITY

Selecting an Appropriate Treatment

A wide variety of treatments have been used in the treatment of obese individuals. These include lay-led community self-help groups (such as TOPS or Overeaters Anonymous), commercial weight loss programs (such as Weight Watchers or NutriSystems), individual dietary or psychological counseling, hospital-based multidisciplinary treatment programs, and multidisciplinary residential treatment programs. Recently it has been proposed that individuals be matched to interventions based on medical risk. Bray (1989) proposed an algorithm for determining medical risk based on increasing BMI and accompanying risk factors (see Figure 12-3). He then suggested a hierarchy of recommended treatment alternatives based on increasing risk.

Brownell and Wadden (1991) have taken this concept a step further, proposing a more elaborate match-

ing procedure (see Figure 12-4). Their model is theoretically appealing, but there are few data available to support the specific client-program matching, proposed in column 3.

A complete review of these approaches is beyond the scope of this chapter. This section will summarize the efficacy of approaches that have particular potential for worksite treatment. In general, long-term treatment results from most approaches have been poor (National Institutes of Health, Technology Assessment Conference Statement, 1992). However, available data also suggest ways by which effectiveness can be increased. In addition, it may not be necessary to get employees down to chart-defined ideal body weights to have significant medical impact and to produce potential long-term savings in corporate medical expenditures.

Behavioral Treatment

An early review by Stunkard and McLaren-Hume (1959) indicated that traditional dietary management of obesity was not very successful. Behavioral therapies, introduced in the early 1970s, focused on changing eating patterns and physical activity and produced substantially better short-term data, as shown in Table 12-1 (Brownell & Kramer, 1989).

In these recent studies, patients were less likely to drop out of treatment, and weight losses were significant, amounting to about one pound per week. Over time, active treatment phases have increased from an average of 8.4 weeks to 16.7 weeks, producing an increase in average weight loss. The rate of weight loss has not changed, but there has been a disturbing increase in attrition. Short-term follow-ups suggested very good results up to six months, and maintenance of weight loss at one year continues to be reasonable, with approximately two-thirds of initial weight loss being maintained. As a result, behavioral modification has become a part of most commercial and professionally-led weight management programs and is considered necessary for effective treatment (Council on Scientific Affairs, 1988; Weinsier et al., 1984).

However, published reports of extended follow-up intervals for individuals who have not continued in

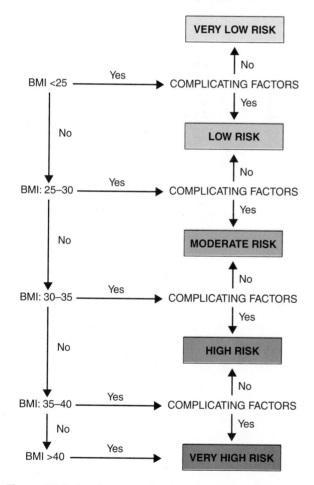

RISK CLASSIFICATION ALGORITHM

Figure 12-3 An algorithm for determining medical risk according to increasing BMI and accompanying risk factors.

Source: G. A. Bray, 1989, Classification and Evaluation of the Obesities, *Medical Clinics of North America* 73:161–84. Reprinted with permission from W. B. Saunders Company.

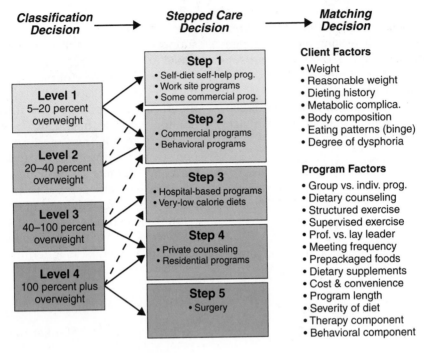

Figure 12-4 A more elaborate matching procedure.

Source: K. D. Brownell and T. A. Wadden, 1991, The Heterogeneity of Obesity: Fitting Treatments to Individuals, *Behavior Therapy* 22(2). Copyright 1991 by the Association for Advancement of Behavior Therapy. Reprinted with permission of the publisher and the author.

Table 12-1 Summary of Data (mean values) from Controlled Trials of Behavioral Therapy Completed Before and During 1974 and During 1978, 1984, and 1986*

	1974	1978	1984	1986
Number of studies included (%)	15	17	15	6
Sample size	53.1	54.0	71.3	93.3
Initial weight (lbs)	163.0	194.0	197.0	210.6
Initial percent overweight	49.4	48.6	48.1	53.4
Length of treatment (weeks)	8.4	10.5	13.2	16.7
Weight loss (lbs)	8.5	9.4	15.4	22.0
Loss per week (lbs)	1.2	0.9	1.2	1.4
Attrition (%)	11.4	12.9	10.6	20.7
Length of follow-up (weeks)	15.5	30.3	58.4	44.0
Loss at follow-up (lbs)	8.9	9.1	9.8	14.5

*All values are means across studies. Studies are those appearing in *Journal of Consulting and Clinical Psychology, Behavior Therapy, Behavior, Research and Therapy,* and *Addictive Behaviors.*

Source: K. D. Brownell and F. M. Kramer, 1989. Behavior Management of Obesity. *Med Clin N. Amer* 73:185–201. Reprinted with permission from W. B. Saunders Company.

treatment have demonstrated a continuous increase in the amount of weight regained. By five years, follow-ups of many behavioral treatments have shown an average return to baseline weights (Stalonas, Perri, & Kerzner, 1984; Wadden, Sternberg, Letizia, Stunkard, & Foster, 1989). These data demonstrate the need for more extended treatment following weight loss to ensure the incorporation of weight management skills. Studies that have attempted to provide more structured maintenance phases have produced better results, although five-year data have not been reported (Perri, McAdoo, Spevak, & Newlin, 1984; Perri, Shapiro, Ludwig, & McAdoo, 1984).

More Aggressive Treatment Options

Because behavioral approaches employing modest dietary restriction (generally 1200 kcal/day balanced diets) do not tend to produce large weight losses, more aggressive treatments have been recommended for the seriously overweight population (BMI ≥ 30) (Brownell & Jeffery, 1987). Such treatments include extreme caloric restriction, such as supplemented very-low-calorie diets, and surgical intervention.

Very-low-calorie diets are defined as regimens of less than 800 kcal/day (Atkinson, 1989). They emerged as an outpatient treatment option in the mid 1970s. Such diets require careful medical screening and ongoing supervision to minimize health risks and should be offered only with accompanying behavioral education (American Dietetic Association, 1990; Wadden, Van Itallie, & Blackburn, 1990). While weight losses that can be achieved on such diets can be impressive, weight regain without behavioral education and ongoing maintenance participation is equally dramatic. Wadden and Stunkard (1986) demonstrated that without behavioral education, participants had regained two-thirds of their weight loss in one year, significantly more than participants who had received either behavioral education alone or the very-low-calorie diet in combination with behavioral education. By five years, however, all groups had regained the majority of the weight they had lost (Wadden et al., 1989). It is clear that for weight loss to be maintained, intervention must extend beyond initial weight loss.

Commercial Weight Management Programs

Numerous commercial weight control programs have been established, particularly during the past decade. Stunkard (1986) has reviewed data on community-based weight management approaches. These include self-help groups such as TOPS (Take Off Pounds Sensibly) and commercial programs such as Weight Watchers. In his evaluation of TOPS, Stunkard found early dropouts lose little weight and longer-term participants who lose more eventually regain it despite continued program participation. Introduction of behavioral education improved dropout rates from 67% to 40%, but the organization did not adopt the behavioral model subsequently.

One of the greatest problems in evaluating commercial programs is the lack of published data. The limited available data suggest that early dropout rates may be appreciable. For example, Volkmar et al. (1981) found that by 12 weeks of treatment only 25% of participants remained in treatment. By 24 weeks, the dropout rate had reached 80%. Attrition of this magnitude obviously compromises any conclusions that can be drawn regarding the success of the intervention. Recent data presented by NutriSystems suggest reasonable maintenance of weight loss, but the generalizability of their data is uncertain due to a highly selected sample and very small sample size (Shapiro, 1991). Weight Watchers, one of the oldest community groups, has published little data demonstrating short-term or long-term weight loss effectiveness. This is of particular concern because Weight Watchers is one of the largest vendors of worksite-based weight control programs.

REVIEW OF WORKSITE WEIGHT MANAGEMENT PROGRAMS

Advantages of Worksite Treatment

A significant proportion of adult Americans in the workforce is either obese or overweight. Estimates range between 26% to as much as 53% (Anderson & Jose, 1987; Efurt, Foote, & Heirich, 1991; Jeffery, Forster, & Schmid, 1989; Siegelman, 1991; Wild, Smith, & Martin, 1992). The worksite seems to offer these people a unique opportunity for efficient and effective obesity management on a much wider scale, and potentially at lower cost, than is possible with clinic-based treatment. From a public health perspective, providing treatment at the worksite enables health providers to reach much larger numbers of individuals who would benefit from treatment compared with private practice. Whereas few of these individuals would be likely to join formal comprehensive programs for weight management, 100% report for work on a regular basis. Worksites, with their "captive" audience, provide an efficient medium for dissemination of health information, monitoring of risk factors, and support of behavioral change. Many worksites have systems already in place that would support educational efforts in the area of weight management. These include company newsletters, interoffice memos, payroll inserts, posters, and bulletin boards, all of which could be used to enhance enrollment in health programs, increase readiness of employees to make lifestyle changes, provide reliable and accurate information, offer incentives, and reinforce efforts. In addition, by enrolling worksites in healthy weight management efforts, it is possible to access those individuals whose current weight does not yet put them at excessive risk but for whom preventive efforts could be most effective in the control of future weight and associated medical risk factors. The importance of maintaining a healthy risk factor profile has been demonstrated by Edington, Musich, Schneuringer, & Edington (1999). He has shown that employees who move from low-risk status (0–1 risk factor) to high-risk status (3 or more risk factors) demonstrate approximately a two-fold increase in health care costs.

Not only is it possible to provide interventions more efficiently at the worksite, but ongoing follow-up of individuals who participate in weight management programs is also easier. Unlike maintenance groups offered in community or clinic-based weight control programs, in which attrition tends to be quite high, people report to work regularly. In fact, one of the most interesting possibilities offered by worksite weight management is the ability to take advantage of the naturally-occurring social supports among coworkers, departments within a company, corporate sites, and the individual corporate "culture" and environment.

Worksite weight management programs offer several advantages for the employee. These include easier access to treatment and ongoing support, greater time efficiency, decreased health risks, and improved quality of life. To the extent that such programs are either partially or fully funded by employers, the employee may also benefit directly by reduction in costs for treatment. Thus, worksite weight management seems to make sense from both public and personal health perspectives. However, there are also potential problems associated with worksite weight management programs. These primarily involve issues of confidentiality. For example, not all individuals wish to be identified as being "in need" of weight management (even though obesity is so obviously visible), and not all individuals feel comfortable being treated in a group including co-workers. Effective worksite programs must remain sensitive to such issues.

Finally, there is a critical question of what form of intervention is most likely to succeed at the worksite. Should worksite models be replications of clinic models, with group treatments being offered onsite? Or should the weight management focus at the worksite be broader, more corporate-culture-based, and perhaps less costly, supporting individuals in maintaining healthier weights without direct intervention in the form of group therapies? For answers to these questions, we must examine the literature.

Models for Worksite Treatment

Although attempts to apply clinical models for the treatment of obesity to the worksite have been reported since the late 1970s, the majority of studies have been reported between 1985 and 1995. Therefore, worksite weight management could be fairly judged to be in its infancy. How effective have these efforts been? A conservative evaluation of the available literature lead to three conclusions. First, as Hennrikus and Jeffery (1996) state in their recent review of the worksite weight management literature, much of the research on worksite weight management has been methodologically weak, making it difficult to reach conclusions about the potential for such interventions. In their review of 44 data-based studies, only 10 (23%) used randomized control designs to evaluate the intervention(s) under investigation. Second, most worksite programs have not produced overwhelming success in their primary goal of weight management. Third, data are not available regarding the impact of participation in worksite weight management programs on overall risk factor management for individuals or populations. Neither are there data relating participation to specific savings in corporate health care expenditures. Unfortunately, we know little more today than we did five years ago. Hennrikus and Jeffery (1996) discuss a set of research priorities for investigators of worksite weight management. These include an increased use of randomized designs, as well as replication across worksites, an expanded set of outcome measures to document impact, and an improved characterization and exploration of worksite factors that could influence weight management outcomes. Finally, there was a dearth of new research in worksite-based weight management during the second half of the 1990s. This likely reflects the limited success of most interventions, whether or not they have been based at the worksite.

A variety of intervention models have been applied at the worksite, but the majority fall within four broad categories. These include clinic-format treatment models (Abrams & Follick, 1983; Brownell, Stunkard, & McKeon, 1985; Dennison, Dennison, & McCann, 1990; Efurt, Foote, & Heirich, 1991; Evans, Harris, McNeill, & McKenzie, 1989; Fowler, Abrams, Peterson, & Follick, 1983; Peterson, Abrams, Elder, & Beaudin, 1985; Pritchard, Nowson, & Marks, 1997; Siggard, Raben, & Astrup, 1996; Stunkard & Brownell, 1980; Sumner, Schiller, Marr, & Thompson, 1986); financial incentive programs, such as payroll deductions and worksite competitions (Brownell, Cohen, Stunkard, Felix, & Cooley, 1984; Cohen, Stunkard, & Felix, 1987; Colvin, Zopf, & Myers, 1983; Follick, Fowler, & Brown, 1984; Forster, Jeffery, Sullivan, & Snell, 1985; Jeffery, Forster, et al., 1992; Jeffery, Forster, & Schmid, 1989; Jeffery, Forster, & Snell, 1985; Seidman, Sevelius, & Ewald, 1984; Stunkard, Cohen, & Felix, 1989); commercial models (Frankle, McIntosh, Bianchi, & Kane, 1986; Miller & Edelstein, 1990);

and comprehensive health promotion intervention at the worksite (Bly, Jones, & Richardson, 1986; Holt, McCauley, & Paul, 1995; Jose & Anderson, 1986). Table 12-2 presents a basic summary of the results of these interventions.

Clinic-format treatment models

Initial worksite weight management efforts involved transferring standard group behavioral modification programs designed for private practice (e.g., Ferguson, 1985) directly into corporate settings. As behavioral programs have improved, these changes have been added to worksite models. Programs have consisted of active treatment phases extending over 8–26 weeks and 8–16 onsite group sessions. Sessions usually are offered during employee time (lunchtime or before/after work) and typically last 45 minutes to one hour. Such programs have been offered to both blue- and white-collar employees in a wide variety of worksites. Table 12-3 shows typical content areas covered in standard behavioral obesity treatment (Stunkard & Berthold, 1985).

As displayed in Table 12-2, end of treatment weight losses for employees completing these interventions was 8.2 pounds (range: 2.4–14.5 pounds) for treatments lasting an average of 13 weeks. However, these results are modified by attrition, which has been a significant problem with use of the clinic model at the worksite. In these studies, attrition by the end of treatment ranged from 21% to 82% with a mean of 47.5%. By making a conservative assumption that employees failing to complete treatment are not likely to have achieved any weight loss, the average weight loss for these types of intervention can be estimated to be only 4.7 pounds.

Most of these programs included neither formal maintenance programs nor follow-up data collection to assess maintenance of weight loss. Of those that conducted follow-ups, the usual follow-up duration was six months. Weight loss maintenance was highly variable, ranging from 0% maintained to over 100% regained, based on completers (mean = 7.9 pounds; median = 5.5 pounds). Adjusting the data for dropouts, the average weight loss maintained was 3.1 pounds (ranging from 0–8.7 pounds).

Table 12-2 **Results of Worksite Weight Management Programs**

Author(s)	Worksite	Intervention
Clinic-based treatments		
Stunkard & Brownell 1980	Union workers N = 40	• Standard Group Behavioral Modification (SGBM) • 16 weeks; 45-minute sessions • Worksite (W) versus clinic (C); Lay-led (L) versus professional (P); Standard weekly (S) versus 4/week, intensive (I)
Abrams & Follick 1983	Hospital employees N = 133	• SGBM • 10 weeks; 30-minute sessions; 4 maintenance sessions held biweekly • Structured (SM) versus unstructured (USM) maintenance • 3- and 6-month follow-ups
Fowler et al. 1983	Hospital employees N = 57	• SGBM (as in Abrams & Follick, 1983) • 1-hour sessions • Lay (L) versus Professional (P) • 8-month follow-up
Brownell, Stunkard, & McKeon 1985	Department store employees N = 132 n = 61 n = 71	• SGBM • 16 weeks; 45-minute sessions • Lay (L) versus professional (P); Standard weekly (S) versus intensive (I); Worksite (W) versus Clinic (C) • 1-year follow-up
Peterson et al. 1985	High-tech industry N = 63	• SGBM • 12 weeks; 1-hour sessions (8 weeks weekly then biweekly for 8 weeks) • Lay (L) versus Professional (P) • 4-month follow-up
Sumner et al. 1986	Insurance company N = 120	• SGBM • 8 weeks (9 sessions); 45-minute sessions • 4 classes • Maintenance classes held every 2–4 weeks
Evans et al. 1989	University employees N = 75	• SGBM • 10 weeks
Efurt, Foote, & Heirich 1991	Manufacturing company; 4 sites N = 690 n = 173 (control) n = 194 n = 150 n = 173	• SGBM • Health Classes (H); Sites 2-4; offered 2 times/year on a variety of topics • Individualized Intervention (HI); Sites 3-4; Menu of options, including telephone guidance; 1:1 consultation; minigroups of 2–7 participants; full groups (as in H)

	Attrition		Weight Change		Maintenance	
LIW	31%	LIW	6.8 lbs.	NA		
LSW	50%	LSW	12.3 lbs.			
PSC	75%	PSC	5.9 lbs.			
PSW	82%	PSW	8.2 lbs.			
End of treatment:	45%	End of treatment:		3-month:		
		USM	10.3 lbs.	USM	6.8 lbs	
End of maintenance:	75%	SM	11.9 lbs.	SM	9.7 lbs	
		End of maintenance:		6-month:		
		USM	13.0 lbs.	USM	3.3 lbs	
		SM	9.0 lbs.	SM	9.0 lbs	
L	70%	L	5.3 lbs.	L	2.0 lbs.	
P	30%	P	9.2 lbs.	P	4.8 lbs.	
Studies and 2/3:		Studies and 2/3:		Studies and 2/3:		
LSW	61.1%	LSW	11.5 lbs.	LSW	10.8 lbs	
	37.5%		6.4 lbs.		5.5 lbs	
LIW	37.5%	LIW	5.5 lbs.	LIW	6.8 lbs.	
	NA		NA		NA	
PSW	36.7%	PSW	9.3 lbs.	PSW	8.1 lbs.	
	29.0%		8.6 lbs.		5.9 lbs.	
PSC	20%	PSC	9.0 lbs.	PSC	7.5 lbs.	
	NA		NA		NA	
For the four classes						
P	76%	P	12.8 lbs.	P	23.8 lbs.	
L	48%	L	13.9 lbs.	L	16.7 lbs.	
	16% / 29%	3.4–7.0 lbs.		NA		
	41% / 59%					
				NA		
	3.8%		6.5 lbs.	NA		
NA		C	+4.2 lbs.	NA		
		H	2.4 lbs.			
		HI	5.0 lbs.			
		HIE	6.4 lbs.			

continued

Table 12-2 Results of Worksite Weight Management Programs—*(continued)*

Author(s)	Worksite	Intervention
Efurt, Foote, & Heirich 1991—*continued*		• Environmental Support; Site 4; site-wide health promotion activities throughout the year • Health classes (H) versus Classes + Individual (HI) versus Classes + Individual + Environmental supports (HIE) versus Control (C)
Dennison, Dennison, & McCann 1990	University employees N = 63	• Computer-assisted groups behavior modification • 8 weeks • Focus on nutrition and exercise goals; reward system for achieving goals
Siggard, Raben, & Astrup 1996	Insurance company in Denmark N = 86	• Nutrition education for maintaining a carbohydrate-rich, low fat diet • 12 weeks; Nutrition education (I) versus Control (C) • 24- and 52-week follow-up
Pritchard, Nowson, & Marks 1997	Business corporation employees N = 66	• SGBM • 12-month intervention; bimonthly sessions • Diet (D) versus Exercise (E) versus Control (C)
Financial Incentive Models		
Colvin, Zopf, & Myers 1983	Medical school staff and students N = 23	• No formal program • Social support (S) versus monetary incentive (I)
Follick, Fowler, & Brown 1984	Hospital employees N = 48	• SGBM • Monetary incentive (I) versus Control (C) • 6-month follow-up
Jeffery, Forster, & Snell 1985	University employees N = 36	• SBGM (optional enrollment) 50% and 75% for two groups (G) • 6-months; 12 sessions held biweekly • Incentive plan based on payroll deductions • 3-month follow-up
Forster et al. 1985	University employees N = 131	• (See Jeffery, Forster, and Snell 1985) • Optional (O) versus required (R) attendance; Group (G) versus self-instructional (S)
Jeffery, Forster, & Schmid 1989	Manufacturing company N = 170 (includes 34 re-enrollees)	• (See Jeffery, Forster, and Snell 1985) • Optional attendance; Required payroll deduction; Two rounds (R) of treatment
Jeffery et al. 1992	Variety of worksite types (n = 32 sites) N = 2041	• (See Jeffery, Forster, and Snell 1985) • 4 rounds of treatment over 2 years
Seidman, Sevelius, & Ewald 1984	Manufacturing company N = 2499	• Competition; 3-month • Minimal behavioral training: one 90-minute session

Attrition		Weight Change		Maintenance	
24%			9.6 lbs.	NA	
23%		I	9.2 lbs.	52 weeks:	
		C	1.8 lbs.	I	69% maintained 5.5 lb loss or greater
12% overall;				NA	
D	22%	D	15.8 lbs.		
E	4%	E	6.6 lbs.		
C	10%	C	+2.3 lbs.		
S	50%	S	3.7 lbs.	S	3.1 lbs.
I	46%	I	9.3 lbs.	I	6.0 lbs.
C	80%	C	8.0 lbs.	"poor at 6 months"	
I	40%	I	7.0 lbs.		
6% overall		G1	8.1 lbs.	"good"	
		G2	17.0 lbs.		
21.4% overall		GR	12.7 lbs.	NA	
		GO	10.0 lbs.		
		SR	11.9 lbs.		
		SO	14.1 lbs.		
R1	6.8%	R1	7.3 lbs.	NA	
R2	6.1%	R2	6.6 lbs.		
NA		4.8 lbs. overall		NA	
30%		8.2 lbs.		NA	

continued

Table 12-2 Results of Worksite Weight Management Programs—*(continued)*

Author(s)	Worksite	Intervention
Brownell et al. 1984	Bank (B) employees N = 176 Manufacturing companies (M) N = 53; 48	• Competition; 12 weeks; 13 weeks; 15 weeks • Behavioral self-help manual • 6-month follow-up
Cohen, Stunkard, & Felix 1987	Manufacturing company N = 131	• Competition; 12 weeks • Behavioral self-help materials • 3 rounds of competition: Group (R1; R3) versus Individual competition (R2)

Stunkard, Cohen, & Felix 1989	Study 1: Banks
	(n = 2 sites) N = 109;
	manufacturing Companies
	(n = 4 sites) N = 895
	Study 2: College, bank, manufacturing
	N = 1001
	Study 3: Banks and manufacturing company
		• Competition (see Cohen, Stunkard, and Felix 1987)
		• Teams within worksite (T) versus Individual (I) versus Worksites as teams (W)
		• Team competition (T) versus Individual competition (I) versus Cooperation (C)
		
		• Follow-up for 3 sites involved in Study 2:
		  ✳ Site 1 (banks): 6 months
		  ✳ Site 2 (manufacturing company): 8 months
		  ✳ Site 3 (banks): 12 months

Commercial Programs		
Frankle et al. 1986	Variety of settings	• Weight Watchers at Work; Balanced deficit diet; Group behavior modification; Lay-led groups • 8 weeks; 1-hour sessions
Miller & Edelstein 1990	Hospital employees N = 32	• Weight Watchers at Work (See Frankle et al. 1986)
Total Health Promotion		
Bly, Jones, & Richardson 1986	Johnson & Johnson N = 2023	• SGBM as part of total health promotion efforts • Live for Life® sites versus control sites
Jose & Anderson 1986	Control Data N = 53 percent (high-risk population)	• SGBM offered as part of total health promotion efforts; Stay Well 6- to 9-week courses
Holt, McCauley, & Paul 1995	AT&T employees	• SGBM offered as part of total health promotion efforts; Total Life Concept program

Attrition		Weight Change		Maintenance	
0.5%		B	13.2 lbs.	B	10.3 lbs.
		M1	11.9 lbs.	M1	NA
		M2	9.9 lbs.	M2	NA
R1	0%	R1	11.2 lbs.	NA	
R2	17%	R2	3.5 lbs.		
R3	3%	R3	8.5 lbs.		
Study 1:		Team competitions produced greater weight loss than individual. Overall losses: approximately 6–12 lbs.		NA	
T	0%				
I	17%				
W	1%				
Study 2:		T	10.8 lbs.	NA	
2.9%		I	4.0 lbs.		
(range: 0–13%)		C	9.0 lbs.		
Study 3:					
Site 1	13%	Site 1	7.0 lbs.	6 month	54%
Site 2	35%	Site 2	5.5 lbs.	8 month	50%
Site 3	42%	Site 3	3.7 lbs.	12 month	27%
NA		7.2 lbs.		NA	
NA		8.0 lbs.		NA	
NA		1.1 lb. average loss for LFL sites versus +0.5 lbs. average gain for non-LFL sites at 2 years		NA	
70%		11.4 lbs. (completers); % overweight employees decreased 27% in experimental sites versus a 36% increase in control sites		NA	
69% from treatment to follow-up		NA; End of treatment weight index (Sheldon): 12.36 for follow-up survey responders and 12.44 for nonresponders		12.35 for survey responders (lower index = higher weight)	

Table 12-3 Behavioral Weight Control Content Areas

Principle	Sample Procedures
Self-monitoring	Keep daily records of food intake and physical activity.
Physical activity	Increase routine physical activities (e.g., walking, use of stairs).
Nutrition education	Decrease intake of fat; increase intake of complex carbohydrates. Learn nutritional and caloric values of foods.
Stimulus control	Make specific plans for structured eating. Remove food from inappropriate storage areas in the house. Maintain a lower-fat food environment at home and work.
Cognitive restructuring	Avoid setting unrealistic goals for weight and behavior changes. Avoid imperatives like "always" or "never."
Support/Rewards	Solicit help from family and friends. Plan specific rewards for achieving specific behavioral or weight loss goals.
Eating behavior	Prepare foods one portion at a time.

Financial Incentives: Deposits and Payroll Deductions

Reinforcement is one of the basic principles in behavior therapies (Stunkard & Berthold, 1985). In attempts to improve attrition rates and increase weight loss, reinforcement procedures have been applied to worksite programs in two basic forms—deposits/payroll deductions and competitions. Colvin, Zopf, and Myers (1983) conducted a comparison of financial incentives for weight loss and a nonincentive control with 23 employees in a medical school setting over 11 weeks. Even without the benefit of a formal behavioral treatment program, incentive participant weight loss averaged 9.2 pounds compared with only 3.7 pounds for controls. These values deteriorated by six months, although incentive participants still maintained twice as much weight loss (6 pounds vs. 3.1 pounds). End-of-treatment attrition also was reduced compared with earlier studies, but it still averaged 46% and 50% for incentive and control participants, respectively.

Follick, Fowler, and Brown (1984) randomly assigned hospital employees participating in a standard 10-week behavioral program to either a financial incentive (based on an initial deposit) or control condition. Deposits were returned on a weekly basis contingent only on attendance and food record compliance, not weight loss. The incentive manipulation significantly decreased program attrition (40% for the incentive group vs. 80% for the control group). Weight loss—which was not rewarded—did not differ among completers for the two conditions (7.0 vs. 8.1 pounds for incentive and control conditions, respectively). Again, including dropouts as treatment failures produces conservative estimates for program impact of only 4.2 and 1.6 pound average weight losses for incentive and nonincentive conditions, respectively.

In a series of studies (Forster et al., 1985; Jeffery, Forster, et al. 1992; Jeffery et al., 1989; Jeffery et al., 1985), Jeffery and colleagues have studied the use of incentives for program compliance combined with optional versus mandatory participation in behavioral education. The basic intervention consists of a six-month weight loss period during which employees agree to have a self-selected standard amount deducted from their paycheck. At bi-weekly weigh-ins, participants receive refunds based upon achievement of weekly weight loss and attendance goals (for mandatory attendance conditions). A pilot study (Jeffery et al. 1985) that involved two groups of 18 university employees, and optional attendance at behavioral sessions (behavioral self-help instructional materials were made available to all participants) produced an attrition rate of only 6% and an average weight loss of 12.3 pounds. Better weight loss was associated with weigh-in attendance ($x^2 = 6.44, p < 0.05$). Employees attending more than six behavioral sessions lost an average of 11.9 pounds compared with 7.2 pounds for those attending fewer than seven sessions.

In an expanded study of 131 university employees, Forster et al. (1985) added mandatory versus optional attendance and group behavioral instruction versus self-instruction to their payroll incentive model. Attendance at sessions averaged 70%. Attrition was 21.4%, with equal dropout rates across conditions and with no significant differences in weight losses between self versus group instruction or between optional versus mandatory attendance. However, similar to their pilot project, attendance at the weigh-ins and group sessions was the strongest predictor of weight loss. Those who attended 10 or fewer weigh-ins lost 4.3 pounds compared with 10.8 pounds for those attending more than 10 weigh-ins. Employees in the group instruction condition who attended more than six sessions lost an average of 16.7 pounds compared with 6.5 pounds for those attending less than seven sessions.

Extending this treatment model to a 485-employee manufacturing company, Jeffery et al. (1989) noted that the program was successful in attracting over 50% of the employees in need of weight reduction. Attrition rates were low (6–7%) for the two six-month intervention cohorts. However, attendance at sessions also was lower (41%) than in their previous study (70%), and average weight losses were less (7.3 and 6.6 pounds, for each cohort, respectively).

Most recently, Jeffery, Forster et al. (1992) reported two-year results of their Healthy Worker Project, a 32-worksite controlled trial for weight management and smoking cessation. The intervention included the payroll incentive procedure, weekly weigh-ins, behavioral self-instructional materials, and optional group sessions. The program proved popular, with 2041 of approximately 10,000 employees participating, but the average weight loss results at two years were disappointing—4.8 pounds for intervention worksites, with no difference in weight loss between intervention and control sites.

Financial incentives based on monetary deposits or self-selected payroll deductions increase attendance and reduce attrition rates compared with control conditions. Their effect on weight loss is questionable given the small losses achieved when dropouts are included in analyses. On the other hand, to the extent that incentives can reduce attrition, they should be included in worksite weight management programs. The protocols used suggest that the amount of the incentive need not be large. Deposits for 12-week programs have ranged between $40 and $60. Jeffery and colleagues used minimum payroll deductions extending over six months ranging from $5–$10 per pay period for a total of $60–$120. While no maximum amounts were imposed, the upper limit for these self-selected deductions was only $30 per pay period (Forster et al., 1985). These amounts are not likely to be prohibitive for a majority of employees and may also be cost-effective for employers to fund or cofund. Incentives have been used primarily to reinforce weight loss and attendance. However, in the future it may not be advisable to continue the former type of incentive given newer guidelines that are almost certain to apply to the use of incentives in health promotion (Society of Prospective Medicine, 1999). Specifically, the Health Insurance Portability and Accountability Act (HIPAA), enacted by Congress in 1996, prohibits the use of premium penalties based on health-status-related factors. This is also likely to apply to the use of other monetary disincentives or incentives. The area that is left open for incentives seems to be that of participation in health promotion regardless of outcomes (Terry, Anderson, & Serxner, 1999).

Financial Incentives: Worksite Competitions

One of the more promising worksite interventions is the use of weight loss competitions either among employees, between groups of employees, or between entire companies. Compared with the clinic group treatment model, worksite competitions can be very cost-effective, particularly when combined with self-instructional materials and volunteer efforts. The first large-scale clinical trial of a weight loss competition was conducted with over 2400 employees of Lockheed who participated in groups of 5–10 during a three-month "Take It Off in 83" weight loss campaign (Seidman, Sevelius, & Ewald, 1984). There was no behavioral intervention except for a single one-hour session at the beginning. Winners received $10 as well as a certificate of achievement and public recognition for reaching their preestablished weight loss goals. Attrition was 30% at three months. Weight loss averaged 9.1 pounds for those attending the weigh-in and 6 pounds for those self-reporting weight loss. No follow-up was conducted.

Cohen and colleagues have conducted a systematic series of investigations of worksite competitions (Brownell et al., 1984; Cohen et al., 1987; Stunkard et al., 1989). Their intervention has combined self-help behavioral materials with weight loss competitions across a variety of worksites. Dropout rates have been low, ranging from 0–17% with an average of 1.5%. The competitions have been effective in recruiting both blue- and white-collar employees. They also have attracted a significant number of nonobese employees. This could create a greater degree of social support within the workplace. The average weight loss for these competitions was about 8.5 pounds. Their data demonstrate that the most effective type of competition is a team rather than individual approach. A team approach helps to generate cooperative efforts among teammates, which enhances the incentive provided by the competition. Stunkard et al. (1989) also have examined the maintenance of weight losses achieved during competitions. Follow-up data at 6, 8, and 12 months indicated a steady and substantial regain across sites. After 12 months, only 27% of initial weight loss was maintained. These data do not compare favorably with the benchmark of 67% maintenance at one year established by clinic-based behavioral approaches (Wadden et al., 1989). It should be noted that these competitions included only minimal behavioral training. Therefore, attempts to decrease program costs may have resulted in decreased success in maintenance.

Commercial Programs at the Worksite

Stunkard (1987) has suggested that commercial programs represented a significant potential avenue for reaching large numbers of individuals, particularly those in need of mild weight loss. These programs can provide an opportunity for learning basic nutrition, exercise, and behavioral skills in a cost-effective and flexible format. It would seem appropriate to extend this concept to worksites by encouraging industry to form partnerships with major commercial providers to offer their programs on site. The largest effort of this kind has been the Weight Watchers International program, "Weight Watchers at Work." Described by Frankle et al. (1986) as an effort to modify the standard Weight Watchers program to fit the special needs of a working population (primarily female), it is an eight-week course stressing healthy eating, exercise, and behavioral principles for groups of 25–30 people. Despite widespread use of this program, few data are available to assess its effectiveness. Frankle et al. (1986) reported that participants averaged a 7.2 pound weight loss over the eight weeks, with 50% losing between 8–11 pounds. No data were given, however, regarding participation rates among overweight employees, attrition, changes in prevalence of overweight in participating companies, or long-term follow-up.

Total Wellness Approaches

Weight management programs also have been offered in the context of organized worksite health promotion programs that integrate them with other programs and corporate environmental changes designed to support healthier lifestyles. Examples of this approach are Johnson & Johnson's Live for Life® program (Bly, Jones, & Richardson, 1986), Control Data's StayWell® program (Anderson & Jose, 1987; Jose & Anderson, 1986; Milliman and Robertson, Inc., 1987), and AT&T's Total Life Concept program (Holt, McCauley, & Paul 1995). These programs represent longstanding corporate health promotion efforts. Both Johnson & Johnson and Control Data began their pilot interventions in 1979. Both programs are currently being marketed to other corporations. Despite the length of time these programs have been in existence and the large number of companies that have already used their approach and materials, there is very little published data available from the perspective of how these programs impact on weight loss and maintenance. Effectiveness of the total health approach on weight loss or on changes in the prevalence in overweight following the introduction of the program remains relatively unknown.

These comprehensive programs are characterized by strong support from management. Specific components generally include initial health risk screenings, follow-up screenings, a menu of lifestyle improvement programs (such as smoking cessation, weight control, exercise and fitness, stress management, nutrition/cholesterol management, and blood pressure intervention), social support, and environmental supports (such as worksite smoking policies, improvements in cafeteria selections, lunchtime seminars, and exercise facilities).

Bly, Jones, and Richardson (1986) published two-year follow-up weight loss results from their study of Live for Life® (LFL) sites compared with control sites. LFL sites showed an average weight loss of 1.1 pounds compared with a 0.5 pound gain for non-LFL sites. No data were reported for participation rates, attrition, changes in the prevalence of overweight, or long-term follow-up of participants in the weight loss intervention.

The StayWell® program (Anderson & Jose, 1987; Jose & Anderson, 1986) includes both instructor-led (6–9 week) and self-study courses for weight management. Anderson and Jose (1987) report an average initial weight loss of 11.4 pounds for employees who completed their self-study course. However, there also was a 70% dropout rate. They report that programs including incentives (books, T-shirts, etc.) for completion of the course have better attrition results, but no data were presented. The StayWell® program was successful in attracting a majority (53%) of the high-risk overweight population. In addition, they report that the percentage of overweight employees in their StayWell® intervention sites decreased by 27% compared with an increase of 36% in control sites. No long-term weight loss maintenance data were available.

The AT&T Total Life Concept program was introduced in 1983 in seven AT&T locations. Following an assessment phase involving the collection of biometric data and the completion of a health risk appraisal, employees were invited to participate in lifestyle change modules that consisted of group sessions lasting 1–1 ½ hours over 4–12 weeks. Environmental support for healthy lifestyles was provided by the company and included healthy food choices in cafeterias and vending machines; walking routes, par courses, and fitness centers; and a health information newsletter. Initial results had revealed positive changes attributable to the program; however, at five years the weight index had worsened compared with preintervention levels (Holt, McCauley, & Paul 1995).

Cost/Effectiveness of Worksite Weight Management Programs

There is no doubt that worksite weight management programs can be offered at much lower cost than more intensive hospital-based or private practice programs. For example, Stunkard et al. (1989) present data comparing a variety of approaches (see Figure 12-5).

It is clear that competitions incur only a fraction of the costs associated with university-based programs. However, there are few data to suggest that they reach the highest-risk obese groups and/or produce successful weight loss and maintenance.

Follow-up of most approaches to weight management suggests that, without ongoing treatment, total regain for many individuals is likely to occur within 5 years of initial weight loss (Stalonas, Perri, & Kerzner, 1984; Wadden et al., 1989). Providing formal ongoing support for weight loss maintenance at the worksite would increase program costs, but this is the only way these programs are likely to produce the kind of sustained lifestyle change that can eventually result in improved health for the employee and decreased health costs for the employer.

No data exist regarding participation in worksite weight management programs and short- or long-term improvements in either health behaviors or related medical risk factors. Published data have focused only on weight losses, changes in percentage overweight, or prevalence of obesity at the worksite. Programs usually do not have strong ongoing maintenance components to support the changes employees begin to make in 8–12 session programs. It is left to conjecture whether healthy behavior changes have produced initial weight loss, whether these

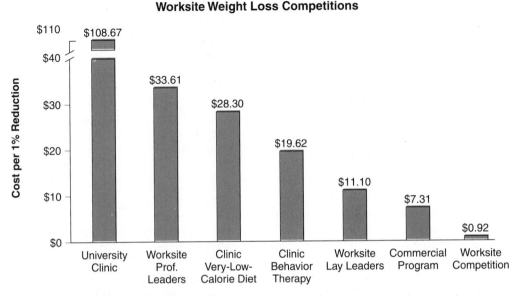

Figure 12-5 Worksite weight management programs can be offered at much lower cost than more intensive hospital-based or private-practice programs.

Source: Reprinted with permission from *Preventive Medicine* 18(1989).

changes will be maintained, or whether they will also result in meaningful long-term changes in associated medical risk factors (such as blood pressure, lipid profiles, or glucose tolerance) that can affect health care costs.

Finally, there are no controlled, prospective trials linking the very modest weight loss results reported in most programs to decreased health costs. Because the results achieved by these low-intensity, no-maintenance programs are less than impressive, financial data confirming the benefits of worksite weight management are not likely to be forthcoming. This does not mean there is no value in offering worksite weight management programs. Research on the behavioral treatment of obesity has identified variables that are likely to control considerable variance in the success of individuals maintaining significant weight loss. These variables are the subject of the next section.

Summary

Within these very modest results are suggestions for how worksite weight loss programs may be im-

proved. Both incentives (deposits or payroll deductions) and the less intensive, more flexible, self-directed approaches (e.g., worksite competitions) have been effective in reducing attrition. In Stunkard and Brownell's (1980) first effort, professionally-led behavioral groups resulted in attrition of 75–82%. With incentives, dropout rates have been cut in half. Competitions have reduced attrition to less than 5%. However, low attrition has potentially been achieved at the cost of success in weight-loss maintenance. It is possible to lose weight over 12-15 weeks by following a rigid diet without making lifestyle changes that would support maintaining a lower weight. For example, Wadden and Stunkard (1986) found that patients placed on a very-low-calorie diet without behavioral training lost an average of 13 pounds during the 4-month treatment. Attrition also was low (15%). However, by the end of one year these individuals were maintaining only 33% of their initial weight loss, a figure similar to the one year follow-up of a worksite competition reported by Stunkard et al. (1989). If individuals are not required to attend group behavioral sessions, skills for maintaining consistent lifestyle change are unlikely to be learned. Consistent with this view, Jeffery and colleagues have noted that weight loss success in their program was associated with attendance at classes (Forster et al. 1985).

The most important lesson to be drawn from the research is that obesity is a chronic medical condition that is very resistant to self-management efforts for lifestyle change. For weight loss to be maintained, long-term treatment is necessary. *Treatment should extend well beyond the weight loss phase of a program.* Worksites provide a unique opportunity to provide structured long-term maintenance programs with incentives for regular attendance.

Building on the experience gathered in community weight management, various investigators have studied the type of leader needed for worksite weight management groups. The results have been mixed. Although Stunkard and Brownell (1980) found that professionally-trained lay leader groups showed significantly lower attrition rates (31–50%) and somewhat greater weight loss at the end of treatment compared with professionally-led groups, Peterson et al. (1985) found that their lay-led groups did not perform as well as professionally-led groups. It may be that it is the program content and format that is more critical than the credential of the individual leading the group, assuming that leaders receive some training specific to assisting others in weight management.

Competitions are among the most promising of the weight loss interventions that have been offered at the worksite. Studies clearly demonstrate superior results for team-based competitions that include cooperative efforts among individuals making changes, compared with individual competitions pitting employees against each other. However, competitions have so far focused only on short-term weight loss. No data are currently available on the efficacy of repeat competitions for those who might benefit from greater weight loss than can be achieved in the typical 12-week competition. There also are no data on competitions focused on behavior changes (e.g., increased physical activity) or long-term maintenance. Given the poor performance of competitions for weight loss maintenance, we suggest that they be used as part of a more comprehensive approach to weight management at the worksite. A competition could be an additional environmental support sponsored by management as an incentive for employees who are also learning behavioral self-management skills for losing weight and maintaining weight loss.

A MODEL FOR EFFECTIVE WORKSITE WEIGHT MANAGEMENT

Overview

As discussed in the previous section, most worksite weight management programs have demonstrated only minimal effectiveness. Therefore, recommendations for programs should be based on approaches and procedures that have both a reasonable theoretical basis as well as data to demonstrate their effectiveness. In constructing an ideal worksite intervention, it is recommended that a parsimonious approach be taken (i.e., including the minimum of procedures to obtain the maximum weight loss and maintenance benefits). This approach has the advantages of being easier to teach to employees and being more cost-effective. The core elements of an effective worksite weight management intervention are summarized in Table 12-4.

The literature provides ample demonstrations of the key lifestyle changes that are associated with maximal success in weight loss and maintenance. These include sustained increases in physical activity (Jeffery et al., 1984; Miller & Sims 1981; Skender et al., 1996; Wadden, Vogt, Foster, & Anderson, 1998), reduced calorie intake (Harvey-Berino, 1999) and reduced fat intake (Astrup, Toubro, Raben, & Skov, 1997; Carmichael, Swinburn, & Wilson, 1998; Lissner, Heitmann, & Bengtsson, 1997; Shick et al., 1998; Westerterp et al., 1996), and ongoing self-monitoring (Boutelle & Kirschenbaum, 1998). However, the literature reviewed earlier on the delivery of weight management programs at the worksite suggests that the traditional approach of offering onsite classes is not likely to be effective for the majority of employees for whom intervention is appropriate. It is time to reevaluate the overall goals for worksite weight management and use this evaluation to provide the main direction for programming decisions.

Table 12-4 Elements of a Recommended Model for Worksite Weight Management

Goals for Intervention:
Maintenance of healthier body weights
Maintenance of lifestyle changes that support healthy body weights
Improvement in overall health profile

Intervention Focus:
Offer stage-based intervention
    For non-action-based intervention:
        Worksite policies to support healthy weight management

            Worksite-based exercise
            Healthful food offerings in cafeterias and vending machines
            Support for participation

    For action-based interventions:
        Self-monitoring of daily food intake and activity
        Reduction of dietary fat
        Increase in high-fiber, nutrient-dense foods—fruits, vegetables, whole grains
        Encourage environmental management to reduce the need for willpower
        Use of health risk appraisal to demonstrate and reinforce health improvement
        Long-term focus

Evaluation:
    Conduct regular evaluations (every 6 months) of key outcome variables:
        Participation
        Program Satisfaction
        Weight Changes
        Improvements in Lifestyle – Physical Activity, Diet
        Health Improvement Changes

Program Goals

Effective worksite weight management programs should be based on clearly specified goals, and progress toward these goals should be measured on a regular basis. Such data collection ensures program accountability while providing valuable information for ongoing program improvement. While weight loss and a reduction in the percentage of overweight employees are primary goals for worksite weight management programs, they are not the only goals worthy of consideration. As discussed earlier, the degree of weight loss achieved need not be great to have a significant impact on health. However, research on relapse following weight loss clearly demonstrates that a longer-term goal of weight loss maintenance should be established for worksite programs. Support

for this goal should include a program that minimally offers extended follow-up, retreatment opportunities, and perhaps financial incentives for maintenance as well.

It is also important that the content of the program maximally support the goal of maintenance. Weight loss maintenance requires lifestyle change, particularly increased leisure and/or work-related energy expenditure, decreased calorie/fat intake, or a combination of these (Duncan, Bacon, & Weinsier, 1983; Jeffery et al., 1984; Kayman, Bruvold, & Stern, 1990; Kendall, Levitsky, Strupp, & Lissner, 1991; Miller & Sims, 1981; Shepard, Kristal, & Kushi, 1991). These behavioral goals also have the advantage of being related to other health promotion goals, such as reduction in risk for cardiovascular disease, cancer, hypertension, and diabetes; therefore, focusing on these

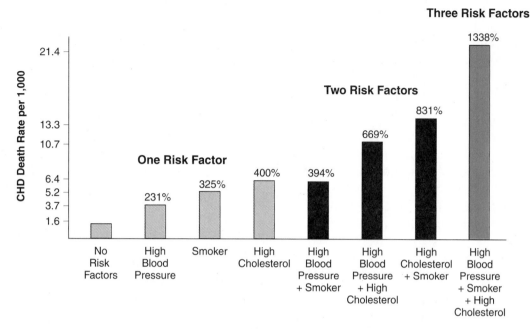

Figure 12-6   Relative risk of coronary heart disease (CHD) mortality. Multiple Risk Factor Intervention Trial—Males, ages 35–57.

Source: Adapted from *Journal of the American Medical Association* 256 (1986):2823–28. Copyright 1986, American Medical Association.

lifestyle changes makes a weight management program more relevant for all employees regardless of degree of overweight.

Perhaps the most important goal for a worksite weight management program is improved employee health. This goal has implications both for the content of weight management programs and for evaluation of their effectiveness. Being overweight constitutes only one health risk factor, but much of the premature illness and death in this country can be attributed to the combined effects of multiple risk factors. These include both elevated medical indicators (such as blood pressure, cholesterol, and triglycerides) and behavioral indicators (such as sedentary lifestyle, high fat diets, excessive alcohol intake, and smoking). The concept is clearly illustrated in data from the Multiple Risk Factor Intervention Trial (Stamler, Wentworth, & Neaton, 1986). As can be seen in Figure 12-6, the combined effect on coronary heart disease mortality for just three risk factors (elevated diastolic blood pressure, elevated cholesterol,

and smoking) produced an increase in risk of 1338% compared with the effects of each risk factor taken singly, which ranged from 231–400%.

Therefore, the most important focus of worksite weight management programs should be on the identification and control of multiple risk factors associated with being overweight, not merely the control of weight.

Finally, research by Prochaska and colleagues (Prochaska & Velicer, 1997) has demonstrated that the majority of individuals who may have a particular health risk, such as overweight, are not likely to be ready to engage in sustained efforts to modify their lifestyles. Individuals progress through a series of stages from not thinking about or acknowledging their risk status (Precontemplation) to considering making a change (Contemplation) to beginning to take action (Preparation) to actively engaging in a lifestyle change effort (Action) to working on issues of longer-term maintenance of change (Maintenance). In addition, most individuals who attempt lifestyle change experience relapses not only in the area of risk they are attempting to change, but also in their readiness to reestablish a change effort. Thus, weight management programs offered at the worksite are likely to capture only a minority of individuals for whom they may be appropriate and are likely to have limited impact. This suggests that a broader goal of establishing a healthier lifestyle, regardless of weight status, might be more successful. By giving an overweight employee multiple targets for change rather than a narrower focus on weight loss, more individuals could be influenced.

A Worksite Intervention That Supports Maintenance of Healthier Weights

The structure of a worksite weight management program can be broken down into two components: informational content and environmental support. The core content gives employees the basic information and procedures necessary for maintaining a healthier weight.

As mentioned earlier, two of the most effective procedures for weight loss involve making food choices to decrease overall fat/calorie intake while substantially increasing physical activity. Breakdowns in these two procedures are also predictive of weight regain (McGuire, Wing, Klem, Lang, & Hill, 1999). Records of calorie intake and expenditure have been shown to be an effective way to accomplish and maintain changes in these areas (Boutelle & Kirschenbaum, 1998).

Increasing Physical Activity

Physical activity may be the single most important aspect of successful weight and health risk factor management. Studies have found it to be one of the best predictors of long-term success in maintaining weight loss (Jeffery et al., 1984; Miller & Sims, 1981; Skender et al., 1996; Wadden et al., 1998). Physical activity burns calories, and this may be the most important reason for increasing daily levels. As an example, for the average sedentary American female who requires about 11 kcal/pound/day to maintain her weight, burning an additional 300 kcal/day can make the task much easier. Racette, Schoeller, Kushner, and Neil (1995) also noted that physical activity had a pos-

itive impact on dietary compliance during weight loss. Finally, data suggest that engaging in physical activity while losing weight may benefit long-term weight management by helping to preserve lean body mass and metabolic rate (Brownell, 1982).

In addition to direct caloric and metabolic effects, regular physical activity can produce such beneficial psychological changes as decreased levels of depression and anxiety and improvements in self-esteem. Such changes can be helpful for maintaining weight loss. In fact, some researchers have suggested that these effects are the main benefit of physical activity for weight control (Foreyt & Goodrick, 1991).

Finally, regular physical activity is associated with many health benefits (see Chapter 10). Their importance is accentuated for overweight individuals because of the association between obesity and elevated medical risk factors. In fact, physical activity may help overweight individuals improve health status and reduce health risk, independent of weight loss.

Data suggest that a minimum level of 2000 kcal of physical activity per week may be desirable for success in weight control (Schoeller et al., 1997; Stifler, Kaplan, & Lindewall, 1985; Wing, 1999;) and for health benefits (Paffenbarger, Hyde, Wing, & Hsieh, 1986). For an individual weighing 150 pounds, 2000 kcal/week would be the equivalent of walking approximately 20 miles during the week, or about three miles per day. While this may sound like an unrealistic goal, with specific program emphasis it is not difficult to accomplish once participants are convinced of its importance (Kaplan, Stifler, Framer, & Scheiber, 1990). There are also data that challenge the conventional wisdom that moderate activity is most effective for long-term weight management. Doucet and Tremblay (1998) argue that more intense exercise is likely to have greater caloric and metabolic effects. This raises the issue of the "fat burning zone." It has been proposed that higher-intensity exercise might not be best for weight control because it is likely to be anaerobic (i.e., it pushes the body beyond its capacity to use oxygen in the production of energy to power the exercise). Under conditions of anaerobic exercise, the body must turn to energy sources (stored glycogen) that do not require oxygen to be metabolized. Energy production from fat metabolism requires oxygen; therefore, exercises that are outside the fat burning zone supposedly would not be useful in weight management. This is only partially correct. Anaerobic activity does burn calories and therefore does factor into weight management; however, by definition, individuals are very limited in their ability to maintain anaerobic activity. Muscle glycogen becomes depleted; waste by-products of anaerobic metabolism build up in muscle tissue, causing soreness; and the individual is forced to stop. So lower-intensity, aerobic activity is preferable for weight management because individuals can do far more of it and have a total caloric deficit effect that is greater. On the other hand, with proper training, including anaerobic activity interspersed with aerobic exercise (e.g., wind sprints incorporated into a jogging training regimen), one's ability to engage in higher intensity physical activity without becoming anaerobic is increased. So in the long run, the best activity regimen for weight control is to become increasingly fit. The caveat is that exercise intensity must be increased gradually to avoid strain on the musculoskeletal and cardiovascular systems of individuals who may begin an exercise program in poor physical condition.

To change physical activity, it is helpful to monitor it on a daily basis. Monitoring physical activity in terms of calorie expenditure is desirable because it places activity choices on the same continuum as food choices and allows individuals to see the relationship among these choices and their weight, over time. Precise energy expenditures for activities depend on a number of factors, including duration, intensity, mechanical efficiency, and perhaps other metabolic factors; reasonable estimates can be made by using a simplified calorie continuum with "anchor points" for low-, medium-, high-, and very-high-intensity activities. Figure 12-7 displays such a system.

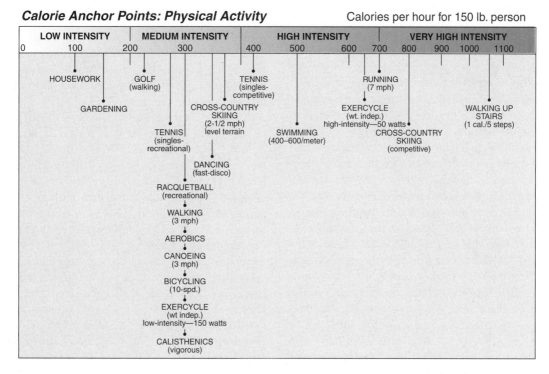

Figure 12-7   Reasonable estimates of energy expenditures for activities can be made by using a simplified calorie continuum with anchor points for low-, medium-, high-, and very-high-intensity activities.
Source: Reprinted with permission from Health Management Resources.

Keeping records of activity calories rather than just logging minutes allows a wide variety of physical activities to be combined meaningfully. For example, with calories as the common denominator, participants can combine a half-mile brisk walk, an hour of doubles tennis, and five flights of stairs climbed at work. Specific daily/weekly exercise calorie goals can be set, and even small amounts of activity can be reinforced as increasing totals for the week.

Regardless of specific activities chosen, maintaining a weekly calorie expenditure that averages over 2000 kcal may require adding in extra walking as part of an overall exercise plan. Walking can be done at almost any time, requires no special equipment other than a good pair of walking shoes, lends itself to small amounts of time throughout the day, and can be done in combination with socializing or even business. A recent survey of participants in a high-risk obesity treatment program who were averaging 2132 kcal/week in physical activity showed that 68% of the self-reported calories in physical activity came from walking (Kaplan et al., 1990).

Should supervised exercise groups be offered at the worksite as part of a weight management intervention? The literature suggests that home-based activity may be more likely associated with success in weight loss (Perri, Martin, Leermakers, Sears, & Notelovitz, 1997). This finding is probably related to several factors, including the increased flexibility in achieving activity goals, lower attrition rates, and an increased compliance with other weight management procedures such as self monitoring of food intake. However, a significant factor in these results was the fact that participants had to travel to the clinic-based facility for exercise. It is possible that a worksite-based facility would have produced better results for a non-home-based intervention. On the other hand, setting up an exercise facility onsite may be financially unrealistic for most companies that would like to support exercise among their employees. Encouraging home-based activity is a cost-efficient strategy for employers. However, they can still encourage greater activity levels at the worksite by supporting low-cost programs such as lunch-time walking groups or activity competitions.

Managing Food Choices to Lower Calorie/Fat Intake

To maintain weight loss, individuals must learn to reduce overall calorie intake (Harvey-Berino, 1999). For most people this can be accomplished most efficiently by decreasing the average fat content of the diet. Not only is fat 2.5 times more calorically dense than carbohydrate or protein, but there is also a growing body of evidence that excess calories from fat may be stored more efficiently than those from protein or carbohydrate (Flatt, 1978). Evidence is growing that low-fat diets are helpful in maintaining weight loss—providing calories are also controlled (Astrup et al., 1997; Carmichael et al., 1998; Lissner et al., 1997; Shick et al., 1998; Westerterp et al., 1996). These results are most likely due to energy deficits created by lower fat diets, but there is also evidence for metabolic factors involving fat oxidation (Larson, Ferraro, Robertson, & Ravussin, 1995).

Like changing exercise habits, changing food choices to reduce both dietary fat and calories requires a monitoring system that displays both food choices and calorie consequences. Using these food records, individuals can set goals, make plans, and evaluate lifestyle changes that can reduce calorie intake while maintaining a reasonable volume and variety of food. Such changes will necessarily be highly individualized.

Keeping food records that will be useful to the task of managing weight requires people to be trained in making accurate food calorie estimations. Without such training, most individuals underestimate energy intake (Hegsted, 1992). Among the obese, the degree of error is positively correlated with BMI (Bandini, Schoeller, Cyr, & Dietz, 1990). Unless record keeping takes place within close proximity to the time of eating, errors are likely to occur. Such errors would be expected to increase with increasing volume of food consumed and in proportion to the fat content of the diet. For example, forgetting to record a high-fat food choice such as 2–3 tablespoons of dressing on a salad (75–100 kcal/T) will result in a greater calorie error than forgetting a low-fat choice (e.g., the salad itself at 10–30 kcal/cup).

Estimating food calories requires skill in judging portion sizes and knowledge of food calorie values based on standard measurements. Without training, people are not good at portion size estimation (Lansky & Brownell, 1982; Rapp, Dubbert, Burkett, & Buttross, 1986). Underestimating portion sizes can result in very substantial calorie errors, particularly of high-fat foods. For example, a standard muffin listed in many calorie books is 165 kcal (1.5 oz.), but the size of muffins sold in bakeries today ranges from 4 to as many as 16 oz. Learning portion size estimation requires practice, but it is a reasonably easy skill to develop.

One example of a simplified system, similar to that presented earlier for physical activity, that can be used to learn calorie values for foods is shown in Figure 12-8 (Stifler, Galante-Schwarz, & McFadden, 1987). In this system, foods are grouped according to general categories including meats, baked goods, vegetables, fruits, beverages, and prepared combinations. Within each of these categories, common foods are arranged by "anchor points" on a calorie continuum based on standard units of measure (per ounce, tablespoon, cup). Participants can estimate calorie

values for nonlisted foods by making comparisons to the anchor point foods.

In general, choosing more foods from the left-hand side of the pages results in decreasing fat content as well, but the goal of changing food choices is to lower fat intake, not to eat a no-fat diet. Thus, individuals should identify favorite higher-fat foods and find ways to include them in their diet while they eliminate those fats that have little importance. For example, if a person has no preference for deep-fat-fried versus broiled chicken, many calories can be saved by having it broiled most of the time. These calories can be used for other favorite foods.

A procedure to help decrease fat is to increase intake of complex carbohydrates, particularly vegetables and fruits, which are calorically less dense than grain products. For many, this is an easier dietary change to make because it means eating more, not less, and can be operationalized as having a minimum of five servings of fruits and vegetables every day (Reynolds, 1991). Increased consumption of these

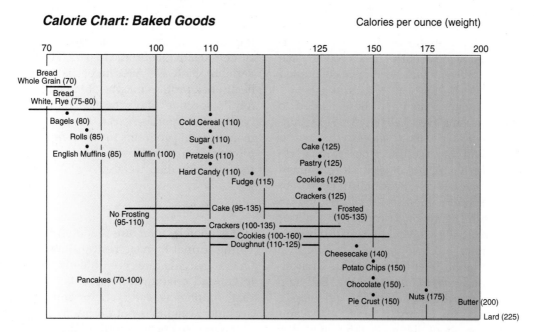

Figure 12-8 A simplified system can be used to learn caloric values for the general categories of foods. This is a sample anchor point page for baked goods.
Source: Reprinted with permission from Health Management Resources.

foods also improves the nutrient and fiber composition of the diet while assisting with weight loss.

Environmental Management

An important ingredient for success in managing weight is establishing an environment that supports weight loss and maintenance. Modern American lifestyles do not support either high levels of physical activity or a low-fat diet. Dieters frequently encounter unexpected environmental problems, such as the coworker who brings a box of doughnuts to the office, the friends who suggest going out for drinks at the end of the day, or two-for-one supermarket specials on favorite foods. Therefore, assertiveness is needed to change those environments over which there is more control, such as the home. Maintaining a home environment in which the average fat content of available food is over 30% decreases the likelihood of maintaining a lower-fat diet. If food records have identified high-fat foods (or other high-calorie foods) that are difficult for an individual to control, common sense dictates that keeping such foods in the home and trying to resist eating them would not be successful. Setting up a supportive environment also means bringing in foods, such as fruits and vegetables, which need to be consumed in greater amounts.

Environmental management can be extended to strategies for increasing physical activity. For example, keeping comfortable walking shoes in the car and at the worksite will increase the opportunity to do more walking. Having a piece of exercise equipment at home (such as an exercycle, treadmill, or stair-stepper) can be helpful for some individuals. Setting up appointments with friends or coworkers to walk or exercise will increase the probability of maintaining a more active lifestyle.

Worksites can be an integral part of an environment that supports weight management. Self-help materials, such as brochures, books, and videotapes, can be kept in an on-site library to assist those wanting to learn more about living healthy lifestyles. Vending machines can provide low-fat alternatives such as low-fat yogurt or fresh fruit. Cafeterias can include lower-fat alternatives for weight-and-nutrition-conscious employees. Calorie and nutrition information can be displayed prominently to assist those interested in making changes in food choices (Dubbert, Johnson, Schlundt, & Montague, 1984). Employees also can set up informal guidelines for foods brought into the workspace or served during meetings.

Program Management

Needs Assessment

Before making a decision to implement worksite-based weight management interventions, it is important to conduct a needs assessment. This enables corporate decision makers to make informed program decisions and involves employees as part of the health promotion process. The assessment would include determining the percentage of employees who might benefit from treatment, the desire for weight management programs at the worksite, and employee preferences regarding treatment locations and times.

Since the benefits of weight management for both employee and corporation are based on overall health improvement, the initial assessment also should include a health risk profile in which weight is only one variable of interest. A recent partial listing of available health risk profiles may be obtained from the Society for Prospective Medicine (1999). Data from repeat health risk appraisals can be used during weight management programs to show employees (and employers) their progress in improving their health as they work on their weight.

Program Format

Unfortunately, there are few data that support providing formal management groups at the worksite. Overall success rates are unlikely to counterbalance initial and ongoing investments. This is not to say that finding ways to help employees maintain healthier weights is not desirable. Nor is this to say that there are not even individuals for whom the cost of providing a good quality, long-term weight management intervention is not reasonable, given their risk status and contribution to the company. Because successful long-term weight management rests on making and maintaining other healthy lifestyle changes in diet and physical activity, it may be more efficient to directly address these areas instead and illustrate the benefits for weight control for those for whom the issue is relevant. This has an added advantage of making whatever program that is offered meaningful to a greater number of employees, thus potentially increasing the penetration of the intervention(s) and the ultimate impact. However, if an intervention focused on weight management alone is desired, there are now alternatives other than the traditional onsite 6 to 8 week long weight management group with little or no follow-up. One possibility is to make an online intervention available. Another is to provide stage-of-change-based self-help materials. Recent work by Wing and Jeffery (1999) suggests that pairing individuals who are attempting to manage their weight with a buddy increases success. Such a buddy system could be implemented using self-help materials and a wellness facilitator who could serve as a central resource for questions. Finally, the weight losses resulting from team competitions are promising, especially given the low implementation costs. However, there are no data that demonstrate that these losses are maintained over time without more structured programming. If health benefits are to be maintained, weight losses also must be maintained. Regardless of which approach is selected, the most important thing an employer can do is to provide a work environment that is supportive of healthy weight management as discussed in the previous section.

Evaluation

Regardless of the type of intervention offered, data on a minimum set of variables likely to predict participant success should be collected and evaluated on an ongoing basis to enhance program effectiveness. Ongoing data collection also enables corporate decision makers to evaluate the success of the program on relevant variables. The variables monitored minimally should include program participation rates, indices of dietary change, physical activity, weight changes, and other health changes (from repeat health risk appraisals). It is also helpful to collect data on program satisfaction, including whether or not participants feel that they have been helped to manage their own weight (self-efficacy).

Group statistics can be summarized at the end of the intervention to demonstrate program impact. Ideally these data should be recalculated at regular intervals following the conclusion of the program. Such analyses can identify populations in need of outreach and reenrollment in other relevant interventions.

Employee issues

One of the most important considerations for worksite weight management is who should participate. The most immediate cost-effective approach is to target those employees at greatest risk for health problems and provide incentives for participation in ongoing treatment to reduce risk. However, such an approach might create problems of employee confidentiality. Although obesity is a visible condition, employees may justifiably be concerned that being identified as a "high-risk" candidate (based on a health risk appraisal) for weight management might result in job discrimination.

On the other hand, an open recruitment policy allows all interested employees to participate regardless of excess weight or associated risk factors. There are additional benefits to such a policy. The more employees that take part in the program, the easier it will be to develop a corporate culture that can support all employees in their efforts to maintain desirable body weights and healthy lifestyles. Groups can be organized that take walks during breaks or at lunch. Decisions can be made not to bring high-fat foods into the workspace. Finally, open recruitment promotes prevention of weight and health problems. Data suggest that individuals continue to gain weight as they age. By middle age, over 50% of the workforce may have a weight problem substantial enough to affect health. By teaching elements of successful weight management to employees who are normal to mildly overweight, these problems may be avoided. Since the focus is on the establishment of healthy lifestyles, even employees who are not overweight can benefit from participation.

Management Issues

For health promotion efforts to be effective, they must have visible and ongoing support of management. Minimally, employees should receive a health risk appraisal and introductory orientations describing the health promotion programs. Participation in these activities should be mandatory, while participation in specific programs (such as weight management) can be optional. It may be possible to develop incentive systems to encourage employees to participate in programs that would be of benefit. Given newer ethical guidelines, care must be taken so that incentives are not punitive and that they are not based on actual changes in risk factors. For example, rebates on health insurance deductibles could be problematic. Individuals could potentially claim discrimination. However, point systems for healthy lifestyle program participation that can be traded in for merchandise, such as caps or coffee mugs, may be helpful. Moreover, data suggest that the incentives offered need not be large. Company-sponsored competitions may be one way to support employee efforts to make lifestyle changes, but the focus needs to be shifted to longer range goals—perhaps the maintenance of weight loss. Other incentives, such as time off work for physical activity, offering classes during work time rather than employee time, or earned extra vacation time based on improvements in health risks, could be developed; however, these would have to be scrutinized carefully to make sure they do not violate HIPAA guidelines. It is recommended that management and employees participate together in developing such incentives.

CONCLUSION

Weight management at the worksite would seem to have much potential for improving employee health and productivity, enhancing job satisfaction, and ultimately reducing corporate health care costs via primary prevention. However, the results of worksite weight management programs have paralleled the initial success rates of earlier clinic-based programs. Short-term modest weight losses can be achieved with a variety of approaches including group behavioral classes and competitions, but maintenance of weight loss has not been demonstrated. In companies that have attempted longer interventions and follow-up intervals, the amount of weight loss maintained by the average participant has been minimal.

In addition, because weight losses achieved have been minimal and maintenance has been lacking, there has been no documentation of the impact worksite weight management programs can have on related health parameters. This is important because if participants can maintain other healthy behaviors (e.g., regular physical activity or lower dietary fat intake), health benefits may be considerable, even if weight losses are small. Once again, the focus of these programs needs to shift from weight control to health management and risk factor reduction.

Depending on the size and resources of a corporation, it may be unrealistic to develop a health promotion department to provide weight management and other lifestyle health programs. A promising solution is for industry to form partnerships with professional or academic groups already possessing the expertise to provide comprehensive programming onsite. Corporate support for a successful partnership would include providing space for the educators and classes, time for employees to participate, and possibly partial coverage of program costs. Health educators who are located onsite increase program visibility and enhance their relationship with participants. Accountability should be established for weight management interventions just as it is with any other division of a corporation. Annual health appraisals of employees can document progress made toward achieving a healthier and less overweight workforce.

References

Abrams, D. B., & Follick, M. J. (1983). Behavioral weight-loss intervention at the worksite: Feasibility and maintenance. *Journal of Consulting Clinical Psychology, 51*, 226–233.

Allison, D. B., Faith, M. S., & Nathan, J. S. (1996). Risch's lambda values for human obesity. *International Journal of Obesity, 20*, 990–999.

Allison, D. B., Fontaine, K. R., Manson, J. E., Stevens, J., & VanItallie, T. B. (1999). Annual deaths attributable to obesity in the United States. *Journal of the American Medical Association, 282*, 1530–1538.

American Dietetic Association. (1990). Position of the American Dietetic Association: Very-low-calorie weight loss diets. *Journal of the American Dietetic Association, 90,* 722–726.

Anderson, D. R., & Jose, W. S. (1987). Employee lifestyle and the bottom line. Results from the StayWell evaluation. *Fitness in Business,* 86–91.

Anderson, J., Brinkman, V., & Hamilton, C. (1991, June). *Changes in serum lipids and blood pressure for obese diabetic persons treated with 800 calories in liquid supplement versus liquid meal replacement and food.* Poster session presented at the 14th International Diabetes Federation Congress, Washington, DC.

Armstrong, B. (1986). Poor employee nutrition can eat up corporate profits. *Corporate Commentary, 2,* 53–54.

Astrup, A., Gøtzsche, P. C., van de Werken, K., Ranneries, C., Toubro, S., Raben, A., & Buemann, B. (1999). Meta-analysis of resting metabolic rate in formerly obese subjects. *American Journal of Clinical Nutrition, 69,* 1117–1122.

Astrup, A., Toubro, S., Raben, A., & Skov, A. R. (1997). The role of low-fat diets and fat substitutes in body weight management: What have we learned from clinical studies? *Journal of the American Dietetic Association, 97* (Suppl.), S82–S87.

Atkinson, R. L. (1989). Low and very low calorie diets. *Medical Clinics of North America, 73,* 203–215.

Bandini, L. G., Schoeller, D. A., Cyr, H. N., & Dietz, W. H. (1990). Validity of reported energy intake in obese and nonobese adolescents. *American Journal of Clinical Nutrition, 52,* 421–425.

Barofsky, I., Fontaine, K. R., & Cheskin, L. J. (1997). Pain in the obese: Impact on health-related quality-of-life. *Annals of Behavioral Medicine, 19,* 408–410.

Bartlett, S. J., Wadden, T. A., & Vogt, R. A. (1996). Psychosocial consequences of weight cycling. *Journal of Consulting and Clinical Psychology, 64,* 587–592.

Beeson, V., Ray, C., Coxon, A., & Kreitzman, S. (1989). The myth of the yo-yo: Consistent rate of weight loss with successive dieting by VLCD. *International Journal of Obesity, 13* (Suppl. 2), 135–139.

Birmingham, C. L., Muller, J. L., Palepu, A., Spinelli, J. J., & Anis, A. H. (1999). The cost of obesity in Canada. *Canadian Medical Association Journal, 160,* 483–488.

Blackburn G. L., & Kanders, B. S. (1987). Medical evaluation and treatment of the obese patient with cardiovascular disease. *American Journal of Cardiology, 60,* 55G–58G.

Blackburn, G. L., Wilson, G. T., Kanders, B. S., Stein, L. J., Lavin, P. T., Adler, J., & Brownell, K. D. (1989). Weight cycling: The experience of human dieters. *American Journal of Clinical Nutrition, 49,* 1105–1109.

Blair, S. N. (1991). *Living with exercise.* Dallas, TX: American Health Publishing.

Blair, S. N., Kohl, H. W., III, Paffenbarger, R. S., Clark, D. G., Cooper, K. H., & Gibbons, L. W. (1989). Physical fitness and all-cause mortality. A prospective study of healthy men and women. *Journal of the American Medical Association, 262,* 2395–2401.

Bly, J. L., Jones, R. C., & Richardson, J. E. (1986). Impact of worksite health promotion on health care costs and utilization. Evaluation of Johnson & Johnson's Live for Life program. *Journal of the American Medical Association, 256,* 3235–3240.

Bouchard, C. (1994). Genetics of obesity: Overview and research directions. In C. Bouchard (Ed.), *The Genetics of Obesity* (pp. 223–233). Boca Raton, FL: CRC Press.

Boutelle, K. N., & Kirschenbaum, D. S. (1998). Further support for consistent self-monitoring as a vital component of successful weight control. *Obesity Research, 6,* 219–224.

Bray, G. A. (1989). Classification and evaluation of the obesities. *Medical Clinics of North America, 73,* 161–184.

Brownell, K. D. (1982). Obesity: Understanding and treating a serious, prevalent, and refractory disorder. *Journal of Consulting and Clinical Psychology, 50,* 820–840.

Brownell, K. D., Cohen, R. Y., Stunkard, A. J., Felix, M. R., & Cooley, N. B. (1984). Weight loss competitions at the work site: Impact on weight, morale and cost-effectiveness. *American Journal of Public Health, 74,* 1283–1285.

Brownell, K. D., Greenwood, M. R. C., Stellar, E., & Shrager, E. E. (1986). The effects of repeated cycles of weight loss and regain in rats. *Physiological Behavior, 38,* 459–464.

Brownell, K. D., & Jeffery, R. W. (1987). Improving long-term weight loss: Pushing the limits of treatment. *Behavior Therapy, 18,* 353–374.

Brownell, K. D., Lissner, L., & D'Agostino, R. B. (1991). Variability of body weight and health outcomes [letter to the editor]. *New England Journal of Medicine* 324: 1745–46.

Brownell, K. D., & Kramer, F. M. (1989). Behavioral management of obesity. *Medical Clinics of North America, 73*, 185–201.

Brownell, K. D., Stunkard, A. J., & McKeon, P. E. (1985). Weight reduction at the work site: A promise partially fulfilled. *American Journal of Psychiatry, 142*, 47–52.

Brownell, K. D., & Wadden, T. A. (1991). The heterogeneity of obesity: Fitting treatments to individuals. *Behavior Therapy, 22*, 153–171.

Bruce, A. C., McNurlan, M. A., McHardy, K. C., Broom, J., Buchanan, K. D., Calder, A. G., Milne, E., McGaw, B. A., Garlick, P. J., & James, W. P. T. (1990). Nutrient oxidation patterns and protein metabolism in lean and obese subjects. *International Journal of Obesity, 14*, 631–646.

Carmichael, H. E., Swinburn, B. A., & Wilson, M. R. (1998). Lower fat intake as a predictor of initial and sustained weight loss in obese subjects consuming an otherwise ad libitum diet. *Journal of the American Dietetic Association, 98*, 35–39.

Castelli, W. P. (1989). A view from Framingham *Current Concepts.* Kalamazoo, MI: Upjohn.

Chen, M. K. (1986). The epidemiology of self-reported fatigue among adults. *Preventive Medicine, 15*, 74–81.

Cleland, R., Graybill, D. C., Hubbard, V., Kahn, L. K., Stern, J. S., Wadden, T. A., Weinsier, R., & Yanovski, S. (1998). *Commercial weight loss products and programs: What consumers stand to gain and lose.* Washington, DC: Federal Trade Commission, Bureau of Consumer Protection.

Cnattingius, S., Bergström, R., Lipworth, L., & Kramer, M. S. (1998). Prepregnancy weight and the risk of adverse pregnancy outcomes. *New England Journal of Medicine, 338*, 147–152.

Cohen, R. Y., Stunkard, A. J., & Felix, M. R. J. (1987). Comparison of three worksite weight-loss competitions. *Journal of Behavioral Medicine, 10*, 467–479.

Colditz, G. A. (1992). The economic costs of obesity. *American Journal of Clinical Nutrition, 55* (Suppl.) 503S–507S.

Colditz, G. A., Willett, W. C., Stampfer, M. J., Manson, J. E., Hennekens, C. H., Arky, R. A., & Speizer, F. E. (1990). Weight as a risk factor for clinical diabetes in women. *American Journal of Epidemiology, 132*, 501–513.

Colvin, R. H., Zopf, K. J., & Myers, J. H. (1983). Weight control among coworkers. Effects of monetary contingencies and social milieu. *Behavior Modification, 7*, 64–75.

Committee on Diet and Health, National Research Council Commission on Life Sciences. (1989). *Diet and Health.* Washington, DC: National Academy Press.

Corrigan, S. A., Raczynski, J. M., Swencionis, C., & Jennings, S. G. (1991). Weight reduction in the prevention and treatment of hypertension: A review of representative clinical trials. *American Journal of Health Promotion, 5*, 208–214.

Council on Scientific Affairs. (1988). Treatment of obesity in adults. *Journal of the American Medical Association, 260*, 2547–2551.

D'Alessio, D. A., Kavle, E. C., Mozzoli, M. A., Smalley, K. J., Palansky, M., Kendrick, Z. V., Owen, L. R., Bushman, N. E., Boden, L., & Owen, D. E. (1988). Thermic effect of food in lean and obese men. *Journal of Clinical Investigation, 81*, 1781–1789.

deGroot, L., van Es, A. J. H., van Raaij, J., Vogt, J. E., Hautvast, G. A. J. (1989). Adaptation of energy metabolism of overweight women to alternating and continuous low energy intake. *American Journal of Clinical Nutrition, 50*, 1314–1323.

deGroot, L., van Es, A. J. H., van Raaij, J., Vogt, J. E., & Hautvast, G. A. J. (1990). Energy metabolism of overweight women 1 mo and 1 y after an 8-wk slimming period. *American Journal of Clinical Nutrition, 51*, 578–583.

Dennison, D., Dennison, K. F., & McCann, S. (1990). Integration of nutrient and activity analysis software into a worksite weight management program. *Health Education, 21.* 4–7.

Ditschuneit, H. (1991). Obesity and related disorders. In G. Ailhaud, B. Guy-Grand, M. Lafontan, & D. Ricquier (Eds.), *Obesity in Europe 91* (pp. 191–200). London: John Libbey.

Doucet, E., & Tremblay, A. (1998). Body weight loss and maintenance with physical activity and diet. *Coronary Artery Disease, 9*, 495–501.

Dubbert, P. M., Johnson, W. G., Schlundt, D. G., & Montague, N. W. (1984). The influence of caloric information on cafeteria food choices. *Journal of Applied Behavior Analysis, 17*, 85–92.

Duncan, K. H., Bacon, J. A., & Weinsier, R. L. (1983). The effects of high and low energy diets on satiety, energy intake, and eating time of obese and nonobese subjects. *American Journal of Clinical Nutrition, 37,* 763–767.

Eaton, S. B., & Konner, M. (1985). Paleolithic nutrition. A consideration of its nature and current implications. *New England Journal of Medicine, 312,* 283–289.

Edington, D. W., Musich, S., Schnueringer, E., & Edington, M. (1999, September). The maintenance of low-risk as an important healthcare strategy. Workshop conducted at the annual meeting of the Society of Prospective Medicine, Colorado Springs, CO.

Efurt, J. C., Foote, A., & Heirich, M. A. (1991). Worksite wellness programs: Incremental comparison of screening and referral alone, health education, follow-up counseling, and plant organization. *American Journal of Health Promotion, 5,* 438–448.

Eisenstein, E. L., Nelson, C. L., Shaw, L. K., Hakim, Z., & Mark, D. B. (1999, November). *Assessing the relationship between obesity and life expectancy in post-acute coronary syndrome patients: A weighty matter.* Paper presented at the American Heart Association Annual Scientific Sessions, Atlanta, GA.

Evans, G. F., Harris, P., McNeill, A. W., & McKenzie, R. D. (1989). Montana State University: An employee wellness program financed by a self-insurance group health plan. *American Journal of Health Promotion, 3,* 25–33.

Faltermayer, E. (1992, March 23). Let's really cure the health system. *Fortune,* 46–58.

Ferguson, J. (1985). *Learning to Eat.* Palo Alto, CA: Bull Press.

Field, A. E., Byers, T., Hunter, D. J., Laird, N. M., Manson, J. E., Williamson, D. F., Willett, W. C., & Colditz, G. A. (1999). Weight cycling, weight gain, and risk of hypertension in women. *American Journal of Epidemiology, 150,* 573–579.

Fielding, J. E., & Piserchia, P. V. (1989). Frequency of worksite health promotion activities. *American Journal of Public Health, 79,* 16–20.

Flatt, J. P. (1978). The biochemistry of energy expenditure. In G. A. Bray (Ed.), *Recent Advances in Obesity Research: II* (pp. 211–228). Westport, CT: Technomic.

Follick, M. J., Fowler, J. L., & Brown, R. A. (1984). Attrition in worksite weight-loss interventions: The effects of an incentive procedure. *Journal of Consulting Clinical Psychology, 52,* 139–140.

Fontaine, K. R., Cheskin, L. J., & Barofsky, I. (1996). Health-related quality-of-life in obese persons seeking treatment. *Journal of Family Practice, 43,* 265–270.

Forbes, G. B. (1990). Do obese individuals gain weight more easily than nonobese individuals? *American Journal of Clinical Nutrition, 52,* 224–227.

Forbes, G., & Welle, S. L. (1983). Lean body mass in obesity. *International Journal of Obesity, 7,* 99–107.

Foreyt, J. P., & Goodrick, G. K. (1991). Factors common to successful therapy for the obese patient. *Medicine & Science in Sports & Exercise, 23,* 292–297.

Forman, M. R., Trowbridge, F. L., Gentry, E. M., Marks, J. S., & Hogelin, G. C. (1986). Overweight adults in the United States: The Behavioral Risk Factor Surveys. *American Journal of Clinical Nutrition, 44,* 410–416.

Forster, J. L., Jeffery, R. W., Sullivan, S., & Snell, M. K. (1985). A work-site weight control program using financial incentives collected through payroll deduction. *Journal of Occupational Medicine, 27,* 804–808.

Foster, G. D., Wadden, T. A., Feurer, I. D., Jennings, A. S., Stunkard, A. J., Crosby, L. O., Ship, J., & Mullen, J. L. (1990). Controlled trial of the metabolic effects of a very-low-calorie diet: Short- and long-term effects. *American Journal of Clinical Nutrition, 51,* 167–172.

Foster, G. D., Wadden, T. A., Kendall, P. C., Stunkard, A. J., & Vogt, R. A. (1996). Psychological effects of weight loss and regain: A prospective evaluation. *Journal of Consulting and Clinical Psychology, 64,* 752–757.

Fowler, J. L., Abrams, D. B., Peterson, G. S., & Follick, M. J. (1983). *Worksite weight loss: Professionally led vs. self-help.* Paper presented at the 4th annual meeting of the Society for Behavioral Medicine, Baltimore, MD.

Frankle, R. T., McIntosh, J., Bianchi, M., & Kane, E. J. (1986). The Weight Watchers at Work Program. *Journal of Nutrition Education, 18* (Suppl.) S44–S47.

Golay, A., Allaz, A., Morel, Y., de Tonnac, N., Tankova, S., & Reaven, G. (1996). Similar weight loss with low- or high-carbohydrate diets. *American Journal of Clinical Nutrition, 63,* 174–178.

Goldstein, D. J. (1992). Beneficial health effects of modest weight loss. *International Journal of Obesity, 16,* 397–415.

Gray, D. S. (1989). Diagnosis and prevalence of obesity. *Medical Clinics of North America, 73*, 1–13.

Gray, D. S., Fisler, J. S., & Bray, G. A. (1988). Effects of repeated weight loss and regain on body composition in obese rats. *American Journal of Clinical Nutrition, 47*, 393–399.

Hammer, R. L., & Fisher, A. G. (1990). Weight regain does not increase relative abdominal adiposity in obese women [Abstract No. 1982]. *Medicine & Science in Sports & Exercise, 68*, (Suppl.) S129.

Harvey-Berino, J. (1999). Calorie restriction is more effective for obesity treatment than dietary fat restriction. *Annals of Behavioral Medicine, 21*, 35–39.

Hegsted, D. M. (1992). Defining a nutritious diet: Need for new dietary standards. *Journal of the American College of Nutrition, 11*, 241–245.

Heitmann, B. L., Lissner, L., Sørenson, T. I. A., & Bengtsson, C. (1995). Dietary fat intake and weight gain in women genetically predisposed for obesity. *American Journal of Clinical Nutrition, 61*, 1213–1217.

Hennrikus, D. J., & Jeffery, R. W. (1996). Worksite intervention for weight control: A review of the literature. *American Journal of Health Promotion, 10*, 471–498.

Heyward, V. H., & Stolarczyk, L. M. (1996). *Applied Body Composition.* Champaign, IL: Human Kinetics.

Holt, M. C., McCauley, M., & Paul, D. (1995). Health impacts of AT&T's Total Life Concept (TLC) program after five years. *American Journal of Health Promotion, 9*, 421–425.

Huang, Z., Willett, W. C., Manson, J. E., Rosner, B., Stampfer, M. J., Speizer, F. E., & Colditz, G. A. (1998). Body weight, weight change, and risk for hypertension in women. *Annals of Internal Medicine, 128*, 81–88.

Hypertension Prevention Trial Research Group. (1990). The Hypertension Prevention Trial: Three-year effects of dietary changes on blood pressure. *Archives of Internal Medicine, 150*, 153–162.

Jeffery, R. W., Adlis, S. A., & Forster, J. L. (1991). Prevalence of dieting among working men and women: The Healthy Worker Project. *Health Psychology, 10*, 274–281.

Jeffery, R. W., Bjornson-Benson, W. M., Rosenthal, B. S., Lindquist, R. A., Kurth, C. L., & Johnson, S. L. (1984). Correlates of weight loss and its maintenance over two years of follow-up among middle-aged men. *Preventive Medicine, 13*, 155–168.

Jeffery, R. W., Forster, J. L., French, S. A., Kelder, S. H., Lando, H. A., McGovern, P. G., Jacobs, D. R., & Baxter, J. E. (1992). *Healthy worker project: Results of a two-year randomized trial of worksite intervention for weight control and smoking cessation.* Paper presented at the 13th annual meeting of the Society of Behavioral Medicine, New York, NY.

Jeffery, R. W., Forster, J. L., & Schmid, T. L. (1989). Worksite health promotion: Feasibility testing of repeated weight control and smoking cessation classes. *American Journal of Health Promotion, 3*, 11–16.

Jeffery, R. W., Forster, J. L., & Snell, M. K. (1985). Promoting weight control at the worksite: A pilot program of self-motivation using payroll-based incentives. *Preventive Medicine, 14*, 187–194.

Jeffery, R. W., Wing, R. R., & French, S. A. (1992). Weight cycling and cardiovascular risk factors in obese men and women. *American Journal of Clinical Nutrition, 55*, 641–644.

Jequier, E. (1990). Energy metabolism in obese patients before and after weight loss, and in patients who have relapsed. *International Journal of Obesity, 14* (Suppl. 1), 59–67.

Jose, W., & Anderson, D. (1986). Control Data: The StayWell program. *Corporate Commentary, 2*, 1–13.

Källén, K. (1998). Maternal smoking, body mass index, and neural tube defects. *American Journal of Epidemiology, 147*, 1103–1111.

Kaplan, G. D., Miller, K. C., & Anderson, J. W. (1992). Comparative weight loss in obese patients restarting a supplemented very-low-calorie diet. *American Journal of Clinical Nutrition, 56* (Suppl.), 290S–291S.

Kaplan, G. D., Stifler, L. T. P. S., Framer, E., & Scheiber, J. (1990). *Developing physically active lifestyles in an obese population.* Poster session presented at the 11th annual meeting of the Society for Behavioral Medicine, Chicago, IL.

Kayman, S. B., Bruvold, W., & Stern, J. S. (1990). Maintenance and relapse after weight loss in women: Behavioral aspects. *American Journal of Clinical Nutrition, 52*, 800–807.

Keenan, N. L., Strogatz, D. S., James, S. A., Ammerman, A. S., & Rice, B. L. (1992). Distribution and correlates of waist-to-hip ratio in black adults: The Pitt County Study. *American Journal of Epidemiology, 135*, 678–684.

Kendall, A., Levitsky, D. A., Strupp, B. J., & Lissner, L. (1991). Weight loss on a low fat diet: Consequence of the imprecision of the control of food intake in humans. *American Journal of Clinical Nutrition, 53,* 1124–1129.

Kissebah, A. H., Freedman, D. S., & Peiris, A. N. (1989). Health risks of obesity. *Medical Clinics of North America, 73*(1): 111–138.

Klem, M. L., Wing, R. R., McGuire, M. T., Seagle, H. M., & Hill, J. O. (1998). Psychological symptoms in individuals successful at long-term maintenance of weight loss. *Health Psychology, 4,* 336–345.

Koplan, J. P., & Dietz, W. H. (1999). Caloric imbalance and public health policy. *Journal of the American Medical Association, 282,* 1579–1581.

Kuczmarski, R. J., Carroll, M. D., Flegal, K. M., & Troiano, R. P. (1997). Varying body mass index cutoff points to describe overweight prevalence among U.S. adults: NHANES III (1988 to 1994). *Obesity Research, 5,* 542–548.

Kuczmarski, R. J., Flegal, K. M., Campbell, S. M., & Johnson, C. L. (1994). Increasing prevalence of overweight among US adults. *Journal of the American Medical Association, 272,* 205–211.

Lansky, D., & Brownell, K. D. (1982). Estimates of food quantity and calories: Errors in self-report among obese patients. *American Journal of Clinical Nutrition, 35,* 727–732.

Larson, D. E., Ferraro, R. T., Robertson, D. S., & Ravussin, E. (1995). Energy metabolism in weight-stable postobese individuals. *American Journal of Clinical Nutrition, 62,* 735–739.

Lissner, L., Heitmann, B. L., & Bengtsson, C. (1997). Low-fat diets may prevent weight gain in sedentary women: Prospective observations from the population study of women in Gothenburg, Sweden. *Obesity Research, 5,* 43–48.

Lissner, L., Odell, P. M., D'Agostino, R. B., Stokes, J., Kreger, B. E., Belanger, A. J., & Brownell, K. D. (1991). *New England Journal of Medicine, 324,* 1839–1844.

Maclure, K. M., Hayes, K. C., Colditz, G. A., Stampfer, M. J., Speizer, F. E., & Willett, W. C. (1989). Weight, diet, and the risk of symptomatic gallstones in middle-aged women. *New England Journal of Medicine, 321,* 563–569.

Manninen, P., Riihimäki, H., Heliövaara, M., & Mäkelä, P. (1996). Overweight, gender and knee osteoarthritis. *International Journal of Obesity, 20,* 595–597.

Markovic, T. P., Fleury, A. C., Campbell, L. V., Simons, L. A., Balasubramanian, S., Chisholm, D. J., & Jenkins, A. B. (1998). Beneficial effect on average lipid levels from energy restriction and fat loss in obese individuals with or without type 2 diabetes. *Diabetes Care, 21,* 695–700.

McGuire, M. T., Wing, R. R., Klem, M. L., Lang, W., & Hill, J. O. (1999). What predicts weight regain in a group of successful weight losers? *Journal of Consulting Clinical Psychology, 67,* 177–185.

Melby, C. L., Schmidt, W. D., & Corrigan, D. (1990). Resting metabolic rate in weight-cycling collegiate wrestlers compared with physically active, noncycling control subjects. *American Journal of Clinical Nutrition, 52,* 409–414.

Metropolitan Life Insurance Co. (1959). New weight standards for men and women. *Statistical Bulletin of the New York Metropolitan Life Insurance Company, 40,* 1–4.

Miller, A., & Edelstein, S. (1990). Establishing a worksite wellness program in a hospital setting. *Journal of the American Dietetic Association, 90,* 1104–1106.

Miller, P. M., & Sims, K. L. (1981). Evaluation and component analysis of a comprehensive weight control program. *International Journal of Obesity, 5,* 57–65.

Milliman and Robertson, Inc. (1987). *Health risks and behavior: The impact on medical costs.* Milwaukee, WI: Author.

Must, A., Spadano, J., Coakley, E. H., Field, A. E., Colditz, G., & Dietz, W. H. (1999). The disease burden associated with overweight and obesity. *Journal of the American Medical Association, 282,* 1523–1529.

National Institutes of Health Consensus Development Panel on the Health Implications of Obesity. (1985). Health implications of obesity. *Annals of Internal Medicine, 103* (6, part 2), 1073–1077.

National Institutes of Health Technology Assessment Conference Statement. (1992). Methods for voluntary weight loss and control.

National Research Council Commission on Life Sciences. (1986). *What is America eating?* Washington, DC: National Academy Press.

NHLBI Obesity Education Initiative Expert Panel on the Identification, Evaluation, and Treatment of Overweight and Obesity in Adults. (1998). Clinical guidelines on the identification, evaluation, and treatment of overweight and obesity in adults – The evidence report. *Obesity Research, 6* (Suppl. 2), 51S–209S.

Nelson, K. M., Weinsier, R. L., James, L. D., Darnell, B., Hunter, G., & Long, C. L. (1992). Effect of weight reduction on resting energy expenditure, substrate utilization, and the thermic effect of food in moderately obese women. *American Journal of Clinical Nutrition, 55,* 924–933.

Norris, J., Harnack, L., Carmichael, S., Pouane, T., Wakimoto, P., & Block, G. (1997). US trends in nutrient intake: The 1987 and 1992 National Health Interview Surveys. *American Journal of Public Health, 87,* 740–746.

Office of Disease Prevention and Health Promotion. (1987). *National survey of worksite health promotion activities: A summary, 1987.* Bethesda, MD: U.S. Department of Health and Human Services.

Paffenbarger, R. S., Hyde, R. T., Wing, A. L., & Hsieh, C. (1986). Physical activity, all-cause mortality, and longevity of college alumni. *New England Journal of Medicine, 314,* 605–613.

Perri, M. G., Martin, D., Leermakers, E. A., Sears, S. F., & Notelovitz, M. (1997). Effects of group-versus home-based exercise in the treatment of obesity. *Journal of Consulting and Clinical Psychology, 65,* 278–285.

Perri, M. G., McAdoo, G., Spevak, P. A., & Newlin, D. B. (1984). Effect of a multicomponent maintenance program on long-term weight loss. *Journal of Consulting and Clinical Psychology, 52,* 480–481.

Perri, M. G., Shapiro, R. M., Ludwig, W. W., & McAdoo, W. G. (1984). Maintenance strategies for the treatment of obesity: An evaluation of relapse prevention training and posttreatment contact by mail and telephone. *Journal of Consulting and Clinical Psychology, 52,* 404–413.

Peterson, G., Abrams, D. B., Elder, J. P., & Beaudin, P. A. (1985). Professional versus self-help weight loss at the worksite: The challenge of making a public health impact. *Behavior Therapy, 16,* 213–222.

Popkin, B. M., & Doak, C. M. (1998). The obesity epidemic is a worldwide phenomenon. *Nutrition Reviews, 56,* 106–114.

Pritchard, J. E., Nowson, C. A., & Marks, J. D. (1997). A worksite program for overweight middle-aged men achieves lesser weight loss with exercise than with dietary change. *Journal of the American Dietetic Association, 97,* 37–42.

Prochaska, J. O., & Velicer, W. F. (1997). The transtheoretical model of health behavior change. *American Journal of Health Promotion, 12,* 38–48.

Quesenberry, C. P., Jr., Caan, B., & Jacobson, A. (1998). Obesity, health services use, and health care costs among members of a health maintenance organization. *Archives of Internal Medicine, 158,* 466–472.

Racette, S. B., Schoeller, D. A., Kushner, R. F., & Neil, K. M. (1995). Exercise enhances dietary compliance during moderate energy restriction in obese women. *American Journal of Clinical Nutrition, 62,* 345–349.

Rand, C. S. W., & Macgregor, A. M. C. (1991). Successful weight loss following obesity surgery and the perceived liability of morbid obesity. *International Journal of Obesity, 15,* 577–579.

Rapp, S. R., Dubbert, P. M., Burkett, P. A., & Buttross, Y. (1986). Food portion size estimation by men with type II diabetes. *Journal of the American Dietetic Association, 86,* 249–251.

Reid, D. J., & Dunkley, G. C. (1989). Weight control in the workplace: A needs assessment for men. *Canadian Journal of Public Health, 80,* 24–27.

Revicki, D. A., & Israel, R. G. (1986). Relationship between body mass indices and measures of body adiposity. *American Journal of Public Health, 76,* 992–994.

Rexrode, K. M., Hennekens, C. H., Willett, W. C., Colditz, G. A., Stampfer, M. J., Rich-Edwards, J. W., Speizer, F. E., & Manson, J. E. (1997). A prospective study of body mass index, weight change, and risk of stroke in women. *Journal of the American Medical Association, 277,* 1539–1545.

Reynolds, T. (1991). "5-a-day for better health" program is launched in Boston. *Journal of the National Cancer Institute, 83,* 1538–1539.

Rippe, J. M., Price, J. M., Hess, S. A., Kline, G., DeMers, K. A., Damitz, S., Kreidieh, I., & Freedson, P. (1998). Improved psychological well-being, quality of life, and health practices in moderately overweight women participating in a 12-week structured weight loss program. *Obesity Research, 6,* 208–218.

Rissanen, A., Heliovaara, M., Knekt, P., Reunanen, A., & Aromaa, A. (1990). Is the burden of overweight on cardiovascular health underestimated? *Diabetes Research and Clinical Practice, 10* (Suppl. 1), S195–S198.

Rubin, R. (1999, September 15). *Costs of obesity.* Paper presented at the annual meeting of the American Obesity Association.

Schoeller, D. A., Shay, K., & Kushner, R. F. (1997). How much physical activity is needed to minimize weight gain in previously obese women? *American Journal of Clinical Nutrition, 66,* 551–556.

Schotte, D. E., Cohen, E., & Singh, S. P. (1990). Effects of weight cycling on metabolic control in male outpatients with non-insulin-dependent diabetes mellitus. *Health Psychology, 9,* 599–605.

Seidman, L. S., Sevelius, G. G., & Ewald, P. (1984). A cost-effective weight loss program at the worksite. *Journal of Occupational Medicine, 26,* 725–730.

Senauer, B., Asp, E., & Kinsey, J. (1991). *Food trends and the changing consumer.* St. Paul, MN: Eagan Press.

Serdula, M. K., Mokdad, A. H., Williamson, D. F., Galuska, D. A., Mendlein, J. M., & Heath, G. W. (1999). Prevalence of attempting weight loss and strategies for controlling weight. *Journal of the American Medical Association, 282,* 1353–1358.

Shah, M., & Jeffery, R. W. (1991). Is obesity due to overeating and inactivity, or to a defective metabolic rate? A review. *Annals of Behavioral Medicine, 13,* 73–81.

Shapiro, S. H. (1991). *Public announcements as a non-surgical approach for maintaining large weight losses.* Paper presented at the North American Association for the Study of Obesity, Sacramento, CA.

Shaw, G. M., Velie, E. M., & Schaffer, D. (1996). Risk of neural tube defect-affected pregnancies among obese women. *Journal of the American Medical Association, 275,* 1093–1096.

Sheppard, L., Kristal, A. R., & Kushi, L. H. (1991). Weight loss in women participating in a randomized trial of low-fat diets. *American Journal of Clinical Nutrition, 54,* 821–828.

Shick, S. M., Wing, R. R., Klem, M. L., McGuire, M. T., Hill, J. O., & Seagle, H. (1998). Persons successful at long-term weight loss and maintenance continue to consume a low-energy, low-fat diet. *Journal of the American Dietetic Association, 98,* 408–413.

Siegelman, S. (1991). Employees fighting the battle of the bulge. *Business & Health, 9,* 62, 63, 66, 68, 70–73.

Siervogel, R. M., Wisemandle, W., Maynard, L. M., Guo, S. S., Roche, A. F., Chumlea, W. C., & Towne, B. (1998). Serial changes in body composition throughout adulthood and their relationships to changes in lipid and lipoprotein levels. The Fels Longitudinal Study. *Arteriosclerosis, Thrombosis and Vascular Biology, 18,* 1759–1764.

Siggard, R., Raben, A., & Astrup, A. (1996). Weight loss during 12 weeks' ad libitum carbohydrate-rich diet in overweight and normal-weight subjects at a Danish work site. *Obesity Research, 4,* 347–356.

Simkin-Silverman, L. R., Wing, R. R., Plantinga, P., Matthews, K. A., & Kuller, L. H. (1998). Lifetime weight cycling and psychological health in normal-weight and overweight women. *International Journal of Eating Disorders, 24,* 175–183.

Skender, M. L., Goodrick, G. K., Del Junco, D. J., Reeves, R., Darnell, L., Gotto, A. M., & Foreyt, J. P. (1996). Comparison of 2-year weight loss trends in behavioral treatments of obesity: Diet, exercise, and combination interventions. *Journal of the American Dietetic Association, 96,* 342–346.

Society of Prospective Medicine. (1999). Guidelines for developers and administrators. In G. C. Hyner, K. W. Peterson, J. W. Travis, J. E. Dewey, J. J. Foerster, & E. M. Framer (Eds.), *SPM Handbook of Health Assessment Tools,* Pittsburgh, PA: The Society of Prospective Medicine & The Institute for Health and Productivity Management, p. xxiii.

Stalonas, P. M., Perri, M. G., & Kerzner, A. B. (1984). Do behavioral treatments of obesity last? A five-year follow-up investigation. *Addictive Behaviors, 9,* 175–183.

Stamler, J., Wentworth, D., & Neaton, J. D. (1986). Is relationship between serum cholesterol and risk of premature death from coronary heart disease continuous and graded? Findings in 356,222 primary screenees of the Multiple Risk Factor Intervention Trial (MRFIT). *Journal of the American Medical Association, 256,* 2823–2828.

Steen, S. N., Oppliger, R. A., & Brownell, K. D. (1988). Metabolic effects of repeated weight loss and regain in adolescent wrestlers. *Journal of the American Medical Association, 260,* 47–50.

Stifler, L. T. P., Galante-Schwarz, L., & McFadden, E. (1987). *The HMR Calorie System.* Boston, MA: Health Management Resources.

Stifler, L. T. P., Kaplan, G. D., & Lindewall, D. (1985). *The role of physical activity in a comprehensive weight control program.* Poster Session presented at the 93rd annual meeting of the American Psychological Association, Toronto, Canada.

Stunkard, A. J. (1986). The control of obesity: Social and community perspectives. In K. D. Brownell & J. P. Foreyt (Eds.), *Handbook of Eating Disorders* (pp. 213–228). New York: Basic Books.

Stunkard, A. J. (1987). The current status of treatment for obesity in adults. In A. J. Stunkard & E. Stellar (Eds.), *Eating and its disorders* (pp. 157–173). New York: Raven Press.

Stunkard, A. J., & Berthold, H. C. (1985). What is behavior therapy? A very short description of behavioral weight control. *American Journal of Clinical Nutrition, 41,* 821–823.

Stunkard, A. J., & Brownell, K. D. (1980). Worksite treatment for obesity. *American Journal of Psychiatry, 137,* 252–253.

Stunkard, A. J., Cohen, R. Y., & Felix, M. R. J. (1989). Weight loss competitions at the worksite: How they work and how well. *Preventive Medicine, 18,* 460–474.

Stunkard, A. J., Harris, J. R., & McClearn, G. E. (1990). Heritability of weight gain and obesity [Letter to the Editor]. *New England Journal of Medicine, 323,* 1069.

Stunkard, A. J., Harris, J. R., Pedersen, N. L., & McClearn, G. E. (1990). The body-mass index of twins who have been reared apart. *New England Journal of Medicine, 322,* 1483–1487.

Stunkard, A. J., & McLaren-Hume, M. (1959). The results of treatment for obesity. *Archives of Internal Medicine, 103,* 79–85.

Sumner, S. K., Schiller, E. L., Marr, E. R., & Thompson, D. I. (1986). A weight control and nutrition education program for insurance company employees. *Journal of Nutrition Education, 18* (Suppl.) S60–S62.

Swinburn, B., Ashton, T., Gillespie, J., Cox, B., Menon, A., Simmons, D., & Birkbeck, J. (1997). Health care costs of obesity in New Zealand. *International Journal of Obesity, 21,* 891–896.

Taylor, C. B., Jatulis, D. E., Fortmann, S. P., & Kraemer, H. C. (1995). Weight variability effects: A prospective analysis from the Stanford Five-City Project. *American Journal of Epidemiology, 141,* 461–465.

Terry, P., Anderson, D. R., & Serxner, S. (1999). Health assessment at the worksite. In G. C. Hyner, K. W. Peterson, J. W. Travis, J. E. Dewey, J. J. Foerster, & E. F. Framer (Eds.), *SPM Handbook of Health Assessment Tools* (pp. 207–215). Irving, TX: The Institute for Health and Productivity Management.

Thompson, D., Edelsberg, J., Colditz, G. A., Bird, A. P., & Oster, G. (1999). Lifetime health and economic consequences of obesity. *Archives of Internal Medicine, 159,* 2177–2183.

Tokunaga, K., Matsuzawa, Y., Kotami, K., Keno, Y., Kobatake, T., Fujioka, S., & Tarui, S. (1990). Ideal body weight estimated from the body mass index with the lowest morbidity. *International Journal of Obesity, 15,* 1–5.

Trentham-Dietz, A., Newcomb, P. A., Storer, B. E., Longnecker, M. P., Baron, J., Greenberg, E. R., & Willett, W. C. (1997). Body size and risk of breast cancer. *American Journal of Epidemiology, 145,* 1011–1019.

Tucker, L. A., & Friedman, G. M. (1998). Obesity and absenteeism: An epidemiologic study of 10,825 employed adults. *American Journal of Health Promotion, 12,* 202–207.

U.S. Department of Health and Human Services, Public Health Service. (1993). National survey of worksite health promotion activities: Summary. *American Journal of Health Promotion, 7,* 452–464.

U.S. Public Health Service. (1999). *Healthy People 2010,* available on Internet.

Van Gaal, L. F., Wauters, M. A., & De Leeuw, I. H. (1997). The beneficial effects of modest weight loss on cardiovascular risk factors. *International Journal of Obesity, 21* (Suppl. 1), S5–S9.

Van Gemert, W. G., Adang, E. M., Greve, J. W. M., & Soeters, P. B. (1998). Quality of life assessment of morbidly obese patients: Effect of weight-reducing surgery. *American Journal of Clinical Nutrition, 67,* 197–201.

Vansant, G. A., Van Gaal, L. F., & De Leeuw, I. H. (1989). Decreased diet-induced thermogenesis in gluteal-femoral obesity. *Journal of the American College of Nutrition, 6,* 597–601.

Venditti, E. M., Wing, R. R., Jakicic, J. M., Butler, B. A., & Marcus, M. D. (1996). Weight cycling, psychological health, and binge eating in obese women. *Journal of Consulting and Clinical Psychology, 64,* 400–405.

Vgontzas, A. N., Bixler, E. O., Tan, T., Kantner, D., Martin, L. F., & Kales, A. (1998). Obesity without sleep apnea is associated with daytime sleepiness. *Archives of Internal Medicine, 158,* 1333–1337.

Wadden, T. A., Foster, G. D., Letizia, K. A., & Mullen, J. L. (1990). Long-term effects of dieting on resting metabolic rate in obese outpatients. *Journal of the American Medical Association, 264,* 707–711.

Wadden, T. A., Sternberg, J. A., Letizia, K. A., Stunkard, A. J., & Foster, G. D. (1989). Treatment of obesity by very low calorie diet, behavior therapy, and their combination: A five-year perspective. *International Journal of Obesity, 13* (Suppl. 2), 39–46.

Wadden, T. A., & Stunkard, A. J. (1986). Controlled trial of very low calorie diet, behavior therapy, and their combination in the treatment of obesity. *Journal of Consulting and Clinical Psychology, 54,* 482–488.

Wadden, T. A., Van Itallie, T. B., & Blackburn, G. L. (1990). Responsible and irresponsible use of very-low-calorie diets in the treatment of obesity. *Journal of the American Medical Association, 263,* 83–85.

Wadden, T. A., Vogt, R. A., Foster, G. D., & Anderson, D. A. (1998). Exercise and the maintenance of weight loss: 1-year follow-up of a controlled clinical trial. *Journal of Consulting and Clinical Psychology, 66,* 429–433.

Weinsier, R. L., Wadden, T. A., Ritenbaugh, C., Harrison, G. G., Johnson, F. S., & Wilmore, J. H. (1984). Recommended therapeutic guidelines for professional weight control programs. *American Journal of Clinical Nutrition, 40,* 865–872.

Weisbrod, R. R., Pirie, P. L., Bracht, N. F., & Elstun, P. (1991). Worksite health promotion in four midwest cities. *Journal Community Health, 16,* 169–177.

Westerterp, K. R., Verboeket-van deVenne, W. P. H. G., Westerterp-Plantenga, M. S., Velthuis-te Wierik, E. J. M., de Graaf, C., & Weststrate, J. A. (1996). Dietary fat and body fat: An intervention study. *International Journal of Obesity, 20,* 1022–1026.

Wild, B., Smith, C., & Martin, J. (1992). Worksite and community health promotion/risk reduction project–Virginia, 1987–1991. *Morbidity and Mortality Weekly Report, 41,* 55–57.

William M. Mercer, Inc. (1999). 1999 national worksite health promotion survey. *American Journal of Health Promotion.*

Williamson, G. F., Kahn, H. S., Remington, P. L., & Anda, R. F. (1990). The 10-year incidence of overweight and major weight gain in US adults. *Archives of Internal Medicine, 150,* 665–672.

Wilson, M. G., DeJoy, D. M., Jorgenson, C. M., & Crump, C. J. (1999). Health promotion programs in small worksites: Results of a national survey. *American Journal of Health Promotion, 13,* 358–365.

Wing, R. R. (1999). Exercise dose-response issues for the overweight adult: How much is enough? *Obesity Research, 7* (Suppl. 1), 5S.

Wing, R. R., & Jeffery, R. W. (1999). Benefits of recruiting participants with friends and increasing social support for weight loss and maintenance. *Journal of Consulting Clinical Psychology, 67,* 132–138.

Wing, R. R., Marcus, M. D., Salata, R., Epstein, L. H., Miaskiewicz, S., & Blair, E. H. (1991). Effects of a very-low-calorie diet on long-term glycemic control in obese type 2 subjects. *Archives of Internal Medicine, 151,* 1334–1340.

Witteman, J. C. M., Willett, W. C., Stampfer, M. J., Colditz, L. A., Sacks, F. M., Soeizer, F. E., Rosner, B., & Hennekens, C. H. (1989). A prospective study of nutritional factors and hypertension among US women. *Circulation, 80,* 1320–1327.

Wolf, A. M., & Colditz, G. A. (1996). Social and economic effects of body weight in the United States. *American Journal of Clinical Nutrition, 63* (Suppl.), 466S–469S.

Wolf, A. M., & Colditz, G. A. (1998). Current estimates of the economic cost of obesity in the United States. *Obesity Research, 6,* 97–106.

Ziegler, R. G., Hoover, R. N., Nomura, A. M. Y., West, D. W., Wu, A. H., Pike, M. C., Lake, A. J., Horn-Ross, P. L., Kolonel, L. N., Siiteri, P. K., & Fraumeni, J. F., Jr. (1996). Relative weight, weight change, height, and breast cancer risk in Asian-American women. *Journal of the National Cancer Institute, 88,* 650–660.

CHAPTER

13

Tobacco Control and Cessation

Nell H. Gottlieb

INTRODUCTION

Tobacco control, including policies limiting exposure to environmental tobacco smoke and cessation programming, is an essential component of worksite health promotion. Tobacco use remains the leading cause of death in the United States. The adult rates of smoking have been steadily decreasing over the past 30 years, although initially declining youth prevalence rates have increased over the past decade, and young adults now have the highest prevalence of all age groups (Centers for Disease Control and Prevention [CDCP], 1999c; Nelson, Kirkendall, et al., 1994).

The context for tobacco control has changed markedly since the 1964 Surgeon General's Report on Smoking and Health, which summarized the evidence that smoking was detrimental to health (U.S. Department of Health and Human Services [USD-HHS], 1964). Beginning in the 1970s, the focus shifted to include exposure to environmental tobacco as a major concern, leading to the diffusion of restrictive tobacco policies in worksites and communities over the past two decades. Large-scale antitobacco efforts have included the earmarking of tobacco excise tax

revenue for smoking prevention programs by five states. The recent settlement of state lawsuits to recover Medicaid costs for tobacco-related illnesses by the tobacco companies has given states an unprecedented amount of income that could be used for tobacco control.

In this chapter we summarize the rationale and context for worksite tobacco control and the implications of such control for worksite health promotion in the twenty-first century. We review the evidence for worksite tobacco use cessation programs and policy impacts. We then introduce an ecological model for worksite programming that includes the individual, group, organizational, community, and governmental levels and discuss worksite tobacco control within that framework.

TOBACCO AND HEALTH

Tobacco is the leading cause of death in the United States (CDCP, 7/30/00b) (see Figure 13-1). In 1990, approximately 400,000 adults—276,000 men and 142,000 women—died from a tobacco-related disease. The number of smoking-attributable deaths by states ranged from 402 in Alaska to 42,574 in California, with a median of 5,619 deaths. Utah had the lowest

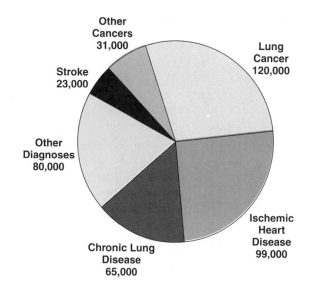

Figure 13-1 Deaths attributable to cigarette smoking—
United States, 1990.

Source: Centers for Disease Control and Prevention. 2000b. Deaths
attributable to smoking, 1990. [On-line]. Available:
http://www.cdc.gov/tobacco/attrdths.htm

mortality rate (218/100,000) and the lowest percentage
of deaths attributable to smoking (13.4%), while
Nevada had the highest mortality rate (478.1 / 100,000)
and the highest percentage of deaths from smoking
(24.0%) (McGinnis & Foege, 1993; Nelson, Kirkendall,
et al., 1994)

As seen in Table 13-1, the relative risks of male current smokers compared to male non-smokers range
from 27.5 for lip, oral cavity, and pharyngeal cancer
and 22.4 for lung cancer to 1.6 for ischemic heart disease over age 65. For female smokers, the highest relative risk in comparison to female non-smokers is for
cancer of the larynx (17.8), followed by lung cancer
(11.9) (Nelson, Kirkendall, et al., 1994). In the mid
1980s, the number of women dying from lung cancer
exceeded that for breast cancer, formerly the top
cause of cancer death among women (CDCP, 1993).
The largest number of deaths attributable to smoking
in 1990 was from lung cancer, followed by ischemic
heart disease (see Figure 13-1).

The benefits of cessation begin within twenty minutes of smoking the last cigarette, with the blood pressure, pulse, and body temperature of hands and feet
returning to normal. As seen in Figure 13-2, this continues with the blood carbon monoxide level decreasing and the oxygen level increasing to normal within
8 hours. By the first three months, circulation improves and lung function increases. At one year, the
ex-smokers excess risk of coronary heart disease is
half that of a smoker, and at five years the lung cancer
death rate for the average former smoker increases by
almost half and at 10 years is similar to that of nonsmokers. At 15 years, the risk of coronary heart disease is that of a non-smoker (American Cancer Society [ACS], n.d.).

Each year, an estimated 3,000 nonsmokers in the
U.S. die from lung cancer as a result of exposure to
secondhand smoke. From 150,000 to 300,000 children
suffer from lower respiratory tract infections. Secondhand smoke has also been implicated as causing heart
disease in adults, with 50,000 cardiovascular deaths
attributable to environmental tobacco smoke annually (U.S. Environmental Protection Agency, 1992;
USDHHS, 2000). The Third National Health and Nutrition Examination Survey (1988–1991) found that
87.9% of the sample of nontobacco users aged 4 and
older had detectable levels of serum cotinine, a biological marker for exposure to secondhand smoke
(Pirkle, 1996).

Smoking during pregnancy is a special case of secondhand smoke. The consequences of smoking during pregnancy include spontaneous abortions, low
birthweight, and sudden infant death syndrome. The
relationship with low birthweight is likely due to in-
trauterine hypoxia, which is due to increased carbon
monoxide in the blood or to reduced blood flow. (US-
DHHS, 1989; USDHHS, 2000)

Tobacco smoke contains over 4,000 chemical compounds, of which at least 43 are known to cause cancer in humans and animals. Table 13-2 shows the primary toxic and cancer-causing components of both
mainstream (inhaled by the smoker) and sidestream
(generated by the smoldering of tobacco products
and the major source of environmental tobacco
smoke [ETS]) smoke. Sidestream smoke contains
more toxic chemicals than mainstream smoke, but it
is inhaled at far lower concentrations. Nicotine is the

Table 13-1 Relative Risks Attributable to Smoking and Estimated Smoking-Attributable Mortality for Current and Former Smokers Compared with Nonsmokers by Disease Category and Sex—United States, 1990

	Relative risk			
	Males		Females	
Disease category (ICD-9)	Current Smokers	Former Smokers	Current Smokers	Former Smokers
Diseases among adults (≥ 35 years of age)				
Neoplasms				
Lip, oral cavity, pharynx (140–149)	27.5	8.8	5.6	2.9
Esophagus (150)	7.6	5.8	10.3	3.2
Pancreas (157)	2.1	1.1	2.3	1.8
Larynx (161)	10.5	5.2	17.8	11.9
Trachea, lung, bronchus (162)	22.4	9.4	11.9	4.7
Cervix uteri (180)	NA	NA	2.1	1.9
Urinary bladder (188)	2.9	1.9	2.6	1.9
Kidney, other urinary (189)	3.0	2.0	1.4	1.2
Cardiovascular diseases				
Hypertensive diseases (401–404)	1.9	1.3	1.7	1.2
Ischemic heart disease (410–414)				
Persons ages 35–64 yrs	2.8	1.8	3.0	1.4
Persons ages ≥65 yrs	1.6	1.3	1.6	1.3
Other heart diseases (390–398, 415–417, 420–429)	1.9	1.3	1.7	1.2
Cerebrovascular diseases (430–438)				
Persons ages 35–64 yrs	3.7	1.4	4.8	1.4
Persons ages ≥65 yrs	1.9	1.3	1.5	1.0
Atherosclerosis (440)	4.1	2.3	3.0	1.3
Aortic aneurysm (441)	4.1	2.3	3.0	1.3
Other arterial diseases (442–448)	4.1	2.3	3.0	1.3
Respiratory diseases				
Pneumonia and influenza (480–487)	2.0	1.6	2.2	1.4
Bronchitis and emphysema (491–492)	9.7	8.8	10.5	7.0
Chronic airways obstruction (496)	9.7	8.8	10.5	7.0
Other respiratory diseases (010–012, 493)	2.0	1.6	2.2	1.4
Diseases among infants (<1 yr of age)				
Short gestation, low birth weight (765)		1.8		1.8
Respiratory distress syndrome (769)		1.8		1.8
Other respiratory conditions of newborn (770)		1.8		1.8
Sudden infant death syndrome (798)		1.5		1.5
Deaths* from burns (E890–E899)		NA		NA

*Estimated to be 50% of deaths on the basis of injury surveillance studies (19).

NA = not applicable.

ICD-9 = *International Classification of Diseases* (9th rev.).

Source: Nelson et al., *Morbidity and Mortality Weekly Report,* 1994.

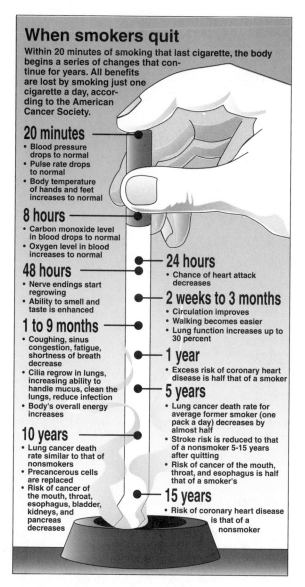

When smokers quit

Within 20 minutes of smoking that last cigarette, the body begins a series of changes that continue for years. All benefits are lost by smoking just one cigarette a day, according to the American Cancer Society.

20 minutes
- Blood pressure drops to normal
- Pulse rate drops to normal
- Body temperature of hands and feet increases to normal

8 hours
- Carbon monoxide level in blood drops to normal
- Oxygen level in blood increases to normal

48 hours
- Nerve endings start regrowing
- Ability to smell and taste is enhanced

1 to 9 months
- Coughing, sinus congestion, fatigue, shortness of breath decrease
- Cilia regrow in lungs, increasing ability to handle mucus, clean the lungs, reduce infection
- Body's overall energy increases

10 years
- Lung cancer death rate similar to that of nonsmokers
- Precancerous cells are replaced
- Risk of cancer of the mouth, throat, esophagus, bladder, kidneys, and pancreas decreases

24 hours
- Chance of heart attack decreases

2 weeks to 3 months
- Circulation improves
- Walking becomes easier
- Lung function increases up to 30 percent

1 year
- Excess risk of coronary heart disease is half that of a smoker

5 years
- Lung cancer death rate for average former smoker (one pack a day) decreases by almost half
- Stroke risk is reduced to that of a nonsmoker 5-15 years after quitting
- Risk of cancer of the mouth, throat, and esophagus is half that of a smoker's

15 years
- Risk of coronary heart disease is that of a nonsmoker

Figure 13-2 Health benefits of quitting.
Source: The American Cancer Society, *The Health Benefits of Quitting*, n.d.

oxygen in red blood cells, are the major contributors to the increased risk of cardiovascular disease among smokers and persons exposed to ETS. Tar, the particulate matter in smoke suspended in organic solvents, has been shown in animals to induce carcinoma after subcutaneous injections and skin cancers after topical injections, with the primary tumor initiators coming from polynuclear aromatic hydrocarbons. The other carcinogens and cocarcinogens in smoke are likely causative agents for specific smoking-related cancers (including lung, larynx, esophagus, pancreas, bladder, and oral cavity) (USDHHS, 1989).

The smoke from cigars is as, or more, toxic than that of cigarettes, and a dose-response relationship has been found for cigar smoking for cancers of the buccal cavity and pharynx, esophagus, larynx, lung, and pancreas; chronic obstructive pulmonary disease; and coronary heart disease. The disease risk has been less than cigarettes, however, due to the patterns of use and the deposition and retention of smoke among cigarette and cigar smokers. Cigar smokers tend to maintain smoke in their mouths rather than inhaling it into their lungs and to smoke less than daily. Primary cigar users have similar mortality ratios (ratio of the death rate in smokers compared to those who have never smoked) to cigarette users for oral cancer and esophageal cancer, much lower ratios for coronary heart disease, chronic obstructive lung disease and lung cancer, and moderately lower ratios for laryngeal cancer. However, when five or more cigars are smoked per day with moderate inhalation, the lung cancer risks approximate those of a one-pack-per-day cigarette smoker. Similarly, risks for coronary heart disease are significantly increased among users of three or more cigars a day or among cigar smokers who inhale (Burns, 1998; Gerlach et al., 1998). Similar relationships are found for pipe smokers (USDHHS, 1989).

Users of smokeless tobacco have increased risk for cancer of the oral cavity and for oral leukoplakias that may develop into carcinomas. The primary carcinogens in smokeless tobacco are tobacco-specific *N*-nitrosamines. The exposure to nicotine from smokeless tobacco is similar in magnitude to that from cigarette smoking. As discussed earlier, nicotine likely plays a

active pharmacologic agent that determines the addictive behavior of the smoker, and nicotine is now recognized as being as addictive as cocaine or heroin (USDHHS, 1989). Nicotine, a central nervous system stimulant, and carbon monoxide, which replaces

Table 13-2 Toxic and Cancer-causing Agents in Mainstream and Sidestream Cigarette Smoke

Smoke Constituents	Type	Unfiltered Cigarette	Filtered Cigarette A	Filtered Cigarette B	Low Tar Cigarette with Perforated Filter
Tar (mg)	C	20.10	15.60	6.80	0.90
		22.60	24.40	20.00	14.10
Nicotine (mg)	T	2.04	1.50	0.81	0.15
		4.62	4.14	3.54	3.16
Carbon monoxide (mg)	T	13.20	13.70	9.50	1.80
		28.30	36.60	33.20	26.80
Catechol (g)	CoC	41.90	71.20	26.90	9.10
		58.20	89.90	69.50	117.00
Benzo(a)pyrene (mg)	C	26.20	17.80	12.20	2.20
		67.00	45.70	51.70	44.80
Nitrosodimethylamine (ng)	C	31.10	4.30	12.10	4.10
		735.00	597.00	611.00	685.00
Nitrosopyrrolidine (mg)	C	64.50	10.20	32.70	13.2
		117.00	139.00	233.00	234.00
Nitrosonornicotine (ng)	C	1007.00	488.00	273.00	66.30
		857.00	307.00	185.00	338.00
4-(methylnitrosamino)-1-(3-pyridyl)-1-butanone	C	425.00	180.00	56.20	17.30
		1444.00	752.00	430.00	386.00

Note: C=carcinogenic, CoC=Co-carcinogenic, T=Toxic

Mainstream smoke   Sidestream smoke

contributory or supportive role in coronary artery and peripheral vascular disease (USDHHS, 1986a; USDHHS, 1989).

PREVALENCE OF TOBACCO USE

Smoking prevalence has decreased among adults from 42.4% in 1965 to 24.7% in 1997. As seen in Figure 13-3, in 1997, 27.6% of men reported currently smoking, compared to 22.1% of women (CDCP, 1993; CDCP, 1999c). However, this decrease has not been shared by all groups within the population. According to the 1997 National Health Interview Survey (CDCP, 1999c), the prevalence of smoking was highest among American Indians/Alaska natives (34.1%) and lowest among Asian/Pacific Islanders (21.6%).

Within each of the ethnic groups, women had lower rates of smoking than men, with the smallest difference among non-Hispanic whites. Overall, smoking rates were lowest for Hispanic women (14.3%) and Asian/Pacific Islander women (12.4%). Smoking prevalence was also associated with education, with 35.4% of adults with 9–11 years of education being current smokers, compared to 11.6% of college graduates. One-third of adults below the poverty level indicated they were current smokers, compared to 24.6% of those at or above the poverty level.

Smoking prevalence also varies by occupation, and this has important implications for smoking cessation programming at worksites. Blue-collar workers, in 1987–1990, had a higher smoking prevalence (39.2%) than white-collar workers (24.2%) and showed a

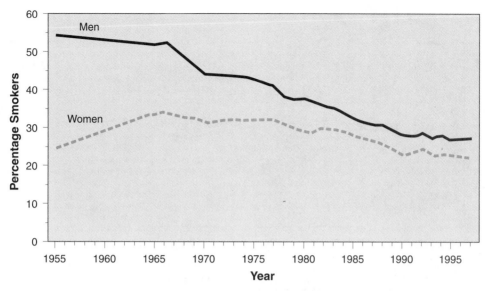

* Before 1992, current smokers were defined as persons who reported having smoked ≥100 cigarettes and who currently smoked. Since 1992, current smokers were defined as persons who reported having smoked ≥100 cigarettes during their lifetime and who reported now smoking every day or some days.

Figure 13-3 Trends in cigarette smoking* among persons aged 18 years and older, by sex—United States, 1955–1997.
Sources: 1955 Current Population Survey; 1965–1997 National Health Interview Survey. Morbidity and Mortality Weekly Report, 1994.

smaller decrease from 1978–1980 of 4.5% compared to the 7.5% decrease among white-collar employees (Nelson et al., 1994a). Among males, smoking prevalence by occupational groups (1987–1990) was highest for transportation operatives (41.6%), nontransportation operatives (40.9%), laborers (40.7%), and craftsmen/kindred workers (39.2%), with farmers and farm managers (18.2%) and professional and technical employees (18.5%) having the lowest rates. Similar patterns were seen for women. Among individual occupational categories, roofers (57.8%) and crane and tower operators (57.4%) and clergy (6.7%) and physicians (5.5%) were at either extreme (Nelson et al., 1994).

Many smokers have stopped. In 1997, almost half (48.0%) of persons who reported ever smoking indicated they were former smokers. The percentage of adults who never smoked increased from 44% in the mid 1960s to 55% in 1997. However, an increased prevalence of smoking has been found among college students (Wechsler et al., 1998), and the 18–25 age

cohort of smokers in 1997 showed a higher prevalence of smoking than in 1995, suggesting that this earlier trend of not ever starting to smoke may not be continuing (CDCP, 1999d).

As seen in Figure 13-4, the rates of smoking among young people declined from the late 1970s to the mid 1980s when the prevalence of smoking during the past month among 12th graders was approximately 30%. Since that time it has increased to 36.5% in 1997 (CDCP, 1999c). The rates are highest for Whites and lowest among Blacks. The 1997 Youth Risk Behavior Survey (grades 9–12) conducted by the Centers for Disease Control found the prevalence of using cigarettes in the past month to be 37.7% for males and 34.7% for females. Non-Hispanic African American youth had the lowest prevalence (22.7%) and non-Hispanic Whites, the highest (39.7%) (CDCP, 1998).

The overall prevalence of smokeless tobacco use among men aged 18 years and older in the U.S. from the 1992–1993 Current Population Survey was 4.0%,

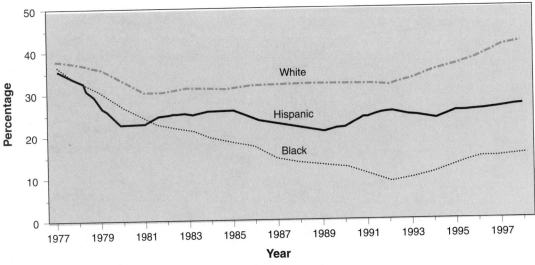

* Smoking is defined as having smoked on ≥1 of the 30 days before the survey.
† Two-year moving averages are used to stabilize estimates.

Figure 13-4 Trends in cigarette smoking among 12th graders, by racial/ethnic group—United States, 1977–1998.
Source: MMAAWR 11/5/99 pg. 990)

with a range of 0.1% in Connecticut to 15.6% in West Virginia (CDCP, 11/14/99d). In 1997, the prevalence in 17 states that assessed smokeless tobacco as part of the Behavioral Risk Factor Survey ranged, among men, from 2.6% in Arizona to 18.4% in West Virginia and, among women, from 0.1% in Virginia to 1.7% in Georgia (Cook et al., 1998). The prevalence of smokeless tobacco use is highest among high school males, with a prevalence of 20% among Whites, 6% among Hispanics, and 4% among Blacks. The prevalence of use varies geographically, with lowest rates in the northeast (CDCP, 1999c). Among youth in grades 9–12, the 1997 prevalence of using smokeless tobacco in the past month was 15.8% for males and 1.5% for females, with Whites having the highest prevalence (12.2%), followed by Hispanics (5.1%) and African-Americans (3.2%) (CDCP, 1998).

The total consumption of cigars was 8 million in 1970. This decreased to 2 million in 1993 but since then has shown a sharp upward trend, reaching 3.6 million in 1997 (CDCP, 1999c). The prevalence of current cigar smoking among men almost doubled from 1990 to 1996, reaching 8.8%. Among women, 1.1% re-

ported they regularly smoked cigars in 1996. The relationship of income and education to use of cigars is opposite to that for cigarette smoking. Among men, the prevalence of current cigar use increased with income and education, with 14.8% of men earning $75,000 and over and 11.4% of college graduates reporting current cigar use (Burns, 1998). In 1997, the proportion of youth in grades 9–12 who reporting using cigars in the past month was 31.2% for males and 10.8% for females, with non-Hispanic Whites having a prevalence of 22.5%, Hispanics, 20.3%, and African Americans, 19.4% (CDCP, 1998).

THE CONTEXT OF TOBACCO CONTROL

The context of tobacco control has changed radically since 1964, when the first Surgeon General's Report on Smoking and Health concluded that smoking was a cause of lung cancer in men and a suspected cause of lung cancer in women. Tobacco control includes the prevention and cessation of smoking and smokeless tobacco use and the restriction of second-hand smoke exposure. Table 13-3 outlines major tobacco

Table 13-3 Significant Events Related to Smoking and Health (1964–1999)

Year	Event
1964	Surgeon General's Report concludes that smoking is a cause of lung cancer in men and a suspected cause in women.
1965	Federal Cigarette Labeling and Advertising Act requires health warnings on all cigarette packages.
1967	Federal Communications Commission rules that the Fairness Doctrine applies to cigarette advertising and that stations broadcasting cigarette commercials must provide equal time to smoking prevention messages.
1970	Public Health Cigarette Smoking Act of 1969 passed, banning cigarette advertising on television and radio.
1972	Surgeon General's Report identifies involuntary (secondhand) smoking as a health risk.
1975	Minnesota enacts the first comprehensive clean indoor air act, restricting smoking in most buildings open to the public.
1977	American Cancer Society sponsors the first national "Great American Smokeout."
1980	Health Objectives for the Nation include a goal to reduce smoking to below 25% among adults by 1990.
1982	Congress temporarily doubles the federal excise tax on cigarettes to 16 cents per pack (extended permanently in 1986 and raised in subsequent years).
1984	Surgeon General's Report focuses on smoking and chronic obstructive lung disease.
	Food and Drug Administration approves nicotine polacrilex gum as a new drug.
1985	Surgeon General's Report covers smoking and occupational exposures.
	Minnesota enacts the first state legislation to earmark a portion of the state cigarette excise tax to support smoking prevention program.
1986	Surgeon General's Report focuses on the health consequences of involuntary (secondhand) smoking.
	Surgeon General's Report documents the health consequences of smokeless tobacco.
1988	Congress bans smoking on domestic airline flights scheduled for two hours or less (extended to six hours or less in 1990).
1991	National Institute for Occupational Safety and Health issues bulletin recommending that secondhand smoke be reduced to the lowest feasible concentration in the workplace.
	National Cancer Institute and American Cancer Society fund 17 states over seven years in the American Stop Smoking Intervention Study (ASSIST).
	Food and Drug Administration approves a nicotine patch as a prescription drug.
1993	Environmental Protection Agency (EPA) classifies environmental tobacco smoke (secondhand smoke) as a "Group A" carcinogen, and representatives of the tobacco industry file suit against the EPA.
1994	Occupational Safety and Health Administration announces proposed regulation to prohibit smoking in the workplace, except in separately ventilated areas.
	Mississippi becomes the first state to sue the tobacco industry to recover Medicaid costs for tobacco-related illnesses.
	Department of Defense (DOD) bans smoking in all DOD workplaces.
1996	The Department of Transportation reports that about 80% of nonstop scheduled U.S. airline flights between the US and foreign points will be smokefree by June 1, 1996.
	FDA approves nicotine gum and two nicotine patches for over-the-counter sale.
1998	The tobacco industry agrees to a 46-state Masters Settlement Agreement, the largest settlement in history, nearly $206 billion.

Source: Adapted from CDC's TIPS – Chronological Review on Smoking 1964-96; Achievements in Public Health: Tobacco Use—United States, 1900-1999.

Table 13-4 Healthy People 2010 Objectives for Tobacco Use from Draft Documents

Objective	1997 Baseline	2010 Target
Tobacco Use in Population Groups		
1. Reduce tobacco use by adults		
a. Cigarette smoking	24%	12%
b. Spit tobacco		Developmental
c. Cigars		Developmental
d. Other products		Developmental
2. Reduce tobacco use by adolescents		
a. Tobacco products	43%	21%
b. Cigarettes	36%	16%
c. Spit tobacco	9%	1%
d. Cigars	22%	8%
3. Reduce initiation of tobacco use among children and adolescents		Developmental
4. Increase the average age of first use of tobacco products by adolescents and young adults.		
a. Adolescents aged 12 to 17 years	12 years	14 years
b. Young adults aged 18 to 25 years	15 years	17 years
Cessation and Treatment		
5. Increase smoking cessation attempts by adult smokers.	43%	75%
6. Increase smoking cessation during pregnancy.	12%	30%
7. Increase tobacco use cessation attempts by adolescent smokers.	73%	84%
8. Increase insurance coverage of evidence-based treatment for nicotine dependency.		
a. Managed care organizations	75%	100%
b. Medicaid programs in states and the District of Columbia	24 states/DC	51 states/DC
c. All insurance		Developmental
Exposure to Secondhand Smoke		
9. Reduce the proportion of children who are regularly exposed to tobacco smoke at home.	27%	10%
10. Reduce the proportion of nonsmokers exposed to environmental tobacco smoke.	65%	45%
11. Increase smoke-free and tobacco-free environments in schools, including all school facilities, property, vehicles, and school events.	37%	100%
12. Increase the proportion of worksites with 50 or more employees with formal smoking policies that prohibit smoking or limit it to separately ventilated areas.	79%	100%

control measures relevant to smoking among adults undertaken since 1964. The following discussion of the context of tobacco control in the U.S. is based primarily on this table, which was drawn from the Center for Disease Control's Tobacco Information and Prevention Source (CDCP, 1999a, 1999b).

The initial response to the first Surgeon General's Report was a requirement for health warnings on all cigarette packages, which was subsequently strengthened. The 1967 Fairness Doctrine required equal time for smoking prevention messages and cigarette commercials, and this counteradvertising was associated

Table 13-4 Healthy People 2010 Objectives for Tobacco Use from Draft Documents—*continued*

Objective	1997 Baseline	2010 Target
Exposure to Secondhand Smoke (continued)		
13. Establish laws on smoke-free indoor air that prohibit smoking or limit it to separately ventilated areas in public places and worksites (States and the District of Columbia)		
a. Private workplaces	1	51
b. Public workplaces	13	51
c. Restaurants	3	51
d. Public transportation	16	51
e. Day care centers	22	51
f. Retail stores	4	51
g. Tribes		Developmental
h. Territories		Developmental
Social and Environmental Changes		
14. Reduce the illegal buy rate among minors through enforcement of laws prohibiting the sale of tobacco products to minors. (Jurisdictions with a 5% or less illegal buy rate among minors.)		
a. States and the District of Columbia	0	51
b. Territories	0	All
15. Increase the number of States and the District of Columbia that suspend or revoke state retail licenses for violations of laws prohibiting the sale of tobacco to minors.	34	51
16. Eliminate tobacco advertising and promotions that influence adolescents and young adults.		Developmental
17. Increase adolescents' disapproval of smoking.		
a. 8th grade	80%	95%
b. 10th grade	75%	95%
c. 12th grade	69%	95%
18. Increase the number of Tribes, Territories, and States and the District of Columbia with comprehensive, evidence-based tobacco control programs.		Developmental
19. Eliminate laws that preempt stronger tobacco control laws.	30	0
20. Reduce the toxicity of tobacco products by establishing a regulatory structure to monitor toxicity.		Developmental
21. Increase the average federal and state tax on tobacco products.		
a. Cigarettes	$0.63	$2.00
b. Spit tobacco	$0.27	$2.00

with a downturn in tobacco consumption. However, in 1970, federal law banned cigarette advertising on television and radio.

The Health Objectives for the Nation, published in 1980, included a goal to reduce tobacco use to below 25% among adults by 1990. There are 24 tobacco use objectives and 28 related objectives from other focus areas in the Year 2010 objectives (see Table 13-4). The tobacco use objective categories are tobacco use in population groups, cessation and treatment, exposure to secondhand smoke, and social and environmental changes. The 2010 goal for tobacco use is to

"Reduce disease, disability, and death related to tobacco use and exposure to secondhand smoke" (US-DHHS, 2000, p.).

The federal excise tax on cigarettes was doubled in 1982 to 16 cents per pack and, as of the end of 1998, was 24 cents per pack. At the end of 1998, all states had an excise tax on cigarettes, with an average tax of 38.9 cents per pack and a range of 2.5 cents per pack in Virginia to one dollar per pack in Alaska and Hawaii. Fewer states (42) have an excise tax on smokeless tobacco products, and the rate is often lower than that for cigarettes (CDCP, 1999a).

In 1985, Minnesota became the first state to earmark a portion of the state cigarette excise tax to support smoking prevention programs. In 1988 California voters passed Proposition 99, a referendum raising the state cigarette tax by 25 cents per pack with 20% of tax revenues earmarked for tobacco control. Other states to enact similar legislation were Massachusetts (1992), Arizona (1994), and Oregon (1996) (CDCP, 1999d; CDCP, 7/30/00e). In California per capita consumption of cigarettes decreased by over 50%, from 126.6 packs in the 1987-88 fiscal year when Proposition 99 was passed to 61.3 packs in the 1998-99 fiscal year (California Department of Health Services, 2000). In Oregon cigarette consumption was decreased by 11.3% in the two years following passage of their voter initiative to increase cigarette excise tax (CDCP, 2000). The reduction of smoking initiation among adolescents, however, has remained an elusive goal (Siegel and Biener, 1997).

Efforts to increase tobacco prevention and control programming to other states include the American Stop Smoking Intervention Study (ASSIST) of the National Cancer Institute and the American Cancer Society, which has provided funding to 17 states, beginning in 1991. In 1994, the Robert Wood Johnson Foundation and the American Medical Association began the "SmokeLess States" grant program to fund local initiatives for tobacco use prevention.

State tobacco control efforts should escalate dramatically with the settlements of lawsuits by the tobacco industry to recover Medicaid costs for tobacco-related illnesses. Mississippi was the first state to sue the tobacco industry in 1994, followed by Texas, Minnesota, and Florida. These states settled individually with the tobacco industry. Then in 1998, the industry, though admitting no wrongdoing, agreed to a 46-state Masters Settlement Agreement for a total of $246 billion. The impact of this settlement on tobacco control among states is not clear at this time. The agreement did not require that this money be used for tobacco use prevention and control. State legislatures are responsible for allocating the settlement dollars, and this money is being used to fund many things, including state indigent health care costs, capital construction projects, and educational funding, as well as tobacco prevention and control. A national foundation, The American Legacy Foundation, was funded to implement nationwide advertising and educational programs and to conduct studies related to reducing youth tobacco use (CDCP, 11/14/99a; National Governor's Association; Campaign for Tobacco Free Kids).

During this time period, the treatment of nicotine addiction has become both more effective and more accessible to the public. Pharmacotherapy coupled with behavioral therapy has become the standard of care for nicotine addiction (see discussion later in this chapter) (Fiore et al., 1996, 2000). In 1984, the Food and Drug Administration approved nicotine gum as a prescription drug, and this was followed by the nicotine patch in 1991. In 1996, nicotine gum and two nicotine patches were approved for over-the-counter sale. This policy change has made it possible for behavior therapists, cessation program facilitators, and the general public to use nicotine replacement therapy as a treatment component.

The other major thread of tobacco policy relevant to adult tobacco exposure and use has been clean air policy. The 1972 Surgeon General's Report identified involuntary, or secondhand, smoke as a health risk. In 1985 the Surgeon General's Report covered smoking and occupational exposures, and the 1986 Surgeon General's Report focused on the health consequences of involuntary smoking. In 1991, the National Institute for Occupational Safety and Health issued a bulletin recommending that involuntary smoke be reduced to the lowest feasible concentration in the workplace. Involuntary smoke became viewed as an environmental issue, and, in 1993, the Environmental Protection Agency classified environmental tobacco smoke (secondhand smoke, or involuntary smoking) as a group A (known human) carcinogen; in 1994 the Occupational Safety and Health Administration proposed regulations (not made final at the time of this writing) to prohibit smoking in the workplace, except in separately ventilated areas.

Minnesota enacted the first comprehensive clean air act in 1985. The U.S. Department of Health and Human Services banned smoking in its facilities in 1987. Smoking was banned on short domestic airline flights in 1988, on flights of six hours or less duration in 1990, and on most U.S. international flights in 1996. The Department of Defense banned smoking in its worksites in 1994. By 1998, 20 states and the District of Columbia had limited smoking in private worksites, although only one state had eliminated exposure to ETS by either banning smoking or limiting it to separately ventilated areas; 41 states and the District of Columbia had laws restricting smoking in state government worksites, with 13 eliminating exposure to ETS (CDCP, 1999a).

Figure 13-5 shows the relationship between adult cigarette consumption and major smoking and health events from 1900–1998. Cigarette consumption rose

relatively steadily until the First Surgeon General's Report on Smoking and Health, decreasing significantly with the Fairness Doctrine antitobacco messages on television, then increasing slightly and beginning a decline that has continued up until the present time.

THE WORKSITE AND TOBACCO CONTROL

Workplaces have been concerned with tobacco control for a variety of reasons. The rapidly increasing costs of health insurance over the past two decades led companies to explore ways to reduce the demand for health care services by employees. Studies showed that smoking employees had excess illness costs (Sofian, McAfee, Doctor, & Carson, 1994; Bertera, 1991; Kirstein, 1983). Increasing productivity to keep pace in the global economy was another concern of industry (Deming, 1982), and smoking was associated with increased absenteeism and reduced productivity (Bertera, 1991; Korsak, 1977; Kirstein, 1983; Weiss, 1983). Warner and colleagues (1996) used a simulation model to examine the economic implications of a worksite cessation program. Using current

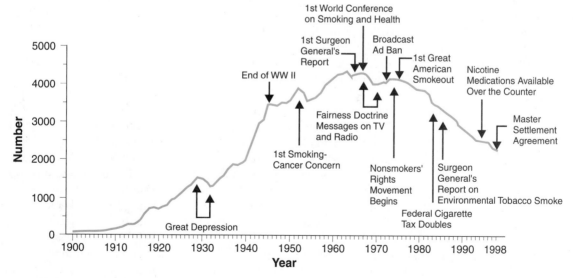

Figure 13-5 Annual adult per capita cigarette consumption and major smoking and health events—United States, 1900–1998 (MMWR 12/5/99, pg 986).

Sources: United States Department of Agriculture; 1986 Surgeon General's Report.

data for the background quit rate, participation and cessation rates of programs, absenteeism, on-the-job productivity, employee turnover rates, and health effects of smoking, they found a positive benefit/cost ratio of 1.75 beginning in Year 5 after the program began that increased to 8.89 after 25 years.

Prior to the late 1980s, the primary reason for restricting smoking at the worksite was for safety of the worker, workplace, and product (e.g., around natural gas or oxygen), or to protect equipment. When research indicated that environmental tobacco smoke was detrimental to the health of those exposed to it, employees began to organize for restrictions on smoking at the worksite. With the EPA ruling that environmental tobacco smoke was carcinogenic, ETS became a major risk and liability issue for worksites, and smoke-free policies became the norm (USDHHS, 1986). The proportion of worksites with restrictive tobacco policies increased from 27% in 1985 to 59% in 1992 and 79% in 1999 (Association for Worksite Health Promotion, USDHHS, & William M. Mercer, Inc., 2000; USDHHS, 1993). In a nationwide household survey conducted in 1992–1993, 81.6% of indoor workers reported that their worksite restricted smoking, with 46.0% reporting their worksite was smoke-free (Gerlach, Shopland, Hartman, Gibson, & Pechacek, 1997). Service workers (34.8%) and blue-collar workers (27.4%) were much less likely to work in a smoke-free site than white-collar workers (53.7%). Workers aged 15–19 (32.1%) and those 20–24 (40.9%) were less likely than other workers to report working in a smoke-free environment (Lerlach et al., 1997).

Hospitals have been the only industry to ban tobacco nationwide, although specific fast-food restaurants have banned smoking and nonsmoking rooms are widely available in motels and hotels (Brownson, Eriksen, Davis, & Warner, 1997). The Joint Commission on Accreditation of Healthcare Organizations (JCAHO) required hospitals to ban smoking in hospital buildings by December 31, 1993, and a 1994 survey found that 96% of hospitals were in compliance, with 41.4% having enacted policies that were more restrictive than that required by the JCAHO. The four most important influences in the decision to go smoke-free were the JCAHO requirement, concern for employee health, public image, and fire safety (Longo et al., 1998).

Another trend in the workplace has been the replacement of fee-for-service health insurance for managed care, which covered over 85% of enrollees among medium and large employers in 1998 (Levitt, Lundy, and Srinivasan, 1998). Assessment of tobacco use and counseling for cessation are key clinical preventive services (USDHHS, 1994), and guidelines were developed by the Agency for Health Care Policy Research (now Agency for Health Care Research and Quality) (Fiore et al., 1996) and recently revised by a consortium of seven federal government and nonprofit organizations (Fiore et al., 2000). The prevalence of assessment of tobacco use is an indicator for the Health Plan Employer Data and Information Set (National Committee for Quality Assurance, 1997). This system is a "report card" that managed care organizations have agreed upon and by which they can be judged by employers. In 1996, 61% of managed care participants received advice to quit from a plan provider (USDHHS, 2000). Benefits managers within worksites should be sure that the managed care organizations with whom they contract have effective tobacco interventions.

Tobacco control is a key component of a comprehensive worksite health promotion program. These programs address a variety of risk and wellness behaviors, several of which, such as stress management, fitness, and nutrition, are supportive of tobacco cessation (O'Donnell, 1994a, 1994b). From a programming perspective, there is more interest among employees in multicomponent programs, especially as the proportion of smokers in a worksite's program decreases.

As community tobacco control efforts increase, companies should link employees to resources in the community such as quit lines, media campaigns, and print interventions, in addition to the already-mentioned counseling within the health care system. For example, the Great American SmokeOut (GASO), a community-wide campaign sponsored by the American Cancer Society (ACS), was begun in 1977. Focused on the worksite with its potential for coworker support, the aim of the SmokeOut is to have smokers quit for a day with the assistance of a buddy. In 1998, an estimated 9 million persons participated in GASO community activities by either smoking less or not at all for 24 hours (CDCP, 1999b). Some divisions of ACS have informally added the goal of tobacco use prevention by youth. In worksites, this might include such activities as coloring contests for children of employees and materials on how to talk with your children about tobacco.

CESSATION INTERVENTIONS

Stages of Change

Behavior change is not an all-or-none event but instead proceeds in stages that include motivational readiness as well as behavioral action. In the first stage, precontemplation, the tobacco user has no intention of quitting in the next six months. In the contemplation stage, the user is seriously considering quitting in the next six months. In the preparation stage, the tobacco user intends to quit within the immediate future (i.e., the next month). The action stage begins with quitting and extends for six months. It is during this period that the individual is at greatest risk for relapse. The maintenance stage begins after the tobacco user has quit for six months and still involves efforts to prevent relapse and to maintain nonuse; it has been estimated to last for five years for smoking. Relapse is the return from action or maintenance to an earlier phase, with the majority returning to contemplation or preparation (Prochaska, Redding, & Evers, 1997; Prochaska & Velicer, 1997).

Based on a number of studies across a variety of behaviors, including smoking, the proportion of the population at-risk in the precontemplation stage has been estimated to be 40%, with 40% in contemplation and 20% in preparation. Most of the programming, however, has been directed toward the 20% who are making plans to quit, using self-help, counseling, or group approaches. We will discuss the behavioral processes used in successful cessation (i.e., movement from preparation into action) in the section following this one. The preparation stage involves a strong commitment to change and belief that one can change the behavior (self-efficacy). The processes of change during action include contingency management, helping relationships, counterconditioning, and stimulus control. (Prochaska & Velicer, 1997)

In this section, we will discuss movement from precontemplation to contemplation and from contemplation to preparation. The pros of changing the behavior are the benefits of changing, and the cons of changing are the costs of changing. For movement out of precontemplation, the pros must increase; for movement out of contemplation the cons must decrease. Experiential processes are important and provide motivation to change. For precontemplators, consciousness-raising about ones' tobacco habit, its effects on oneself and others, and the feelings of fear and anxiety that go with the behavioral risk are key to movement to contemplation. For contemplators, who are considering quitting, self-reevaluation of their self-image with and without tobacco use and how tobacco use fits with their core values will help move them to prepare for quitting. Interventions based on these processes include media campaigns, personal testimonies, factual information, confrontation, values clarification, and personal resolution (Prochaska, Redding, & Evers, 1997).

Components of Cessation Programs and their Effectiveness

In this section, we turn to the cessation programs designed for the tobacco user in the action stage. We will concentrate on interventions for smoking cessation because cigarette smoking is the most prevalent form of tobacco use and by far the most outcomes research has been conducted on smoking cessation interventions. However, the USDHHS Public Health Service-sponsored Clinical Practice Guideline recommends that users of smokeless tobacco should be encouraged to quit and treated with the same psychosocial cessation interventions recommended for smokers (Fiore et al., 2000). Insufficient evidence was found for the use of pharmacological treatments, although nicotine replacement may be useful for smokeless tobacco cessation (Fiore et al., 1996).

Methods for smoking cessation must address the determinants of smoking and quitting. Psychological, social, and economic factors interact with biological factors to determine tobacco use, and these must be addressed in cessation efforts (Fisher, Lichtenstein, Haire-Joshu, Morgan, & Rehberg, 1993). There are two basic categories of methods for smoking cessation: behavioral counseling/education and nicotine replacement therapy. They have been shown to have additive effects, and a combined approach is clearly preferable to either alone (Fiore et al., 2000; Schwartz, 1987; USDHHS, 1988; Wetter et al., 1998). They may be delivered through a variety of channels, including group cessation clinics, physician counseling, telephone quit lines, self-help video and bibliotherapy. These intervention programs should be viewed, however, in the overall context of community tobacco control, in which social norms and regulation controlling access, cost, and restrictions on tobacco use provide powerful influences for tobacco use onset and cessation.

Table 13-5 provides key methods and principles underlying effective smoking cessation interventions. The first phase of a cessation program, preparation for quitting, begins with the mobilization of client motivation and commitment. Clients review reasons for quitting and the benefits of cessation. Incentive systems contingent on clinic attendance, cessation, or both may be established. Records of number of cigarettes smoked and the circumstances in which the smoking occurred (e.g., time, place, persons present, and feelings) are kept in order to identify patterns of smoking and, as part of self-management training, to discover the client's typical cues for smoking. Clients then set a quit date, ideally within two weeks. Planning ahead for that date allows the smoker to develop plans for coping with situations that might provoke relapse and builds commitment. Quitting abruptly, or "cold turkey," appears to be more effective than gradual withdrawal, which has been found to prolong the period of urges to relapse. Self-management training includes identification of individuals' cues for smoking, the identification of substitutes for smoking and alternative nonsmoking behaviors, and stress management training (e.g., relaxation or physical activity). To mobilize social support outside of the treatment setting, the client can practice identifying supportive individuals and requesting their assistance. (Edmundson, McAlister, Murray, Perry, & Lichtenstein, 1991; Fiore et al., 1996, 2000; Fisher et al., 1993).

The second phase, quitting, includes extinguishing conditioned cravings to smoke by the clients' avoiding smoking in response to their typical cues for smoking. Aversive conditioning procedures may be used to reduce the attractiveness of smoking or to make cigarette smoke itself aversive. Rapid smoking, inhaling every 6–8 seconds in the clinic until nausea is imminent, and satiation, doubling or tripling the rate of at-home smoking, have been found to increase cessation rates. However, because these techniques can pose a health risk in some persons and clients require monitoring during treatment, they have not been widely used. (Edmundson et al., 1991; Fiore et al., 1996, 2000; Fisher et al., 1993.)

Nicotine replacement methods should be initiated on the client's quit day and as indicated. Precautions should be taken, however, with pregnant smokers and with patients with cardiovascular diseases. For first-line pharmacotherapy, the Public Health Service (PHS)-sponsored Tobacco Cessation Guideline (Fiore et al., 2000) recommends (without rank-order) five Federal Drug Administration (FDA)-approved pharmacotherapies for smoking cessation: buproprion SR, nicotine gum, nicotine inhaler, nicotine nasal spray,

Table 13-5 Phases and Methods in Tobacco Cessation Programs

Preparation
- Building motivation
- Self-monitoring
- Setting a quit date / going cold turkey
- Self-management training

Quitting
- Extinguishing conditioned responses
- Aversive conditioning
- Pharmacotherapy

Maintenance
- Coping skills training
- Social support
- Follow-up sessions or phone calls
- Weight, diet, or nutrition management
- Exercise or fitness programming
- Pharmacotherapy

Sources: E. B. Fisher et al., *Annual Review of Medicine*, 1993; D. W. Wetter et al., *American Psychologist*, 1998; and Edmundson E., McAlister A., Murray D., Perry C., and Lichtenstein E. (1991).

and the nicotine patch. Two second-line pharmacotherapies, clonidine and nortriptyline, have not been approved by the FDA for tobacco dependence treatment but may be used, under a physician's direction, with patients for whom the first-line medications are contraindicated or for patients who have been unable to quit with first-line medications (Fiore et al., 2000).

Of over-the-counter medications, both the 16- and 24-hour nicotine patch and nicotine gum have been shown to be effective. Patch therapy has been associated with higher compliance (a new patch is placed each day on a relatively hairless location between the neck and waist) and requires less training by the clinician or facilitator than the gum (which is to be intermittently chewed and "parked" between the cheek and gum for 30 minutes, using at least one piece every 1–2 hours). However, clients may prefer the gum or have previously failed with the patch. About 15–20% of successful abstainers have been found to use the gum a year or longer. Although weaning should be encouraged, the continued use of the patch or gum is preferable to a return to smoking, as the nicotine replacement products do not contain non–nicotine toxic substances, produce strong surges in blood nicotine level, or produce strong dependence (Fiore et al., 1996, 2000).

Along with pharmacotherapy, a number of behavioral strategies are important for maintenance of cessation. Coping skills training includes transferring the self-management skills to maintenance by avoiding cues to smoke and using substitutes and other behaviors (such as deep breathing, cinnamon sticks, and water) instead of smoking in the presence of cues and urges to smoke. Anticipating high-risk situations and planning coping strategies for dealing with these situations are an important component of coping skills training. Other relapse prevention skills include coping with slips or lapses so that they do not become full relapses but merely mistakes from which the individual can learn. Social support for quitting can come from professionals and from family and friends in the smoker's environment. Developing buddy systems and involving significant others can be part of the cessation program (Curry & McBride, 1994; Fiore et al., 1996, 2000).

Follow-up sessions and phone calls can provide social support, encouragement, and assistance with coping skills for high-risk situations. Especially for clients with concern about weight gain with cessation, weight control training, diet management, and physical activity programs may be helpful. The latter may also assist with tension relief and anxiety. However, the evidence of effectiveness for these modalities is lacking. In fact, the PHS-sponsored Guideline suggests that smokers should not engage in strict dieting to counteract weight gain during a quit attempt until they are confident they will not return to smoking and that nicotine gum may be used to delay weight gain (Curry & McBride, 1994; Edmundson et al., 1991; Fiore et al., 1996, 2000).

The PHS-sponsored Tobacco Cessation Guideline did not recommend acupuncture based on five studies and did not reexamine hypnosis, which had been found in an independent review by the Cochrane Group to have insufficient evidence to be supported as a treatment for smoking cessation (Abbot, Stead, White, & Ernst, 1999). Stepped care for treatment delivery and individually tailored interventions using the transtheoretical model were not recommended in the Guideline due to insufficient data. Additional research will be required to establish efficacy of these behavioral treatments (Fiore, 2000).

The discussion above has been based in large part on the Public Health Service-sponsored Tobacco Cessation Guideline published in 2000, which was based on reviews of approximately 6,000 randomized trials of tobacco-use cessation interventions (Fiore et al., 2000). The primary audiences of the guideline are primary care clinicians, smoking cessation specialists, and health care administrators, insurers, and purchasers. Although the guideline was designed for health care settings, the findings provide information for cessation interventions in other settings. The findings should be considered along with those presented next for worksite cessation programs. The recommendations for health care provider practice and insurance coverage are also important for worksites as they should be considered in company contracts with managed care organizations and coordinated planning of on-site and health care smoking cessation activities.

The meta-analyses conducted for the PHS-Sponsored Tobacco Cessation Guideline found individual counseling (estimated abstinence rate of 16.8%) to be more effective than group (13.9%) or proactive telephone counseling (13.1%) or self-help programs (12.3%), which had a small but significant effect compared to no intervention (10.8%). Increasing the number of these counseling formats being used for a single individual had a dose-response effect, from an estimated abstinence rate of 15.1% (one format), to 18.5% (two formats), to 23.2% (for three or four formats). Although minimal contact sessions (lasting less than 3 minutes) increase cessation rates over no-treatment controls (estimated abstinence rate of 13.4% vs. 10.9%), a strong dose-response relationship was found between counseling intensity and success, with rates of 16.0% for 3–10 minutes of counseling and 22.1% for sessions lasting more than 10 minutes. In terms of number of person-to-person treatment sessions, the rates increased from 12.4% for 0–1 sessions, to 16.3% for 2–3 sessions, 20.9% for 4–8 sessions, and 24.7% for greater than 8 sessions. Nicotine replacement therapy or sustained release (SR) buproprion was recommended for all patients except those for whom this would be a health risk. Rates compared to placebo were 30.5% versus 17.3% for bupropion SR, 23.7% versus 17.1% for nicotine gum, 22.8% versus 10.5% for the nicotine inhaler, 30.5% versus 13.9% for nicotine nasal spray, and 17.7% versus 10.0% for the nicotine patch. The most effective types of counseling and behavioral therapy were rapid smoking (19.9% estimated abstinence rate), other aversive smoking (17.7%), general problem solving (16.2%), and extra-treatment social support (16.2%) (Fiore et al., 2000).

In addition to the recommendations regarding type and content of cessation interventions, the Guideline recommends that clinicians should routinely assess the smoking status of all patients and intervene with every patient who smokes and that smoking cessation counseling and pharmacotherapy should be provided as paid services for subscribers of health insurers/managed care (Fiore et al., 2000).

Effectiveness of Worksite Smoking Cessation Interventions

Fisher and colleagues (1990) conducted a meta-analysis of long term (over 12 months) quit rates from 20 controlled cessation trials at worksites. The weighted average follow-up quit rate over all interventions was 13%. Interventions that lasted from 2–6 hours (18%), that involved the use of some employee time as well as work time (18%), that were from smaller (100–249 employees) worksites (16.5%), and that included heavier smokers (16%) had the largest estimated quit rates.

A review by Eriksen and Gottlieb (1998) of 52 evaluations of smoking cessation programs between 1968–1994 found group programs to be more effective than minimal treatment programs. The 37 group interventions had a median cessation rate of 23% compared to 10.1% for the 19 minimal programs, the majority of which were self-help manual-based interventions. Seven studies of competitions showed high participation rates, with a median of 47%, and large cessation rates (median 65%). Five studies using incentives for cessation showed a median participation rate of 26% and a median quit rate of 20%. In each of these categories, however, better-controlled studies and those that used the worksite as the unit of analysis showed lower cessation rates. The quality of the research methodology for this worksite cessation literature was rated suggestive for group and incentive interventions, indicative for minimal interventions, competitions, and medical interventions, and acceptable for the testing of treatment components.

Heaney and Goetzel (1997) reviewed the outcomes of multicomponent worksite health promotion programs published between 1978 and 1996. Smoking was included as an outcome in the majority of the studies included. Decreases in smoking were found for 12 of the 19 studies that examined smoking as a specific outcome. The authors concluded that programs that provided behavioral counseling along with worksite-wide programming were most likely to provide changes in health behaviors, particularly smoking and diet.

Worksite Smoking Policies

There are two basic types of worksite smoking policies. Smoke-free policies prohibit smoking in company facilities and vehicles and can be extended to include the property or grounds of the employer. Alternatively, policies may limit smoking to separately ventilated smoking rooms. Although both types of policies comply with most laws and ordinances, smoke-free policies have several important advantages. They greatly reduce ETS exposure for all employees, provide the best health and safety benefits for employees, may reduce the number of cigarettes smoked and encourage smokers to quit, decrease maintenance costs, are easier to administer and enforce, and have a low implementation cost. These policies require smokers to alter their behavior and may be inconvenient for smokers. If not properly managed, smokers may be disproportionately absent from their work stations. On the other hand, separately ventilated areas allow smokers to continue to smoke, while reducing nonsmokers' exposure to ETS. However, they may have adverse effects on smokers' health, often require expensive modification to buildings, and may not adequately protect nonsmokers from ETS exposure (CDCP, Wellness Council of America, American Cancer Society, n.d.).

Seven components have been recommended by experts for inclusion in a smoking policy: a) the purpose for the policy (harmful effects of ETS on health); b) a tie between the ETS policy and both cessation support and recognizable corporate values; c) a clear statement of where smoking is prohibited; d) a clear statement of where smoking is permitted (if anywhere); e) a clear statement on enforcement and consequences of noncompliance; f) a clear statement of support to be provided for employees who smoke; and g) the name and phone number of a person who can answer questions about the policy. Other tobacco products, such as chewing tobacco and snuff, may also be handled in the policy if these products are used by employees. However, this will require a different rationale than protection of employees from ETS, such as the impact on consumers and on young people (as in

professional baseball) (CDCP, Wellness Council of America, American Cancer Society, n.d.).

In a review of 29 studies conducted between 1983 and 1994 of the effect of worksite restrictive smoking policies, Eriksen and Gottlieb (1998) found consistent evidence of a reduction in cigarette consumption at work, with a median reduction of 3.4 cigarettes per day. The results were less consistent regarding whether there was a decrease in overall cigarette consumption, with 12 of the 29 studies reporting some decrease and 3 reporting either no decrease or an increase. The evidence for a decrease in smoking prevalence was inconclusive. Half of the 14 studies that examined it found no change, and the six that did find a change showed a median prevalence decrease of 5%. Lower levels of environmental nicotine vapor and salivary cotinine levels of nonsmokers were found in worksites with bans than with restrictoins or no policy, as were self-reports of increased air quality and decreased exposure to smoke (Eriksen & Gottlieb, 1998). Chapman and colleagues (1999) calculated the impact of smoke-free policies on tobacco consumption in Australia and in the United States, and then extrapolated to the impact if workplaces were universally smoke-free. They concluded that smoke-free workplaces are currently responsible for a 1.8% decrease in cigarette consumption in Australia (602 million cigarettes) and 2% in the United States (9.7 billion cigarettes). They suggested that if all worksites were smoke-free, the percentages would increase to 3.4% in Australia (1.14 billion cigarettes) and 4.1% in the United States (20.9 billion cigarettes).

An Ecological Approach to Tobacco Control Programming

Figure 13-6 provides an ecological view of tobacco control, in which individuals and their smoking behavior are embedded within groups which in turn are embedded within organizations, community, and government. Each of the higher levels can shape the levels below them and in turn be influenced by them. For example, a government's clean air act will influence norms for smoking within a community,

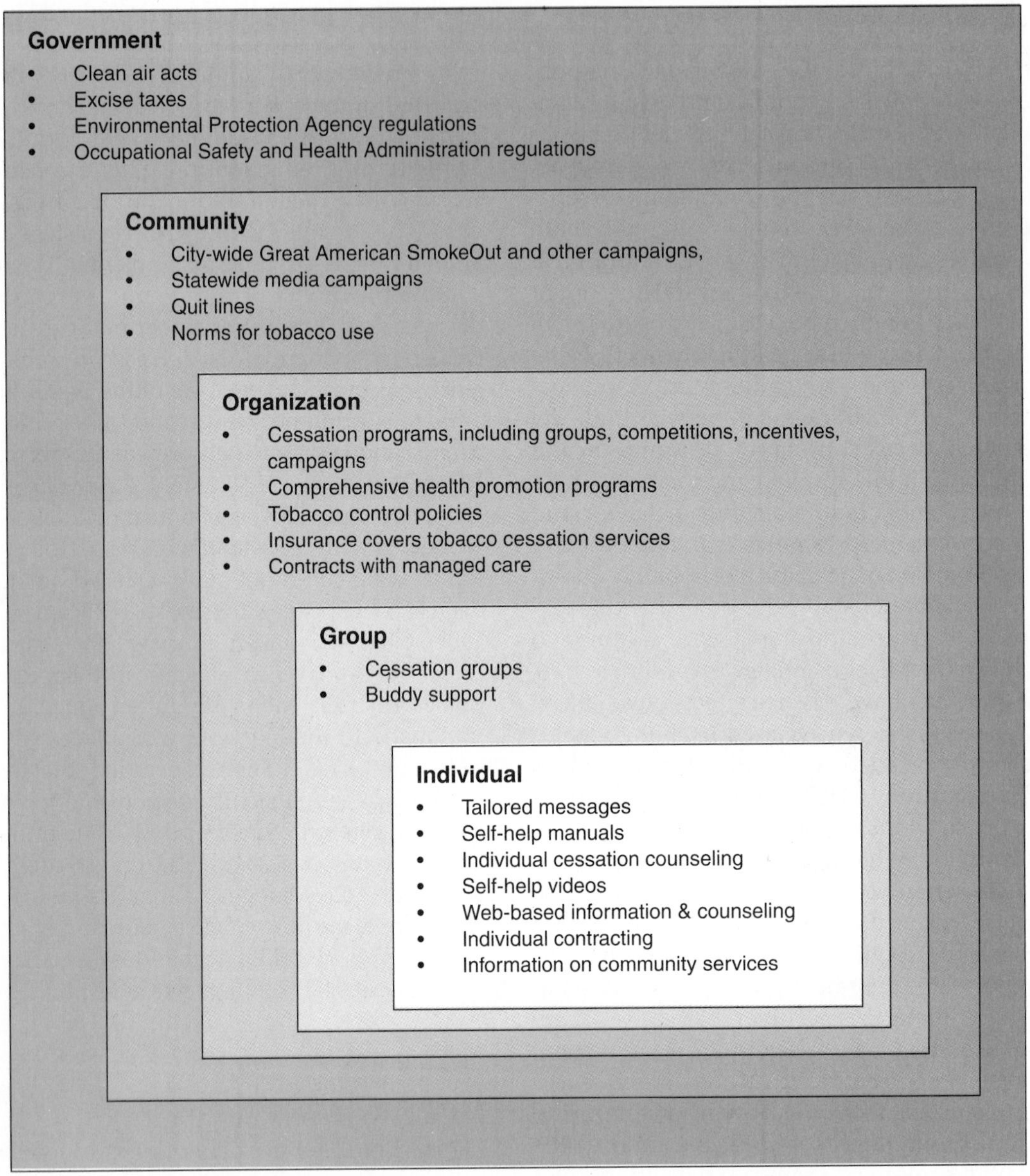

Government
- Clean air acts
- Excise taxes
- Environmental Protection Agency regulations
- Occupational Safety and Health Administration regulations

Community
- City-wide Great American SmokeOut and other campaigns,
- Statewide media campaigns
- Quit lines
- Norms for tobacco use

Organization
- Cessation programs, including groups, competitions, incentives, campaigns
- Comprehensive health promotion programs
- Tobacco control policies
- Insurance covers tobacco cessation services
- Contracts with managed care

Group
- Cessation groups
- Buddy support

Individual
- Tailored messages
- Self-help manuals
- Individual cessation counseling
- Self-help videos
- Web-based information & counseling
- Individual contracting
- Information on community services

Figure 13-6 Ecological approach to tobacco control programming.

whether smoking is prohibited in restaurants and worksites, and individual smoking behavior. Individuals, voluntary health agencies, and corporate political action committees may all influence whether legislators vote for clean air legislation. Worksite health promotion and tobacco cessation programming and tobacco control policies are important determinants of employee smoking cessation and restriction of smoking.

From the standpoint of a worksite health promotion coordinator who wishes to develop a sound tobacco control program, the first step is to conduct needs and assets assessments at each of the ecological levels diagrammed in Figure 13-6, with a specific focus on employees at the worksite organization. Suggestions for indicators in such an assessment are included in Table 13-6. At the employee level, it is important to know the prevalence of use of cigarettes, smokeless tobacco, cigars, and pipes; the stage of change for each of the tobacco use behaviors a person has; and, if the user is interested in quitting, his or her preference for quitting method. This can be obtained through an expanded health risk appraisal or an employee questionnaire.

At the organizational level, existing documents related to the policies for tobacco use should be examined and observation made of where employees and visitors currently smoke at the worksite. Specific places for smoking to be allowed/prohibited and observed include in offices, in designated smoking rooms, in other places inside the buildings, just outside the front door, in the parking lot, in designated smoking areas outside, in vehicles, and in other places outside (CDCP, Wellness Council of America, American Cancer Society, n.d.). The health benefits contract should be analyzed to see if tobacco cessation services are covered, and managed care contracts should be queried concerning the rate of tobacco assessment by their health care providers in the Health Plan Employer Data and Information Set (HEDIS) and what cessation interventions they offer to subscribers. Cessation interventions currently offered by the company should be analyzed for effectiveness, using expert reviews (including the PHS-sponsored Tobacco Cessation Guideline [Fiore et al., 2000]) and participation levels. A culture audit of "how we do

Table 13-6 Needs and Assets Assessment for Worksite Tobacco Programming

Individual
- Tobacco (all types) prevalence
- Proportion of tobacco users at each stage of change
- Tobacco users' preference for quitting method/program

Organization
- Tobacco policies
- Benefits coverage of tobacco cessation
- Managed care contractors' rates of assessment and counseling for smoking
- Managed care contractors' tobacco cessation offerings
- Organizational culture related to tobacco
- National prevalence within occupation/industry

Community
- Anti-tobacco media
- Cessation campaigns, such as the Great American SmokeOut
- Cessation resources, including quit lines, cessation programs of voluntary agencies and other private entities
- Campaign to establish smoke-free worksites
- Tobacco-related activities in other sectors, including schools and health care
- Norms for tobacco use

Government
- Local, state, and national laws and regulations related to tobacco use and their enforcement

things here" (e.g., "At our company, people don't smoke" or "At our company, smokers get together for breaks outside the building") could provide information about what is expected of employees regarding smoking (Allen & Bellingham, 1994). Norms differ within industries, measured by the prevalence rates for smoking among different occupations (Nelson et al., 1994a). For example, in the gas pipeline industry, smokeless tobacco use is more prevalent than in the general population, probably because of safety issues and longstanding restrictive smoking policies (Gottlieb, Weinstein, Baun, & Bernacki, 1992).

It is in the community and government levels that much of the tobacco control activity supported by the tobacco settlement monies and other national initiatives will be taking place, and it is important to link individual worksite programming to these resources. States and other governmental and nongovernmental organizations will be offering various tobacco prevention and control interventions, including telephone quit lines and clearinghouses, countermarketing, and youth prevention programs and focusing on enforcement of restrictions on minors' access to tobacco products and on smoking (clean air acts) (CDCP, 1999e, 7/30/00a; National Governors' Association; Campaign for Tobacco Free Kids). At the community level, worksite health promotion programs should develop a list of cessation resources (self-help, group, telephone counseling, and web-based programs), including those of the voluntary health agencies, hospitals, government, and other private entities. Activities in other sectors may also reach employees—such as assessment, counseling, and referral by health care providers and school programs that target employees' children. The program coordinator should also be aware of the specifics of national, state, and local legislation and regulations affecting worksites in particular and employees in general.

The needs and asset assessment data become the foundation for worksite tobacco control program planning. The program mix will depend on the proportion of employees using different types of tobacco, their stages of change for each, and their preferred quitting methods. Although most tobacco users are in the stages of precontemplation and contemplation, almost all worksite tobacco programming in the past was directed to the needs and issues of smokers who were in preparation, leading to low recruitment rates. For smokers in precontemplation and contemplation, for example, the company newsletter and broadcast e-mail messages may be used to publicize facts about smoking and health and the benefits of quitting. Family members can be encouraged to talk with their smoking members concerning the effect that smoking has on them. Awareness activities at the worksite can be coordinated with community campaigns such as the Great American SmokeOut and antitobacco media.

For employees who are ready to engage in the process of quitting, print and video self-help materials may be made available through a company resource center library; community cessation services, including web-based information, counseling, and quit lines can be publicized to employees; and individual counseling and referral can be offered by the health promotion coordinator. Role model stories of employees who have quit that include the techniques they have used and the benefits they received from quitting, can be provided in the company newsletter. Support from friends and families for smokers trying to quit can be recruited using strategies such as newsletter articles on how to help a person quit or formal contracts spelling out actions the supporter will take to assist the smoker as part of a program. The decision of whether to offer a cessation group on-site should be made depending on the number of employee smokers who indicate they wish to quit in a group and the availability of effective cessation groups in the community.

At the company level, a coordinated initiative for tobacco control would consist of cessation programs and activities by the health promotion program, complementary programs through the health promotion program (e.g., stress management and physical fitness) and through the employee assistance program, a comprehensive tobacco policy with equitable enforcement, health benefits coverage that includes tobacco cessation services, and managed care offerings that include assessment and counseling for tobacco cessation. These will require an organized effort to coordinate and lay aside any "turf" issues by the managers of these units.

Community and statewide antitobacco media campaigns, quit lines, and other cessation services are also important resources for the company employees and health promotion program. Health promotion coordinators should be involved in planning committees to design and implement programs that benefit the community. Legislation with impacts on tobacco prevention and control and government regulations are also key determinants of individual tobacco use and, with media, set community norms for tobacco use. Company and professional association political action groups can work to influence state and national policies to decrease tobacco use and exposure to secondhand smoke, and health promotion coordinators can take an active role in these efforts. By working at the community, state, and national levels, as appropriate, and by taking advantage of tobacco control activities outside of the worksite, a health promotion coordinator can maximize the policy and program resources available and develop an ecologically sound tobacco control program for his or her organization.

CONCLUSION

There have been many changes affecting worksite tobacco control in the past decade. Large-scale meta-analyses have provided guidelines for cessation efforts. There is better understanding of cessation as proceeding in stages, with interventions required for precontemplators and contemplators as well as for smokers in preparation and action. Tobacco policy has become an essential element of occupational health and safety. Large-scale anti-smoking campaigns and other prevention and cessation resources are being diffused through state dedication of tobacco excise taxes to tobacco prevention and control and through funds from the tobacco company settlements with states.

It is important that contemporary worksite health promotion programs build their tobacco control programs to take advantage of this context. We suggest an ecological approach to programming, in which smokers at the worksite are provided the most effective behavior change options and in which their behavior change is supported by other activities and policies within the worksite, their health care organization, and their community. This requires the health promotion coordinator to take an active role in working with the corporate departments handling policy and health care benefits and to reach out through community coalitions and professional associations to contribute to tobacco control at the community and society levels.

References

Abbot, N., Stead, L., White, A. B. J., & Ernst, E. (1999). Hypnotherapy for smoking cessation (Cochrane Review). The Cochrane Library. 1999; (1).

Allen, J., & Bellingham, R. (1994). Building supportive cultural environments. In M. P. O'Donnell, & J. S. Harris (Eds.), *Health promotion in the workplace* (2nd ed., pp. 204–216). Albany, NY: Delmar.

American Cancer Society (n.d.). *The health benefits of quitting* (Publication No. T792.12). [Brochure]. Atlanta, GA: American Cancer Society.

Association for Worksite Health Promotion, U.S. Department of Health and Human Services, & William M. Mercer, Inc. (2000). *1999 national worksite health promotion survey*. Northbrook, Illinois: Association for Worksite Health Promotion and William M. Mercer, Inc.

Bertera, R. L. (1991). Effects of behavioral risks on absenteeism and health care costs in the workplace. *Journal of Occupational Medicine, 33*(11), 1119–1124.

Brownson, R. C., Eriksen, M. P., Davis, R. M., & Warner, K. E. (1997). Environmental tobacco smoke: health effects and policies to reduce exposure. *Annual Review of Public Health, 18,* 163–165.

Burns, D. M. (1998). Cigar smoking: overview and current state of the science. *Smoking and tobacco control* (Monograph No. 9, NIH Publication No. 98-4302, pp. 1–20). Washington, DC: U.S. Department of Health and Human Services.

California Department of Health Services/Tobacco Control Section. (1988). *A model for change: the California experience in tobacco control*. Sacramento, CA: Author.

California Department of Health Services (Accessed 10/23/00). Adult smoking trends in California. [On-line]. Available: www.dhs.cahwnet.gov/cdic/ccb/TCS/documents/ CTUpdate.pdf.

Campaign for Tobacco Free Kids. State Tobacco Settlement. (Accessed 6/29/00). [On-line]. Available: http://www.tobaccofreekids.org/ reports/settlements.

Centers for Disease Control and Prevention. (1993). Mortality trends for selected smoking-related and breast cancer—United States, 1950–1990. *Morbidity and Mortality Weekly Report, 42*(44), 857, 863–6.

Centers for Disease Control and Prevention. (1998). Tobacco use among high school students— United States, 1997. *Morbidity and Mortality Weekly Report, 47* (12), 229–233.

Centers for Disease Control and Prevention. (1999a, June 25). State laws on tobacco control—United States, 1998. *Morbidity and Mortality Weekly Report Surveillance Summary.*

Centers for Disease Control and Prevention. (1999b, November 5): Great American Smokeout—November 18, 1999. *Morbidity and Mortality Weekly Report, 48*(43), 985.

Centers for Disease Control and Prevention. (1999c, November 5): Tobacco use—United States 1900–1999. *Morbidity and Mortality Weekly Report, 48*(43), 986–993.

Centers for Disease Control and Prevention. (1999d, November 5). Cigarette smoking among adults—United States, 1997. *Morbidity and Mortality Weekly Report, 48*(43), 993–996.

Centers for Disease Control and Prevention (1999e). *Best Practices for Comprehensive Tobacco Control.* Atlanta, GA: U.S. Department of Health & Human Services.

Centers for Disease Control and Prevention. (Accessed 11/14/99a): *Chronology: Significant developments related to smoking and health 1964–1996. Tobacco information and prevention source.* [On-line]. Available: http://www.cdc.gov/tobacco/chron96.htm.

Centers for Disease Control and Prevention. (Accessed 11/14/99b): *Achievements in public health: Tobacco use—United States, 1900–1999. Tobacco information and prevention source.* [On-line]. Available: http://www.cdc.gov/tobacco/achievements99.htm.

Centers for Disease Control and Prevention. (Accessed 11/14/99c). *Fact sheet: Cigarette smoking-related mortality. Tobacco information and prevention source.* [On-line]. Available: http://www.cdc.gov/tobacco/mortali.htm.

Centers for Disease Control and Prevention. (Accessed 11/14/99d). *Current smokeless tobacco use among men aged 18 years and older—United States, 1992–1993. Tobacco information and prevention source.* [On-line]. Available: http://www.cdc.gov/tobacco/achievements99.html.

Centers for Disease Control and Prevention. (Accessed 7/30/00a). *State and national tobacco control data. State tobacco activities tracking and evaluation system.* [On-line]. Available: http://www.cdc.gov/tobacco/stat&natdata.htm.

Centers for Disease Control and Prevention. (Accessed 7/30/00b). *Deaths attributable to smoking, 1990.* [On-line]. Available: http://www.cdc.gov/tobacco/attrdths.htm.

Centers for Disease Control and Prevention Accessed 7/29/00. Office on Smoking and Health, Wellness Council of America, American Cancer Society, CDCP (10/23/00). *Making your workplace smokefree. A decision maker's guide.* [On-line]. Available: http://www.cdc.gov/tobacco/etsguide.html.

Chapman, S., Borland, R., Scollo, M., Brownson, R. C., Dominello, A., & Woodward, S. (1999). The impact of smoke-free workplaces on declining cigarette consumption in Australia and the United States. *American Journal of Public Health, 89,* 1018–1023.

Cook, J., Owen, P., Bender, B., Senner J., Davis B., et al. (1998). State-specific prevalence among adults of current cigarette smoking and smokeless tobacco use and per capita tax-paid sales of cigarettes—United States, 1997. *Morbidity and Mortality Weekly Report, 47*(43), 922–926.

Curry, S. J., & McBride, C. M. (1994). Relapse prevention for smoking cessation: Review and evaluation of concepts and interventions. *Annual Review of Public Health, 15,* 345–366.

Deming, W. E. (1982). *Quality, productivity, and competitive position.* Cambridge, MA: Massachusetts Institute of Technology Press.

Edmundson, E., McAlister, A., Murray, D., Perry, C., & Lichtenstein, E. (1991). Approaches directed to the individual. In *Strategies to control tobacco use in the United States: A blueprint for public health action in the 1990's* (NIH Publication No. 92-3316, pp. 147–199). Washington, DC: U.S. Department of Health and Human Services.

Eriksen, M. P., & Gottlieb, N. H. (1998). A review of the health impact of smoking control at the workplace. *American Journal of Health Promotion, 13*(2), 83–104.

Fiore, M. C., Bailey, W. C., & Cohen, S. J. (1996). *Smoking Cessation* (Clinical Practice Guideline No. 18; AHCPR Pub. No. 96-0692) Rockville, MD: U.S. Department of Health and Human Services.

Fiore, M. D., Bailey, W. C., & Cohen, S. J., (2000, June) *Treating tobacco use and dependence. Clinical Practice Guideline.* Rockville, MD: U.S. Department of Health and Human Services.

Fisher, E. J., Glasgow, R. E., & Terborg, J. R. (1990). Worksite smoking cessation: A meta-analysis of long-term quit rates from controlled studies. *Journal of Occupational Medicine, 32*(5), 429–439.

Fisher, E. B., Lichtenstein, E., Haire-Joshu, D., Morgan, G. D., & Rehberg, H. R. (1993). Methods, successes, and failures of smoking cessation programs. *Annual Review of Medicine, 44,* 481–513.

Gerlach, K. K., Cummings, K. M., Hyland, A., Gilpin, E. A., Johnson, M. D., & Pierce, J. P. (1998). Trends in cigar consumption and smoking prevalence. *Smoking and tobacco control* (Monograph No. 9, NIH Publication No. 98-4302, pp.). Washington, DC: U.S. Department of Health and Human Services.

Gerlach, K. K., Shopland, D. R., Hartman, A. M., Gibson, J. T., & Pechacek, T. F. (1997). Workplace smoking policies in the United States: results from a national survey of more than 100,000 workers. *Tobacco Control, 6,* 199–206.

Gottlieb, N. H., Weinstein, R. P., Baun, W. B., & Bernacki, E. J. (1992). A profile of health risks among blue-collar workers. *Journal of Occupational Medicine, 34*(1), 61–68.

Heaney, C. A., & Goetzel, R. Z. (1997). A review of health-related outcomes of multi-component worksite health promotion programs. *American Journal of Health Promotion, 11*(4), 290–308.

Kirstein, M. M. (1983). How much can business expect to profit from smoking cessation? *Preventive Medicine 12:*358–81.

Korsak, A. (1977). Job absenteeism among habitual smokers. *World Smoking and Health, 2*(2), 15–17.

Levitt, L., Lundy, J., & Srinivasan, S. (1998, August). *Trends and indicators in the changing health care marketplace chartbook.* Prenlo Park, CA: The Henry J. Kaiser Family Foundation.

Longo, D. R., Feldman, M. M., Kruse, R. L., Brownson, R. C., Petroski, G. F., & Hewett, J. E. (1998). Implementing smoking bans in American hospitals: results of a national survey. *Tobacco Control, 7,* 47–55.

McAfee and Sofian. (1988).

McGinnis, J. M., & Foege, W. H. (1993). Actual causes of death in the United States. *Journal of the American Medical Association, 270,* 2209–12.

National Committee for Quality Assurance. (1997). HEDIS 3.0/ 1998 Measurement Specifications. [Computer Software] Washington, DC: National Committee for Quality Assurance.

National Governor's Association. Tobacco Settlement. (Accessed 6/29/00) [On-line]. Available: http://www.nga.org/ health/tobacco.asp.

Nelson, D. E., Emont, S. L., Brackbill, R. M., Cameron, L. L., Peddicord, J., & Fiore, M. C. (1994).

Cigarette smoking prevalence by occupation in the United States. A comparison between 1978–1980 and 1987 to 1990. *Journal of Occupational Medicine, 36*(5), 516–25.

Nelson D. R., Kirkendall, R. S., Lawton, R. L., Chrismon, J. H., Merritt, R. K., Arday, D. A., & Giovino, G. A. (1994, June 6). Surveillance for smoking-attributable mortality and years of potential life lost, by State—United States, 1990. *Morbidity and Mortality Weekly Report, 43* (No. SS-1), 1–8.

O'Donnell, M. P. (1994a). Designing workplace health promotion programs. In M. P. O'Donnell & J. S. Harris (eds.), *Health Promotion in the Workplace* (2nd ed., pp. 41–65). Albany, NY: Delmar.

O'Donnell, M. P. (1994b). Employers' financial perspective on health promotion. In M. P. O'Donnell & J. S. Harris, (eds.), *Health Promotion in the Workplace* (2nd ed., pp. 69–88). Albany, NY: Delmar.

Prochaska, J. O, Redding, C. A., & Evers, K. E. (1997). The Transtheoretical Model and stages of change. In K. Glanz, F. M. Lewis, & B. K. Rimer (eds.), *Health Behavior and Health Education: Theory, Research, and Practice* (2nd ed., pp. 60–84). San Francisco: Jossey-Bass.

Prochaska, J. O., & Velicer, W. F. (1997). The transtheoretical model of health behavior change. *Am. J Health Promot. 12*(1): 38–48.

Schwartz, J. L. (1987). Review and evaluation of smoking cessation methods: The United States and Canada, 1978-1985 (NIH Publication No. 87-2940). Washington, DC: U.S. Department of Health and Human Services.

Schwartz, J. L. (1992). Methods of smoking cessation. *Medical Clinics of North America, 76*(2), 451–476.

Siegel, M., & Biener, L. (1997). Evaluating the impact of statewide anti-tobacco campaigns: The Massachusetts and California tobacco control programs. *Social Issues, 53*(1), 147–168.

Sofian, N. S., McAfee, T., Doctor, J., & Carson, D: Tobacco control and cessation. In O'Donnell, M.R., and Harris, J. S. (eds): *Health Promotion in the Workplace,* 2nd ed. Delmar: Albany, NY, (1994), p. 346.

USDHHS. (1964). *Smoking and health: Report of the Advisory Committee to the Surgeon General of the Public Health Services.* Washington, DC: U.S. Government Printing Office.

USDHHS. (1986a). *The health consequences of using smokeless tobacco. A report of the Advisory Committee to the Surgeon General* (NIH Publication No. 86-2874). Washington, DC: Author.

USDHHS. (1986b). *The health consequences of involuntary smoking. A report of the Surgeon General* (DHHS Publication No. 87-8398). Washington, DC: U.S. Government Printing Office.

USDHHS. (1988). *The health consequences of smoking: Nicotine addiction. A report of the Surgeon General* (DHHS Publication No.) Washington, DC: U.S. Department of Health and Human Services.

USDHHS. (1989). *Reducing the health consequences of smoking: 25 years of progress. A report of the Surgeon General* (DHHS Publication No. 89-8411). Washington, DC: U.S. Department of Health and Human Services.

USDHHS. (1993). *1992 national survey of worksite health promotion activities: Summary report.* Washington, DC: U.S. Department of Health and Human Services.

USDHHS. (1994). *Clinician's handbook of preventive services.* Washington DC: U.S. Government Printing Office.

USDHHS. (2000). *Healthy People 2010* (Conference ed., vols. 1–2). Washington, DC: U.S. Government Printing Office. [On-line]. Available: http://www.health.gov/healthypeople/document. (7/29/00).

U.S. Environmental Protection Agency. (1992). *Respiratory health effects of passive smoking: Lung cancer and other disorders.* Washington, DC: EPA/600-6-90/006F.

Warner, K. E., Smith, R. J., Smith, D. G., & Fries, B. E. (1996). Health and economic implications of a work-site smoking cessation program: A simulation analysis. *Journal of Occupational and Environmental Medicine, 38*(10), 981–92.

Wetter, D. W., Fiore, M. C., Gritz, E. R., Lando, H. A., Stitzer, M. L., Hasselblad, V., & Baker, T. B. (1998). Agency of Health Care Policy and Research Smoking Cessation Clinical Practice Guideline: Findings and implications for psychologists. *American Psychologist, 53*(6), 657–669.

CHAPTER

14

Medical Self-Care

Paul E. Terry

INTRODUCTION

The practice of taking care of common health problems undoubtedly dates back to the origins of *Homo sapiens;* it is an attribute that likely explains our natural selection and perhaps even our survival as a species. The search for home remedies began with native tribes plying wide varieties of oils, roots, herbs, and tonics to relieve pain and offer comfort. To this day, in ever shrinking parts of the world, native cultures continue to heal their sick with time-honored home-based treatments. Indeed, even in the western world, under the guise of alternative therapy, a growing diversity of people practice medicine with impunity. While there is nothing new about medical self-care, there is a growing cadre of professionals dedicated to assisting people with self-care. In turn, there is a litany of new products and services devised to support self-care of health problems.

The advent of medical self-care education, with its attendant self-care books, training sessions, and subsequent on-line decision support materials, corresponds to the changes in United States health policy priorities. Where lifestyle and individual responsibil-

ity were the watchwords of the 1970s and early 1980s, there is now a movement toward population health and managed care models of health insurance reimbursement. However, it took little time for policy makers to realize that the promise of citizens and patients taking control of their lifestyles was not only difficult but took considerable time to accomplish. Still worse, the cost savings from health promotion would take years, if ever, to materialize. Accordingly, the policy momentum in the late 1980s into the 1990s, and likely well into the second millennium, has shifted to a quest for short-term cost containment. It is in this era that medical self-care education, along with its correlated concepts of disease and demand management, has grown and will thrive in the future.

Definition of Medical Self-Care

Because medical self-care education resides in a crossroads between medical care and personal health management, it is reasonable to define medical self-care according to the precepts of these related fields. The medical side of the definition is the easy side to describe; it is connected to medicine, which is the science of diagnosing, treating, and curing disease. The self-care part of the definition is somewhat more obscure because it is a field spawned from consumer and market need, fueled by entrepreneurs, and substantiated by medical providers. Since the field of self-care education derives from an agreed-upon cohort of behavioral theories or empirical studies, Hibbard has noted that the "study of self-care has been characterized by a lack of conceptual clarity"(Hibbard, 1999).

Taking care of oneself is, after all, as natural as avoiding walking off a cliff. Where is the need for education and/or conceptual frameworks in that? Given there are no professional societies or consensus panels dedicated to determining a definition for medical self-care, borrowing from a close cousin discipline is a fair substitute. In a consensus panel dedicated to defining health education, Green and others (1988) define health education as "any combination of learning experiences designed to facilitate voluntary actions conducive to health." Until such time that self-care education has an authoritative panel dedicated to its identity, for this chapter, medical self-care education will be defined as any combination of learning activities designed to facilitate the personal diagnosis, treatment, and cure of illness.

A critic less schooled in the principles of personal empowerment and individual responsibility that attend the field of health promotion could view this definition of medical self-care as practicing medicine without a license. To address this concern, it is important to distinguish between medical self-care for chronic conditions versus acute emergency versus self-limiting conditions. Teaching others the ability to distinguish between these conditions and discern what can be treated alone and what needs professional attention is at the heart of medical self-care education. Acute, emergency conditions that require medical attention benefit from self-care education that teaches people how to identify life-threatening problems and act quickly. When conditions are self-limited, they will go away without medical intervention. Self-care education has a role in providing comfort. For chronic health conditions, those lasting six months or longer, self-care education offers therapeutic as well as comforting benefits. Involving patients in self-care of chronic health problems is, after all, the most critical component of treating problems that have no cure.

Even though self-care education in the past ten years has addressed a broad range of acute and chronic conditions, the primary reason for its utility in an era of health care cost containment has related to keeping people out of the doctor's office. Accordingly, self-care education that teaches people to care for acute self-limited conditions—those that will go away without a doctor's visit—has been the most studied and popularized type of program.

Purpose of this Chapter

For acute conditions, self-care education seeks to assist medical consumers in identifying problems that will go away on their own; these are "self-limited" conditions such as colds, back pain, or fevers. Self-care education also deals with conditions that could become worse without medical intervention, such as bacterial infections or fractures. Self-care education teaches people to know when Mother Nature should take her course and when it is time to see the doctor. This chapter reviews the literature related to self-care education and seeks to assist the health promotion practitioner in distinguishing between programs of self-care, "demand management," and disease management. The first section of this chapter offers a conceptual framework for self-care education. Issues of patient preferences and the interaction between consumer satisfaction and effective educational strategies will be discussed.

A major priority for worksite health promotion, aside from the primary goal of improving employee health, has been that of reducing health care costs. This comes at a time of hyperconsumerism. The combination of an aging population, with the accompanying increased health problems, and the information age, especially easy access to health information on the Internet, is creating runaway health care utilization patterns. These trends speak to the need for self-care education. The second section of this chapter offers the practitioner practical program information from leading studies and projects in self-care education. This section is divided by the major chronic health conditions so that the practitioner can assess similarities and differences between self-care strategies.

At the same time employers are scrutinizing the cost of care provided to their employees, retaining employees in an era of low unemployment has become a paramount concern. Accordingly, the quality of medical care has become a major issue in evaluating employee benefits. Worksite health promotion practitioners have typically offered self-care education as an adjunct to health care or, more often, altogether separately from the employees' relationship to their health care providers. The final section of this chapter will illustrate how employees who become patients see their physician as the primary and preferred authority, a concept often counter to the typical self-care education delivery mechanisms, which bypass the medical community. In addition, the final section will review the effectiveness of traditional group education programs, medical self-care books, and emerging strategies for teaching self-care education.

Self-Care Education Conceptual Framework

Teaching about self-care or preventive services appreciably improves outcomes related to overall care (Weingarten, Stone, & Green, 1995); conversely; those dissatisfied with care regularly name the lack of the provision of information as a primary complaint (Williams & Calman, 1991). Still, there are marked discrepancies between what patients value and what physicians think is important during routine office visits (Gerteis, Edgman-Levitan, & Walker, 1993; Hall & Dornan, 1988; Laine, Davidoff, Lewis et al., 1996). Laine and colleagues (1996), for example, showed that both physicians and patients named professional expertise as the most valued aspect of the clinical encounter, a statistically significant level of agreement in values. However, Laine also showed that patients ranked getting information as the second most important aspect of a visit, while physicians rated it a distant sixth in importance. Moreover, even when physicians are advised that the provision of information is a care preference of the patient they are seeing, they are no more likely to provide it (Sanchez-Menegay & Stalder, 1994). There is some evidence that patient satisfaction rates are higher when patient information is sponsored by a medical group rather than other sources (such as a university). When surveys assessing patient satisfaction were sent via the letterhead of a medical practice; for example, six of seven scores related to the patient's satisfaction with the care they received were higher than scores from a survey sent by a university (Etter,

Perneger, & Rougemont, 1996). Another study showed that patients are most satisfied when they consider the physician a partner in exchanging information rather than an authority who controls the relationship (Anderson & Zimmerman, 1993).

Because satisfaction with care is strongly associated with the quantity and quality of patient education that physicians provide (Abramowitz, Cote, & Berry, 1987; Robbins, Bertakis, & Helms, 1993; Savage & Armstrong, 1990; Schauffler, Rodriguez, & Milstein, 1996; Weingarten et al., 1995), health systems need to find new ways to involve physicians in self-care education. Unfortunately, even though patient education is highly valued by patients, they seldom ask physicians to provide additional instructions (Kalet 1994). This inability to ask for more education seems to persist regardless of a patient's health status (Zapka, Palmer, & Hargraves, 1995).

In another study of the relationship between patient satisfaction and health education, patients were significantly more likely to be satisfied with their physician if the physician had discussed one or more health education topics with them in the past three years (Schauffler, Rodriguez, & Milstein 1996). Since satisfaction with care is closely linked to positive clinical outcomes, studies on employee satisfaction advance the employer's goal of reducing costs. It is likely that using self-care education to increase customer satisfaction will work best when it is an integrated, rather than a separate part, of the health system. The section on self-care and medical services use later in this chapter describes a study that tests such integration between self-care and medical services.

Creating Employee and Medical Provider Partnerships

In addition to the health care quality improvement benefits of self-care education described in the section above, training in medical self-management has been shown to positively affect health care consumerism. (Gifford et al., 1998; Nelson et al., 1984; O'Reilly, 1994). Lectures and demonstrations concerning the use of health services not only moderate use, as will be seen in the following section, but produce improvements in health knowledge, skills performance, skills confidence, and even life quality (Nelson et al., 1984).

Using one of the most intensively medically managed conditions—HIV/AIDS—as an example, Gifford and colleagues (1998) demonstrated the tremendous value of making the patient a partner in health care decision making. In a randomized controlled study, 71 men with symptomatic HIV/AIDS were taught wide-ranging disease self-management and physician-patient communication skills. The main outcome measure comparing the intervention and control groups was symptom status. The treatment group was significantly more successful in controlling symptoms and showed increased self-efficacy for managing symptoms that occurred. Similar positive effects of self-management education on self-efficacy and psychosocial functioning have been shown for patients with heart disease (Clark 1992). Another study showed that in addition to increasing consumer competence, self-care education through a pharmacy of a U.S. Army health system significantly increased commitment to seek preventive services and improved opinions about the health care system (Steinweg, Killingsworth, Nannini, & Spayde, 1998). Employees who are active, informed consumers, then, tend to have better outcomes and view the health system more positively. The following section describes the extent to which such employees can also reduce health care costs.

SELF-CARE EDUCATION PROGRAM OPTIONS

Self-care resources are proliferating and, particularly with the growth of the Internet, access to increasingly comprehensive and detailed health information is likely to expand exponentially. Are people using these resources, and does self-care education affect utilization? The answer to the first question is yes; the answer to the second question is more equivocal. Concerning use of self-care resources, Hibbard and her colleagues assessed the use of self-care resources in three communities and found that self-care books were a fairly commonly used resource and use of nurse phone-lines were another common means of acquiring health information (Hibbard, Greenlick, et al., 1999). It is instructive to note that this study found statistically significant but, from a programming perspective, rather modest variation in community use

of self-care, with 49% of respondents in one town and 41% in another town using a self-care book within the last few months. At the time of this study, only 8% of the respondents in each of the communities had used a computer for health or medical information in the last few months.

The question of how self-care affects utilization is more difficult because it varies by the type of health condition and the nature of the population. As will be described later in this chapter, self-care education of chronic conditions has generally favorable effects on consumer satisfaction and certain health outcomes but less predictable effects on medical system utilization. It can be argued that, for many chronic conditions, an educated patient will learn to use the health system more often. However, for conditions that will resolve on their own, education is likely to be the most cost-effective and consumer-friendly way to reduce unnecessary use of health services. The following sections discuss rationale for, and the benefits of, commonly used self-care education resources.

Self-Care Books

Medical self-care books have served as the staple educational resource for a wide variety of self-care education programs in the workplace and in other settings. Such books are available in bookstores, from private publishers, medical associations, and nonprofit health care organizations. Self-care books typically focus on the most common self-limiting health conditions but often include content related to chronic conditions and recommended preventive services as well. To help consumers in making decisions about self-care, books use decision guides or symptom lists that offer clear directions for the type of self-care recommended.

A variety of visual icons have been employed by self-care publishers to assist consumers in making difficult choices related to management of symptoms of illness. Figure 14-1 shows a page from the book *Well-Advised*, a self-care book created by the Institute for Research and Education, HealthSystem Minnesota, in cooperation with the StayWell Company. Note that the "Decision Guide Key" on this page related to caring for cuts offers a clear guideline for

Signs of infections usually don't appear until at least 24 hours after the injury. Bacteria need time to grow and multiply. If you have fever, swelling, redness or a red streak, increased pain, or pus oozing from the wound, call your doctor.

Family Practitioner

Decision Guide Key

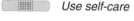 *Use self-care*

 Call doctor's office for advice

 See doctor

 Seek help now

 Emergency, call 911

CUTS

Simple cuts can become not-so-simple infections, so it is important to know how to treat them properly.

Minor cuts damage only the skin and the fatty tissue beneath it. They usually heal without permanent damage. More serious cuts may damage muscles, tendons, blood vessels, ligaments, or nerves, and these cuts should be examined by a doctor.

The three major concerns in treating a cut or wound are:
- Stop the bleeding. Apply direct pressure to the wound.
- Clean the cut or wound thoroughly. This will help avoid infection.
- Bandage the wound. To promote healing, bring the edges of the skin together with tape or stitches.

SELF-CARE STEPS FOR CUTS

The next time you get a cut from a nail, a knife, or even a piece of paper, follow these steps.

Stop the Bleeding
- Cover the wound with a gauze pad, or a thick, clean piece of cloth. Use your hand if nothing else is available.
- Press on the wound hard enough to stop the bleeding. Don't let up on the pressure even to change cloths. Just add a clean cloth over the original one.
- Raise the wound above heart level, unless this movement would cause pain.
- Get medical help immediately if blood spurts from a wound or bleeding does not stop after several minutes of pressure.

Clean the Wound
- Wash the cut with soap and water or use hydrogen peroxide (3 percent solution). Don't use Mercurochrome, Merthiolate, or iodine. They are not necessary and can be very painful.
- Make sure no dirt, glass, or foreign material remains in the wound.

Bandage the Wound
- Bandage a cut (rather than seeing a doctor for stitches) when its edges tend to fall together and when the cut is not very deep.
- Use "butterfly bandages," strips of sterile paper tape, or adhesive strip bandages. Change them daily.
- Apply the bandage crosswise, not lengthwise. This will bring the edges of the wound into firm contact and promote healing.

Are stitches needed?
See a doctor for stitches or other care as soon as possible if:
- The wound is deep and gapes widely, is very dirty or irregular, or can't be held together with a bandage.
- A deep cut is located on an elbow, knee, finger or other area that bends.
- The cut is on the finger or thumb joint, palm of the hand, face, or other area on which you would like to minimize scars.
- The cut damages bones or muscles or feels numb.
- The victim is a young child who is likely to pull off the bandage.
- Bleeding cannot be controlled after applying pressure for 20 minutes.
- The cut was caused by an obviously dirty object or a foreign object is embedded in the wound.
- The victim's tetanus booster is not up-to-date.

Figure 14-1 Well-advised/self-care for common problems

Source: Reprinted with permission from Well Advised ©, a self-care book created by The Institute for Research and Education, HealthSystem Minnesota, in cooperation with The StayWell Company.

deciding when a symptom can be treated with self-care, when a call to the doctor's office is warranted, when to see the doctor, or when to seek help immediately. When self-care is recommended, books such as *Well-Advised* offer detailed lists of home remedies.

Group Education Programs and Self-Care Resources

It is unlikely that educational materials alone will change behavior and save employers money; rather, the preponderance of health education and self-care literature indicates that a comprehensive, integrated approach to teaching self-care is most likely to be effective (Pelletier, 1993). Many organizations provide self-care education books as a part of an ongoing plan of health care consumer education. Books may be distributed at one-hour programs or brief in-service self-care practices. Instruction may include common first aid, how to use decision guides, or information about how to establish a relationship with a primary care provider. Self-care education campaigns can include promotion of a nurse-information

line or instructions on how to access health information on the Internet. As the studies of self-care programs detailed earlier in this chapter indicate, changes in knowledge and awareness are an important but insufficient approach to changing behavior. Self-care education programs work best when they are part of an ongoing plan to educate and empower employees to manage their own health. Table 14-1 outlines the types of educational approaches appropriate for the different kinds of conditions a worksite is seeking to improve.

Impact of Self-Care Education Programs

An education program that is intended to reduce inappropriate use of a complex and alluring health system should include skills development as well as efforts to change consumer attitudes. Medical self-care is much more than first aid and knowing when to put on a bandage. The workplace health promotion practitioner embarking on employee self-care education should consider the types of self-care programs out-

Table 14-1 Self-Care Education Program Framework. Preferred Strategy Index: 1 = Primary Strategy, 2 = Supportive Strategy, 3 = Ineffectual.

Condition/ Strategies	Individual Counseling and clinical Visits	Group Programs	Newsletter	Self-Care Books, Videos, Pamphlets	Internet References/ Expert Systems	Support Groups/ Virtual Chat Rooms	Phone Counseling and Education Services
Acute-self-limiting conditions	3	2	2	1	1	2	1
Acute-emergent conditions	1	3	2	2	1	2	1
Chronic diseases	1	1	3	2	2	1	2
Lifestyle change/ unhealthy habits	2	1	3	2	3	1	2
Location variables:							
Worksite-based self-care	3	1	2	1	2	2	1
Community-based self-care	2	2	3	1	3	3	2
Health care-based self-care	1	3	2	1	2	2	1

lined in this section when setting goals appropriate for his/her company employees.

Numerous studies show that educating employees about medical self-care, particularly about home remedies for symptom management of self-limiting conditions, can be effective in reducing unnecessary clinic visits (Fries et al., 1993; Roberts et al., 1983; Terry & Pheley, 1993; Vickery et al., 1983; Vickery et al., 1988). On the average, these programs yielded three dollars saved for every one dollar invested in self-care education. Considered another way, these studies reduced unnecessary visits between 7% and 17%, depending on the health conditions being evaluated. Self-care education programs have traditionally been delivered directly to consumers as a way to offer standardized consumer information about self-management of common health problems (Lorig et al., 1985; Lynch, & Vickery et al., 1993; Terry, 1994). While self-care education strategies have been shown to be cost-effective (Fries et al., 1993, Kemper, 1982), less is known about the effect of self-care education on satisfaction with the health care system and the effects of education on informed medical decision-making once an employee is under a doctor's care (McClellan, 1986; Schauffler & Rodriguez, 1996; Shank, Murphy, & Schulte & Mowry, 1991). JAMA Council 1990.

Pundits have speculated about the day when "your employer becomes your doctor," predicting that the economic stakes for the purchasers of health care would encroach on the time-honored authority of the physician as mediator of health decisions. Workplace self-care education programs traditionally bypass the physician, with consumers receiving medical self-care instruction at the workplace, in group programs, or via direct mail (Barry, 1980, Vickery et al., 1989). Little is known about effects of self-care education on the physician's gate-keeping behavior and whether it complements or competes with managed care systems intent on eliminating unnecessary health care services (Ley, 1982).

For the worksite health practitioner, deciding to use materials alone versus working through health providers to improve health care consumerism is a choice having only modest supporting evidence. For example, a materials-based self-care program offered to 5,200 employees resulted in utilization reduction of

0.8, down to 2 visits per household per year (Vickery et al., 1983). Another study of self-care instruction in a prepaid ambulatory care center tested a five-minute program for persons who wanted to see a health professional. The cost of an outpatient visit compared to the cost of a "self-care center" visit saved seven dollars for each one dollar invested in the program. Savings over two years were estimated at over $46,000 (Zapka & Averill, 1979). A similar study showed how self-care education might affect satisfaction with health services as well as utilization. Differences in decreased visit rates corresponded to the intensity of the intervention in experimental groups, yielding significant decreases in minor illness visits of 17–35%, with estimated cost savings from $2.50 to $3.50 for each dollar spent on the educational intervention (Terry & Pheley, 1993; Macmillan, 1986).

Many employees and physicians fear they may be neglecting a potentially serious health threat when illness symptoms persist. To examine this concern, Vickery and colleagues (1989) studied the utilization practices of participants who had been educated about self-care for common problems and had fewer subsequent clinic visits. By tracking post-intervention claims data, this study demonstrated that the short-term utilization reduction effects of education did not result in delayed care seeking for truly problematic conditions. For very common self-limiting conditions, such as a cold, it is important that the reduction in utilization can be explained by the intervention alone. For example, one randomized controlled study showed decreases of 44% in unnecessary visits for upper respiratory tract infections after brief self-care education. Instruction and materials were provided whenever members of the experimental group were in the clinic (Roberts et al., 1983). A greater than 40% decrease in visits is a truly remarkable and positive outcome when the programmer can be confident that it will not lead to additional problems for the patient.

Examining the Cost-Impact of Consumer Education

The above data suggest that educating consumers about managing self-limiting conditions will, on the average, save a company money. However, self-care education may also play a role in increasing appropriate utilization for certain types of health conditions. In a randomized controlled study of over 14,000 managed care members, Terry and Pheley (1993) found the use of self-care education materials reduced unnecessary utilization of services for certain conditions (such as colds and flu) but increased visits for such conditions as fever and sore throat. This selective increase in utilization would have been a positive finding had it been the intended purpose of the intervention. It is true, for example, that in some cases untreated fevers or sore throats can lead to more serious problems. However, for most consumers, fever and sore throat can be well-managed at home. The authors suggested that special care needs to be taken in how self-care messages are presented to achieve the desired outcome.

The potential for self-care education to lead to more appropriate utilization, rather than to reduced overall utilization, was also demonstrated in a community-based study. After a community-wide intervention in which residents were provided a self-care book and advised about access to a nurse-phone service, Hibbard (1999) reported that use of a self-care manual was as likely to increase utilization as it was to reduce utilization. The intervention community was more likely to access a self-care book, but there were no significant differences in the use of a phone service. The conscientious consumer considering risks and benefits may be making a perfectly reasonable choice to visit and rule out the possibility of having a more serious illness. Education, then, depending on the goals of the program developers, can be a means of increasing utilization.

Most self-care education books, and many other consumer education materials, teach about the need for preventive exams along with instructions about self-care of common problems. For most populations, preventive services such as mammograms, colon exams, flu shots, cholesterol tests, and other such exams are underutilized. It is as likely that encouraging use of these services will lead to more clinical visits as it is that discouraging doctor visits for a cold or flu will decrease clinical visits. In the end, an effective self-care education may simply be a "zero sum game" with the decrease in unneeded visits canceling out the increases in appropriate visits.

Specific Applications of Self-Care on Consumer Choice

Employer purchasers of health care have used measurement of health care quality as a device for negotiating lower rates and increasing competition among medical providers. Employee satisfaction with doctors has been one of the measures that companies can use to monitor health service quality. As noted above, self-care education programs have typically bypassed health systems. Worksite health promotion programs that are trying to maximize the role of their medical providers in improving employee health need to consider how to engage, rather than go around, doctors. It is likely that employees will be responsible for an increasing proportion of their health care coverage. Consumer choices will be made based upon both satisfaction with health services and the perceived added value available at health institutions. Self-care education can be one of those value-added services from employees. Table 14-2 summarizes the best studies concerning the relationship of consumer satisfaction and health outcomes.

A study to examine the difference between self-care education that is provided via traditional consumer-direct approaches and education provided during routine office visits was conducted to examine how doctors can improve the effectiveness of self-care education (Terry & Healy, 1999). This is the only study presently available to help practitioners decide about the merits of involving health systems in employee self-care education versus other consumer-direct approaches. Using a randomized controlled study design, self-care education interventions were tested, including physician-initiated education that introduced a medical self-care book during routine office visits and the distribution of a medical self-care book via the mail. The study attempted to assess how these two different methods of self-care education affect consumer satisfaction with clinical services and employee practices in using home remedies for self-limited conditions. The research hypothesis held that patients presented with physician-initiated self-care education would be more satisfied with the information provided and

Table 14-2 Self-Care Education and Consumer Satisfaction

Author(s)	Title	Sample Size	Evaluation Period	Findings
Williams & Calman (1991)	Key Determinants of Consumer Satisfaction with General Practice	454 surveys returned	2 months	Persons were generally satisfied with their physicians (95%), but some could not discuss personal problems with their physician (38%). Yet others were dissatisfied with the level of information (26%), and some were dissatisfied with the length of time with their physician (25%).
Weingarten et al. (1995)	A Study of Patient Satisfaction and Adherence to Preventive Care Practice Guidelines	3,249 patients selected. An average of 2,570 completed 3 surveys on patient satisfaction	5 months	Patients were generally satisfied with their physician's care (mean of 4.2 on a scale of 1 to 5, 5 being most satisfied). Patients who received or were offered mammography, vaccines, and exercise counseling sessions were more satisfied with their medical care than those patients who did not.
Robbins et al. (1993)	The Influence of Physician Practice Behaviors on Patient Satisfaction	100 new patients	Not indicated	Total visit-specific satisfaction was positively related to previsit satisfaction and to time spent on health education, physical examination, and discussion of treatment effects. There was a negative effect to spending time on history taking.
Zapka et al. (1995)	Relationships of Patient Satisfaction with Experience of System Performance and Health Status	3,151 patients	Not indicated	Analyses demonstrate that patient reports of the quality of processes of care or system performance are significantly related to satisfaction independently of perception of health status.
Abramowitz et al. (1987)	Analyzing Patient Satisfaction: A Multianalytic Approach	841 patients	Not indicated	Among three professional groups (physicians, house staff, and nurses), patients reported high satisfaction marks to the groups paying attention to the patients' concerns and explaining procedures and treatment.
Savage & Armstrong (1990)	Effect of a General Practitioner's Consulting Style on Patients' Satisfaction: Controlled Study	200 patients	Not indicated	Patients who were able to control the consultation were highly satisfied on all outcomes measured, but those who were diagnosed with physical problems or who received prescriptions were more noticeable in satisfaction.
Anderson & Zimmerman (1993)	Patient and Physician Perceptions of their Relationship and Patient Satisfaction: A Study of Chronic Disease Management	134 male patients	1 year	Patients with lower levels of education were most satisfied and physicians who viewed the relationship as a patient-physician partnership had more satisfied patients than those who viewed the relationship as physician controlled.

have greater intentions to use home care for self-limiting conditions compared to those with a direct-mail-based consumer education approach.

To assess the effects of providing a self-care book during routine patient visits, questionnaires were administered two weeks subsequent to office visits and were also distributed after "usual care" visits in which the physician did not provide the book or formally discuss medical self-care. Sites were rotated between the direct mail approach, the physician delivery approach, and usual care. The results of this study indicated that patients were significantly more likely to be satisfied with their medical visit when they received self-care education and a self-care book. When comparing those who received the book from the doctor with those who received the book at home, in 11 of 14 items, those receiving the book from the doctor were significantly more likely to be satisfied. Satisfaction variables such as "my physician is a good communicator," "my physician explains things clearly," or "my physician does a good job of educating me" indicated the positive benefits of receiving the book during a routine office visit. Employers seeking to differentiate between health care providers and to increase the quality of care offered to employees need to be proactive in seeking health systems with these value-added services. Patient education is an often-overlooked variable in distinguishing quality, but it is one of the most valued parts of the employee's interaction with the health system. This study adds credibility to an employer's search for those health systems that offer effective education as an integral part of quality clinical care.

SELF-CARE AND MANAGING DEMAND FOR HEALTH SERVICES

Self-care education is one of several managed health care cost containment and health improvement concepts. Other approaches, such as "demand management," "disease management," or "health management" are similar in their goals but different with respect to the disease states they address. As with self-care education, these managed health care concepts are not guided by an empirically derived theoretical

framework or by professional standards as much as they have evolved from health care market needs. Table 14-3 lists some suggested theoretical and practical differences between these health services. In spite of these differences, there are several actions that practitioners use in common in all of these demand reduction approaches:

- Assessing educational needs, health risks, health interests, health status, and readiness for change
- Development of educational content for health decision support and design of systems for working with health systems to improve their ability to educate consumers
- Health education services delivery (such as phone-based, Internet-based, materials-based, group programs, or individual instruction in health improvement and disease management)
- Using quality improvement methods to reduce unnecessary utilization of health services
- Program evaluation for quality improvement and education system redesign

Ongoing assessment of individual employee behaviors and health system utilization patterns, along with periodic population-based health assessment, is used in managed health programs in order to plan and target programs to employees who will benefit most. Health assessment tools also offer essential information about which clinical and education activities are needed most by a company's employees. Targeted education interventions have been shown to be most effective in attracting program participation. For managed health programs, cost-containment is a primary objective; accordingly, identification and surveillance of high risk patients, focused education, and routine follow-up are common elements to all such demand management efforts to reduce unnecessary visits and improve health outcomes. While the orientation of most managed health services is toward reduction in utilization and the presumed cost savings this can yield in the short term, programs to increase utilization of preventive services are often of interest to health care purchasers.

Table 14-3 Differentiating Self-Care and Health Management Programs

Programs	Primary Related Theories	Cost and Prevalence of Conditons Addressed	Time Needed for Program Impact	Resource Use Implications
Medical Self-Care Education	- Sick-role theory - Theory of Reasoned Action - Health Belief Model	Low cost, high pre-valence of conditions; primarily self-limiting conditions (e.g., colds, flu, fevers, headaches, earaches)	Short-term impact (hours to a few days before effect changes)	Good evidence of cost-effectiveness
Demand Management Programs	- Health Belief Model - Expectancy Theory	Moderate to high cost, moderate prevalence conditions; of both self-limiting and chronic conditions (e.g., backaches, chronic pain syndrome, adult asthma)	Short to intermediate term impact (weeks to months before effect changes)	Weak or no evidence of cost-effectiveness; suggestive evidence supporting individual case management
Disease Management Programs	- Transtheoretical Model (Stages of Change) - Organizational Change Theories - Value Expectancy Frameworks	High cost, high prevalence of conditions; primarily chronic conditions (e.g., diabetes, congestive heart failure, pediatric asthma, hyperlipidemia)	Intermediate to long-term impact (months to years before effect changes)	Suggestive evidence of cost-effectiveness for select conditions (such as CHF, pediatric asthma); cost increases likely for many conditions
Health Promotion/ Disease Prevention Programs	- Social Learning Theory - PRECEDE/PROCEED Framework - Transtheoretical Model (Stages of Change) - Social Marketing	Lifestyle conditions, (e.g., smoking, diet, exercise, clinical preventive services such as immunizations, blood pressure measurement)	Long-term impact (many years before effect changes)	Good evidence of long-term cost-effectiveness for select conditions such as exercise, early detection of hypertension; equivocal evidence for obesity, diet

Preventive Services Utilization

Self-care education includes teaching about appropriate use of preventive services such as routine breast or colon exams, up-to-date immunizations, or timely knowledge of lipid levels. Such education programs have been shown to increase consumer knowledge of the need for preventive services (Terry, 1994). There are many studies that show that reminder systems, for example, increase compliance with recommended prevention schedules. One study (Terry, 1994) showed a materials-based approach to self-care education can serve to increase employee knowledge of the often-changing schedules that are recommended by professional societies and expert panels. Patients of a family practice office at Park Nicollet Clinic were randomly assigned to an experimental group receiving an instruction manual on preventive services and a control group receiving unrelated health information. A 22-item questionnaire on preventive health services that measured respondents' age-adjusted risks and knowledge of risk-based screening guidelines was sent to both experimental and control groups. The treatment group was significantly more accurate in reporting the risk-based guidelines of the U.S. Preventive Services Task Force than the control group. Specifically, the intervention group was 2–13 times more likely to indicate when an exam was not recommended; however, the percentage of total respondents reporting that screening was not recommended was relatively small, with only 18 percent identifying correct exam schedules.

Worksite health programs increasingly target their most prevalent disease risks for cost containment. Examining prevention services related to such conditions, while garnering less attention, can result in substantial savings. Selective changes in prevention visits can also improve management of chronic health conditions. One of the most common preventive services, taking blood pressure measurements, also may have the most variation in quality of any preventive exam. When blood pressure readings are not taken with strict adherence to the standards of the American Heart Association, false high readings can often lead to costly and unnecessary medical management of a condition that may not even exist. A study of the Hypertension Management Program at Park Nicollet shows the value of standardized approaches to measurement in detecting hypertension (Pheley et al., 1995). Of 275 patients referred for screening, 78% had normal blood pressure. When patients are referred to such a program for screening, it usually means the doctor suspects hypertension based on their readings and wishes confirmation. Since most primary care practices do not have access to such a hypertension management screening service, it is likely that many patients begin treatment rather than confirmatory screening. The data from the Park Nicollet study suggests that the use of screening techniques using multiple methods ensures that patients will not be treated unnecessarily.

This study of hypertension management practices also indicated the value of disease self-management education in helping patients control their blood pressure. At entry into the management phase of the Park Nicollet program, which is a nurse-based education and counseling service, only 17% of patients had blood pressure within controlled limits. By the twelve-month follow-up, this proportion had increased to 44% (p < 0.001), compared to 27% in comparison groups. The 6 mm Hg average decrease in systolic blood pressure found in this study is associated with a 34% reduction in strokes and a 24% reduction in heart disease, according to epidemiological evidence. These types of early detection and ongoing management programs, then, have both short-term and long-term cost impacts. Worksite health promotion program leaders need to consider both the short-term cost containment potential of examining preventive services as well as the long-term impact of improving management of chronic conditions.

Self-Care and Common Chronic Conditions

Managed care has progressed through several stages of maturation in its goal of improving the health of members. Starting with employee health education, moving into increasing preventive services rates, and advancing to population health management, worksite health promotion programs, particularly those who partner with managed care companies, are at a crossroads while demand management and self-care education are converging on specific chronic conditions (Terry, 1998). Keeping people who have chronic conditions healthy likely represents the next level of sophistication for companies that have already realized whatever gains they could get from utilization management and casework. The following sections highlight exemplary approaches to management of chronic disease states. It is noteworthy that chronic disease management has been a subject of scientific inquiry for many years, as the references in the following section will attest. Still, we are presently in an era in which "disease management" programs are being introduced as innovative approaches to care. One should consider then whether the programs outlined in the following section of this chapter, with their care guidelines and patient-centered educational approaches, were ahead of their time or whether present claims concerning disease management simply represent "old wine in new bottles." Table 14.4 outlines

Table 14-4 Self-Care Education and Chronic Health Conditions

Author	Title	Sample Size	Evaluation Period	Findings
Clark et al. (1992)	Impact of Self-Management Education on the Functional Health Status of Older Adults with Heart Disease	758 persons met criteria; 324 agreed to participate; 246 complete program	1 year	Program group members at the end of the 12-month program experienced less illness than the control group.
Montgomery, Lieberman, Singh, & Fries (1994)	Patient Education and Health Promotion Can Be Effective in Parkinson's Disease: A Randomized Controlled Trial (Propath Advisory Board)	290 patients involved in study: 140 in the intervention group; 150 in the control group	6 months	Medical utilization was significantly lower in the intervention group versus the control group.
Gifford et al. (1998)	Pilot Randomized Trial of Education to Improve Self-Management Skills of Men with Symptomatic HIV/AIDS	71 men: 34 received educational intervention; 37 received usual care	7 sessions	The symptom severity index decreased in the experimental group and increased in the control group. A trend of more exercise was higher in the experimental group versus the control group.
Anderson et al. (1995)	Patient Empowerment: Results of a Randomized Controlled Trial	64 patients met criteria: 22 placed in intervention group; 23 were placed in control group	12 weeks	Intervention group showed gains in 4 of 8 self-efficacy subscales. There were no differences between groups on the remaining 4 subscales.
Campbell, Redman, Moffitt, & Sanson-Fisher (1996)	The Relative Effectiveness of Educational and Behavioral Instruction Programs for Patients With NIDDM: A Randomized Trial	241 patients total, split into 4 groups: Minimum instruction–59; Individual visits–57; Group educational courses–66; Behavioral program–59	1 year	Individual and group education programs had higher attrition rates than the behavior and minimal programs. Behavior program showed a greater reduction in diastolic blood pressure and a greater reduction in cholesterol risk factor ratio over 3 months compared to the other programs.
Fries, Carey, & McShane (1997)	Patient Education in Arthritis: Randomized Controlled Trial of a Mail-Delivered Program	375 program participants; 434 control participants	6 months	Function, decreased pain, global vitality, and joint count were improved in the program group. The number of days missed from work or confined to the home also decreased by 52%.

(continued)

Table 14-4 Self-Care Education and Chronic Health Conditions

Author	Title	Sample Size	Evaluation Period	Findings
Mazzuca et al. (1997)	Effects of Self-Care Education on the Health Status of Inner-City Patients with Osteoarthritis of the Knee	211 inner-city patients applied; 165 complete the trial	1 year	At the conclusion of the trial, the educational program group had lower scores for disability and resting knee pain.
Fries, Bloch, Harrington, Richardson, & Beck (1993)	Two-Year Results of a Randomized Controlled Trial of a Health Promotion Program in a Retiree Population: The Bank of America Study	4,712 Bank of America retirees separated into three groups: intervention group, risk appraisals, and claims data	2 years	Overall health risk scores improved by 12% at the end of one year and by 23% at the end of the second year compared to the controlled group.
Kruger, Helmick, Callahan, & Haddix (1998)	Cost-Effectiveness of the Arthritis Self-Help Course		4 years	At the end of 4 years, the pain of arthritis decreased by 20%.
Lorig, Mazonson, & Holman (1993)	Evidence Suggesting that Health Education for Self-Management in Patients with Chronic Arthritis has Sustained Health Benefits while Reducing Health Care Costs	343 subjects	6 weekly two-hour sessions	Pain had declined by a mean of 20% and visits to the physician by 40%.
Nelson et al. (1984)	Medical Self-Care Education for Elders: A Controlled Trial to Evaluate Impact	330 elders	13 sessions	Medical self-instruction produces substantial improvements that were sustained for one year in health knowledge, skills performance, and skills confidence; stimulates many attempts to improve lifestyle; and generates improvements in life quality.
Vickery, Lolaszewski, Wright, & Kalmer (1998)	The Effect of Self-Care Interventions on the Use of Medical Services Within a Medicare Population	560 subjects in experimental group; 449 in control group	1 year	A decrease of 15% in total medical visits was found in the experimental group as compared with the control group. Medical visit decreases resulted in savings of $36.65 per household in the experimental group.

some of the best research related to self-care of chronic conditions.

Asthma

Educating patients and making them an active partner in the health care team is critical to the successful management of asthma. Because of the high prevalence of asthma and the very high costs associated with recovering from poorly managed asthma, it is a condition that is garnering considerable attention from employers and health systems. The National Asthma Education Program, an initiative from the late 1980s, named four major asthma management components: pharmacologic therapy, lung function measurement, patient education, and environmental modifications (Bone, 1993). These recommendations form the foundation of "step-care" approaches, which are considered the best way to prevent unnecessary hospitalization of patients with asthma.

Increases in the morbidity and mortality from asthma have been blamed, in part, on the history of poor patient compliance with recommended treatment regimens. A tenet of community health education is to simplify the regimen for consumers. Step-care strategies simplify asthma management by educating patients about therapeutic alternatives and gradually increasing medication doses until management is achieved. As it relates to cost-containment and productivity in the workplace, when self-care of asthma improves (as may be accomplished by adjusting treatment doses and correctly using peak flow meters) asthma outcomes, such as fewer missed work days, will also improve.

A number of studies clearly demonstrate asthma self-care education works. One widely recognized controlled trial comparing individual and group education was designed to improve poor self-management practices among patients (Wilson et al., 1993). Patients with moderate to severe asthma were randomly assigned to one of three groups ranging from six to eight members per group. One group received classroom instruction, group support, behavioral contracting, and at-home activities. The second group received individual instruction delivered in

three to five customized counseling sessions drawing from the same content as the small group education. The third group was a control group receiving either an asthma workbook or no education.

Significant improvements in use of a metered dose inhaler were achieved by groups one and two at a five-month follow-up, and improvements in symptom measures for these two groups occurred by the one-year follow-up. Physician evaluation of study participants indicated that asthma status was measurably improved for 52% of those in group education compared to 44% and 42% improvement in the counseling group and control group, respectively. The study also showed the small group education to be somewhat more effective than the individual counseling and that both forms of education were significantly more effective than the control groups. Educated patients had fewer symptom days (19% treatment vs. 27% control), a reduction in acute visits per year, and lower overall hospitalization rates.

While many studies indicate the benefits of self-care instruction in asthma management, the effect of education on changes in morbidity and mortality remains controversial. To address this concern, one study focused on the role of asthma self-management in behavior of patients during an acute severe asthma attack (Kolbe, Vamos, Fergusson, Elkind, & Garrett, 1996). This cross-sectional study used a comprehensive questionnaire to associate asthma knowledge with self-reported behavior during asthma attacks. Knowledge scores were positively correlated with medical care factors and the likelihood of the patient having a written action plan for asthma management. The key variables that are associated with self-care education (an action plan, use of peak flow meters, and a supply of medications) were positively associated with behaviors appropriate to an asthma attack. The authors noted that, while their findings lent support to asthma education initiatives, they still found a troublesome gap between knowledge of asthma management and the rate at which patients were doing the right things during asthma attacks. This result reinforces the need to design chronic disease-based self-care education programs that emphasize behavior changes as well as improved knowledge.

Arthritis

Even though self-management education programs for chronic conditions such as arthritis have been shown to be effective, there remains skepticism concerning the salience of such interventions (Katz, 1998, Riemsma et al., 1997). To address this concern, Lorig and colleagues studied the effects of self-management programs four years after the intervention (Lorig, Mazonson, & Holman, 1993). Using self-administered instruments designed to measure health service utilization, health status, and psychological states, sustained improvement was shown in the intervention groups while no similar gains were found in the control group. Specifically, those who had been taught arthritis self-management skills had 40% fewer doctor visits and 20% reduction in self-reported pain. Patient savings were estimated to be $648 for rheumatoid arthritis patients and $189 for osteoarthritis patients.

As stated earlier in this chapter, it is difficult to defend disease management as a cost-savings strategy when such large populations are presently undertreated for conditions such as arthritis. James Fries, one of the most prolific authorities in self-care education, designed a study to determine if mail-delivered arthritis self-management programs could positively affect patient outcomes and decrease medical costs (Fries, Carey, & McShane, 1997). In this randomized controlled trial, at three-month intervals retirees in the intervention group received health assessment questionnaires and individualized, computer-processed letters recommending self-care practices. After six months, intervention group participants had 16% fewer doctor visits than the control group. Numerous health measures improved, including decreased pain, improved functional status, increased vitality, increased exercise, and higher self-efficacy scores. The authors noted that their findings were similar to those attained through traditional group education programs. Considering the many barriers to involving patients in traditional education programs, the success of a mail-delivered approach holds great promise for self-care education in an era of cost controls by health providers.

Developing and implementing self-management programs for chronic arthritis has led to the examination of several other alternative delivery approaches. For example, most often patient education is provided one-on-one by the costliest of medical providers—the doctor. Targeting inner-city patients with osteoarthritis of the knee, a self-care education program delivered by an arthritis nurse specialist was designed to test the effects of a concise intervention (Mazzuca et al., 1997). The education participants received individualized 30- to 60-minute education sessions and brief phone contacts after one and four weeks. The intervention group had significantly lower scores for resting knee pain and disability, and, like the Fries study described above, the magnitude of effects compared favorably to more time-consuming and labor intensive programs. Studies such as these, showing the cost-effectiveness of arthritis self-management programs, are critical to the continued funding and development of self-care education. Some would still argue, however, that the costs are justified from the patients' perspective rather than the purchaser's, or broad health policy setting, perspective. To counter this concern, a study of the Arthritis Self-Help Course (ASHC), a six-week program sponsored by the Arthritis Foundation, was conducted to assess the long-term cost benefits from a societal perspective (Kruger, Helmick, Callahan, & Haddix, 1998). A decision model was developed to assess per-person program costs along with estimated physician costs, pain related costs, and time and transportation costs. The ASHC was analyzed over a four-year time horizon and computed to save $320 per patient from a "societal" perspective and $267 from a health care perspective (while society is concerned with costs related to productivity, health care focuses on the costs of illness). Perhaps it seems intuitively obvious that when patients are taught self-care they will use fewer health care resources. The results of these well-designed and -executed arthritis studies should convince even the shrewdest health policy antagonist that self-care education is an investment, not merely an added cost.

Diabetes

Among the costliest of the chronic conditions, both to treat and if left undertreated, is diabetes. Both in terms of patient education time and treatment intensity, diabetes is among the most difficult to manage and the most complex to self-manage (Assal, Jacquemet, & Morel, 1997, Howard, Barrett, Chan, & Wolf, 1986). Perhaps that is why "the formula of who is to teach what, when, and how and how to assess suitable outcome seems to be the Holy Grail of diabetes education." (Flack, 1990). Accordingly, diabetes educators are likely to be certified as diabetes educators while health professionals conducting disease self-management programs for other conditions are often not "certified" experts. Similarly, for programs in diabetes education to be officially recognized, the American Diabetes Association (ADA) has a process of self-evaluation and documentation for organizations that wish to meet their National Standards for Diabetes Patient Education Programs (Funnell & Haas, 1995).

Diabetes education, unlike self-care education, has formal sanctions and standards intended to reduce practice variation and to increase effectiveness in patient education. Several of the national standards are designed to elicit patient self-care behavior. Standard 18, for example, requires that "an individualized education plan, based on the assessment, will be developed in collaboration with each patient." Explicit throughout the guidelines is the concept of diabetes as a lifelong management challenge and the need for periodic reassessments and education. Standard 20 states "the program will offer appropriate and timely educational intervention based on periodic reassessments of health status, knowledge, skills, attitudes, goals, and self-care behaviors." Self-care education for diabetes, perhaps more than any other chronic condition, needs to be grounded in a continuous feedback cycle. Just as medical management of the condition is required for life, learning about changes in physical functioning and metabolic responses to other changes (such as exercise level, diet, and insulin use) is also a lifetime challenge.

To highlight the keen interaction between self-management behaviors and the occurrence of hypoglycemia in insulin-dependent diabetic patients, Clarke and his colleagues studied the effects of a blood glucose awareness-training program (Clarke et al., 1997). Using a handheld computer, subjects measured their blood glucose level and then recorded

whether their food, exercise, or insulin had been missed or were greater, less than, or about the same as usual. When glucose readings were low, meals were more likely to have been missed; high readings corresponded to missed bouts of exercise. Low glucose levels also corresponded to more insulin and more exercise. The findings suggested that many patients have poor awareness, or "symptom perception," related to blood glucose levels. However, patients who paid careful attention to their recent activity levels, insulin dose, or amount of food eaten, were able to anticipate fluctuations in their individual blood glucose profiles. Self-care education for diabetic patients becomes a balancing act, with blood glucose monitoring becoming the fulcrum on which changes in insulin, food, and exercise regimens are monitored.

Given the intricacy of diabetes self-care and the high health stakes involved in effective management, patient education needs to account for the patient's self-efficacy as much as for the patient's knowledge and skills. To this end, a six-week patient empowerment program was studied in a randomized controlled trial to assess if participation in the program would improve attitudes toward diabetes as well as lower blood glucose levels (Anderson et al., 1996). The study found that the intervention group had a statistically significant improvement based on self-efficacy and attitude subscales, along with significant reductions in glycated hemoglobin levels, compared to the control group. Such a finding lends support to the need for including psychosocial supports and education in the self-care portfolio for people with diabetes. One of the most commonly accepted devices (both socially and behaviorally) for facilitating positive self-care is the diabetes self-management record. Records are checklists for diabetes self-management that include dates, times, and sometimes a point system for behaviors such as exercise, reading food labels, checking meat portion size, abstaining from beverages with added sugar, and many other diabetes control goals. One study used a record with 39 adults to self-monitor behaviors such as exercise, glucose control, fat consumption, sugar/carbohydrate consumption, and other eating practices (Bielamowicz, Miller, Elkins, & Ladewig, 1995). Diabetes management scores were higher among the record-keeping group than the control group, and the behaviors were maintained at least six weeks postintervention.

The American Dietetics Association's national standards in diabetes education positively influenced the content of diabetes education programs offered throughout the country. However, considerable obstacles remain for organizations attempting to improve self-care education for their employees or patients (Mangan, 1997). Employers can play an instrumental role in advancing the quality of diabetes management by advocating reimbursement of quality service. For example, the inclusion of an annual eye examination for people with diabetes to detect diabetic retinopathy has been included in the Health Plan Employer Data and Information Set (HEDIS). This is a tool that was developed to make health plans more accountable to employer purchasers. Many managed care companies will reimburse diabetes education only if it occurs at ADA-recognized medical practices or hospitals. As with their advocacy for HEDIS-related accountabilities, employers can, and have, steered their employees toward centers of excellence in diabetes care. Nevertheless, there remains wide variability in the level of intensity of education and the effectiveness associated with different approaches. Similarly and as with the arthritis management studies, there is some evidence that it is difficult to distinguish between the effects of educational versus behavioral instruction. One randomized controlled trial, for example, assigned diabetics to one of four programs that included individual visits, group instruction, behavioral programming, or a combination of these (Campbell et al., 1996). Using measures such as glucose control, cholesterol levels, blood pressure, and program satisfaction, there were virtually no differences between groups related to key measures such as glucose control and obesity; reductions were observed in all patients in all programs. This finding supports the conclusions from similar studies that the level of intensity of patient instruction will not necessarily explain improvements in outcomes.

For employers referring their employees for service or providing such services at the workplace, the intensity of the educational approach should be carefully considered. Many studies show the effectiveness of a comprehensive educational approach while neglecting to show the attrition rates of the program. Simply put, the less time it takes to get through a program, the more likely employees are to complete the program. In worksite self-care education programs, there is always a tradeoff between time and intensity. A less intensive program that attracts and retains many participants will likely yield greater health benefits than a comprehensive program in which only a few people are willing to participate.

Self-Care and Other Chronic Conditions

The most prevalent chronic conditions, such as arthritis, asthma, and diabetes, have benefited from the longest history of self-care education; however, many other conditions have proved to be ameliorated through self-care (Clark et al., 1992; Gonzalez, Steiner, Lum, & Barrett, 1999, Montgomery et al., 1997, Steinweg et al., 1998). As with other chronic conditions, the complexity of the problem and the severity of the symptoms are important variables in determining the type of self-care education needed. A study of uncomplicated acute bronchitis in adults showed that a comprehensive education program did not improve patient self-care behavior significantly more than a minimal intervention (Gonzalez et al., 1999). One of the variables examined in this study was antibiotic use. Certain self-care behaviors, such as use of cough suppressants and analgesics, were not affected by the comprehensive program. Still, there was a significant decline in antibiotic prescription use at the comprehensive intervention site. Because of the increasing resistance of many microorganisms to infection, employers need to be concerned, as the health profession is, about unnecessary antibiotic use. Therein lies the difficulty in determining the benefits of self-care education. Often, behaviors that the program prevents from occurring are as important as new behaviors or skills that participants can demonstrate. This, of course, is the conundrum for prevention programs generally; how do we quantify problems we avoid? Clearly, randomized controlled trials offer the most promise for getting such answers.

The difficulty in quantifying certain benefits of self-care education also reinforces the need to study the most cost-efficient ways to educate employees and still achieve results. An exemplary study of patients with Parkinson's disease shows how a minimal intervention can have demonstrated benefits (Montgomery, Lieberman, Singh, & Fries, 1994). This randomized controlled trial used a through-the-mail approach to provide patient information, customized letters from physicians, and computer-generated disease assessments. The intervention group had significantly increased exercise, reduced side effects, and decreased Parkinson's symptoms. As important, from an employer's perspective, the education groups decreased time off work and increased quality-of-life scores.

WORKPLACE SELF-CARE PROGRAM IMPLEMENTATION STRATEGIES

Like other health improvement initiatives in the workplace, there are many planning and program development issues that are unique to employee-directed health improvement campaigns. Planning a worksite self-care program is a process of clarifying the values of the organization, identifying needs of employees, and aligning resources with needs. A self-care plan usually includes an assessment of health care costs, outlines a comprehensive array of self-care intervention techniques, and has an evaluation component. This section discusses these planning components and suggests resources that are available to the workplace health promotion program planner.

Data Sources for Employee Health Services Utilization

While many organizations have developed questionnaires designed to assess health services utilization (Hibbard, Greenlick, Jimison, Kunkel, & Tusler, 1999), there is little evidence that these tools reliably predict future utilization. The biggest problem is the employee's unreliable recollection of frequency of visits and reasons for visits. Some organizations have worked with health care providers to audit medical records; regrettably, health care provider accuracy in recording details of interest to educators in the medical record is also very inconsistent.

The most relevant source of data about the health services utilization that can be affected by self-care education is claims data that can be provided by insurance companies or benefits consulting firms. Pharmaceutical claims costs are also a source of data that can be of interest to employers attempting to understand the need for employee self-care education. Many companies monitor their highest inpatient or outpatient medical cost claims, their top 10–20 pharmaceutical claims, or both. For example, most large organizations have observed the dramatic increase in costs related to Prozac and other depression medications. Similarly, after very aggressive consumer-direct marketing by one pharmaceutical manufacturer of an allergy medication, many employers have noted the unexpected and costly increase in their allergy medication claims costs. Table 14-5 outlines studies that demonstrate the cost-effectiveness of self-care education for self-limiting conditions.

Assessing Avoidable Medical Costs

The key issue in claims analysis is accurately distinguishing between controllable versus uncontrollable medical claims costs. A closely related issue relates to the time horizon an organization chooses in its attempts to contain medical costs. Identifying increases in cancer and heart disease-related claims, for example, can be as readily explained by the aging of the population as by the lifestyle changes occurring, or not occurring, in the population. The dilemma in trying to associate increasing or decreasing costs to health program interventions relates to the resistance most employers have to randomized, controlled experiments using their employees. Without control groups, however, it is unlikely that program leaders can attribute gains or losses in claims costs to their program interventions. There is such a multitude of other variables that can explain changes in health costs, including changes in medical benefits, secular trends, new medical guidelines, costly new therapies, etc., that health programs can only be expected to explain a small proportion of total change.

Self-care education is one health improvement approach that can address cost savings in the short-term; consequently, many of the scientific arguments

Table 14-5 Self-Care Education and Acute Health Conditions

Author(s)	Title	Sample Size	Evaluation Period	Findings
Gonzales, Steiner, Lum, & Barrett (1999)	Decreasing Antibiotic Use in Ambulatory Practice.	2,462 adults included in baseline; 2,027 adults included in study	3 months baseline; 3 months study	Full intervention site saw a decline in antibiotic prescription rates (74% to 48%). Control group went from 78% to 76%, and the limited intervention group went from 82% to 77%.
Wilson et al. (1999)	A Controlled Trial of Two Forms of Self-Management Education for Adults with Asthma	323 adult patients randomly assigned to one of four groups: small group education, individual teaching, control group with a workbook, and a control group with no workbook	Records taken in a 3-year period	Self-management educational programs showed improvements in the control of asthma symptoms, metered dose inhaler (MDI) techniques, and environmental control practices.
Kemper (1982)	Self-Care Education: Impact on HMO Costs	900 HMO members	1 year	Of the families who participated, 86% said the workshop improved health care for their families, and 81% said they read at least half of the handbook.
Lorig, Kraines, Brown, & Richardson (1985)	A Workplace Health Education Program that Reduces Outpatient Visits	5,200 employees	15 months	Visit rates for households insured only by Blue Cross of California were reduced by 17%, or 2.0 visits per household per year. For all the participants, the reduction was 7.2%.
Fleming, Giadrello, Andersen, & Andrade (1984)	Self-Care: Substitute, Supplement, or Stimulus for Formal Medical Care Services?	A child younger than 17 years from each randomly selected U.S. household.	2 years	Those who used non-prescribed home treatment (NPHT) were less apt to contact a physician than were those who did not use NPHT ($p < 0.05$).

for the need for randomized controls need not be invoked. If a program aimed at a specific, self-limiting condition results in significant decreases in costs related to the treatment of that condition within a few months, then arguments that other variables can explain the changes are abated. When a comparison group is available, such as another department or company with similar demographics, short-term changes can even more reliably be attributed to the intervention. Program planners need to work with their insurance providers to assess the extent to which claims can be sorted by codes that relate only to specific conditions of interest. For example, if an employer wants to reduce allergy- or sinusitis-related costs, it is important to know whether the insurance provider can isolate these costs. Herein lies yet another practical dilemma for the program evaluator. Insurance companies will likely be able to dedicate the resources needed for this analysis for their large, self-insured employer customers; however, it may be difficult, if not impossible, for a small health insurance purchaser to conduct such a detailed analysis. At the same time, the large employer is likely to have many facility locations and/or many insurance providers. Coordinating claims analyses for these multiple sites from multiple insurance carriers can be complex and, therefore, costly.

Appropriate Employee Use of Preventive Services

Earlier sections of this chapter have noted the likely overlap between self-care education for self-limiting conditions and education for use of preventive services. Assessing need in an employed population should balance the short-term cost-containment benefit of self-care education with the longer-term health benefit of self-care from use of preventive services. Just as disease management may as often increase as decrease health care costs, self-care using preventive exams may also increase costs in the short term. For example, most organizations that have analyzed claims related to services such as mammograms, influenza immunizations, Pap smears, and pelvic exams have been able to determine that certain of their employees or certain locations underutilize these services. Table 14-6 shows the most recent studies describing the cost impact of educational efforts to ameliorate emergent conditions.

It would not be unusual to find that less than 50% of women are up-to-date on mammograms or that less than 50% of men and women are current in their recommended colon exams. There is no argument against the claim that early detection of cancer saves lives; however, there is often debate about the cost savings that will result from a population-wide screening and prevention education campaigns. In-

creasing these exam rates will inevitably cost more for the conscientious employers looking out for the long-term health of employees. Countering these costly investments in long-term self-care with short-term investments in self-care education that reduce unnecessary medical visits may be the only way to keep a balanced approach to employee self-care budget neutral.

THE EMPLOYEE'S ROLE IN DISEASE MANAGEMENT

There are subtle but distinct differences between medical self-care education and a new trend coined as "disease management." Like self-care education, disease management is more of an industry than a professional discipline and more like a business line than a field of study. Still, those drawn to develop and deliver disease management programs are typically schooled in medicine, education, and management so it has many similarities to self-care. An important distinction relates to the disease specialization inherent in disease management programs. Disease management programs tend to segment a condition while self-care education has traditionally offered comprehensive education programs and products that could assist individuals and their families in a broad array of health decisions. The specialization also represents a weakness for disease management programs in that few physicians deal with chronic conditions in isolation. The prospect of segmenting patients based on one condition and referring them into a program runs counter to the tenets of primary care.

Most primary care providers see their role as coordinator of care, particularly for the common occurrence of comorbidity in their patients. Turning patients over to a specialist may also be counter to many reimbursement systems wherein the physician is rewarded for productivity as measured by the number of patients seen. In spite of such barriers, disease management is a growing industry moving from an estimated $60 million in revenue in 1997 to over $350 million in 1999 (Moran, 1999). Still, disease management is far from a mature discipline. There are virtually no prospective studies of the effectiveness of such programs, and there remains tremendous variability in the quality of the program offerings.

Table 14-6 Self-Care Education and Emergent Health Conditions

Author(s)	Title	Sample Size	Evaluation Period	Findings
Terry & Pheley (1993)	The Effect of Self-Care Brochures on Use of Medical Services	Intervention group-7439 Control group-7478	1 year	Less utilization of medical visits for colds was found in the intervention group. Less utilization for earaches coupled with a reduction in medical costs, was also found in the intervention group.
Stergachis et al. (1990)	The Effect of a Self-Care Minimal Intervention for Colds and Flu on the Use of Medical Services	12,353 persons in experimental group 7,774 persons in control group	3 months	Upper respiratory infection medical visits resulted in a 14% decrease in the experimental group compared to the control group.
Steinweg et al. (1998)	The Impact on a Health Care System of a Program to Facilitate Self-Care	283 were enrolled in the Self-Care Intervention Program (SCIP) 191 returned surveys	6 months	Increased knowledge of personal health issues, treating minor illnesses, practice of healthy behaviors, and a commitment to seek preventive medicine.
Estabrook (1979)	Consumer Impact of a Cold Self-Care Center in a Prepaid Ambulatory Care Setting	Intervention: 74 Comparison: 104	1 month	Knowledge of criteria for seeking professional care was greater than in non-users. 20% sought professional care, and 6% anticipated seeking care for future colds.
Roberts et al. (1983)	Reducing Physician Visits for Colds Through Consumer Education	Intervention: 433 families Control: 444	6 months	The test families made 44% fewer unnecessary visits than the control families.
Zapka & Averill (1979)	Self-Care for Colds: A Cost-Effective Alternative to Upper Respiratory Infection Management	URI visits to clinicians per 1,000 members	5 years	The operating cost ratio of an outpatient visit was 14.7/1. Savings over a 2-year period are estimated at over $46,000.
Moore, LoGerfo, & Inui (1980)	Effect of a Self-Care Book on Physician Visits	785 families divided into 3 groups	1 year	The average number of visits decreased by 24% in group 3, by 21% in group 2, and 16% in group 1.
Vickery et al. (1983)	Effect of a Self-Care Education Program on Medical Visits	2,833 households	1 year	Statistically significant decreases on total medical visits and minor illness visits. Decreases averaged 17% and 35%.

Accordingly, the role of the consumer in deriving benefits from disease management offerings is a vital one, a role that is often taught through medical self-care education. Thus, it can be argued that while disease management brings new content to consumer choice in health care, self-care education has offered the framework for active decision-making.

CONCLUSION

Worksite health promotion has proven to be a valuable instrument for improving employee health, and self-care education has become an integral part of effecting the costs-savings that keep such programs viable for business. Programs that focus too much on individual behavior change as the critical element in health improvement risk overlook the more reliable predictors in a healthy workforce. As convincing as the above data are that self-care education can save money and improve health care delivery, the more telling contributors to employee health relate to social and cultural forces that shape an employee's interests and intentions. Self-care education will be a Band-Aid solution in organizations that do not have a concurrent commitment to creating joy and inclusiveness in the workplace. Moreover, for companies that are disconnected from the health concerns of the broader community, self-care education will be equivalent to offering first aid to a chronic pain patient; the solution may even exacerbate the problem. For companies that keep self-care and health promotion in balance, self-care can be one of the most practical and sought-after components of their employee health benefits.

References

Abramowitz, S., Cote, A., & Berry, E. (1987). Analyzing patient satisfaction: A multianalytic approach. *QRB Quality Review Bulletin, 13*(4), 122–130.

Anderson, L. A., & Zimmerman, M. A. (1993). Patient and physician perceptions of their relationship and patient satisfaction: A study of chronic disease management. *Patient Education and Counseling, 20*(1), 27–36.

Anderson, R. M., Funnell, M. M., & Butler. (1995). Patient empowerment: Results of a randomized controlled trial. *Diabetes Care, 18*(7), 943–949.

Assal, J. P., Jacquemet, S., & Morel, Y. (1997). The added value of therapy in diabetes: The education of patients for self-management of their diseases. *Metabolism, 46* (12, Suppl. 1), 61–64.

Barry, P., (1980). *Self-care programs: Their role and potential.* [Monograph]. Chapel Hill, SC: Health Services Research Center, University of North Carolina.

Bielamowicz, M. K., Miller, W. C., Elkins, E., & Ladewig, H. W. (1995). Monitoring behavioral changes in diabetes care with the diabetes self-management record. *Diabetes Educator, 21*(5), 426–431.

Bone, R. C. (1993). The bottom line in asthma management is patient education. *American Journal of Medicine, 94*(6), 561–563.

Campbell, E. M., Redman, S., Moffitt, P. S., Sanson-Fisher, R. W. (1996). The relative effectiveness of educational and behavioral instruction programs for patients with NIDDM: A randomized trial. *Diabetes Education, 22*(4), 379–386.

Clark, N. M., Janz, N. K., & Becker, M. H. (1992). Impact of self-management education on the functional health status of older adults with heart disease. *Gerontologist, 32*(4), 438–443.

Clarke, W. L., Cox, D. J., & Londer-Frederick, L. A. (1997). The relationship between nonroutine use of insulin, food, and exercise and the occurrence of hypoglycemia in adults with IDDM and varying degrees of hypoglycemic awareness and metabolic control. *Diabetes Educator, 23*(1), 55–58.

_____. Education for health: A role for physicians and the efficacy of health education efforts, Council on Scientific Affairs. *Journal of the American Medical Association, 263*(13), 1816–1819.

Estabrook, B. (1979). Consumer impact of a cold self-care center in a prepaid ambulatory care setting. *Medical Care, 17,* 1139–1145.

Etter, J. F., Perneger, T., & Rougemont, A. (1996). Does sponsorship matter in patient satisfaction surveys? A randomized trial. *Medical Care, 34*(4), 327–335.

Flack, J. R. (1990). Effect of diabetes education on self-care metabolic control and emotional well-being. *Diabetes Care, 13*(10), 1094.

Fleming, G. et al. (1984). Self-care: Substitute, supplement, or stimulus for formal medical care services? *Medical Care, 22*(10), 950–966.

Fowles, J. B., & Craft, C. (1996). Patient/Physician Communication Profile. In J. McGee, N. Goldfield, K. Riley, & J. Morton (Eds.), *Collecting Information from Health Care Consumers.* Gaithersburg, Maryland: Aspen.

Fries, J. F., Koop, C. E., & Beadle, C. E. (1993). Reducing health care costs by reducing the need and demand for medical services. The Health Project Consortium. *New England Journal of Medicine, 329,*(5), 321–325.

Fries, J. F., Bloch, D. A., Harrington, H., Richardson, N., & Beck, R. (1993). Two-year results of a randomized controlled trial of a health promotion program in a retiree population: The Bank of America Study. *American Journal of Medicine, 94*(5), 455–462.

Fries, J. F., Carey, C., & McShane, D. J. (1997). Patient education in arthritis: Randomized controlled trial of a mail-delivered program. *Journal of Rheumatology, 24*(7), 1378–1383.

Funnell, M. M., & Haas, L. B. (1995). National standards for diabetes self-management education programs. *Diabetes Care, 18*(1), 100–116.

Gerteis, M., Edgman-Levitan, S., & Walker, J. O. (1993). What patients really want. *Health Management Quarterly, 15*(3), pp. 2–6.

Gifford, A. L., Laurent, D. D., Gonzales, V. M., Chesney, M. A., & Lorig, K. R. (1998). Pilot randomized trial of education to improve self-management skills of men with symptomatic HIV/AIDS. *Journal of Acquired Immune Deficiency Syndromes and Human Retrovirology, 18*(2), 136–144.

Glasgow, R. E., Eakin, E. G., & Toobert, D. J. (1996). How generalizable are the results of diabetes self-management research? The impact of participation and attrition. *Diabetes Educator, 22*(6), 573–574, 581–582, 584–585.

Gonzalez, R., Steiner, J. F., Lum, A., & Barrett, P. H. Jr. (1999). Decreasing antibiotic use in ambulatory practice: Impact of a multidimensional intervention on the treatment of uncomplicated acute bronchitis in adults. *Journal of the American Medical Association, 281*(16), 1512–1519.

Hall, J. A., & Dornan, M. C. (1988). What patients like about their medical care and how often they are asked. *Social Science Medicine, 27*(9), 935–939.

Hibbard, J. H. (1999, October 21). Presentation at The Sixth Annual Park Nicollet Health Conference: Breaking Through Boundaries, Minneapolis, MN.

Hibbard, J. H., Greenlick, M., Jimison, H., Kunkel, L., & Tusler, M. (1999). Prevalence and predictors of the use of self-care resources. *Evaluation and the Health Professions, 22*(1), 107–122.

Howard, M., Barrett, C., Chan, M., & Wolf, F. M. (1986). Retention of knowledge and self-care skills after an intensive in-patient diabetes education program. *Diabetes Research and Clinical Practice, 2*(1), 51–57.

Katz, P. P. (1998). Education and self-care activities among persons with rheumatoid arthritis. *Social Science Medicine, 46*(8), 1057–1066.

Kemper, D. W. (1982). Self-care education: Impact on HMO costs. *Medical Care, 20*(7), 710–718.

Kemper, D. W., Lorig, K., & Mettler, M. (1993). The effectiveness of medical self-care interventions: A focus on self-initiated responses to symptoms. *Patient Education and Counseling, 21*(1-2), 29–39.

Kolbe, J., Vamos, M., Fergusson, W., Elkind, G., & Garrett, J. (1996). Differential influences on asthma self-management knowledge and self-management behavior in acute severe asthma. *Chest, 110*(6), 1463–1468.

Kruger, J. M., Helmick, C. G., Callahan, L. F., & Haddix, A. C. (1998). Cost-effectiveness of the arthritis self-help course. *Archives of Internal Medicine, 158*(11), 1245–1249.

Laine, C., Davidoff, F., Lewis, C., et al. (1996). Important elements of outpatient care: A comparison of patients' and physicians' opinions. *Annals of Internal Medicine, 125*(8), 640–645.

Ley, P. (1982). Satisfaction, compliance, and communication. *British Journal of Clinical Psychology, 21*, 241–254.

Lorig, K. R., & Holman, H. (1993). Arthritis self-management studies: a twelve-year review. *Health Education Quarterly, 20*(1), 17–28.

Lorig, K. R., Kraines, R. G., Brown, B. W. Jr., & Richardson, N. (1985). A workplace health education program that reduces outpatient visits. *Medical Care, 23*(9), 1044–1054.

Lorig, K. R., Mazonson, P. D., & Holman, H. R. (1993). Evidence suggesting that health education for self-management in patients with chronic arthritis has sustained health benefits while reducing health care costs. *Arthritis and Rheumatism, 36*(4), 439–446.

Lynch, W. D., & Vickery, D. M. (1993). The potential impact of health promotion on health care utilization: An introduction to demand management. *American Journal of Health Promotion, 8*(2), 87–92.

Mangan, M. (1997). Diabetes self-management education programs in the Veterans Health Administration. *Diabetes Educator, 23*(6), 687–692, 695.

Mazzuca, S. A., Brandt, K. D., Katz, B. P., & et al. (1997). Effects of self-care education on the health status of inner-city patients with osteoarthritis of the knee. *Arthritis and Rheumatism, 40*(8), 1466–1474.

McClellan, W. (1986). The physician and patient education: A review. *Patient Education and Counseling, 8,* 151–163.

Montgomery, E. B., Jr., Lieberman, A., Singh, L., & Fries, J. F. (1994). Patient education and health promotion can be effective in Parkinson's disease: A randomized controlled trial. PROPATH Advisory Board. *American Journal of Medicine, 97*(5), 429–435.

Moore, S. H., LoGerfo, J. P., & Inui, T. S. (1980). Effect of a self-care book on physician visits. A randomized trial, *Journal of the American Medical Association, 243,* 2317–2320.

Moran, M. (1999). Disease management spreading. *American Medical News, 42*(15), 1, 37–38.

Nelson, E. C., Mettigo, L., & Schmurr, P. (1984). Medical self-care education for elders: A controlled trial to evaluate impact. *American Journal of Public Health, 74*(12), 1357–1362.

O'Reilly, M. (1994). Don't seek medical help for minor problems, Ontario pilot project tells patients. *Canadian Medical Association Journal, 151*(2), 201–202.

Pelletier, K. R. (1993). A review and analysis of the health and cost-effective outcome studies of comprehensive health promotion and disease prevention programs at the worksite: 1991–1993 update. *American Journal of Health Promotion, 8*(4), 50–62.

Pheley, A. M., Terry, P., & Pietz, L. (1995). Evaluation of a nurse-based hypertension management program: Screening, management, and outcomes. *Journal of Cardiovascular Nursing, 9*(2), 54–61.

Riemsma, R. P., Taal, E., Brus, H. L., Rasker, J. J., & Wiegman, O. (1997). Coordinated individual education with an arthritis passport for patients with rheumatoid arthritis. *Arthritis Care Research, 10*(4), 238–249.

Robbins, J. A., Bertakis, K. O., & Helms, J. L. (1993). The influence of physician practice behaviors on patient satisfaction. *Family Medicine, 25,* 17–20.

Roberts, C. R., Imrey, P. B., Turner, J. D., Hosokawa, M. C., & Alster, J. M. (1983). Reducing physician visits for colds through consumer education. *Journal of the American medical Association, 250*(15), 1986–1989.

Sanchez-Menegay, C., & Stalder, H. (1994). Do physicians take into account patients' expectations? *Journal of General Internal Medicine, 9*(7), 404–406.

Savage, R., & Armstrong, D. (1990). Effect of a general practitioner's consulting style on patients' satisfaction: A controlled study. *British Medical Journal, 301,* 968–970.

Schauffler, H., Rodriquez, T. & Milstein, A. (1996). Health education and patient satisfaction. *Journal of Family Practice, 42*(1), 62–68.

Shank, J. C., Murphy, M., & Schulte-Mowry, L. (1991). Patient preferences regarding educational pamphlets in the family practice center. *Family Medicine, 23*(6), 429–432.

Sirles, A. T. (1988). Self-care education, parent knowledge, and children's health care visits. *Journal of Pediatric Health Care, 2*(3), 135–140.

Steinweg, K. K., Killingsworth, R. E., Nannini, R. J. & Spayde, J. (1998). The impact on a health care system of a program to facilitate self-care. *Military Medicine, 163*(3), 139–144.

Stergachis, A., Newmann, W. E., Williams, K. J., & Schnell, M. M. (1990). The effect of a self-care minimal intervention for colds and flu on the use of medical services. *Journal of General Internal Medicine, 5*(1), 23–28.

Terry, P. E. (1994). The effect of a materials-based intervention on knowledge of risk-based clinical prevention screening guidelines. *Journal of Occupational Medicine, 36*(3), 365–371.

Terry, P. E. (1998). How mature is your organization's prevention effort? Four stages of managed care health promotion. *Healthcare Forum Journal, 41*(5), 54–58.

Terry, P. E., Abelson, D., & Kind, A. (1995). *Well-Advised—A Practical Guide to Everyday Health Decisions.* Mosby Consumer Health, Boston, MA.

Terry, P. E., & Healy, M. (1999, February 23). *Comparing a physician delivered and consumer-direct approach to self-care education.* Paper presented at the Minnesota Health Services Research Conference.

Terry, P. E., & Pheley, A. (1993). The effect of self-care brochures on use of medical services. *Journal of Occupational Medicine, 35*(4), 422–426.

Vickery, D. M., Lolaszewski, T. J., Wright, E. C., & Kalmer, H. (1989). A preliminary study of the timeliness of ambulatory care utilization following medical self-care interventions. *American Journal of Health Promotion, 3,* 27–31.

Vickery, D. M., Lolaszewski, T. J., Wright, E. C., & Kalmer, H. (1988). The effect of self-care interventions on the use of medical services within a Medicare population. *Medical Care, 26,* 580–588.

Vickery, D. M., Kalmer, H., & Lowry, D. (1983). Effect of a self-care education program on medical visits. *Journal of the American Medical Association, 250*(21), 2952–2956.

Vickery, D. M, & Lynch, W. D. (1995). Demand management: Enabling patients to use medical care appropriately. *Journal of Occupational and Environmental Medicine, 37*(5), 551–557.

Weingarten, S., Green, A., & Stone, E. (1995). A study of patient satisfaction and adherence to preventive care practice guidelines. *American Journal of Medicine, 99*(6), 590–596.

Williams, S. J. & Calman, M. (1991). Key determinants of consumer satisfaction with general practice. *Family Practice, 8,* 237–242

Wilson, S. R., Scamagas, P., & Herman, D. F. (1993). A controlled trial of two forms of self-management education for adults with asthma. *American Journal of Medicine, 94*(6), 564–576.

Zapka, J., & Averill, B. W. (1979). Self-care for colds: A cost-effective alternative to upper respiratory infection management. *American Journal of Public Health, 69*(8), 814–816.

Zapka, J., Palmer, H., & Hargraves, L. J. (1995). Relationships of patient satisfaction with experience of system performance and health status. *Journal of Ambulatory Care Management, 18*(1), 73–83.

CHAPTER

15

Stress Management

Lawrence R. Murphy

INTRODUCTION

A host of occupation-specific studies and national surveys over the past thirty years have converged to yield the conclusion that job stress is a major problem for many workers. The landmark studies of Kahn, Wolfe, Quinn, Snoek, and Rosenthal (1964) on role relationships and stress and *Job Demands and Worker Health* by Caplan, Cobb, French, van Harrison, and Pinneau (1975) laid the groundwork for an intensive research effort to understand the health and safety consequences of job stress. Since then, hundreds and hundreds of research studies have linked a wide range of work conditions to physical and mental ill-health, including workload, machine-pacing, lack of control, rotating shift work, and lack of promotion potential, to name a few. Moreover, the frequent and sometimes indiscriminate downsizing and restructuring by many U.S. companies over the past 15 years led to heightened stress due to increased workload, multi-skilling, job insecurity, and changes in the psychological contract between workers and employers with respect to employment stability.

How prevalent is job stress at the national level? Several indicators suggest that job stress is a significant problem for many workers. For example, in the 1999 Gallup Labor Day Poll, which involved interviews with a randomly selected sample of 641 employed adults, workers expressed the most dissatisfaction with the level of stress at work, job security, and pay (Gallup, 1999). Less than 50% of workers reported being "completely satisfied" with their job security, their bosses, workload, and opportunity to learn new things. At the same time, 9 out of 10 workers reported being generally satisfied with their current jobs. Another study, the 1997 National Study of the Changing Workforce, interviewed a nationally representative sample of 2,877 workers (Bond, Galinsky, & Swanberg, 1998). The results indicated that about 25% of employees felt stressed "often or very often," and 13% had difficulty coping with the demands of everyday life. Twenty-six percent reported being emotionally drained by their work, and 36% felt "used up" at the end of the workday. Similarly, many employees are affected by negative spillover from their jobs into their personal lives. Twenty-eight percent reported not having the energy to do things with their families or other important people in their lives.

Earlier nationwide studies, such as the 1985 National Health Interview Survey, reported that workers rated mental stress as the most frequent health-endangering condition at work, second only to loud noise (Shilling & Brackbill, 1987).

The national significance of the problem of work stress also is reflected in the increasing role of the federal government in this area. For example, in 1984, the National Institute for Occupational Safety and Health (NIOSH) listed psychological disorders (e.g., stress) as one of their Top Ten Leading Work-Related Diseases and Injuries (Millar, 1984) and later formulated a national prevention strategy (Sauter, Murphy, & Hurrell, 1990). NIOSH joined with the American Psychological Association to host scientific conferences on job stress in 1990, 1992, 1995, and 1999. In 1996, NIOSH developed a National Occupational Research Agenda and listed the "organization of work" (which includes job stress) as one of its 15 priority research areas (National Institute for Occupational Safety and Health, 1996). Most recently, NIOSH published a document entitled *Stress at Work*, which defines the problem in lay terms and offers concrete suggestions for companies on ways to prevent and manage job stress (National Institute for Occupational Safety and Health, 1999).

In the United Kingdom, the Health and Safety Executive produced a series of reports on job stress and, most recently, a review of organizational stress interventions (Parkes & Sparkes, 1998) and discussion booklets on stress at work (Health and Safety Executive, 1995, 1998a, 1998b). The Finnish Institute for Occupational Health publishes an occupational stress questionnaire, complete with user instructions (Elo, Leppänen, Lindström, & Ropponen, 1993). The European Foundation for the Improvement of Living and Working Conditions published two documents dealing with job stress and stress prevention for use by member countries (Cooper, Liukkonen, & Cartwright, 1996; Kompier & Levi, 1994). In Australia, COMCARE sponsored national conferences on job stress in 1993 and 1996 and published a series of documents to help organizations address the problem of job stress (COMCARE, 1997a, 1997b).

Accurate figures on the costs of job stress are difficult to come by, but estimates have ranged upwards of $150 billion per year in the United States. However, one recent study provides concrete data on this issue. Goetzel et. al. (1998) examined the relationship between modifiable health risks and actual medical expenditures for 46,026 employees working for six large U.S. employers. The data consisted of health risk appraisal surveys (used to calculate risk scores) and insurance claims for inpatient and outpatient medical services (used to assess medical expenditures). The results indicated that the health risks most highly associated with health care expenditures were depression and high stress. Overall, about 19% of workers reported to be troubled by stress "Almost always." Workers reporting high stress had annual medical expenditures that averaged 46% higher than those of moderate- or low-stress workers. Workers who reported high depression *and* high stress ". . . were found to be 147% more costly than their counterparts without those risks" (Goetzel et. al., 1998, p. 653). The authors interpreted their findings to mean that depressed and highly stressed workers may seek medical attention more frequently and develop more serious illnesses. This study confirmed prior work that identified a relationship between job stress and symptoms of stress, health care costs, and health care claims (Manning, Jackson, & Fusilier, 1996). The study combined survey data with health insurance record data to examine the link between stress and health care use. Multivariate statistical analyses revealed that 16% of the variance in health care costs and 21% of the variance in the frequency of health care claims could be explained by job stress measures.

The increased salience of job stress, and the cost estimates noted above, has stimulated interest in ways to prevent stress—or at least to manage it better. The purpose of this chapter is to review the research evidence on the effectiveness of various interventions to reduce or manage stress at work and to offer suggestions on how to design comprehensive, effective stress interventions at the workplace.

This chapter is divided into 5 sections: a review of job stress/health research, a description of the two basic approaches to stress prevention (organizational change and individual stress management) and the effectiveness of each approach, a listing of key elements of a comprehensive stress intervention program, and a discussion of the relationship between job stress and other health promotion programs. A concluding section suggests that research on job stress and stress intervention be broadened to focus on organizational health, defined as worker well-being plus organizational effectiveness.

THE RELATIONSHIP BETWEEN JOB STRESS AND HEALTH

Over the past 25 years, a large list of job and organizational factors have been identified as causes of stress, and various models showing how job stress leads to ill health have been proposed. The model in Figure 15-1 is a simplified, generic model that contains the key elements found in most models in the field (e.g., Cooper and Marshall, 1976; Israel, Baker, Goldenhar, Heaney, & Schurman, 1996). The center of the model shows that the worker appraises job factors that, depending on the valence of the appraisal, lead to acute reactions, which in turn can lead to ill health. Individual factors and nonwork factors, shown at the top and bottom of the model, can influence the process at all steps. Table 15-1 provides examples of factors in each box of the model.

Research dating back to the 1920s and 1930s linked stress to a wide range of physical and mental health conditions, many more than the few examples shown

in Table 15-1. In the early 1930s, Hans Selye discovered that a wide variety of noxious stimuli (which he later referred to as stressors), such as exposure to temperature extremes, physical injury, and injection of toxic substances, evoked an identical pattern of physiological changes in laboratory animals (Selye, 1936). In each case, the cortex of the adrenal gland became enlarged, the thymus and other lymphatic structures became involuted, (i.e., shrank in size) and deep-bleeding ulcers developed in the stomach and intestines. These effects were "nonspecific," that is, they occurred regardless of the particular exposure and were superimposed on any specific effects associated with the individual agents. Later, Selye described this somatic response as the general adaptation syndrome (GAS) and defined stress as the nonspecific response of the body to any demand (Selye, 1946). His mention of "nervous stimuli" among the stressor agents capable of eliciting the GAS had an energizing effect on those working in the field of psychosomatic medicine.

Cannon (1929) had earlier laid the groundwork for an understanding of how emotions affect physiological functions and disease states in his description of the "fight or flight" response. This response, evoked by potentially dangerous situations, includes elevated heart rate and blood pressure, a redistribution of blood flow to the brain and major muscle groups

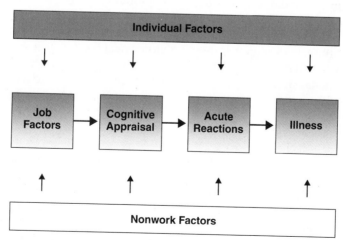

Figure 15-1 General job stress/health model.

Table 15-1 Examples of Factors in Each Component of General Job Stress/Health Model

Job Factors	Cognitive Appraisal	Acute Reactions	Illness	Individual Factors	Nonwork Factors
Organizational practices • Reward systems • Supervisory practices • Promotion potential *Job features* • Workload • Workpace • Worker control • Physical comfort *Culture/climate* • Employee growth • Innovation • Trust • Integrity *Interpersonal* • Supervisors • Coworkers	• Perception of events as threatening • Perceived demands exceed capacity to perform • Perceived lack of ability to adapt to external demands	*Psychological* • Nervousness • Frustration • Burnout *Physiological* • Muscle aches • Blood pressure • Catecholamines • Immune function • High blood lipids *Behavioral* • Sleep disturbances • Substance use	• Chronic anxiety • Chronic depression • Coronary heart disease	• Personality traits • Coping skills	• Family stress • Financial concerns • Number of children

and away from distal body parts, and a decrease in vegetative functions. Perhaps equally important, Cannon (1935) advanced the concept of "physiological homeostasis" and developed an engineering concept of stress and strain. In particular, Cannon proposed the notion of critical stress levels that were capable of producing strain in the homeostatic mechanisms. Although he used the term somewhat casually, Cannon, like Selye, conceived of stress as involving physical as well as emotional stimuli.

In view of the widespread and pernicious effects of stress on many bodily systems, it is not surprising that stress causes or exacerbates a wide range of health conditions. These include heart disease and stroke, high blood pressure, impaired immune function, headache, backache, diabetes, substance use/abuse, eating disorders, anxiety, and depression. Stress also has been linked to family problems, accidents/injuries, sleep disturbances, and even cancer (Cooper and Marshall, 1976; Quick and Quick, 1984; Seyle, 1946).

How stressors get translated into acute health reactions and, eventually, health consequences, is determined more by a person's perception of the stressor than its objective nature. Lazarus (1966) described cognitive appraisal as the psychological process that translates objective events into stressful experiences. The importance of this formulation lies in its recognition that subjective factors can play a much larger role in the experience of stress than objective factors. Indeed, any given objective event can at once be perceived in a positive way by one person yet as stressful by another (one person's meat is another person's poison).

Stress also is believed to impair work performance, but there is less empirical data to support this relationship. This is true for several reasons. First, there is the difficulty of how to measure performance or productivity. In any one job, many different measures could be used but no single measure really seems to capture all aspects of productivity. For instance, in secretarial work, one could measure the number of keystrokes per hour or the number of phone calls answered, but neither of these would capture the true nature of the work. Annual performance appraisal ratings could be used, but these ratings do not vary enough between employees to be useful; industrial psychologists have known for years that performance appraisals are subject to a range of rating errors, such as halo, leniency, and central tendency (Jewell & Siegale, 1990). A similar scenario could be sketched for other potential measures of productivity.

Nevertheless, a relationship between stress and performance is believed by many to exist based on studies which indicate that:

1. Job stress increases the risk of accidents/injuries at work because of lower concentration and increased distractibility (Murphy, Dubois, & Hurrell, 1986).
2. Job stress leads to higher absenteeism and turnover, which ultimately results in lower productivity and higher costs to organizations (Quick & Quick, 1984).
3. Job stress leads to lower satisfaction and morale, which in turn impairs worker motivation and performance (Quick & Quick, 1984).

TYPES OF STRESS INTERVENTIONS

There are two basic types of interventions that have been used to address stress at work: organizational change and stress management.

Organizational Change

The first approach is to take action(s) to modify or eliminate the sources of stress in the work environment and thus reduce their negative impact on the individual. In this approach, stress is viewed as the consequence of the "lack of fit" between the capacity and needs of the individual and the demands of the work environment. Thus, the main focus of organizational stress interventions is to adapt or change the environment to "fit" the individual worker.

Two conceptual models are frequently used to design organizational change interventions at the work-

place, the Job Characteristics Model (Hackman & Lawler, 1971; Hackman & Oldham, 1976) and the Demand/Control Model (Karasek, 1979). Both of these models predict that interventions to enrich jobs (i.e., increase worker control and the meaning and variety of job tasks) will result in positive health and performance outcomes. The Job Characteristics Model offers five key dimensions of work:

1. *Skill variety*–the extent to which a worker's job requires the use of numerous skills or talents in order to perform the job successfully
2. *Task identity*–jobs in which the worker is able to perform a complete, identifiable piece of work, starting with raw materials and ending with a product that is ready to be used by a customer or another person in the company or group
3. *Task significance*–the impact that a person's work has on other people, either inside or outside the company
4. *Autonomy*–worker has the freedom to decide how the job will be done, what procedures will be used, and how the tasks will be scheduled
5. *Feedback*–the extent to which a worker can tell whether the job is being performed effectively while actually performing the job

These dimensions are measured using the Job Diagnostic Survey, and scores on each dimension are calculated. According to the model, the motivating potential score (MPS) of a job is calculated by averaging scores on the first three characteristics then multiplying the result by scores on the autonomy and feedback dimensions. The formula is shown below:

$$MPS = \left[\frac{(\text{skill variety} + \text{task identity} + \text{task significance})}{3} \right] \times \text{autonomy} \times \text{feedback}$$

Karasek's Demands/Control Model focused on two dimensions of the job, psychological job demands and the amount of worker control, or autonomy. As shown in Figure 15-2, high strain (or stress) results when job demands are high and worker control is low. Jobs with high demands but also high control are called "active" jobs, which should be health-protective or health promoting rather than stressful.

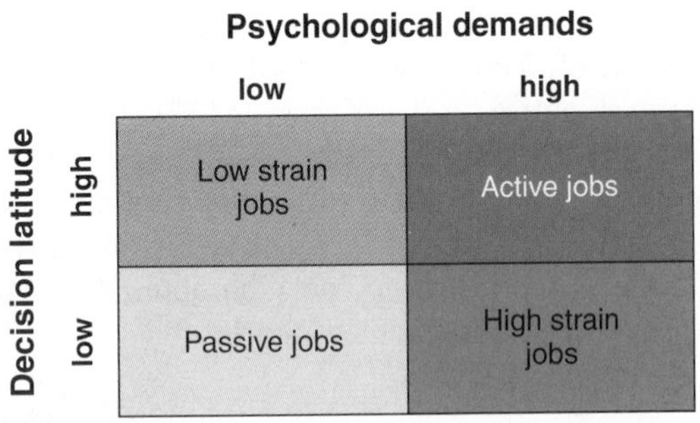

Psychological demands

Figure 15-2 Process model for stress intervention.
Source: Adapted from C. R. Stoner & F. L. Fry, *Personnel*, 1983.

There are several other models of job stress and health that identify characteristics of stressful jobs, so there are many job and organizational factors that could be targeted for change to reduce worker stress. For example, Elkin and Rosch (1990) offered the following 10 strategies:

- Redesign the task
- Redesign the work environment
- Establish flexible work schedules
- Encourage participative management
- Include the employee in career development planning
- Analyze work roles and establish goals
- Provide social support and feedback
- Build cohesive teams
- Establish fair employment policies
- Share the rewards

The National Institute for Occupational Safety and Health (NIOSH) advanced another set of recommendations for reducing job stress (Sauter, Murphy, & Hurrell, 1990) as part of a national strategy for the prevention of work-related psychological disorders. These are not dissimilar from the prior list.

- *Workload and work pace* should be commensurate with the capabilities and resources of workers, avoiding underload as well as overload. Provisions should be made to allow recovery from demanding tasks or for increased control by workers over characteristics such as work pace of demanding tasks.

- *Work schedules* should be compatible with demands and responsibilities outside the job. Recent trends toward flextime, a compressed workweek, and job sharing are examples of positive steps in this direction. When schedules involve rotating shifts, the rate of rotation should be stable and predictable.
- *Roles and responsibilities* at work should be well-defined. Job duties need to be clearly explained, and conflicts in terms of job expectations should be avoided.
- *Ambiguity* should be avoided in opportunities for promotion and career or skill development and in matters pertaining to job security. Employees should be clearly informed of imminent organizational developments that may affect their employment.
- Jobs should provide *opportunities for personal interaction,* both for purposes of emotional support and for actual help as needed in accomplishing assigned tasks.
- Tasks should be designed *to be meaningful and to provide stimulation and an opportunity to use skills.* Job rotation or increasing the scope (enlargement/enrichment) of work activities are ways to improve narrow, fragmented work activities that fail to meet these criteria.
- Workers should be given *opportunities to provide input to decisions* or actions that affect their jobs and the performance of their tasks.

Evidence of Effectiveness

Studies evaluating the benefits of organizational interventions on employee health and well-being are not common in the research literature, and those that have been performed have produced mixed results. Two examples of stress intervention studies are provided below to give the reader a sense of how such interventions are implemented and the type of outcome measures typically utilized.

Example #1: Autonomous Work Groups

Wall, Kemp, Jackson, and Clegg (1986) studied the effects of new management structures and practices designed to support a well-developed form of autonomous group working at a newly built factory in the United Kingdom. Autonomous work groups of 8–12 employees were formed, all of whom were expected to carry out each of the tasks involved in the production process. Group members were collectively responsible for allocating jobs among themselves, reaching production targets, recording productivity data, ordering raw materials, training new recruits, and other routine work activities. In addition to informal interactions between group members, formal weekly group meetings were held to discuss performance and job allocation. The new work organization was evaluated in a quasi-experimental design, and measurements were taken at three intervals (Time 1–6 months; Time 2–18 months; and Time 3–30 months after the start of production at the new site). It was predicted that the implementation of autonomous work groups would have favorable effects on perceived autonomy, job satisfaction, work motivation, organizational commitment, mental health, performance, and turnover. While the results indicated a significant increase in job satisfaction, there were no effects on work motivation, organizational commitment, mental health, or performance. Furthermore, contrary to prediction, labor turnover increased under autonomous work conditions.

Example #2: Role Ambiguity

Schaubroeck, Ganster, Sime, and Ditman (1993) evaluated an intervention to reduce role ambiguity among middle managers in the business services division of a large university. Recent reorganizations had created confusion and ambiguity regarding individual roles and relationships among the various departments within the division. Symptoms of stress included high reported stress levels, psychosomatic disorders, and frequent sick days. A role clarification intervention was designed that began with charting the responsibilities of the managers and their departments and ended with individual role negotiation sessions between each manager and his or her subordinates. Groups of subordinates were randomly assigned to treatment and wait list (control) conditions, and measures of employee stress symptoms were taken several months after implementation. Although the intervention significantly reduced employee perceptions of role ambiguity, it had little impact on employee health symptoms or the frequency of sick leave usage.

While some early reports found positive effects of organizational change interventions on worker distress (Jackson, 1983; Wall & Clegg, 1981), more recent studies have failed to demonstrate significant effects (e.g., Heaney et al., 1993; Landsbergis & Vivona-Vaughan, 1995; Schaubroeck, et al., 1993; Wall, et al., 1986).

Indeed, the most recent review of the organizational stress intervention literature concluded that such interventions are not particularly effective for reducing worker stress levels (Parkes & Sparkes, 1998). This review is particularly well done and offers a thoughtful analysis of the reasons why organizational interventions have had limited effectiveness. For instance, since a fundamental tenet of stress is that change of any type is stressful, then interventions that focus on job redesign or organizational change may increase worker stress in the short-term. This would argue for longer evaluation periods to accurately assess benefits. Second, the change may decrease stress for some workers (the ones who see the change as positive) but increase stress for other workers (those who see the change as negative). This suggests the need for evaluation protocols that include subgroup analyses or which attempt to identify workers who were positively and negatively affected by the interventions. In the same way, organizational change may decrease stress for one group of workers but increase stress for other worker groups.

A final possible reason was suggested recently by Payne, Wall, Borrill, and Carter (1999). Using a large sample of health care workers, the authors demonstrated that psychological strain moderated the relationship between work characteristics and work attitudes (i.e., job satisfaction). That is, the relationship was lower for high-stress than low-stress workers. The authors suggested that stress interventions first should help workers deal with their high strain (through individual-oriented strategies) before attempting to change the stresses in the work environment.

This is not to say that companies should not attempt organizational change interventions. The mixed findings from the research literature may simply reflect the fact that organizational interventions are far more complex to design and evaluate than stress management programs. For example, it is almost impossible to perform a true experiment in a work setting, with random assignment of workers to conditions and control of extraneous factors. Organizations are dynamic entities, and concurrent (and uncontrollable) changes often occur alongside the planned interventions. During postintervention evaluation, it is difficult to untangle the respective roles of the planned intervention and other changes that may have taken place.

Stress Management Training

The second major approach reduces stress by providing workers with specific skills to recognize stress and take steps to reduce its harmful psychological and physiological effects. Stress management is particularly useful in dealing with stressors that cannot be changed. Such training can also prove helpful to individuals to deal with stress in nonwork-related areas of life. However, the role of stress management is essentially one of damage control, addressing the consequences rather than the sources of stress that may be inherent in the organization's structure or culture. Stress management is concerned with improving the adaptability of the individual to the environment.

Common stress management techniques include progressive muscle relaxation, meditation, and cognitive-behavioral skills training. *Progressive muscle relaxation* involves learning to identify small amounts of tension in a muscle group and practicing releasing tension from the muscles. The underlying theory is that, since relaxation and muscle tension are incompatible states, reducing muscle tension levels indirectly reduces autonomic activity and, consequently, anxiety and stress levels. In *biofeedback* training, an individual is provided with continuous information, or feedback, about the status of a physiological function and, over time, learns to control the activity of that function. The electrical activity produced when muscles contract is transformed into a tone, whose pitch rises and falls with muscle activity levels. Using the feedback tone as an indicator of muscle tension level, individuals learn how to reduce muscle activity levels

and create a state of relaxation. Numerous forms of *meditation* have been developed, but the one most widely used in work settings is a secular version developed by Herbert Benson (Benson, 1976). Meditation involves sitting upright in a comfortable position with eyes closed, in a quiet place, and mentally repeating a word or sound (e.g., "one" or "calm") while maintaining a passive mental attitude. The meditation is performed twice per day. Finally, *cognitive-behavioral skills* refer to an assortment of techniques designed to help participants modify their appraisal or thinking processes about the stressfulness of situations and to develop skills for managing stressors. One such technique is called stress inoculation. This training involves three stages: education (learning about how the person has responded to past stressful experiences); rehearsal (learning various coping skills techniques, such as problem solving, relaxation, and cognitive coping); and application (the person practices the skills under simulated conditions guided by the therapist).

A "typical" stress management study that one may find in the published literature is summarized in Table 15-2.

Table 15-2 Components of Typical SMT Study

Stress programs are preventive and seek to improve worker awareness and recognition of stress. In this sense, the label "stress management" is misleading since workers with apparent stress problems are solicited.

Programs are usually offered to workers in white-collar occupations.

Training typically takes place in small groups over a period of two to eight weeks and includes education, some type of relaxation exercise, and may additionally include meditation, biofeedback, and/or a cognition-focused technique.

Few studies compared the relative effectiveness of different training techniques. Thus, although doing something appears to be better than doing nothing, the specific technique that is used may not matter.

Evaluation has been based upon individual-oriented measures (e.g., anxiety) that have been assessed over a short posttraining period (e.g., 3–6 months).

Evidence of Effectiveness

There have been many reviews of the stress management literature over the years (DeFrank & Cooper, 1987; Heaney & van Ryn, 1990; Ivancevich, Matteson, Freedman, & Phillips, 1990; Murphy, 1984, 1988; Newman & Beehr, 1979), including some very recent ones (Bunce, 1997; Murphy, 1996; van der Hek & Plomp, 1997). The summary presented here is based primarily on the review by Murphy (1996) but supplemented with new information presented in later reviews as appropriate.

Overall, the evidence suggests that such stress management interventions can reduce some symptoms of stress in the short-term, but they result in little or no change in job satisfaction, work stress, or blood pressure. Progressive muscle relaxation is associated with significant effects on physiological measures but little change on other outcome measures. This result is consistent with the focus of training on somatic aspects or symptoms of stress. Perhaps because of its restrictive focus on somatic aspects of stress, muscle relaxation was progressively less effective in producing changes on psychological, somatic, and organizational outcomes. Muscle relaxation was often used in combination with one or more other stress-management techniques, as noted later in this article.

Cognitive-behavioral skills training was the single intervention technique used most frequently in stress-management studies and produced the most consistent effects on psychological outcomes, especially anxiety. This is not surprising given that this training focuses on understanding and altering the cognitive aspects of stress (i.e., thinking patterns) and acquiring stress-coping skills. This training also seemed to produce effects on job/organizational outcomes (e.g., job satisfaction), perhaps by helping workers deal with irrational thoughts ("everything I do must be perfect"), thereby improving job satisfaction.

Combination strategies produced significant effects on *each* health outcome measure, and significant results also were seen on job/organizational measures in more than 60% of these studies. The most common combination of techniques was muscle relaxation with cognitive-behavioral skills training. Conceptually, the combination of these two techniques creates a dual focus on cognitive and somatic aspects of stress and involves the development of specific coping techniques. It appears that this particular blend of training techniques is the most effective type of stress-management intervention.

The reason for the superiority of combination techniques may be two-fold. First, the combination of muscle relaxation and cognitive-behavioral skills training provides workers with a balance of somatic and cognitive skills, and this combination may be more effective across more types of outcome measures than either technique alone. For example, muscle relaxation alone was effective for physiological outcomes and cognitive-behavioral skills training was effective for psychological outcomes, so the combination of the two should increase the overall range of effective results. A second possible reason for the effectiveness of combination training centers around the fact that, because more than one skill is taught, there may be fewer participants who fail to learn at least some stress-management skills. In the empirical studies that reported the success rates of participants, it was common to find that about one-third of participants fail to learn a particular stress-management technique. By using a combination of techniques, one might improve participant success rates and, hence, the overall effects on the outcome measures. However, too few published studies report success rates to test this hypothesis.

What's a Practitioner to Do?

If you've made it this far in the chapter, you're probably wondering what exactly can be done to reduce worker stress that has a reasonable chance of success? That's a very good question!

To answer the question, recommendations on what would constitute a successful stress intervention were abstracted from the most recent four reviews of this literature (Israel, et al., 1996; Kompier, Geurts, Gründemann, Vink, & Smulders, 1998; Murphy, 1996; Parkes & Sparkes, 1998). Next, the list of recommendations was compiled, and areas of agreement across the lists were identified. Agreement was found on four recommendations, which are presented in detail below:

- Use a conceptual model to guide program design and evaluation
- Include an assessment of the sources of stress at work
- Include workers in the design, implementation, and evaluation of the program
- Attend to individual and organizational factors in terms of both job stressors and outcomes

Use a Conceptual Model

A conceptual model defines the types of stressors present in the workplace and their relationship to employee well-being. It provides guidance in the targeting of stress intervention strategies (individual vs. work group vs. organizational), how to implement the intervention, and how to evaluate its effectiveness. A number of authors have proposed stress intervention models (Heaney & van Ryn, 1990; Israel et. al., 1992; Ivancevich et al., 1990; Newman & Beehr, 1979; Stoner & Fry, 1983), but these have been underutilized by practitioners and researchers alike.

Given the importance of adopting a conceptual model for stress interventions, a detailed description of one model follows. The model offered by Stoner and Fry (1983) is noteworthy for its clear presentation of job stress and stress prevention and its focus on developing a corporate policy on stress that can include individual, organizational, or combined actions. It was a groundbreaking article in many ways, not the least of which was its discussion of stress at the corporate policy level more than 15 years ago. This would be remarkable even today, where many companies avoid the topic of stress, in part because of their fear that discussions of job stress may prompt employees to file worker compensation claims for stress-related illness. Other reasons that companies avoid the topic of job stress are that they don't know what to do about employee stress or they think employee stress is a personal, not work-related, problem.

Figure 15-3 shows three stages in the overall process for establishing a corporate policy on stress:

monitoring, analysis, and action. The model is laid out as a decision-tree or flow chart, which moves from left to right. The first stage, monitoring, focuses on tracking a well-defined set of undesirable stress symptoms, such as increased absenteeism and turnover, deteriorating performance, increased accidents, impaired concentration, and poor communications. The monitoring can be carried out at various levels within the organization (e.g., business unit, division/department, work group).

If the monitoring reveals negative changes in the levels of stress outcomes, that triggers the second stage which involves the analysis of the nature and scope of the problem. Although the root causes can span a wide range of possibilities, Stoner and Fry (1983) offered a set of job conditions that commonly lead to undesirable stress outcomes. These are shown in Table 15-3.

Next, the scope of the problem is determined; are the stress outcomes limited to a few workers in one work group, or is an entire work group (or department) being affected?

The final stage is the action stage in which corrective policy is formed based on the sources of stress and scope of the problem. For example, if the outcomes are limited to a single worker, then an individual corrective policy should be pursued. This involves three steps: a) the worker is made aware of the undesirable outcome, the sources of stress, and options that are available to them, such as education, training, and counseling, b) a corrective plan is formulated, and c) the plan is monitored to assure its success. Table 15-4 shows examples of corrective policies at the individual level.

If the stress outcomes are more widespread in a work group, then individual corrective policies would be inappropriate and corrective action at the 'organizational' is required. Table 15-5 shows a list of corrective policies at the organizational level. These actions are typically larger scale and more expensive than individual actions, and require a more detailed assessment of the sources of stress in the work environment.

Finally, the feedback loop shown in Figure 15-3 indicates that this is an ongoing process, not a one-time event. The ongoing nature of the process is important;

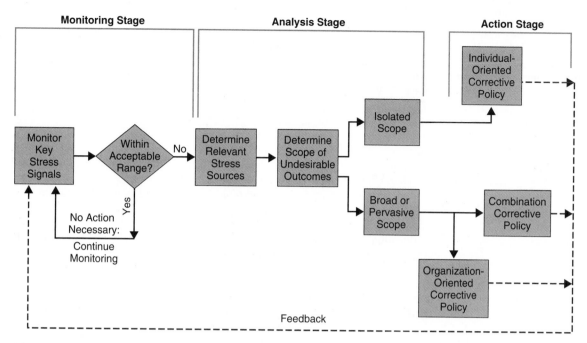

Figure 15-3 Overview of the process for establishing an effective corporate policy on stress.

Table 15-3 Causes of Organizational Stress

Common Stressors	Suggested Causes
Person/job misfit	Job demands skills/abilities that the worker does not possess. Job does not provide opportunity for the worker to utilize skills/abilities.
Role conflict	The formal organization's conception of expected behavior contradicts the worker's conception of expected behavior. The informal group's conception of expected behavior contradicts the worker's conception. The individual worker has two (or more) conflicting influences.
Role ambiguity	Worker is uncertain or unclear about how to perform on the job, what is expected in the job, and/or the relationship between job performance and expected consequences (e.g., rewards).
Role overload	Worker is asked to do more than time permits (time pressure).
Fear/responsibility	Worker is afraid of performing poorly or failing. Worker feels pressure for high achievement. Worker has responsibility for other people.
Working conditions	The job environment is unpleasant; there is improper regulation of temperature, excessive noise, inadequate lighting, etc. On the work floor, the mode of operation may unnecessarily produce pacing problems, social isolation, etc. The machine design and maintenance procedures create pressure. The job involves long or erratic work hours.
Relationships	Individual workers have problems relating to superiors, peers, and/or subordinates. Workers have problems working in groups.
Alienation	Limited social interaction; workers don't participate in decision making.

Table 15-4 Action Programs at the Individual Level

Common Stressors	Corrective Policy	Possible Action Programs
Person/job misfit	Placement	Relocate, transfer
	Training	Set up program to develop skills
	Education	Set up program to enhance aptitude and ability
Role conflict	Communication	Establish clear description of worker's role and help worker realize how he or she can fulfill this role
	Training	Set up programs to build/develop skills that will enable the worker to fulfill role
Role ambiguity	Communication	Clearly explain the nature of job and expectations
Role overload	Training/education	Develop skills to weaken cause of job incompetence; set up time-management programs
Fear/responsibility	Training	Develop skills to address problem areas confidently
	Counseling	Help the worker deal with underlying fears
Working conditions	Counseling	Help individual deal with behavioral issues
	Communications	Help worker understand justification for work process and how he or she fits into overall process
Relationships	Training	Set up encounter- and team-building sessions
	Counseling	Deal with personality conflicts, social isolates, etc.
	Communication	Develop better communication within groups; help workers learn to relate more effectively to each other
Alienation	Counseling	Help workers deal with their feelings
	Communication	Provide avenues for upward communication, participation, and involvement

too many organizations mistakenly view stress intervention as a one-shot effort. In point of fact, stress intervention is a dynamic process that changes as the organization changes and evolves.

Attend to Both Individual and Organizational Factors

Teaching workers stress management skills is necessary and serves a useful purpose, but it deals with only part of the problem. The workplace can be a source of important stressors, which can be identified and targeted for change. Ideas for how to reduce the sources of stress at work should flow naturally from an assessment of job and organizational factors in the work environment. Examples of organizational change interventions were presented earlier in this chapter but additional examples can be found in

Cooper et al. (1996), Jackson (1983), Kompier et al. (1998), Murphy (1995), National Institute for Occupational Safety and Health (1999), and Parkes and Sparkes (1998). Focusing one or a few stressors for change and not introducing too many changes simultaneously also has been recommended (Parkes & Sparkes, 1998).

Include Workers in the Design and Evaluation of Stress Interventions

There is sufficient research attesting to the importance of worker involvement in organizational change efforts and to the importance of the process (i.e., *how* the intervention is done), as well as the content of such interventions. In most stress intervention studies, consultants make all of the decisions regarding program

Table 15-5 Corrective Policies and Action Programs at the Organizational Level

Common Stressors	Corrective Policy	Possible Action Programs
Person/job misfit	Job redesign	Set up job enrichment programs
	Personnel evaluation	Improve selection and placement procedures
	Training	Institute job-related skills training
Role conflict	Training	Provide counseling to explore causes of conflict
	Communication	Examine and reduce misunderstandings that may cause conflict
	Job redesign	Schedule (for example, flextime, 4-day weeks, job sharing, and so forth) to deal with particular conflict areas (that is, working woman vs. family, work vs. leisure)
	Personnel evaluation	Improve selection and placement (transfer, for example)
Role ambiguity	Communication	Provide more accurate job descriptions
	Structure	Define responsibilities and authority structure more precisely
Role overload	Job redesign	Change work floor, layout, or process
	Structure	Rewrite job descriptions
Fear/responsibility	Training	Train in decision-making skills
	Communication	Provide counseling programs for dealing with underlying problems
Working conditions	Job redesign	Change physical conditions and make changes in work routine (rotate jobs, change hours of work, give relaxation breaks, and "stress day" off, for example)
Relationships	Training	Develop human relation skills; provide training to build more cohesive, team-oriented work groups
	Communication	Set up various counseling programs
Alienation	Training	Help with career planning
	Job redesign	Provide job enrichment programs
	Structure	Utilize formal structural design that is most conducive to situation and individual needs (for example, use project or matrix format)
	Rewards	Alter methods and timing of payment; aim incentives more directly at workers' needs and expectations
	Communication	Permit participation by workers

design, assessment tools, interventions, and evaluation protocols. It is recommended that worker groups (e.g., joint labor-management committees) are positioned at the center of the decision-making process, and stress intervention experts are relocated to the periphery. Increasing worker participation and involvement in stress interventions will shift some of the emphasis to the process, without ignoring either the content or outcomes of training. Reynolds and Shapiro (1991) have made a convincing case for examining process variables as well as outcome variables in stress intervention research.

Measure the Sources of Stress in the Work Environment

Without an accurate assessment, one can only guess which are the most important stressors to target for change. If an assessment is to be done, how is it accomplished? Four levels of assessment are described below from the simplest to the most sophisticated levels.

1. *Informal discussions with workers.* Asking employees about the quality of their work life and stressful aspects of their jobs/tasks is a reasonable first step, especially for small companies. Opening a channel

of communication between employees and employee representatives will produce a rich source of information about stress and its perceived sources, as well as ideas for reducing stress. Such communication also legitimizes stress as a topic for discussion.

2. *Formal group discussions.* Group discussions provide an opportunity to assess individual and group stressors, such as coworker relationships, teamwork, and group norms. Group discussions tend to be more formal than Level 1 assessments but can provide more in-depth information on job stress. Additionally, group discussions are an excellent mechanism for brainstorming stress interventions with the people who know the most about their jobs: the workers.

3. *Questionnaire survey.* A questionnaire can obtain information from large numbers of workers about their perceptions of work, and it can be administered at later points in time to assess changes and detect emerging trends. Information obtained from Level 1 and 2 assessments are excellent starting points for developing questionnaire items. Questionnaires have been the most widely utilized data collection method in job stress studies. However, unless care is taken in the construction of the questionnaire, the results may not be reliable or valid. A knowledge of survey methodology is needed to properly design, administer, analyze, interpret, and provide feedback based on the results of a questionnaire. Such survey expertise is usually available from social scientists at local universities. Standardized questionnaires for measuring stress are discussed in the next level.

4. *Standardized questionnaire.* A standardized questionnaire is designed to yield reliable (i.e., repeatable) and valid (i.e., accurate) information and usually contains norms for comparison with a reference group, such as other occupations or the general public. Many questionnaires have been developed to measure job stress and stress reactions, and most are quite long (over 100 items). Most measure employee perceptions of job characteristics, including workload, autonomy, workpace, roles, and responsibility, as well as health symptoms and illness conditions. As noted above, a questionnaire can be administered at a later point in time to assess changes

in stressors and stressor/health relationships and to detect emerging trends.

Due to their popularity in job stress research, examples of commonly used questionnaires to measure job stress are described here. The *Occupational Stress Indicator* (Cooper, Sloan, & Williams, 1988) is based on the Cooper and Marshall (1976) stress model and consists of six scales (plus a number of subscales) that measure sources of stress at work, coupled with scales measuring Type A behavior, locus of control, job satisfaction, mental and physical health, and employee coping strategies. A number of studies have established the reliability of the *OSI*, as well as predictive and concurrent validity (Cooper, Sloan, & Williams, 1988). The *Occupational Stress Inventory* (Osipow & Davis, 1988) measures a wide range of job stressors, employee resources for coping with stress, and mental and physical strains. The various subscales have demonstrated good test-retest reliability, and occupational norms are available. Plotting standardized scores on each subscale produces a "stress profile" for workers. The *Generic Job Stress Questionnaire* (Hurrell & McLaney, 1988) was developed by the National Institute for Occupational Safety and Health (NIOSH). This instrument assesses many different job stressors, as well as stress reactions or strains. Most of the scales were adapted from prior scales with known reliability and validity. This instrument was designed to be modular; organizations can select individual scales, or the entire instrument can be used. Normative data on this questionnaire are currently being gathered. Another commonly used instrument, *The Work Environment Scale* (Moos, 1981), was not developed to assess job stress; rather, it was designed to assess the general work climate. It contains 90 items that make up 10 subscales and uses a *True-False* response format. The subscales have demonstrated good reliability and validity and have been used often by researchers over the past 15 years. Norms are available for a limited number of occupations.

What About Specific Program Elements?

The discussion above dealing with the common elements of a successful stress intervention did not address the issue of which specific program content should be included (i.e., muscle relaxation, cognitive-behavioral training, meditation, etc). Actually, the techniques selected seem to be of less importance than how the intervention is designed and implemented. If the four recommendations noted are followed, then a list of fundamental elements of a stress management intervention would include the following:

- Educational materials about the nature and sources of stress at work and how stress influences physical and mental health
- Some type of relaxation exercise that workers can learn in order to lower tension levels and create a state of mental and physical relaxation (progressive muscle relaxation, cue-controlled relaxation, meditation, etc.)
- Materials and/or training in cognitive-behavioral skills to help workers alter inappropriate thinking patterns or unhealthy behaviors
- Referral to community agencies (e.g., local mental health center) so that more serious clinical problems can be addressed

Relationship of Stress Management to Other Health Promotion Programs

Given the wide variety of stressors that exist in the workplace and that stress has been linked to many lifestyle behaviors, it is not unreasonable to suppose that stress could influence the success of other health promotion programs. How might this influence occur? First, if the job(s) in question is stressful, then stress at work can counter the beneficial effects of other health promotion programs. For instance, since stress has been linked to high blood pressure, if a worker participates in a company-sponsored hypertension treatment program but also has to deal with stress at work on a regular basis, then opposing forces are acting on the worker to reduce blood pressure on the one hand but increase it on the other. In the same way, a company-sponsored stress management program can be expected to produce little or no improvements in well-being if, after each training session, the worker returns to the same stress-producing work environment.

Indeed, job stress may be a moderator of the success of many health promotion programs. A concrete example will illustrate this point. Imagine two workplaces, both with a similar set of health promotion programs. One site (X) has poorly designed jobs, excessive workload, low worker control, and an organizational culture characterized by lack of trust and unsupportive supervisors. The other site (Y) has a more positive, supportive culture, and has redesigned jobs and workflow (via increasing worker autonomy) so as to reduce excessive workload. Because worker stress will be high at site X, the beneficial effects of its health promotion programs will be attenuated by the increased symptoms of, say, anxiety and sleep disturbances. These in turn might lead workers to not enter or to drop out of smoking cessation programs or perhaps to neglect proper nutrition or dietary regimes (common outcomes of stress). At site Y, on the other hand, the low stress levels at work might tend to promote or accentuate the value of health promotion programs by not fostering poor lifestyle habits. The attenuation hypothesis is testable and may explain why many health promotion programs produce less than optimal health benefits on a consistent basis.

SHIFTING ATTENTION FROM JOB STRESS TO ORGANIZATIONAL HEALTH

Action to reduce stress at work is usually prompted by some organizational problem or crisis (for example, escalating rates of sickness, absence, or labor turnover). Consequently, actions tend to be driven by a desire to reduce costs (i.e., problem-driven negative motives) rather than the desire to maximize potential and improve competitive edge (i.e., gains-driven positive motives). The danger of this type of approach is that once sickness, absence, or labor turnover rates stabilize at an acceptable level, interventions may lose their impetus and be considered no longer necessary. Organizations need to consider stress prevention not only as a means of cost reduction or containment, but also as a means of maintaining and improving organizational health and increasing productivity. The costs of stress and the collective health and wealth of organizations and their workers is of great importance to society as a whole.

A proactive approach would involve efforts to improve the overall health of both the worker and the organization and has recently been described as a "healthy work organization approach" (Murphy, in press; Sauter, Lim, and Murphy, 1996). The basic premise is that it is possible to improve worker well-being and organizational effectiveness. Research on healthy work organizations takes place at the intersection of worker well-being and organizational effectiveness and seeks to identify those job and organizational factors that predict *both* health and performance outcomes.

The notion of improved worker well-being plus organizational effectiveness is not novel; it has been discussed in one form or another in the organizational behavior, health promotion, and job stress literatures. For example, Pfeiffer (1987) suggested expanding traditional health promotion programs to include attention to work group- and organizational-level factors. The model offered by Pfeiffer (1987) was well-articulated and specific and listed three key components: individual health, team health, and organizational health. *Individual health* is affected by heredity, the environment, lifestyle, and the medical care system. *Team health* focuses on the execution of assigned work, quality of services provided, nature of the work environment, and health and satisfaction of team members. Poor team health occurs when a team is forced to work short-handed or when the team discourages individual participation in decision-making. *Organizational health* is a function of the interrelationship of the psychosocial work environment (i.e., the accepted or prescribed culture and norms), the quality of its

products and services, the administrative systems that regulate day-to-day performance (e.g., policies, procedures, and programs), and the employees themselves. Organizational health requires coordination of occupational health and safety, human resources, health promotion, medical services, and training/development functions.

Table 15-6 shows examples of the type of interventions at each level that could be used to improve health and organizational effectiveness.

Another example comes from the organizational behavior literature. In his book *The Healthy Company*, Rosen (1991) developed a values-based organizing system for managing and developing human assets. This system consists of 13 dimensions, closely intertwined and mutually reinforcing, which would maximize individual and organizational health and performance. A description of the 13 dimensions is shown in Box 15-1. Notice that a definition of each dimension is provided for a) the organization and b) the employee. The goal for creating a healthy company is to improve scores on these dimensions for both the organization as a whole and individual workers.

Finally, the National Institute for Occupational Safety and Health is developing a model of healthy work organizations based on analyses of employee survey data from a large manufacturing company (Murphy & Lim, 1997; Sauter, Lim, & Murphy, 1996). Questionnaire data on management practices, organizational culture/climate, core values, job satisfaction, work stress, and organizational effectiveness from over 15,000 workers from 1993–1997 were analyzed to identify those factors that were related to both worker

Table 15-6 Examples of Intervention Types

Individual Health	Work Team Health	Organizational Health
Stress management	Communication skills	Job security
Smoking cessation	Occupational health and safety	Compensation
Exercise	Stress management	Health promotion programs
Nutrition	Employee involvement	Corporate medical
Weight management	Conflict resolution	Educational assistance
Employee assistance programs	Job training	Employee training and development

Note. Adapted from G. J. Pfeiffer, *Occupational Health and Safety*, 1987.

BOX 15-1 DIMENSIONS OF A HEALTHY WORK ORGANIZATION

Open Communications

Organization openly communicates about its condition, its operations, the choices it faces, and its plans; sharing occurs at all levels.

Individuals respect the confidence of such information and participate in honest and forthright dialogue.

Employee Involvement

Organization recognizes the value of employee participation in achieving organizational objectives, actively seeks employee involvement and leadership in decision making, planning, work design, and problem solving.

Individuals participate actively, contribute ideas, take responsibility for decisions, participate in teams, and assume leadership roles.

Learning and Renewal

Organization provides continuous opportunities for all of its people to learn, update, and expand their knowledge and skills and to contribute to organizational innovation and learning

Individuals commit to life-long learning, sharing knowledge, and developing multiple skills and flexible competencies, and are responsive to opportunity.

Valued Diversity

Organization sees diversity as a source of stimulation and enrichment, assures equality of employment and opportunity, promotes tolerance, censures discrimination and prejudice, and provides opportunity for all to use their unique talents and capacities to perform to their potential.

Individuals take responsibility for bringing their unique beliefs, talents, and experiences to the workplace, working effectively with the prevailing culture, valuing the differences and uniqueness of others, sharing responsibility for tolerance and the censure of discrimination and prejudice.

Institutional Fairness

Organization promotes and protects privacy, equity, respect, and dissent as rights available to all employees.

Individuals observe the policies and practices of the organization and share responsibility for improving the quality of work relations.

Equitable Rewards and Recognition

Organization has a motivational system that reinforces its values as well as maximizes employee potential; recognizes the contributions of individuals, rewards performance, and shares profits and ownership.

Individuals give full value in their work for the enterprise and accept the organization's multiple financial obligations.

Common Economic Security

Organization recognizes that its economic security and that of its employees are one and the same; vigorously seeks a common security.

Individuals recognize that individual security is directly linked to long-term success of the organization and share commitments and burdens.

People-Centered Technology

Organization seeks and applies technologies that eliminate bad jobs, provide safe and ergonomically sound work, and enhance human capabilities and satisfaction.

Individuals adapt to new technologies, learn how to use new tools, and support innovation and technological changes that yield competitive advantage.

Health-Enhancing Work Environments

Organization works to promote physical and psychological health in the work place, encourages employee pursuit of health, and takes steps to protect them from catastrophic costs of illness.

(continued)

Individuals take personal health seriously, observe safety rules, share the cost of managing health and illness; actively seek to maintain optimum fitness for work.

Meaningful Work

Organization inspires pride and a sense of purpose; creates jobs that have variety, integrity, and significance; and commits to high quality, ethically sound products and services.

Individuals strive to achieve high levels of quality, ethical behavior, and customer satisfaction.

Family/Work/Personal Life Balance

Organization supports the employees' need to balance work, family, and personal life.

Individuals actively seek to balance their commitment to work, family, and personal life needs.

Community Responsibility

Organization leads and invests in public interests, provides benefit to the social well-being of the community and nation.

Individuals share public responsibilities as active citizens and as volunteers to social good.

Environmental Protection

Organization commits itself to preserve and restore environmental health and engages in ecologically sound practices.

Individuals share similar personal commitments and responsibilities and assist the organization in fulfilling its commitment.

Source: Healthy Companies, Inc., *Work Environment Survey. Final Report to the National Institute for Occupational Safety and Health,* 1994.

well-being and organizational effectiveness. Key characteristics associated with organizational health were:

- Workers rewarded for performance
- Open, two-way communication
- Worker growth and development (training)
- Trust and mutual respect
- Strong commitment to core values
- Strategic planning to keep the organization competitive and adaptive
- Workers are aware of how their work contributes to the business

THE MISSING INGREDIENT

The reader should note the presence of two factors in each of the healthy work organization models that are not common or typical in job stress models, namely, *organizational climate* and *commitment to core values.* Taken together, they comprise the organizational culture, which refers to the shared values and beliefs that underlie a company's identity; it can be thought of as the "personality" of the organization. Culture is often set by beliefs of the company founder and codified as a set of policies, rules, and regulations about how the company does business and accomplishes its objectives. It is often measured by employee perceptions of what it is like to work for the company (i.e., the "climate") and by the core values.

Organizational climate refers to the shared perceptions of employees about the way in which their workplace functions. Climate can describe specific areas of work (such as safety climate and climate for customer service); but, in each case, climate is about employee perceptions of how the workplace operates. "Core values are the organization's essential and enduring tenets—a small set of general guiding principles not to be confused with specific cultural or operating practices and not to be compromised for financial gain or short-term expediency." (Collins and Porras, 1994, p. 73). Core values are typically short, probably no more than five or six in number, and they do not come and go with the trends and fads of the day. They are authentically "core" in that they would not change even if the business environment penalized a company for holding such values. All organizations have core values, whether stated or unstated, and they function like the soul of the organization. When values are well-integrated into organizational life, they contribute mightily to organizational effectiveness. For example, in their study of successful companies, Collins and Porras (1994) found that visionary companies are driven by a core ideology that consists of core values and a purpose.

The absence of measures of organizational culture may explain why organizational stress intervention studies have failed to produce significant improvements in worker distress levels. The reasoning runs something like this: the organizational culture provides the background or context in which workers perform their job duties. If the culture is rigid and inflexible, does not foster cooperation and support, and does not encourage training and development, then any changes made at the job level to reduce stress will be counteracted by the negative work climate (e.g., "they really don't care about me, only about improving production or looking good to the public").

The same can be said for core values. Many organizations have developed core values that, at least on paper, are thought to guide the organization's functioning. However, when management actions do not align with their core values (i.e., not "walking the walk"), it results in stress for employees, and management loses credibility. Every reader can identify with the frustration experienced when dealing with people who say one thing but do another, whose actions are inconsistent with their words. It is just as frustrating to deal with an organization that has core values but operates as if they don't or aren't routinely applied in day-to-day organizational life. Besides frustration, the lack of predictability creates ambiguity among workers, which was noted earlier in this chapter as a classic source of stress at work.

Example #1: Culture and Financial Performance

Several studies provide empirical evidence to support the importance of culture/climate on worker stress levels. Bruner and Cooper (1991) used self-report data from 93 senior marketing managers coupled with objective financial data in 14 electronics companies in

the U.S. They selected organizations to represent two groups based on financial performance: 'strong' companies (with positive earnings and increasing revenues) and 'weak' companies (with financial losses and declining revenues). They examined two corporate-level stressors (corporate culture and frequency of change events), three individual factors (education, tenure, and Type A behavior), and three role-related stressors (range of responsibilities, supervisory requirements, and length of workweek).

The following hypotheses were proposed:

- The corporate culture will be less flexible, more inward-looking, and less cooperative in organizations which are losing money.
- There will be more 'corporate change events' in weak performing companies.
- Role stressors will be indistinguishable between the strong and weak company groups.
- Indicators of mental ill-health, poor job performance, and job dissatisfaction will be higher in the financially weak companies.
- Perceived stress will be higher in the financially weak companies.

Analyses of the data revealed support for each of the hypotheses except the last one. Perhaps the most interesting result was that the measures of culture/climate and financial performance were more highly correlated with perceived stress than were the individual and role-related factors. This suggests that a) the culture/climate is an important factor to consider in job stress studies, and b) interventions that focus on job- or task-specific factors (such as role relationships) but ignore culture/climate may be "missing the boat."

Example #2: Culture and Safe Work Behavior

Another example that illustrates the influence of organizational culture/climate on worker perceptions and behavior comes from the safety literature (Gershon, Murphy, Felknor, Vesley, & DeJoy, 1995; Murphy, Gershon, & DeJoy, 1996). Health care workers are exposed to a variety of health-endangering factors at work, including physical agents, chemical agents, infectious diseases, and psychosocial stressors. A recent occupational exposure for health care workers is HIV/AIDS. In occupational settings, health care workers are exposed to HIV/AIDS primarily via needlestick injuries and secondarily by contaminated blood/body fluid splashes to the eyes or mucous membranes.

A study was undertaken to discover the best predictors of health care workers following recommended work practices to reduce occupational exposure to blood-borne pathogens. A wide range of factors were measured, including demographics, job tenure, education/training, personal risk-taking, workload, role ambiguity, work stress, and safety climate. Safety climate measured the general level of safety awareness, management commitment to safety, and level of cooperation among workers and management to reduce safety problems. Examples of items in this scale were "Where I work, employees, supervisors, and managers work together to insure the safest possible working conditions," and "In my organization (or office, or facility), all reasonable steps are taken to minimize hazardous job tasks and procedures." Analyses revealed that safety climate was a key predictor of which health care workers followed the recommended safe work practices and was a far stronger predictor of compliance with safe work practices than personal factors like age or risk-taking tendencies. Thus, efforts to reduce occupational exposure to blood-borne pathogens should include attention to the overall safety climate, one factor that comprises the organizational culture.

CONCLUSION

The studies described above provide empirical evidence to support the notion that organizational culture and climate at work are important determinants of worker perceptions and behavior. This suggests that workplace interventions to reduce stress should attend to culture/climate issues, either directly as an integral part of the intervention or secondarily as a powerful moderator of how the intervention will be perceived (and received) by workers and its ultimate effectiveness.

The importance of company culture has been noted by well-known writers in the business litera-

ture, including Peters and Waterman (*In Search of Excellence,* 1992), Blanchard and O'Connor (*Managing by Values,* 1997), Collins and Porras (*Built to Last,* 1994), and Kotter (*Corporate Culture and Performance,* 1992). Each of these authors emphasized the pivotal role of culture and commitment to core values as key to an organization's success in the marketplace. Similar recommendations for improving the effectiveness of stress interventions can be found in the writings of job stress researchers from Great Britain (Cooper & Williams, 1994), Finland (Lindstrom, 1994), Sweden (Aronsson, 1996), the Netherlands (Kompier et. al., 1998), and Australia (Hart & Wearing, 1999).

Far less research has been published on how organizations can change their culture and better integrate their core values into the daily work routine. However, a few thoughts can be offered. First, the organization's culture cannot be changed directly through edicts or policies, but these are necessary to begin the process. The culture changes as the organization aligns its actions and decisions to comply with its stated policies and goals. For example, if an organization decides that it would like to create a culture for innovation, then it should set goals, establish policies and procedures, and initiate actions that reflect its commitment to innovation. This might mean some or all of the following:

- Defining innovation, explaining why the organization thinks it is important, and disseminating this information to workers at all levels
- Emphasizing innovation at all meetings and in company correspondence
- Providing training for all workers and supervisors on innovation, with examples of innovative ideas used in other companies (i.e., benchmarking)
- Adding innovation to employee job descriptions as a basic element of all jobs
- Establishing the structure and processes needed to support employee innovation (e.g., time off from routine job duties to allow employees to develop new and better ways of doing things)
- Providing concrete examples of how supervisors can foster innovation
- Adding an element to supervisors' performance appraisal on fostering employee innovation

• Setting up incentive programs that reward or recognize employee innovation

The same logic applies to commitment to core values. Commitment to core values is judged by the actions and decisions of upper and middle management, so care needs to be taken to insure that the organizations' actions are in line with the values. Such decisions could include everything from placement and selection to job training to decisions about the processes to be used for restructuring and reorganizing. For example, if *Dignity* is a core value and involves treating all workers with dignity and respect, then it should permeate management actions and decisions. It should be evident in things like employee performance appraisal; hiring, firing, and placement; how management handles restructuring

and reorganization; performance reward systems; and supervisor support for workers. A recent article (Taft, Hawn, Barber, & Bidwell, 1999) offered a concise description of the specific steps involved in embedding the core values into everyday work life in a hospital setting (see Box 15-2).

Another example comes from the retail sales industry. In a remarkable case study of the turnaround of Sears led by CEO Arthur Martinez, Sears undertook a complete revamping of the way it did business. Sears involved 80,000 employees in a process that involved first identifying six core values then formulating a statistical model that linked core values to employee satisfaction, which in turn, was related to increased customer satisfaction and greater profit (Rucci, Kirn, & Quinn, 1998). The statistical model revealed that a 5-point improvement in employee atti-

BOX 15-2 ONE HOSPITAL'S EFFORT TO CREATE A VALUES-DRIVEN ORGANIZATIONAL CULTURE

A recent article in the journal *Health Care Management Review* provided a detailed, step-by-step description of how one hospital attempted to identify, define, and embed their core values into the everyday work experience. The major phases of the "Values Initiative" are shown below:

Phase 1: Values Identification
• 50 volunteers in 5 groups
• Team brainstorming yields preliminary lists of 29 values
• Storytelling illustrates and personalizes the identified values

Phase 2: Values Consolidation
• 15 volunteers from all Phase 1 teams
• New team consolidates 29 preliminary values to final list of 9 core values

Phase 3: Values Integration: Focus on Embracing Values at Department and Team Levels
• Holding leadership workshops

• Holding staff meetings over 3-month time period
• Choosing "Team Captains" to lead ongoing, informal sessions among staff to help assimilate values into daily life

Phase 4: Values Infrastructure: Keeping the Values Alive by Formally Incorporating Them Into the Hospital's Values
• Interviewing process
• Hiring process
• Orientation process
• Staff training
• Job descriptions
• Performance evaluations (first for leaders, then for staff)
• Employee surveys
• Publications
• Team processes

Source: S. Taft, K. Hawn, J. Barber, & J. Bidwell. *Health Care Management Review,* 1999.

BOX 15-3 EXAMPLE OF A HEALTHY ORGANIZATIONAL CULTURE

Orren Pickell Builders
Bannockburn, Ill.; Years in
business: 27; Employees: 80;
Units closed in 1998: 25+

Orren Pickell is an engineer, of sorts. Not of things, but of teams of people. He sees each person—including himself—as an individual set of strengths and weaknesses, and he works to fit jobs to employees, not the other way around.

At the same time, he pushes his crew to pursue fresh ideas and unfamiliar skills—whatever it takes to become better. The result is a hard-earned reputation as an employer of choice in the Chicago area.

"You just know in your gut there's a benefit to maintaining people's passion for their work."

—Anthony Perry, VP, design

Keeping the energy flowing is central to the company's dynamism. Consequently, Pickell, the president, welcomes anything that keeps people motivated and moving forward. That's why the builder encouraged a young architect to get his state license, and paid him a bonus for doing so.

"We are committed to securing for our employees an environment of personal achievement, growth, and advancement." Pickell's head of design, Anthony Perry, recalls the time Orren took the division on a riverboat tour to discuss the architectural features of the Chicago skyline. And last summer, Orren hired a well-known architectural renderer to give the staff a three-day seminar. "Any time we can hook into things like that," Perry says, 'it makes people have a zest for what we do."

Pickell's philosophy is to hire people with positive attitudes, integrity and talent, and willingness to learn. He provides on-the-job training, including assigning new hires in their first three to six months to work with his most experienced employees. Pickell believes that apprenticeship is the company's most important training.

The builder's hiring process is lengthy, with job candidates facing an interview panel of as many as six people. Perry recalls when he was hired six years ago. "It's sometimes frustrating to job applicants. We're very slow to hire. It's only because we're really careful," he says.

"It all comes down to picking the right people and helping them pick the right people," Pickell believes. "You have to have an exceptional group of people, who are working to offset their weaknesses. I wouldn't call myself an exceptional manager, but I surround myself with people who are."

---

tudes led to a 1.3 point improvement in customer satisfaction that led to a 0.5% improvement in revenue growth. Clearly, companies that integrate their values so that they permeate every aspect of work could see tangible benefits on a variety of performance and financial indicators. Additional examples of how companies try to "live out" their core values can be found in Harmon (1996) and in Anderson (1997).

The World Wide Web is fast becoming an excellent source for information on what companies are doing to foster healthy organizational cultures. Many companies have webpages showing a mission statement, core values, and strategic objectives, as well as information on current health and safety programs. Industry-specific websites also offer good information on successful companies. *Builder Online* (builder. hw.net/monthly/1999/mar/covstry/index.htx) recently published a list of eight great home-building companies to work for. Interviews with management and employees at each company provide indications of why each company is so successful (see Box 15-3 for an example).

Employees are rewarded for showing initiative, particularly if they take on projects no one else seems to want. One worker earned herself a nice bonus when she assumed the task of managing all the design contests that the company enters. That's a small price to pay for a vastly improved process, believes the company.

To learn from the experience and knowledge of others, team members periodically rotate through other departments. By maintaining person-to-person contact, the routine facilitates the handoff of a customer through the building process, as a sales associate introduces the customer to the architect, who in turn acquaints the home buyer with the estimator, and so on. In that chain, says Perry, "No one wants to let anyone down. No one wants to be the weak link."

So when Pickell does spot a mistake, he brings the group together and reminds them of the impact of all their actions on the end product and on the customer. Identifying who made the mistake would be beside the point.

On the other hand, when an employee's or a department's performance is good, Pickell makes sure it is recognized. "Every department tries to blow the customer away," he says. "When they do, we bring that to everyone's attention."

Driving these initiatives is Pickell's focus on reducing job stress. By using the "latest and greatest technology," he says, the company is giving workers the tools to do 80 percent of their jobs by rote. Its software gives people a punch list every week. That puts sense and order into their work and leaves them just 20 percent to manage.

"There's nothing like experience to keep the stress level down. If you can be profoundly better than everyone else, you're going to make more money." And if you offer a less stressful environment with a 40-hour workweek, he says, you have your pick of job applicants.

He has seen his philosophy pay off. "You can walk down the hall here and see how people treat each other. You can see it in the help they give each other, the lack of selfishness."

That translates into superior service, says Pickell. "I don't have unhappy customers."

Finally, *Fortune* magazine annually publishes their list of the 100 Best Companies to Work For (www.pathfinder.com/fortune/bestcompanies/index2.html), with links to each company's home page. The 100 Best companies are selected based on several types of information, one of which is a 32-page survey that measures company philosophies, policies, programs, and practices influencing the management of people in their organizations. Ten primary subject categories are measured, including Recruiting/Hiring/Orientation, Development and Learning, Rewards and Recognition, Health and Well-Being, Financial Security, Organizational Culture, and Unique People Practices. Visiting the websites of these 100 companies and examining their policies, programs, and practices should provide sufficient ideas for organizations that are interested in creating successful organizational cultures. The overlap of the subject categories used to select the 100 Best Companies To Work For with the list of healthy work organization characteristics presented earlier should not be lost on the reader.

References

Anderson, C. (1997). Values-based management. *Academy of Management Executive, 11,* 25–46.

Aronsson, G. (1996). Psychosocial issues at work: current situation and trends in Sweden. In *Proceedings of Occupational Health and Safety in Progress: Northern-Baltic-Karelian Regional Symposium.* Lappeenranta, Finland: Finnish Institute of Occupational Health.

Benson, H. (1976). *The relaxation response.* New York: William Morrow.

Blanchard, K., & O'Conner, J. (1997). *Managing by values.* San Francisco, CA: Berrett-Koehler.

Bond, J. T., Galinsky, E., & Swanberg, J. E. (1998). *The 1997 national study of the changing workforce.* New York: Families and Work Institute.

Bruner, B. M., & Cooper, C. L. (1991). Corporate financial performance and occupational stress. *Work and Stress, 5,* 267–287.

Bunce, D. (1997). What factors are associated with the outcome of individual-focused worksite stress management interventions? *Journal of Occupational and Organizational Psychology, 70,* 1–17.

Cannon, W. B. (1929). *Bodily changes in pain, hunger, fear, and rage.* Boston: C. T. Branford.

Cannon, W. B. (1935). Stresses and strains of homeostasis. *American Journal of Medical Science, 189,* 1–14.

Caplan, R. D., Cobb, S., French, J. R. P., Jr., VanHarrison, R. V., & Pinneau, S. R., Jr. (1975). *Job demands and worker health: Main effects and occupational differences* (DHEW NIOSH Publication No. 75-160). Washington, DC: U.S. Government Printing Office.

Collins, J., & Porras, J. (1994). *Built to last: Successful habits of visionary companies.* New York: HarperBusiness.

COMCARE Australia (1997a). *The management of occupational stress in Commonwealth agencies - A joint ANAO/COMCARE better practice guide for senior managers.* [On-line]. Available: http://www.comcare.gov.au/publications/betterpract/fs-cover.html.

COMCARE Australia (1997b). *The management of occupational stress in Commonwealth agencies - Implementing an occupational stress prevention program.* [On-line]. Available: http://www.comcare.gov.au/publications/implementosp/fs-cover.html.

Cooper, C. L., Liukkonen, P., & Cartwright, S. (1996). *Stress prevention in the workplace: Assessing the costs and benefits to organizations.* Dublin, Ireland: European Foundation for the Improvement of Living and Working Conditions.

Cooper, C. L., & Marshall, J. (1976). Occupational sources of stress: A review of the literature relating to coronary heart disease and mental ill health. *Journal of Occupational Psychology, 49,* 11–28.

Cooper, C. L., Sloan, S. J., & Williams, S. (1988). *Occupational stress indicator management guide.* Windsor: NFER-Nelson.

Cooper, C. L., & Williams, S. (1994). *Creating healthy work organizations.* Chichester: Wiley.

DeFrank, R. S. & Cooper, C. L. (1987). Worksite stress management interventions: Their effectiveness and conceptualization. *Journal of Management Psychology, 2,* 4–10.

Elkin, A. J., & Rosch, P. J. (1990). Promoting mental health at the workplace: The prevention side of stress management. *Occupational Medicine State of the Art Reviews, 5*(4), 739–754.

Elo, A.-L., Leppänen, A., Lindström, K., & Ropponen, T. (1993). *Occupational stress questionnaire.* Finnish Institute for Occupational Health, Helsinki, Finland.

Gallup Poll: (1999, September 3). American workers generally satisfied, but indicate their jobs leave much to be desired. Workers are least satisfied with stress and pay levels (by Lydia Saad). Princeton, N.J.: The Gallup Organization.

Gershon, R. M., Murphy, L. R., Felknor, S., Vesley, D., & DeJoy, D. (1995). Compliance with universal precautions among health care workers. *American Journal of Infection Control, 23,* 225–236.

Goetzel, R. Z., Anderson, D. R., Whitmer, R. W., Ozminkowski, R. J., Dunn, R. L., Wasserman, J., & the Health Enhancement Research Organization (HERO) Research Committee. (1998). The relationship between modifiable health risks and health care expenditures. *Journal of Occupational and Environmental Medicine, 40,* 843–854.

Hackman, J. R., & Lawler, E. E. (1971). Employee reactions to job characteristics. *Journal of Applied Psychology Monograph, 55,* 259–268.

Hackman, J. R., & Oldham, G. R. (1976). Motivation through the design of work: Test of a theory. *Organizational Behavior and Human Performance, 16,* 250–279.

Harmon, F. G. (1996). *Playing for keeps: How the world's most aggressive companies use core values to manage, energize, and organize their people and promote, advance and achieve their corporate missions.* New York: John Wiley & Sons.

Hart, P. M., & Wearing, A. J. (1999). Using employee opinion surveys to identify control mechanisms in organizations. In W. J. & A., Grob, (Eds.), *Control of human behaviour, mental processes and consciousness* (pp. 145–171). Mahwah, NJ: Lawrence Erlbaum.

Health and Safety Executive. (1995). *Stress at work: A guide for employers.* Suffolk, United Kingdom: HSE Books.

Health and Safety Executive (1998a). *Help on work-related stress - A short guide.* Suffolk, United Kingdom: HSE Books.

Health and Safety Executive (1998b). *Managing work-related stress: A guide for managers and teachers in schools.* Suffolk, United Kingdom: HSE Books.

Healthy Companies, Inc. (1994). *Work environment survey. Final report to the National Institute for Occupational Safety and Health.* Washington, D.C.: Healthy Companies, Inc.

Heaney, C. A., Israel, B. A., Schurman, S. J., Baker, E. A., House, J. S., & Hugentobler, M. (1993). Industrial relations, worksite stress reduction, and employee well-being: A participatory action research investigation. *Journal of Organizational Behavior, 14,* 495–510.

Heaney, C. A., & van Ryn, M. (1990). Broadening the scope of worksite stress programs: A guiding framework. *American Journal of Health Promotion, 4,* 413–420.

Hurrell, J. J., Jr. & McLaney, A. M. (1988). Exposure to job stress: A new psychometric instrument. *Scandinavian Journal of Work Environment and Health, 14,* 27–28.

Israel, B. A., Baker, E. A., Goldenhar, L. M., Heaney, C. A., & Schurman, S. J. (1996). Occupational stress, safety, and health: Conceptual framework and principles for effective prevention interventions. *Journal of Occupational Health Psychology, 1,* 261–286.

Ivancevich, J. M., Matteson, M. T., Freedman, S. M., & Phillips, J. S. (1990). Worksite stress management interventions. *American Psychologist, 45,* 252–261.

Jackson, S. E. (1983). Participation in decision making as a strategy for reducing job-related strain. *Journal of Applied Psychology, 68,* 3–19.

Jewell, L. N., & Siegall, M. (1990). *Contemporary industrial/organizational psychology.* St. Paul, MN: West.

Kahn, R. L., Wolfe, D. M., Quinn, R. P., Snoek, J. D., & Rosenthal, R. A. (1964). *Organizational stress: Studies in role conflict and ambiguity.* New York: Wiley.

Karasek, R. A. (1979). Job demands, job decision latitude, and mental strain. *Journal of Occupational Behavior, 24,* 285–307.

Kompier, M. A. J., Geurts, S. A. E, Gründemann, R. W. M., Vink, P., & Smulders, P. G. W. (1998). Cases in stress prevention: The success of a participative and stepwise approach. *Stress Medicine, 14,* 155–168.

Kompier, M., & Levi, L. (1994). *Stress at work: Causes, effects, and prevention.* Dublin, Ireland: European Foundation for the Improvement of Living and Working Conditions.

Kotter, J. (1992). *Corporate culture and performance.* New York: Free Press.

Landsbergis, P. A., & Vivona-Vaughan, E. (1995). Evaluation of an occupational stress intervention in a public agency. *Journal of Organizational Behavior, 16,* 29–48.

Lazarus, R. S. (1966). *Psychological stress and the coping process.* New York: McGraw-Hill.

Lindstrom, K. (1994). Psychosocial criteria for good work organization. *Scandinavian Journal of Work Environment and Health, 20,* 123–133.

Manning, M. R., Jackson, C. N., & Fusilier, M. R. (1996). Occupational stress and health care use. *Journal of Occupational Health Psychology, 1,* 1–10.

Millar, J. D. (1984). The NIOSH-suggested list of the ten leading work-related diseases and injuries. *Journal of Occupational Medicine* (letters), 26 (5), 340–341.

Moos, R. (1981). *Work environment scale.* Palo Alto, CA: Consulting Psychologists Press.

Murphy, L. R. (1984). Occupational stress management: A review and appraisal. *Journal of Occupational Psychology, 57,* 1–15.

Murphy, L. R. (1988). Workplace interventions for stress reduction and prevention. In C. L. Cooper & R. Payne (Eds.), *Causes, coping, and consequences of stress at work,* pp. 301–339. Chichester: John Wiley and Sons.

Murphy, L. R. (1995). Managing job stress: An employee assistance/human resource management partnership. *Personnel Review, 24,* 41–50.

Murphy, L. R. (1996). Stress management in work settings: A critical review of the research literature. *American Journal of Health Promotion, 11,* 112–135.

Murphy, L. R. (2000). Models of healthy work organizations. In L. R. Murphy & C. L. Cooper (Eds.), *Healthy and productive work: An international perspective* (pp.). London: Taylor and Francis, p. 1–11.

Murphy, L. R., DuBois, D., & Hurrell, J. J. (1986). Accident reduction through stress management. *Journal of Business and Psychology, 1,* 5–18.

Murphy, L. R., Gershon, R. M., & DeJoy, D. (1996). Stress and occupational exposure to HIV/AIDS. In C. L. Cooper (Ed.), *Handbook of Stress Medicine.* Boca Raton, Florida: CRC Press, p. 177–190.

Murphy, L. R., & Lim, S. Y. (1997). Characteristics of healthy work organizations. In P. Seppälä, T. Luopajärvi, C.-H. Nygård, & M. Mattila (Eds.), *From experience to innovation* (Vol. 1, pp. 513–515). Helsinki, Finland: Finnish Institute of Occupational Health.

National Institute for Occupational Safety and Health. (1996). *National occupational research agenda* (DHHS [NIOSH] Publication No. 96-115). Washington, DC: U.S. Government Printing Office.

National Institute for Occupational Safety and Health (1999). *Stress at work* (DHHS [NIOSH] Publication No. 99-101). Washington, DC: U.S. Government Printing Office.

Newman, J. D., & Beehr, T. (1979). Personal and organizational strategies for handling job stress: A review of research and opinion. *Personnel Psychology, 32,* 1–43.

Osipow, S. H. & Davis, A. S. (1988). The relationship of coping resources to occupational stress and strain. *Journal of Vocational Behavior, 32,* 1–15.

Parkes, K., & Sparkes, T. J. (1998). Organizational interventions to reduce work stress. Are they effective? A review of the literature. Suffolk: United Kingdom HSE books.

Payne, R., Wall, T. D., Borrill, C., & Carter, A. (1999). Strain as a moderator of the relationship between work characteristics and work attitudes. *Journal of Occupational Health Psychology, 4,* 3–14.

Peters, T., & Waterman, R. H., Jr. (1982). *In search of excellence: Lessons from America's best-run companies.* New York: Warner Books.

Pfeiffer, G. J. (1987, October). Corporate health can improve if firms take organizational approach. *Occupational Health and Safety,* 96–99.

Quick, J. C., & Quick, J. D. (1984). *Organizational stress and preventive management.* New York: McGraw-Hill.

Reynolds, S., & Shapiro, D. A. (1991). Stress reduction in transition: Conceptual problems in the design, implementation, and evaluation of worksite stress management interventions. *Human Relations, 44,* 717–733.

Rosen, R. H. (1991). *The healthy company. Eight strategies to develop people, productivity, and profits.* Los Angeles: Jeremy P. Tarcher.

Rucci, A., Kirn, S., & Quinn, R. (1998, January/February). The employee-customer-profit chain at Sears. *Harvard Business Review,* 82–97.

Sauter, S. L., Lim, S. Y., and Murphy, L. R. (1996). Organizational health: A new paradigm for occupational stress research at NIOSH. *Japanese Journal of Occupational Mental Health, 4,* 248–254.

Sauter, S. L., Murphy, L. R., Hurrell, J. J. Jr. (1990). A national strategy for the prevention of work-related psychological disorders. *American Psychologist, 45,* 1146–1158.

Schaubroeck, J., Ganster, D. C., Sime, W. E., & Ditman, D. (1993). A field experiment testing supervisory role clarification. *Personnel Psychology, 46,* 1–25.

Selye, H. (1936). A syndrome produced by diverse noxious agents. *Nature, 138,* 32.

Selye, H. (1946). The general adaptation syndrome and diseases of adaptation. *Journal of Clinical Endocrinology, 6,* 217–230.

Shilling, S., & Brackbill, R. M. (1987). Occupational health and safety risks and potential health consequences perceived by U.S. workers. *Public Health Reports, 102,* 36–46.

Stoner, C. R., & Fry, F. L. (1983, May/June). Developing a corporate policy for managing stress. *Personnel, 66,* 76.

Taft, S., Hawn, K., Barber, J., & Bidwell, J. (1999). Fulcrum for the future: The creation of a values-driven culture. *Health Care Management Review, 24,* 17–32.

van der Hek, H., & Plomp, H. N. (1997). Occupational stress management programs. A practical overview of published effect studies. *Occupational Medicine, 47,* 133–141.

Wall, T. D., & Clegg, C. W. (1981). A longitudinal study of group work redesign. *Journal of Occupational Behavior, 2,* 31–49.

Wall, T. D., Kemp, N. J., Jackson, P. R., & Clegg, C. W. (1986). Outcomes of autonomous workgroups: A long-term field experiment. *Academy of Management Journal, 29,* 280–304.

CHAPTER

16

Employee Assistance Programs

R. Paul Maiden
Donald B. Levitt

INTRODUCTION

Employee assistance program (EAP) experts estimate that 20% of any workforce is affected by personal problems that can influence work performance. They also agree that problems that occur at home tend to show up in the workplace and that work-related pressures often follow employees home and have a negative influence on family life. The premise of EAPs is a simple one. Employees struggling with personal problems need help to deal with these problems—preferably before they have a negative impact in the workplace. Work is a major source of ego identity and is the primary source of our economic security. It is also where we spend the bulk of our waking hours. It is thus in the employer's best interest to help employees resolve personal problems that might affect their work.

But why should an employer offer an EAP when many already provide health care benefits for mental health and substance abuse problems? Why don't employees just use these benefits to get the help they need and thus avoid having their personal problems affect their work? Often times an individual does not know where to turn for help when they need it. They typically rely on word of mouth or recommendation from a friend or family member. Emotional and psychological problems continue to carry a degree of social stigma, and people generally tend to avoid dealing with them until either they reach a crisis point or they become the recipient of institutional interventions (e.g. hospitalization for mental illness, coerced into treatment after being charged with driving under the influence, domestic violence, gambling debt, etc.).

EAPs offer two essential services. The first of these services is counseling for employees regarding personal concerns. While many employee problems can be resolved by a professional EAP counselor in just a few sessions, many other EAP clients are referred by the EAP counselor to specialized and/or longer term professional treatment or other assistance for legal, financial, and child/eldercare issues. For these latter cases, the EAP often continues to maintain contact with the client during and even after the course of treatment or assistance to ensure that the employee's problem is being appropriately treated and resolved. In situations requiring extended absence from the job, the EAP counselor will help the employee with reintegrating into their job.

EAPs are generally "positioned" or presented to employees as providing assistance for a wide range of personal concerns (from the very serious to the more minor "problems of daily living"). They are conceptualized as dealing with any personal problem that will impact job performance and, equally important, any personal problem that can *potentially* impact performance. Consequently, the EAP is generally less stigmatized in the community than professional treatment, and for many employees it is their first encounter with a mental health professional. Thus employees are more likely to seek help from the EAP even when they would not go directly to a mental health professional in the community. Once the employee meets with the EAP counselor, the counselor can help the employee overcome any reticence about seeking professional treatment. Based on the EAP counselor's professional assessment of the client's concerns, he/she can help the employee get appropriate professional help or assistance in the community. In this way EAP counseling helps overcome the barriers of stigma and appropriate treatment as noted earlier. Having access to an EAP also eliminates the need to "therapist shop." Instead, the EAP counselor assesses the needs of the client, often provides short-term interventions, or provides direction in selecting appropriate continued assistance.

The second essential service offered by an EAP is consultation to supervisors, personnel representatives, and union stewards regarding employee job performance problems that may be related to employee personal problems. When an employee continues to have attendance, performance, or conduct problems—even after having received mentoring and counseling from his/her superior and having been advised repeatedly that such behavior is unacceptable—it is very often the case that the employee is unable to improve behavior due to a personal problem. Under these circumstances, the EAP counselor can help the supervisor, personnel representative, or union steward to hold the employee accountable for acceptable behavior while at the same time referring the employee to the EAP. This process of *constructive confrontation* of the employee helps maintain the workplace focus on job performance while at the same time providing strong motivation for the employee to seek help. When the employee is in a state of psychological denial, as is often the case, this motivation can often help the employee overcome the denial that has prevented him/her from seeking assistance.

An EAP, then, helps the employer maintain an efficient workforce and helps employees resolve personal problems that might affect their work. This chapter is designed to provide an introduction to EAPs for health promotion professionals or other human resource professionals who would like to work more closely with an existing EAP or who have been given the responsibility of arranging the implementation of an EAP within their company.

The first section of this chapter provides an overview of the basic principles and concepts of EAPs, addressing such questions as: What comprises the core components of EAP counseling and consultation? How are EAPs managed and delivered in the workplace? What have been the actual outcomes of EAP practice?

The second section addresses some special issues that are of particular relevance to contemporary EAPs, such as specific populations, substance abuse, drug testing, fitness for duty, critical incident stress debriefing, and managed care.

The third section looks at the relationship between EAPs and health promotion in the workplace, examining the conceptual and practical advantages of linking or integrating EAP and health promotion.

BASIC PRINCIPLES OF EAPs

Types and Prevalence of Employee Personal Concerns

What kinds of personal concerns have a negative effect upon employee attendance and performance? Just about any kind of personal concern can have an impact on the workplace. If the employee is spending time at work worrying about the problem, making phone calls to try to resolve the problem, or falling asleep because he/she was up all night worrying, arguing, or drinking, that person is obviously unable to do the best job possible. Typical employee concerns span a wide range of matters, including marital discord, family dysfunction, alcohol use, drug use, dependent care, anxiety and depression, stress, legal issues, job and career issues, finances, and health.

Certainly not everybody who is dealing with a personal concern of this type (which includes just about all of us at some point in time!) has the concern affect his/her work, so why should EAPs be involved in helping employees with all of these problems? Even when the problem is not currently affecting the workplace, many of these problems will eventually get worse and then affect the workplace if they are not resolved. Thus by addressing problems early and preventing more serious problems, EAPs help to maintain a more fully functioning workforce.

Because the intensity of a personal concern, and thus its impact on the workplace, can vary so greatly, it is difficult to determine how many employees have their work negatively affected by personal concerns. Looking at studies that examine the prevalence of alcohol, drug, and mental health problems can, however, give some idea of the prevalence of employee personal concerns that affect work.

Alcohol and drug abuse is the leading cause of preventable and premature illness, disability, and death in the United States (U.S. Department of Health and Human Services [USDHHS], 1995). The total economic cost for alcohol abuse in both tangible and intangible costs was estimated by the U.S. Department of Health and Human Services to be $100 billion in 1992. The total economic cost in lost productivity each year to the U.S. because of alcohol abuse is $65.5 billion. Drug abuse costs our nation $33.3 billion each year in lost productivity alone. In 1990 the U.S. spent $200 billion in medical services, law enforcement, lost productivity, property damage, and insurance claims directly related to alcohol and drug abuse. Costs of treatment are only one percent of the $200 billion yearly cost (USDHHS, 1995).

An estimated 100 million Americans drink alcohol. According to a 1995 report released by the National Institute of Alcohol Abuse and Alcoholism, 13,760,000 U.S. adults (7.41% of persons 18 and older) met standard diagnostic criteria for alcohol abuse or alcohol dependence during 1992. Many alcoholics are teens, one-third to one-half are women, and three million are 60 or over.

The 1994 National Household Survey on Drug Abuse found 6% of those age 12 and older drank five or more drinks per occasion on five or more of the past 30 days. Heavy alcohol use was most common among males, adults in the 18 to 25 age bracket, the unemployed, and those who did not graduate from college (USDHHS, 1995). Heavy use of alcohol also puts users at high risk of contracting HIV or other sexually transmitted diseases (STDs). Over 25% of a sample of undergraduate college students engaged in unsafe sexual activity under the influence of alcohol. Over 50% of heavy drinkers reported they had sex with someone they would not ordinarily have become involved with (Rathus, Nevid, & Fichner-Rathus, 1997).

In 1993, an estimated 11.7 million Americans were illicit drug users. Marijuana accounts for approximately 77% of current illegal drug use. According to the 1994 Household Survey, 31% reported marijuana use in their lifetime, 18 million (9%) reported use in the past year, and 10 million (5%) reported use in the month prior to the survey. The second most popular form of drug abuse is nonmedical use of psychotherapeutic drugs—tranquilizers, sedatives, stimulants, and analgesics. Respondents in the 26–34 age group (the most likely wage earners) had the highest level of lifetime use of any group. The third most popular "drug of choice" in the 1994 Household Survey was cocaine, used by 10% of people in this age group during their life, 1.7% in the past year, and 0.7% currently. There are an estimated 1.3 million cocaine users (National Institute on Drug Abuse [NIDA], 1995).

An estimated 50 million (24%) of Americans were smokers in 1993. This number has declined from 60 million (31%) smokers in 1985. Among youths ages 12–17, rates of smoking have stabilized at about 10%. Current smokers are also more likely to be heavy drinkers and illicit drug users. Among smokers in 1993, 11% were heavy drinkers (drinking five or more drinks per occasion on 5 or more days over a 30 day period) and 12% were illicit drug users (NIDA, 1995).

Alcohol and drugs at work

The Institute for a Drug-Free Workplace (1994) estimates that some 75% of drug users in the U.S. are employed. Nearly 60% of this group work for businesses with 500 or fewer employees. The Institute also estimates that 15% of the American work force is drug-addicted or alcoholic. Alcohol and drugs are estimated to cost $91 billion in on-the-job accidents each year. Workers with alcohol problems generate eight times more medical costs and their families have medical costs seven times greater than average.

A comprehensive program at Burlington Northern Railroad reduced the rate of employees testing positive on a random drug screen to just 0.4% of the total workforce. They credit this reduction to testing variations for safety-sensitive employees in compliance with the 1988 Drug-Free Workplace Act and U.S. Department of Transportation regulations, regular supervisor training, random drug testing for all employees, Operation Stop (an awareness and peer support program), and a Parent-to-Parent program. This railroad's complete behavioral health care expenditures dropped from 12% to 7.25% of all their insurance claims (Grinstein & Oliver, 1994).

Depression

Depression disorders represent the single largest component of all behavioral health care claims, accounting for more than half of all behavioral health care medical plan claims (Contin & Burton, 1995). One out of every eight people suffers from depression at some point in his or her life, accounting for a large portion of the nation's $44 billion annual psychiatric bill (Bengen-Seltzer, 1995). Depression disorders were discovered to account for 52% of all employees on behavioral short-term disability from 1989 to 1992 (Bengen-Seltzer, 1995). An MIT study (Kouzis, 1994) found that the cost of depression, depression-related absenteeism, and diminished productivity for business was more than $36 billion—an average of $3,000 per depressed worker, or roughly $1.8 million per year for a company employing 10,000 people. The average number of days absent from work for an emotional reason range from 3.2 to 9.4. Depression is associated with the greatest number of absences, followed by high distress. The average cost for depression is greater than that owing to all conditions except cancer and cardiovascular problems (Kouzis, 1994). Studies also show that when a patient has one episode of depression, there is a 50% probability that he or she will experience a second episode (Mesaro, 1995).

Absenteeism and Productivity

Unscheduled absenteeism rose 3.46% in 1995 and has increased another 14.1% since 1992 (Medical Benefits, 1995). The mean absenteeism rate across all business sizes and industry segments was 2.78%, meaning that for every 100 work hours, employers pay an average of 2.78 hours of absence per employee (Unscheduled absence survey, 1995). The manufacturing industry showed the highest increase at 15% while absenteeism decreased in the finance/banking and service industries. Firms employing 100 to 249 people suffered a 22.2% jump in unscheduled absences while larger corporations of 5,000 to 9,999 employees lost as much as 1.58 million to absenteeism (Unscheduled absence survey, 1995).

This same absenteeism survey also found that personal illness accounts for 45% of total absenteeism, while unscheduled absences due to time spent with family issues accounts for 27% of absenteeism. Other unscheduled absences were due to personal needs (13%), an employee's belief that he/she is owed time off (9%), and stress (6%). It is estimated that unscheduled absenteeism costs employers as much as $669 per employee per year.

Employers agree that attendance (66%), productivity (63%), and psychological well-being (61%) are all harmfully affected by employees' personal problems (Medical Benefits, 1995).

When considering this issue of prevalence, one must also consider the number of employees who have family members who are struggling with serious personal problems like depression or substance abuse. When a family member is struggling with a serious personal problem, the employee is almost always affected by this problem. Thus the number of employees whose work is impacted by the personal concerns of family members must be added to the number of employees affected by their own personal concerns. This results in an even higher number of employees whose work is directly or indirectly affected by personal problems. This impact of the family member upon the employee is one of the reasons for providing EAP services to family members as well as to employees.

History of Company Responses

In the early part of the twentieth century, a small number of companies established employee counseling or social service programs designed to help employees resolve personal concerns. The roots of the modern EAP, however, date back to the "occupational alcohol programs" that were implemented at a number of large companies (often in the corporate medical department) in the 1940s. These programs were generally based on the principles of Alcoholics Anonymous (established in 1935) and frequently utilized employees who were themselves members of AA to provide informal assistance in the workplace.

While these early programs often trained supervisors to look for signs of employee alcohol abuse, by the late 1960s the focus began to shift toward a greater emphasis upon the employee's job performance. That is, rather than asking the supervisor to determine whether or not an employee was abusing alcohol (i.e., to diagnose the problem), the supervisor was trained to focus exclusively on the employee's performance and conduct. Any referral to the occupational alcohol program was to be made on this basis. This emphasis on job performance helped the supervisor avoid falling into the role of personal counselor, which would be incompatible with the role as supervisor. This emphasis also provided two additional advantages:

1. Employees could be identified and referred for assistance based on poor job performance even before their personal problems became obvious (i.e., early case finding).
2. The identification of job performance problems provided additional leverage for encouraging employees, who may have been denying their personal problems, to seek assistance.

In the early 1970s the National Institute on Alcohol Abuse and Alcoholism (NIAAA) funded occupational program consultants as well as demonstration and research grants to help establish what they referred to as "employee assistance programs." NIAAA

assumed that broadbrush EAPs, which address a wide range of personal concerns, were more effective than programs that were limited to alcohol and drug abuse. This was because

1. Other types of personal concerns can also affect job performance (as noted previously regarding depression).
2. Other types of personal concerns can lead to alcohol or drug abuse if they are not resolved.
3. Employees who may not seek assistance for their alcohol or drug addiction because of the stigma attached to these addictions may nonetheless seek help for other personal problems and thus eventually be directed to the proper assistance for their addiction (Backer & O'Hara, 1991; Bureau of National Affairs, Inc., 1987; Scanlon, 1991; Trice & Sonnenstuhl, 1986; Thompson, 1990).

The late 1970s also saw the blossoming of external providers of EAP services—an alternative to the internal provision of these services, which had been the standard model. The provision of EAP services by external vendors grew dramatically in the 1980s due to vendors' ability to serve small employers as well as large employers with multiple smaller sites. By 1985, fully one-third of the EAPs serving large employee populations (i.e., more than 500 employees) were provided by external contractors (Blum & Roman, 1987).

While external vendors of EAP services generally provide satisfactory counseling services for self-referred employees and family members, being an outside contractor has led some external vendors to neglect the consultation component of EAPs. That is, some external EAP vendors have lost sight of the role of EAPs in the context of poor job performance. While job performance-related cases may be fewer in number than self-referrals, they are the cases that are most troublesome and costly for the employer and are at the very foundation of EAP theory and practice. This emphasis is reflected in the Employee Assistance Professionals Association's definition of an EAP as

"a worksite based program designed to assist in the identification and resolution of productivity problems associated with employees impaired by personal concerns . . ." (Employee Assistance Professionals Association, Inc., 1990, p. 31).

This emphasis is also reflected in the widely accepted "core technology" of EAPs, which encourages EAP practitioners to

> "move vigorously against those who would subsume the EAP specialty as just another species of clinical practice" (Roman and Blum, 1988, p. 18).

Core technology has been defined as a way

> "to identify those unique functions of EAPs that differentiate them from other human-resource activities in the workplace" (Roman and Blum, 1988, p. 18).

THE CORE TECHNOLOGY OF EAPs

The evolution from the early occupational alcoholism to the contemporary employee assistance program occurred because of the continued adherence to two fundamental principles: strict confidentiality used to protect the employee and use of the performance criterion as the basis for provision of service. Maintaining confidentiality conveys that the EAP provides a trusted service to the employee. Use of the performance criterion acknowledges the existence of work performance standards and the legitimate expectation of the employer to have them met. Both parties have access to the EAP when work performance drops below acceptable standards if these two principles have been applied (Smits & Pace, 1992).

As a workplace-focused program, EAPs are unique in serving multiple clients at any given time (Blair, 1995). The employee, family member, supervisor, union representative, work organization as a whole, community, and any other single entity or combination of the above may benefit from EAP worksite intervention. Remembering a commitment to multiple clients is imperative in keeping a neutral position within the workplace. As neutral problem solvers, it is easier to balance the needs of multiple clients, provide advocacy when needed, and maintain confidentiality (Blair, 1995).

Between 1985 and 1988, Roman and Blum (1988) undertook a project involving on-site visits to 439 EAPs. In a continuing effort to identify the unique functions of EAPs that differentiate them from other human-resource activities in the workplace, Roman and Blum found their observations supported their earlier findings. Six distinct core technologies were found that fell into two categories: those primarily involved in a liaison between the EAP and supervisory management and those primarily involved in a liaison between the EAP and benefits management.

Supervisory Management Components

Identification of Employees' Behavioral Problems Based on Job Performance

Job performance is the sole criterion for the identification of troubled employees. Job expectation, job quality, quantity and timeliness of performance, attendance, relationship with coworkers or clients, or drinking and drug use may be linked to job-related conditions that could identify troubled employees. Supervisors are expected to rule out job conditions as the possible source for performance problems (Core Technology 1).

Provision of Expert Consultation to Supervisors, Managers, and Union Stewards on How to Take the Appropriate Steps in Utilizing Employee Assistance Policy and Procedures

Consultation uses the EAP counselor in the role of "gatekeeper" to assist in making decisions as to whether a problem is an appropriate EAP referral. Supervisors are helped to distinguish between problems resulting from other job conditions and those that merit referral to the EAP. Proper use of the EAP and other labor-relations policies can be conveyed to supervisors through the EAP consultation process (Core Technology 2).

Availability and Use of Constructive Confrontation

Rarely mentioned as a strategy for intervention outside the workplace, constructive confrontation deals with an employee's denial of job-based problems. Using the probability of adverse job actions or eventual termination, the technique requires the supervisor to confront an employee about evidence of job problems. The EAP is offered to the worker as a therapeutic intervention and as an alternative to job loss (Core Technology 3).

Benefits Management Components

Linkages with Counseling, Treatment, and Other Community Resources

Focusing on the individual case, the EAP must have created external linkages with the community to refer the employee for treatment and/or counseling services. EAP professionals' knowledge of the availability and quality of community resources is imperative. These include:

- The development of agreements for posttreatment follow-up of the employee should be discussed when forming these linkages (Core Technology 4).
- The creation and maintenance of linkages between the work organization and counseling, treatment, and other community resources (Core Technology 5).
- Creation and utilization of a management information system is vital to provide the best possible service for the work organization in monitoring employee use of services relative to their clinical condition and job performance (Core Technology 6).

EAPs must balance both aspects of linkages. Mental health service providers must adjust to the needs and structure of the company. At the same time, the company must adjust expectations of the employee during and after treatment to reflect an understanding of the realities of the interventions and disorders involved.

The EAP focus on employees' alcohol and drug abuse or other personal problems offers the most significant promise of producing recovery and genuine cost savings for the organization in terms of future performance and reduced benefits usage.

Though EAPs address substantially more work-related problems than the occupational alcoholism programs of the past, they are still the primary agents of change for employees with substance abuse problems. Without EAP advocacy, punitive practices and procedures only turn the problem back to the family and community. Job performance is often ignored

and only EAPs offer constructive solutions to deal with substance abuse in the workplace.

The six core technologies of Roman and Blum (1988) are greatly enhanced through a counseling component, present in many EAPs today. When a job performance problem is detected, a supervisor may be reluctant to make an EAP referral for fear of stigmatizing the employee. A short-term counseling or brief therapy component deals with a variety of problems in the present, rather than as had been done in the past with longer term psychodynamic therapy. Brief treatment counseling, focusing on current job performance or work-related behavior is more appropriate in the work setting. Organizational time constraints and limited resources make EAP counseling a vital element in the workplace. Short-term (six to eight sessions) counseling is ego-supportive to the employee and/or eligible dependent by focusing on current issues rather than past experiences. Substance abuse problems also have a greater probability of early detection, as employees are more likely to use the EAP counseling program for issues other than work performance problems.

An EAP counseling component facilitates proper assessment and increases the likelihood of obtaining appropriate treatment from micro- and macrolinkages. Additionally, short-term counseling can contain costs and restrain the need for more extensive services. Lechnyr (1993) cites a study by Select Care Health Maintenance Organization (HMO) of 31 mental health providers in which the average number of therapy sessions over a three-year period was only 5.4 visits for all providers. A different study by Capital Health Care HMO also reported that subscribers desiring mental health treatment in 1990 averaged five therapy sessions. Lechnyr (1993) concludes that most individuals require only a few sessions to obtain problem resolution. Though EAPs have been criticized for increasing mental health costs for referring employees and/or eligible dependents for treatment, the adoption of a short-term counseling component actually reduces mental health costs to the employer, since the employee's insurance is only utilized when long-term treatment is required. Instead of mental health services being over-utilized, Lechnyr (1993) proposes that society is more aware how to achieve a better, healthier life. Having no additional cost to the employee is also an attractive feature of the service and encourages self-referral.

EAP DIRECT SERVICES: COUNSELING AND CONSULTATION

Counseling

Type of Referrals to the EAP

How do employees or family members get to the EAP counselor? There are three basic methods of referral to EAP (see Table 16-1). The first is self-referral. In this instance, the employee or family member has heard about the program through program advertising or by word of mouth. Because this person recognizes that he/she has a problem and needs help, he/she simply contacts the EAP counselor. A variation of this pure self-referral occurs when an employee has shared a personal problem with a peer, supervisor, or other member of the workplace and is then encouraged to seek assistance from EAP. Self-referral is the easiest and most common type of referral to EAP counseling.

The second type of referral to EAP counseling is a job performance referral. In this case, an employee's poor performance or conduct is not responding to supervisory coaching and counseling (i.e., there is a job performance problem that is not improving). In response to this situation, the employee's supervisor goes through a process of constructive confrontation in which the employee is confronted with, and held accountable for, job performance. At the same time, the employee is referred to the EAP counselor. For union-represented employees, a union steward may be part of this process. When confronted directly regarding poor job performance, many employees who would not otherwise have done so will accept the referral to the EAP counselor. The job performance referral is most likely to be used when the employee is denying (to himself/herself, others, or both) the existence of any problem. Such denial is most common in cases of chemical dependency or other addictions.

A referral from the medical department can be similar to a job performance referral in that it can be based on holding the employee accountable. In this instance, rather than holding the employee accountable for adequate performance and conduct, the medical professional can hold the employee accountable for being fit for duty. That is, the medical professional can advise the employee that he/she will not be allowed to return to work until the personal/medical problem is under control. At the same time, the employee is referred to EAP for assistance regarding that problem.

The third type of referral is a peer referral. A peer referral occurs most frequently in workplaces where employees spend most of their time without a supervisor being present. If a supervisor is not present to observe poor performance or conduct, there is unlikely to be a job performance referral. When an employee's performance or conduct is unacceptable under these circumstances, the employee's coworkers can confront the employee and encourage the employee to seek EAP counseling. While this referral does not carry the concurrent threat of discipline as does the job performance referral, such peer pressure can be a powerful force in motivating behavior (Molloy, 1985).

The percentage of each type of referral depends on the structure and emphasis of the program. Many EAPs have 85–95% self-referrals. For a small number of EAPs, the majority of referrals are based on job performance. In recent years there has been a general decline in the percentage of job performance referrals, perhaps reflecting a decreasing program emphasis on alcohol and drug abuse in favor of a broadbrush approach to EAPs (Googins, 1989).

The Counseling Process

Once the employee and/or family member contacts the EAP counselor, a multistage counseling process begins (see Table 16-2).

Table 16-1 Types of Referrals to the EAP

Self-referral (and encouraged self-referral)

Job Performance referral (and medical referral)

Peer referral

Table 16-2 The Steps of EAP Counseling

- Assessment
- Motivational counseling
- Short-term problem solving
- Treatment matching
- Follow-up
- Return to work
- Aftercare

Assessment

The first task for the counselor is assessment of the problem. A thorough assessment includes assessment of the presenting problem; the onset and history of the presenting problem; current family, social, and work functioning; physical health; and a personal and family history of psychological functioning, substance abuse, and treatment.

Frequently the concerns expressed by the client are superficial manifestations of a different or a more serious problem. A thorough assessment helps the counselor to understand the problem in its broadest context. For example, a husband and wife might come to the counselor complaining of problems in their marriage. But a thorough assessment reveals that the couple is having marital problems because the husband is abusing alcohol. Without the thorough assessment the couple might have entered marriage counseling and never gotten the help they needed.

Motivational Counseling

In cases where the counselor comes to understand the problem and the appropriate treatment differently than does the client, the counselor tries to help the client see the problem in a new way. This motivational counseling process may include educating the client regarding the nature of the problem, confronting the client with evidence of the problem, and describing for the client what the treatment is and how it could help.

Short-Term Problem Solving

Some client concerns can be resolved by meeting with the EAP counselor for short-term problem solving. Many EAPs limit short-term problem solving to two

or three sessions, while other EAPs provide up to ten or more sessions of short-term counseling. If the counselor believes that the problem cannot be resolved in the short-term sessions provided by the EAP, the client is referred to treatment or other assistance in the community immediately after the completion of the EAP assessment. The EAP counselor would not intentionally provide short-term counseling and then refer the client for treatment because this would be disruptive for the client. Nonetheless, sometimes short-term counseling reveals more serious problems that require a referral to treatment.

Client concerns that are often appropriate for short-term EAP problem solving include situations in which the client is having difficulty adjusting to a life event (e.g., new job, career "plateauing," new child, relocation, death in the family), the client is unfamiliar with appropriate resources (e.g., eldercare, a foreign employee unfamiliar with local customs and services), or the client lacks specific coping skills. Typical coping skills include parenting, assertiveness, dealing with difficult people (e.g., supervisors or coworkers), and relaxation techniques for stress management. These types of situations are particularly appropriate for short-term EAP problem solving, either because they can be resolved in just a few sessions or because they require assistance with resources rather than counseling. Situations that involve issues specific to that particular workplace (e.g., corporate reorganization, plateauing, coping with a difficult supervisor) may also be more appropriately handled by the EAP rather than being referred to treatment in the community.

(The teaching of coping skills, as noted earlier, can be considered a secondary preventive technique; i.e., the intervention prevents the development of a more serious problem. These same types of coping skills can also be used by the EAP as a primary preventive technique. For example, many EAPs present lectures or workshops for employees and/or family members regarding specific coping skills).

Treatment Matching

Once the decision is made to pursue treatment or other assistance in the community, the EAP counselor then goes through the process of treatment matching based on the nature and severity of the problem, the existence of family or social support, and the patient's history of previous treatment. There are, of course, a wide variety of treatments and other assistance available in most communities. With respect to mental health and substance abuse treatment, the variety of treatment settings includes inpatient, residential, halfway house, day/night treatment, intensive outpatient, outpatient, and self-help recovery groups. The range of providers includes psychiatrists, psychologists, social workers and other mental health professionals, as well as paraprofessionals who are themselves recovering from one of these personal problems. Other types of assistance that may be required by clients include legal, dependent care, or educational assistance.

In order to provide the best assistance possible for the client, the EAP counselor must be familiar with the specific providers of these services in the community. The EAP counselor should visit and evaluate each treatment provider and determine that provider's area of expertise, credentials, approach to treatment, and willingness to work with the EAP. Over time and with experience in using these providers, the EAP counselor finds out which providers are best able to help the EAP clients.

When selecting a provider of treatment or assistance with the client, the EAP counselor must first match the client's problem and need for assistance with an appropriate type of provider. Having done this, the EAP counselor then considers factors such as location, cost, and insurance reimbursement. Because the EAP counselor works in the best interests of both the employee/client and the employer, the counselor generally seeks to find the most cost-effective treatment or assistance (i.e., treatment or assistance that will be both effective and appropriately priced).

A guiding principle that helps the EAP counselor meet the demands of both effectiveness and cost control is that of *least restrictive treatment*. In a clinical sense, it is generally in the client's best interest to be in the least restrictive treatment setting appropriate for that specific situation. For example, it is better to be in intensive outpatient treatment than in residential or inpatient treatment if the intensive outpatient

treatment can be effective. Being in an unnecessarily restrictive treatment setting can reduce the patient's sense of self-responsibility, which can in turn hinder recovery. At the same time, an overly restrictive treatment setting can greatly increase treatment costs.

While "least restrictive treatment" is a generally agreed-upon theoretical principle, the actual criteria for various levels of treatment continue to be a matter of considerable debate in EAP and managed-care circles. For example, in a study of 227 alcohol-abusing employees who were randomly assigned to either inpatient treatment followed by Alcoholics Anonymous versus Alcoholics Anonymous as the only treatment versus a choice of options, the employees who received inpatient treatment had a better recovery rate at two-years follow-up (Walsh et al., 1991). Even though intensive outpatient chemical dependency treatment was not a widely available option when this study was conducted (1982–1987) and thus its efficacy could not be evaluated, this study does suggest that determining which treatment will be least restrictive and yet effective for the patient is not a simple matter.

After the EAP counselor and the client have agreed to a specific plan of treatment or assistance, the client then contacts the treatment provider. At this point, the EAP counselor—with the client's written permission—may also contact the treatment provider in order to provide information regarding the findings of the EAP assessment. For job performance referral cases, the EAP counselor will also provide detailed information regarding the nature of the workplace problems the client was experiencing. This information regarding workplace problems helps the treatment provider confront the client with the reality of the workplace problems.

Follow-up

After the client actually pursues treatment or assistance, the EAP counselor provides follow-up. During this phase the EAP counselor communicates periodically with the client to express support and ensure that the client is receiving effective treatment and is satisfied with the treatment. With the client's permission, the EAP counselor also maintains communication with the treatment provider as another means of ensuring that proper treatment is being rendered. The frequency of communication with the client and with the treatment provider varies depending on the nature and severity of the problem, whether the client was self-referred or referred due to job performance problems, or whether the EAP counselor is responsible for approving the payment of insurance benefits or is simply responsible for facilitating proper treatment and recovery.

Return to Work

When treatment requires the employee to go on sick leave (e.g., residential or inpatient treatment), the employee's return to work can be particularly difficult and stressful, especially if the employee was experiencing job performance problems before entering treatment. To help with this transition, the EAP counselor can serve as a link between the workplace and the treatment setting while the employee is in treatment. With the employee's permission the EAP counselor can help the supervisor understand the challenges being faced by the employee at this time and learn how to provide clear expectations for the employee while also being supportive when the employee returns to work. At the same time, the EAP counselor can help the employee address his/her own concerns about returning to work (e.g., what to tell coworkers about the absence).

Aftercare

For cases of chemical dependency, chronic psychiatric disorder, or other cases prone to relapse, the EAP counselor can support the client's participation in aftercare even after the completion of formal treatment. To prevent relapse, many chemical dependency clients benefit by participation in ongoing self-help groups such as Alcoholics Anonymous, Narcotics Anonymous, Al-Anon, etc. Some psychiatric patients require long-term treatment with medication. By maintaining periodic contact with the client during this time, the EAP counselor can encourage the client's ongoing involvement in this activity and can be alert to signs of impending relapse (Backer & O'Hara, 1991; Plant, 1987; Thompson, 1990; Turner, 1985).

Confidentiality

Given the social stigma frequently associated with personal concerns, confidentiality is a bedrock of EAP counseling. Clients must be assured that personal information will not be shared with anyone without written permission except as required by law (e.g., cases of potential homicide, suicide, or child abuse). Counseling records must be maintained in a secure fashion with restricted access. Personal counseling information should not be part of the employee's personnel file. Finally, the EAP counseling office must be in a location that allows easy access yet maintains an appropriate level of privacy.

EAP Case Management

There is an increasing body of literature suggesting that addressing alcohol and other drug problems is a critical component of interventions directed at improving employment-related outcomes for alcohol and other drug-using welfare recipients. Data from four national studies (Young & Gardner, 1997) suggest that the proportion of welfare recipients in need of substance abuse treatment or intervention range from 15–39%. Under the recent Temporary Aid to Needy Families (TANF) law, participation in the workforce by welfare recipients is mandatory, with a goal of economic self-sufficiency and with a lifetime eligibility limit of five years (Albelda, 1999). Therefore, there is considerable pressure on all of the serving agencies to promote early, lasting workforce engagement among welfare recipients.

The EAP model is increasingly recognized as being a cost-effective way to address employee-related problems in the workplace, resulting in increases in performance productivity and reductions in tardiness/absenteeism and turnover. However, traditional EAP services are not as well suited for alcohol and drug abuse problems because the services are often short-term in nature (e.g., 3–5 "visits," or sessions, per referral), and they are less often available among small businesses where the majority of TANF participants are likely to be employed.

An innovative variation on the traditional EAP is proposed that provides support to welfare-to-work participants in two ways (Malden, 1998). First, it provides support to TANF participants who are not job-ready due to their use of alcohol and other drugs. Second, it provides long-term (1–2 years) support to welfare-to-work participants in the workplace through biweekly client contact and aftercare directed at relapse prevention. This "case management" EAP model would employ a gender-sensitive assessment (the large majority of welfare recipients are women) and would work collaboratively with Work First service providers, such as state child and family services case managers, therapists, and substance abuse counselors.

The case management model expands traditional EAP services to provide support to former welfare recipients who are identified as having problems with the abuse of alcohol and drugs that might interfere with their job performance. The case management EAP model would provide services within a framework that views addiction as a complex, progressive social problem which has biological, psychological, sociological, and behavioral components. The underlying premises of the case management model EAP are that a) substance abuse is a chronic, relapsing condition requiring long-term support and has impacts on many aspects of a woman's life, thus requiring a holistic approach to treatment; b) there are special needs of women substance abusers so gender-specific services that include such issues as child care, domestic violence, etc. are needed; and c) an integrated approach to substance abuse treatment and work is required, thereby linking the two experiences to reinforce sobriety and maximize success at work and ensure ongoing employment.

The case management model EAP is designed to promote job retention by enhancing the offerings of the traditional EAP with the four enhanced services (Maiden, 1999):

1. The case manager would assume a more proactive approach in his or her involvement with the welfare-to-work participant. The aim of the case management EAP is to provide long-term follow-up services to the new employee to monitor adjustment to the work environment and to provide assistance in resolving work-related or personal problems that might negatively impact employment retention. Case management follow-ups would typically be provided on a biweekly basis to all welfare-to-work participants for at least one calendar year following job placement. Follow-up contacts could occur by telephone or in person, depending on the needs of the participant and to be determined at the discretion of the EAP case manager and supervisor.

2. The EAP case manager would provide general support and mentoring to enhance the welfare-to-work participant's transition from welfare to permanent employment. Mentoring has been found to be a critical component in helping women and minorities make significant advancements in the corporate world. The mentoring program is designed to provide support, direction, skill-building, and encouragement to overcome obstacles related to the workplace.

3. The EAP case manager would monitor participants' involvement in job performance through a defined process of introductory supervisor training and ongoing management consultation involving both the direct supervisor and the participant. The intent of the introductory training is to educate the supervisor about the welfare-to-work initiative and to sensitize them to some of the issues specific to the welfare population. Ongoing management consultation would be available to supervisors on an as-needed basis should participants encounter work or personal problems that may threaten job retention. In addition to optional consultation services, the EAP case manager would also conduct monthly follow-ups with supervisors to monitor work-related issues, including timeliness, attendance, compliance, conformity to work norms, response to supervision, coworker interaction, and performance and productivity. The intent is to detect and resolve potential problems and minimize the occurrence of disciplinary action. Informed consent of the welfare-to-work participant would be necessary for supervisor follow-up.

4. In addition to providing access to traditional EAP services, a broader range of EAP services would be provided that could include ongoing counseling and expanded referrals to community resources, such as locating suitable transportation and housing and other services that would promote employment retention.

In many ways, the case management model EAP proposed here brings employee assistance professionals in the United States full circle as they enter a new century. In the late 1800s and early 1900s, welfare secretaries worked primarily with the working poor and other at-risk populations. Since their introduction to the workplace, they have made significant inroads and progress. Through the development of welfare-to-work initiatives, the employee assistance field is presented with a substantial opportunity to assist former welfare recipients to move towards successful employment and self-sufficiency and, hopefully, away from poverty and dependency.

Employee assistance programs have made substantial inroads into the American workplace in both the private and public sector alike. As indicated here, they have undergone a number of evolutionary changes—from occupational alcoholism programs to the broader employee assistance; from identification of alcoholics requiring tertiary care to training, education, health promotion, and wellness with a primary care focus; from assessment and referral to short-term counseling; from helping to manage absenteeism and accidents to health care cost containment and managing quality of care; and from reactive crisis counseling to proactive critical incident stress debriefing. While EAPs have become an accepted part of the human resource management function in the majority of large workplaces, there is still considerable progress to be made to bring EAPs to small businesses where most of the American workforce is employed. This poses many challenges to the EAP field and will require continued innovation and creativity on the part of EAP professionals in the future.

EAP Counselor Credentials

EAP counselors who practiced during the early history of EAP often were recovering from alcohol or drug addiction. Their own personal experience with recovery was their primary credential for helping others. In today's world of EAPs, however, most counselors have at least a master's level degree in a mental health profession, as well as practical experience in chemical dependency and mental health clinical settings. In addition to clinical knowledge and experience, it is important for the EAP counselor to have at least a basic understanding of the workplace environment in which their clients are working. Finally, while the Certified Employee Assistance Professional (CEAP) certification administered by the Employee Assistance Professionals Association (EAPA) reflects a basic level of knowledge in the EAP field and is an important credential for EAP practitioners, this certification alone does not indicate a professional level of clinical training and expertise.

The Consultation Process

In addition to providing counseling for employees and their family members, EAP counselors also provide consultation at two levels:

1. Consultation to supervisors, personnel representatives, and union stewards about employees with persistent poor performance or conduct problems that might be related to a personal problem
2. Consultation to the work organization regarding issues affecting groups of employees

Consultation to Supervisors

Why is consultation needed when a supervisor has an employee whose poor performance or conduct may be related to a personal problem? Why don't supervisors simply do what they are supposed to do as supervisors: hold the employee accountable for satisfactory performance and conduct and impose discipline if the employee does not improve?

Supervisors in these situations are stuck between two unattractive alternatives. If they hold the employee accountable, the process of progressive discipline could lead to the employee's ultimate dismissal, which may not be in the employer's best interest. Furthermore supervisors often feel that holding an employee accountable when the employee might be struggling with a personal problem may exacerbate the employee's personal problem. The opposite alternative—not holding the employee accountable—is equally unattractive.

When caught in this dilemma, most supervisors will try to cover for the employee. That is, they will try to ignore or minimize the problem, or even do some of the employee's work themselves—at least until the employee can be transferred to another department. This process of covering for the employee does not improve the workplace situation, nor does it improve the employee's personal problem.

Covering for the employee actually makes the personal problem worse. This process of covering for the employee is called *enabling*. By covering for the employee, the supervisor enables the employee to avoid the negative consequences of his/her behavior. This in turn reduces the employee's motivation to seek assistance for the problem, thus allowing it to get progressively worse. Even though enabling is clearly not in the supervisor's (or the employee's) best long-term interest, many employees in this situation become very good at manipulating their supervisor into being indecisive or inconsistent—making it even more difficult for the supervisor to stop the enabling.

EAP counselors can consult with supervisors, personnel representatives, and union stewards under these circumstances to help them handle the situation in a manner that benefits both the employer and the employee. After listening to a description of the employee's behavior and job performance and the steps that the supervisor has taken so far, the EAP counselor can help the supervisor decide if the employee should be held accountable and, at the same time, be referred to the EAP counselor. If a referral to the EAP counselor is appropriate, the counselor can help the supervisor make this referral in a professional and effective fashion and can help the supervisor feel comfortable with taking this action.

The central element of a supervisory referral is constructive confrontation. Because many employees who have a personal problem affecting their work tend to deny or minimize the extent of the workplace problem, it is often necessary for the supervisor to confront the employee with specific evidence of poor job performance or conduct. During this confrontation, the supervisor should focus exclusively on work-related issues and should avoid making references or accusations or giving advice regarding the employee's suspected personal problems. The supervisor is not an expert in diagnosing personal problems but is an expert in observing workplace performance and conduct. The supervisor should stick to that area of expertise. Furthermore, if the supervisor attempts to

discuss the employee's personal problem, the employee may become defensive and accuse the supervisor of meddling in the employee's personal life, thus drawing attention away from the workplace issue.

This kind of supervisory confrontation can also be constructive if the supervisor follows up the confrontation with a referral to the EAP counselor. In the context of the confrontation the employee will often accept the referral. In many companies the employee's decision to accept or reject the referral is strictly voluntary. The employee is held accountable for performance and conduct regardless of whether or not the referral is accepted. In other companies the employee's refusal to accept the referral may trigger negative consequences for the employee (Blair, 1987b; Scanlon, 1991; Thompson, 1990).

Consultation to the Organization

While the phrase "personal problems" has been used in this chapter to refer to employee problems that negatively affect performance or conduct but are not the result of employer or workplace deficiencies (e.g., inadequate training or equipment), one should not conclude that all personal problems are solely the result of a personal psychological or behavioral problem and thus can only be modified by addressing the individual. To the contrary, many personal problems are actually the result of a dysfunction in the person's larger social system. For example, family therapy is based on the principle that an individual's personal problems are often the result of dysfunctional family norms and dynamics.

Social systems at work can also affect personal problems. For example, the cultural norms in a workgroup, worksite, or corporation regarding alcohol and drug use and regarding the role of the supervisor in addressing alcohol and drug use can affect employees' personal problems regarding alcohol and drug use (Googins, 1989). Similarly, job characteristics or work conditions (e.g., unclear objectives, organization restructuring) can create the personal problem of employee stress.

Given that some personal problems are created or affected by the workplace, the EAP has a role in providing consultation to workgroups, worksites, and the corporation regarding workplace policies (e.g., alcohol and drug policies), organizational dynamics (e.g., unsupportive supervisory practices), and changes (e.g., downsizing) that can negatively affect employee well-being.

The Workplace Context

EAP counseling and consultation services are most successful when they take place in a supportive workplace context. One way to create a supportive workplace context is to have a written policy that makes it clear that EAP-related activities are confidential and that employee use of the EAP will not jeopardize the employee's job security or promotional opportunities. Making such policy statements available to all employees in a written format increases employee and supervisor confidence in the program and thus encourages use of the program.

The workplace context should also include adequate sick leave and health care benefits for mental health and chemical dependency problems. The lack of these benefits makes it more difficult for employees to obtain such treatments if they are recommended by the EAP counselor.

Finally a supportive workplace context includes visible demonstrations of support by management and, where appropriate, union leadership. Such support can be manifested in program funding, employee and supervisor training opportunities, verbal or written support as part of the program promotion activities, and other similar activities.

Models of Program Management and Delivery

The choice of an appropriate EAP model for a specific employee population (see Table 16-3) depends on factors such as goals of the program, size, demographics,

Table 16-3 EAP Program Models

- Internal program
- External program
- Union program (member assistance program)
- Joint labor-management program

location(s) of the employee population, and the level of employee trust regarding personnel-related activities. Some of the advantages and disadvantages of various models are described next.

Internal programs, because they provide an EAP counselor who is a company employee and who has an office right at the worksite, offer excellent access for employees and supervisors. The employees and supervisors see the EAP counselor in the hallways, cafeteria, etc.; know where the counselor's office is; and may feel comfortable dropping in or making an appointment. As a company employee, the EAP counselor knows what it is like to work in that company and therefore can easily understand the work-related concerns of both employees and supervisors.

If employees do not trust personnel-related activities in the company, however, the employees may also not trust an internal EAP counselor. This, of course, will reduce employee utilization of the EAP. Another potential disadvantage of an internal program is the possibility that the company will not have sufficient expertise to administer the program.

While external programs occasionally provide an on-site counselor, most often the EAP counselor's office is in a location away from the worksite. This allows the EAP counselor to see employees from a variety of companies in the same counseling office. This also increases the perception of confidentiality for some employees.

External programs originally flourished in serving smaller employee populations where it was not economically feasible to have an internal counselor. In recent years, however, external programs have become increasingly popular for large employers as well. The external programs are attractive to employers because they are more convenient to establish and administer. They do not require any internal expertise, and they can flexibly meet the needs of a shifting employee population working at a variety of locations.

One potential disadvantage of external programs is that, because they serve a variety of companies, they may not customize their service to meet the needs of a specific company. For example, the external EAP counselor may not be adequately familiar with a specific company's approach to discipline or with the company's health insurance benefits. This lack of knowledge may hinder the process of counseling or consultation. For this reason, it is important to have a specific internal person be the liaison between the company and the external vendor to assure that the external vendor customizes the services to an adequate degree.

Some labor unions have established union EAP programs, sometimes known as "member assistance programs," to serve their members. This EAP model helps the EAP to gain the trust of the union-represented employees who know that the program is sponsored by the union and does not have company involvement. Union EAPs focus on helping union members and their families resolve personal problems but generally do not include the consultation component of EAPs that focuses on work performance.

Some companies and unions have joined together to develop joint labor-management EAP programs. This EAP model also is likely to have the trust of union-represented employees and can make it clear to the employee who is having problems in the workplace that neither the company nor the union will support poor performance—and yet both are supportive of recovery (Blair, 1987a; Blum & Roman, 1987).

Program Promotion

An EAP, like any other program or service, must be advertised and promoted in order to attract clients. Unlike many other services, however, potential EAP clients often have a number of fears and concerns regarding this service. Thus the program promotion must do more than simply make the client aware of the service; the promotional activities must address the client's fears and concerns.

In promoting the EAP to employees and family members, the three major concerns to address are confidentiality, stigma, and cost. With respect to confidentiality, it is important that all promotional activities accurately describe the program's policy regarding confidentiality. Other aspects of the program that relate to confidentiality (e.g., location of the counselor's office) can also be used to assure the client on this issue.

Because of the stigma attached to serious personal problems like chemical dependency or psychiatric illness, it is helpful to "position" the program as the broadbrush model, an option available to help clients with a wide range of personal problems, including the normal problems of daily living we all encounter. This approach helps "destigmatize" the EAP and makes it easier for clients to feel comfortable using the service.

Client concerns regarding cost also need to be directly addressed in promotional materials. While most EAP services are free to the client, the client is often referred to treatment in the community, which may require some level of client payment. These potential costs should be made clear in promotional materials.

While it is generally easy for employees to understand the nature of the counseling service, explaining the consultation component of the EAP to supervisors, personnel representatives, and union stewards is a more complex challenge. EAP consultation actually provides a whole new approach to handling a difficult workplace problem (i.e., holding the employee accountable and making a referral to the EAP). Promotion of the consultation service must explain this new approach. Given this complexity, promotion of the consultation service usually includes in-person training sessions during which the program principles and procedures are explained. The goals of this training are to help the clients understand how the consultation can help them do their job, understand their own role in the process, and have confidence that the proposed model of intervention will be effective.

Similar to promotion of the counseling service itself, the issues of stigma and confidentiality must also be addressed. With respect to stigma, many corporate cultures will view an employee job performance problem as an indication of a failing on the part of the employee's supervisor (i.e., supervisors should be able to keep their employees "in line"). When this belief is the corporate norm, supervisors are embarrassed and afraid to admit that one of their subordinates is having a problem. To overcome this stigma, promotion of the consultation service should make it clear that top management recognizes that employees' personal problems can negatively affect job performance and that the company encourages supervisors to use the consultation service to help in addressing these problems.

To further support use of the consultation service, supervisors should also be advised that use of the consultation service is confidential. This confidentiality further helps the supervisor overcome the stigma that may be associated with having a subordinate who has a job performance problem (Thompson, 1990).

Quality Assurance and Program Evaluation

An Employee Assistance Program, like any type of service, needs to be monitored to ensure that the service is being delivered as designed and that program goals are being achieved. Typical areas for quality assurance activities regarding the process of program delivery include program communications and promotional activities, breadth and quality of community treatment resources, customer perception of confidentiality, and continuing education of the EAP staff.

One of the most common means of reviewing the quality of an EAP is through a monthly or quarterly program utilization report. This report provides statistical data regarding factors such as client demographics, sources of client referrals to the EAP, clients' presenting problems and assessed problems, and disposition of clients. These data help determine if there are weaknesses in the process that brings clients into the system and provides them with assistance. While this approach can provide information regarding a program's changing utilization over time, the wide variation in employee demographics and EAP program designs make it difficult to develop utilization norms against which programs can be evaluated.

Another common method of quality assurance consists of client satisfaction surveys. In this method, employees and family members who use the EAP are asked to complete a satisfaction survey immediately following EAP counseling, several months following use of the service, or both. Similarly, supervisors and others who receive consultation from the EAP regarding employee job performance issues can also be asked to complete a satisfaction survey.

With respect to the actual EAP direct services, some EAPs—in addition to regularly scheduled case supervision or case conferences—randomly select a percentage of cases to review for appropriateness of clinical service and organizational interaction. This can be a concurrent review, implemented while the case is still in progress, and/or a retrospective review, which occurs after the case is closed. Often this review is conducted by clinicians other than the EAP counselors in order to provide a fresh perspective on the case. As was mentioned previously, there is considerable disagreement regarding objective criteria for the selection of level of treatment. Consequently the evaluation of clinical services is based more on clinical judgment than on objective criteria.

In addition to quality assurance activities, EAPs also should look at program outcomes to determine if the program goals are being achieved. Different EAPs can have different program goals, so a clear understanding of the specific program goals is required before one can determine which outcomes to measure. Common areas for EAP evaluation include looking at the impact of the EAP on health care costs, absenteeism, and accidents. Looking at specific outcomes of this type can allow the EAP to look at the cost-benefit relationships of the program. Another common cost-related factor often measured is the cost-effectiveness of the program (i.e., the cost to achieve specific desirable outcomes) (Durkin, 1985; Jones, 1987; Maynard, 1990; Selvik, 1987; Spicer, Owen, & Gjerdingen, 1990). While some EAPs evaluate these outcome measures by comparing their levels for EAP clients before EAP intervention and after EAP intervention, the best evaluation studies also compare these outcome measures with employees who have not used the EAP. An example of this type of evaluation, conducted at the McDonnell Douglas Corporation, is described in the next section.

It is interesting to note that EAPs have not generally attempted to measure how many clients who used the EAP actually resolved their personal problems. The lack of measurement in this area probably derives from the original concept of EAPs as a service that referred clients to community treatment providers and left it up to the providers to be responsible for clinical outcomes. In recent years, as many EAPs have become more directly involved in the process of approving health care benefits for mental health and substance abuse treatment, the EAP's interest in measuring clinical outcomes has greatly increased.

Research Regarding EAP Effectiveness: Do EAPs Work?

While EAPs may seem to be a good idea and have many ardent supporters, what is the research evidence regarding EAP effectiveness? Have EAPs provided any added value to the employer, or would the EAP clients have resolved their problems and returned to normal productivity to the same degree and at the same rate even if EAPs did not exist? By reviewing the research literature regarding EAP effectiveness, looking at the strengths and limitations of this research, and examining some of the difficulties inherent in EAP outcome studies, the following section attempts to provide some answers to these questions.

The Employee Assistance Professionals Association (EAPA), speaking in terms of ultimate cost-benefit for the employer, provides an unequivocally affirmative response to this issue.

> "Do employee assistance programs work? Yes,
> EAPs can recover big bucks from the loss column—
> something on the order of $5–7 for every $1
> invested in the EAP" (Employee Assistance
> Professionals Association, Inc., 1991).

EAPA's conclusion is based on a considerable number of studies that have reported positive outcomes regarding the impact of EAPs on direct and indirect health-related costs, productivity (including absenteeism, accidents, and disciplinary action), and resolution of the client's presenting problems. See, for example, a summary of 11 outcome studies conducted between 1976 and 1981, reviewed by the Hazelden Foundation (Bureau of National Affairs, Inc., 1987), and a review of three outcome studies conducted between 1980 and 1985 (Mastrich & Beidel, 1987). Several reviews of this research literature, however, have questioned the quality of these studies and thus the validity of their conclusions.

For example, a review of nineteen EAP outcome studies conducted from 1957 to 1980 concluded

> "We were unable to find any evaluation of OAPs
> (occupational alcoholism programs) that
> represented a reasonable approximation of the
> minimal research design" (Kurtz, Googins, &
> Howard, 1984).

Major limitations noted regarding these studies included an unrepresentative sample, the lack of a control or comparison group, unreliable outcome measures, and an inadequate follow-up period.

The National Institute on Drug Abuse (NIDA) has reported similar conclusions in more recent publications. Referring to EAPs as one of the corporate responses to workplace drug abuse, NIDA noted that

> "missing . . . is the systematic research database . . .
> on the efficacy of various workplace-based
> strategies to reduce drug use and its consequences"
> (Gust & Walsh, 1989).

Also,

> "research on EAP evaluation has been extremely
> limited—primarily descriptive or promotional—
> and without much rigor in evaluation methodology
> or design" (Tompkins, 1991).

Looking at a fairly typical EAP outcome study can help to illustrate these points.

Detroit Edison

The Detroit Edison Company EAP measured changes in work performance for employees referred to and counseled by the EAP during a six-month period (Nadolski & Sandonato, 1987). Of the ninety-seven employees who entered the EAP during that time period, thirty were eliminated from the study due to retirement, death, voluntary termination, transfer to a different supervisor, or for reasons of confidentiality. The measures of work performance were lost time, health insurance claims, discipline, accidents, and work productivity. Data were collected covering the six months before entering EAP and for the time period between seven and twelve months after entering EAP. The results of this study reported an improvement in all outcome measures.

Some limitations of this study are described below.

Study Sample

Thirty-one percent of the potential subjects for this study were eliminated from the study sample. This large of a percentage of subjects who were systematically excluded from the study creates the possibility of an unrepresentative study sample. That is, conclusions regarding the effectiveness of the EAP may not apply to this program's clients in general. Furthermore, most of the criteria used to eliminate subjects (i.e., retirement, death, voluntary termination, and transfer) may be related to unresolved employee personal concerns, and thus the employees who were eliminated may reflect to a large extent the poor outcomes of the EAP.

Study Design

This study did not include a control group or a comparison group, and thus it is impossible to determine if the changes shown by the study sample were the result of EAP activity or if they would have occurred without an EAP. For example, many employees with personal problems ultimately resolve their problems and improve their work performance without any professional help, or they receive professional treatment without EAP involvement. Unless the study sample of those who used the EAP are compared to similar employees who did not use the EAP, it is impossible to draw any conclusions regarding the impact of EAP activities.

Outcome Measures

A strength of this study was that four of the five outcome variables were objective and measurable. These outcome measures were collected during the time period between seven and twelve months after entering EAP in order to allow time for patient recovery and to eliminate the costs of treatment incurred immediately after entering EAP.

Despite the quality of the outcome measures, collecting data only between seven and twelve months after the intervention may not provide a sufficiently long follow-up period. As pointed out by one review,

> "It is difficult to determine what represents a reasonable follow-up period because research on that issue is not available. However, the one year period frequently used in evaluation may be too brief to measure sustained behavioral change" (Kurtz, Googins, & Howard, 1984).

By not collecting outcome data during the first six months following EAP intervention—a time during which lost time, health insurance claims, and work productivity are likely to be negatively affected—this study does not give a true and complete picture of the outcomes of the EAP intervention.

Analysis of Results

This study reports the percent improvement for each outcome measure. For example, days of lost time were reduced from 476 to 341—a reduction of 29%; health insurance claims were reduced from $36,472 to $27,122—a reduction of 26%. Without statistical analysis it is impossible to determine if these changes were statistically significant or if they were due simply to chance. Several more examples of results for which statistical significance is questionable are the reported 13% improvement in written disciplinary action (from eight to seven written disciplines), the reported 40% improvement in suspensions (from five to three suspensions), and the 100% improvement in demotions (from one to zero).

While this study by Detroit Edison is one of the better EAP outcome studies because of its adequate sample size, objective outcome measures, and pre-/postmeasurements, the methodological problems with the study are too great to conclude that the observed changes were significant or that they were the result of EAP intervention. Table 16-4 provides a summary of seven recent outcome studies. All of these studies have major design limitations that compromise the validity of their conclusions.

McDonnell Douglas

One published EAP outcome study has overcome many of the limitations noted regarding the previous studies. From 1985 to 1988 the McDonnell Douglas Corporation worked with an external consulting firm to conduct a multiyear analysis of absenteeism costs and employee and family health care costs associated with employees who used the EAP compared to employees who sought mental health and/or chemical dependency treatment but did not use the EAP (*The ALMACAN*, 1989). Each

Table 16-4 EAP Outcome Studies

Reference	Employer	N	Outcome Measure	Research Design	Time Frame	Comparison Group	Success Rate	Major Limitations
Bruhnsen and DuBuc 1988	University of Michigan Medical Center	122 (182 eliminated)	sick-time costs	pre-/post-test	6 months pretest 6 months posttest	none	60% reduced costs 6% no change 34% increased costs	Sampling strategy unspecified. No control group. Follow-up period brief.
Yandrick 1992	Campbell Soup Company	not reported	behavioral health costs	posttest only	varied over calendar year	previous calendar year	behavioral health costs reduced by 28%	No pretest measure. Sample size not reported. Comparison group may not have been representative of treatment group.
Yandrick 1992	Orange County Public Schools	125 EAP 25 non-EAP	medical costs sick leave	pre-/post-test	1 year pretest 1–4 years posttest	25 non-EAP	Average client cost-reduction from $3,173 to $982 in 4 years. Average sick leave reduction from 58.5 hours to 13.9 hours.	Sampling strategy unspecified. Comparison group may not have been representative of treatment group.

Table 16-4 EAP Outcome Studies

Reference	Employer	N	Outcome Measure	Research Design	Time Frame	Comparison Group	Success Rate	Major Limitations
Yandrick 1992	Virginia Power	not reported	behavioral and non-behavioral medical costs for client and family	pre-/post-	4 years pre- 4 years post-	non-EAP users of behavioral health benefits	EAP total medical costs were 23% lower than non-EAP. Behavioral costs were 17% less and non-behavioral costs 32% less	Sample size unreported. Comparison group may not have been representative of treatment group.
Yandrick 1992	McDonnell Douglas Helicopter Co.	1,876	behavioral helath costs	posttest only	varied over calendar year	2 previous calendar year	behavioral health costs reduced by 34% and 13% in each of 2 years	No pretest measures. Comparison groups may not have been representative of treatment groups
Yandrick 1992	Proctor & Gamble—Oxnard	not reported	behavioral health costs	posttest only	varied over calendar year	1 previous calendar year	behavioral health costs reduced by 61%	Undefined sample size. No pretest measure. Comparison groups may not have been representative of treatment group.
Yandrick 1992	General Dynamics—Forth Worth	12 in aftercare 17 dropouts from aftercare	absenteeism and termination	pre-/post-	3 months pre- 3 months post-	17 dropouts from aftercare	6 fewer days absent per quarter and 50% less termination	Small sample size. Comparison group may not have been representative of treatment group.

study subject, both employees who used the EAP (n = 13,898) as well as those who did not use the EAP, was matched to a cohort control group of ten other McDonnell Douglas employees along the variables of age, sex, marital status, geographic location, family size, and job code. Depending on the year the employee entered the EAP, outcome data were collected from zero to three years pre-EAP and from zero to three years post-EAP. This study concluded that absenteeism costs for the employee and mental health and chemical dependency treatment costs, as well as total medical costs, for the employee and the family were less for those employees who used the EAP when compared to employees who received mental health and/or chemical dependency treatment but did not use the EAP. A savings-to-investment ratio of 4:1 was reported.

This study was superior to the previously noted studies in that it had a large sample size, it used strictly objective outcome measures, it had up to a three-year pre- and postmeasure time frame, and it used a matched comparison group. Even this study, however, has a number of significant limitations (described next).

Study Sample

The published report indicated

> "Only those EAP cases were included in which the EAP counselor provided written verification that the client was complying with the treatment plan" (*The ALMACAN*, 1989, p. 18–26).

EAP clients who do not comply with treatment plans are often unsuccessful in their recovery and consequently may have high rates of absenteeism and/or health care utilization in the future. Systematically excluding these study subjects may distort the validity of the findings.

Study Design

Employee and family mental health and chemical dependency and other health care costs were compared between EAP clients and non-EAP clients using two methods. One method of comparison used per capita costs. The second method compared the ratio of expenditures between EAP clients and their cohort group versus non-EAP clients and their cohort group. For example, the EAP population may have had x times the amount of costs as their cohort group while the non-EAP population may have had y times the amount of costs as their cohort group. The difference between x and y was then used as the measure of difference between EAP and non-EAP clients. This latter method was intended to control for confounding demographic variables.

The report indicated that EAP and non-EAP clients did indeed differ significantly along several demographic variables. For example

> "Single and divorced employees sought EAP help for psychiatric conditions, while married employees were far more likely to access treatment outside of the EAP" (*The ALMACAN*, 1989, p. 22).

And

> "EAP clients for mixed substance abuse and psychiatric conditions were significantly younger than those employees who chose not to access the EAP" (*The ALMACAN*, 1989, p. 22).

The per capita costs used in the first method of comparison do not control for these differences between the EAP and non-EAP clients. The second method of comparison used the cohort groups to control for these differences, but even this method is seriously limited. For example, older substance abusers are likely to have been abusing substances longer than younger substance abusers. Comparing these older non-EAP substance abusers to their older cohort does not control for length of abuse, which may have a strong impact upon treatment outcome and total medical costs. That is, it may be that even if these older clients did go through EAP, they may still have had worse outcomes due to the length of abuse.

Analysis of Results

This study did not indicate the statistical methods used to determine the reported significance of the results.

Impediments to EAP Outcome Studies

Why are there so few high-quality EAP outcome studies? Four reasons are listed here.

1. Corporations do not generally evaluate their human resource functions for effectiveness and do not have or will not devote adequate resources to do so.
2. EAP professionals generally believe in EAP and therefore are reluctant to assign clients to non-EAP control groups.
3. Clinical professionals have not usually emphasized data collection and analysis.
4. Concerns regarding maintaining confidentiality can hinder data collection and reduce the likelihood of using external professional researchers (Kurtz, Googins, & Howard, 1984).

Do EAPs Work?

What conclusions can be drawn regarding EAP effectiveness? As noted earlier, there are many studies that show that EAPs have a positive impact on health costs, productivity, and problem resolution. The quality of this evidence is weak due to impediments previously noted, and it may very well remain weak for these same reasons. Until EAP outcome studies of better quality are conducted, programmatic decisions regarding EAPs will need to be based on the existing inconclusive evidence. (It should be noted that this situation is not unlike many other areas of corporate human resources and occupational health.)

Program Costs

The cost of providing an EAP depends to a large extent on the level of staffing necessary to deliver the specific type of program and scope of services being considered. For example, the level of staffing and thus the cost of the EAP will vary greatly depending on whether the direct services include strictly assessment and referral or if they also include short-term problem solving, follow-up, and utilization management. The cost is also dependent upon whether the direct service is delivered onsite, offsite, or by telephone. Different employee populations can differ greatly in their willingness to use the EAP (i.e., the

EAP utilization rate) and thus require greatly differing levels of staffing.

EAP programs can also vary greatly with respect to the scope of indirect services offered. Some EAPs provide extensive employee orientation and program promotion activities, customized data management, and liaison activities with personnel and medical departments, while other EAPs do not provide these services.

Finally the total number of employees served and the geographic distribution of the employees also affect staffing ratios and thus program costs.

All of these variables notwithstanding, the Employee Assistance Professionals Association estimates that one full-time EAP counselor can serve between 2,500 and 4,000 employees (Employee Assistance Professionals Association, Inc., 1992). (This staffing ratio applies to EAP services only. It does not include managed-care activities. Administrative support staff are also not included in this staffing ratio.) The level of salary and benefits for an EAP counselor depends upon the counselor's credentials and experience and, to a certain degree, upon the region of the country in which the EAP counselor works.

In addition to staffing costs, an EAP also has costs arising from administration, office space and telephones, staff training and development, data management, insurance, program training and promotional materials, and (for external EAP vendors) marketing.

Given all of the variables, it is difficult to arrive at a meaningful average cost for an EAP. Nonetheless a general range of costs for EAP services would be from $18 to $36 per employee per year (Bureau of National Affairs, Inc., 1987).

A SHIFT TO CLINICAL OUTCOME MEASURES

Numerous studies have been conducted to measure the cost/benefit of EAPs. The last decade, however, has seen a shift from cost/benefit measures to clinical quality measures. One reason this shift occurred is due to a recognized inability in the EAP field to conduct the more sophisticated outcomes research. Another reason for this shift has been the dramatic growth of managed health care and the introduction of managed behavioral care into the employee assistance field. Payers are no longer satisfied with lowering health care costs, although initially, this was the primary focus of managed care. In the early 1990s, "total quality management" became the buzzword in American industry. Quality assurance and outcome indicators are now the norm in corporate America. EAPs are also now recognized as a viable ancillary to human resource management in the American workplace.

Heretofore, quality of care was considered synonymous with professional training and licensing of mental health professionals with little or no monitoring of either their practices or their clinical effectiveness. The introduction of managed care protocols such as precertification and utilization review and the increase in competition due to the development of preferred provider networks has resulted in heightened attention to the clinical performance of mental health professionals. The result has been a shift in cost of care to a focus on quality of care. However, one major recent study suggests that, at least initially, EAPs subject to clinical effectiveness outcomes will not fare as well as they did in their ability to demonstrate program cost effectiveness.

Masi (Jacobson & Cooper, 2000) reports findings from some 4,000 clients who provided EAP services between 1984 and 1998. Company size ranged from 300 to 500,000+. Principles of total quality management and six sigma criteria (99% error free) were applied to conceptualize a quality measurement protocol. The case records were peer reviewed by a blue ribbon panel of mental health experts (clinical social workers, psychologists, and psychiatrists) using a protocol developed by Masi Research Consultants with the assistance of a Harvard University psychometrician. Measurable items included the accuracy and quality of demographic data collected, processing of the initial contact by the EAP client (responsiveness, informed consent, confidentiality, etc.), case documentation, clinical services provided (e.g., assessment, short-term counseling), accurate identification and processing of clients considered at risk for violence, and quality of short-term counseling, referrals, and client follow-up. Other items included efficacy of short-term counseling, level of clinical supervision, and the peer reviewers' summary of strengths and weaknesses of each case reviewed. A 50-item instrument using a combination of Likert scale and closed-ended questions was developed. Case documentation and clinical services rendered comprised the two main sections of the protocol.

According to Masi (Jacobson & Cooper, 2000), both the quality of documentation and clinical services were "surprisingly low." The average overall documentation score was only a 2.98 out of a possible 5.00, which Masi considered "below average" and an indication that documentation did not meet required standards. Areas of deficiency included either missing or incomplete "Statement(s) of Understanding" about EAP services, as well as missing or incomplete "Release of Information Forms." Other areas suggesting a "below average" quality of service were missing case notes, limited or inadequate documentation, and comingling of client charts from the same family. Further, overall tracking of referrals for additional service and client follow-up was poorly documented.

Clinical reviews were equally discouraging and garnered a rating of 2.81 out of a possible 5.00. Short-term counseling averaged 3.32 sessions per client based on an eight-session model. Masi considered this well below the norm, and stated that 65–70% of the cases should be seen at least 4 to 4.5 sessions each. Alcohol and drug cases represented 18.9% of total clients seen, as compared to general workforce statistics of 25%. Based on clinical case reviews, of the total number of clients who needed additional medical and/or psychiatric care, only 37.6% received these services. Referral follow-up was not done (or not recorded) on 50% of the clients referred for outpatient care because of the lack of completed "Release of Information" forms. For those clients who did sign a release form, follow-up data indicated that only 52.5% of the clients used the referral, suggesting that 47.5% of the clients determined by the EAP to be in need of further treatment did not get any. Masi (Jacobson & Cooper, 2000) concludes her findings by stating:

"It is apparent that quality of care (in EAPs) is often over-looked and neglected. The findings reflect the limitations evident in today's clinical mental health practice . . . The mental health field has been lackadaisical about quality for far too long. A demand for total quality

improvement/management and the assurance of quality services has arrived and will remain a force to be contended with in the new millenium. Companies and private practitioners need to be asking themselves if they really are providing the highest quality of care because the demand for quality services is steadily increasing and clients and client companies alike will no longer settle for anything less . . ."

SPECIAL ISSUES

Specific Populations

As an increased number of EAPs have been established, it has become clear that the EAP in any specific work setting must be customized to fit the needs of that work environment and the diverse needs of all employees in that environment.

One major workplace characteristic that has required a modification of the traditional model is the lack of close supervision and the resulting difficulty in holding employees accountable for satisfactory performance. Examples of jobs that may not have close supervision include transportation workers (e.g., railroad employees, long-distance drivers, airline pilots, and flight attendants) and health professionals (e.g., physicians, nurses, dentists, pharmacists, psychologists). Both of these areas of work also pose significant hazards to the general public if the employee is impaired.

Given the importance of intervening with impaired employees in these safety-sensitive work settings and the usual lack of close supervision in these settings, a model of EAP intervention that relies on peers rather than supervisors has been developed. In the "peer intervention" model, when an employee's performance is impaired—thus putting the public at risk—coworkers confront the employee and strongly encourage the employee to seek assistance from the EAP. Such encouragement may include the threat of reporting the employee to the supervisor or to a licensing board. In some EAPs that utilize peer intervention, employee volunteers are specially trained in the peer intervention process. Programs that utilize peer intervention also encourage self-referrals and the traditional supervisory referral when it is feasible

(Bureau of National Affairs, 1987; Molloy, 1985; Rivard, 1990; Scanlon, 1991; Sonnenstuhl & Trice, 1988).

Other occupations require similar modifications to traditional EAP practice. An executive, for example, may not have much interaction with his/her supervisor and may have more resources to cover up the problem (e.g., subordinates and secretaries) than do other employees (Shirley, 1985). In some occupations it may be particularly difficult to terminate an employee for poor performance (e.g., tenured professors, some public sector employees), and thus the supervisor's constructive confrontation may not carry much of a threat for the affected employee.

Police and fire departments have many employees who work without close supervision and who pose a threat to the public if they are impaired. These departments are also often a "closed society" that may not allow outsiders (i.e., the EAP counselor) to get close to the employees. For this reason some of these departments use a police officer or fire fighter from the ranks as the EAP counselor so that the employees know that the EAP counselor understands the job stressors and workplace culture of the department (Bureau of National Affairs, Inc., 1987).

While various occupations require modifications to the traditional model of EAP, employee diversity also requires special attention to ensure that the EAP is appropriate for all employees in the workplace. Today's workforce is becoming increasingly diverse with respect to ethnicity, culture, gender, age, disability, and sexual orientation. The traditional models of EAP were based primarily on a white male workforce and thus may require new strategies that can include the entire workforce.

Employees who are part of this new workforce diversity may encounter special stressors arising from overt or covert discrimination (e.g., the "glass ceiling," which prevents the employee's promotion beyond a certain level). Furthermore, they may have values and expectations regarding counseling that make it difficult for them to enter into EAP counseling and/or professional treatment (e.g., feeling that family problems should not be shared with anyone outside of the family).

Given these factors, EAPs must make sure that their program promotion, counseling, referral, and follow-up activities are provided in a manner that is sensitive to the employees and encourages use of the service. To achieve this sensitivity, the EAP staff should take steps to become familiar with the diverse demographic groups in the workplace. Having EAP staff members who are themselves members of diverse demographic groups helps to create a staff and office that are comfortable for all employees. The EAP must also be able to refer to treatment providers who can be sensitive to the needs of a diverse work force (Hooks & Weinstein, 1991; Smollen, 1991; Walker, 1991).

Substance Abuse in the Workplace

EAPs were originally developed to address the problem of employee alcoholism and, later, other drug abuse. Employee chemical dependency continues to be a major problem, thus it continues to be a primary focal point for EAPs. Because of the importance of this problem at the workplace, special legislation, education and training, employee testing, and ongoing support for recovery have been developed.

To understand all of these special activities targeted at chemical dependency, one must first understand the disease concept of alcohol and other drug abuse. As has been previously noted, our society has traditionally considered alcoholics to be irresponsible, immoral, weak, or psychologically disturbed. The founding of Alcoholics Anonymous in 1935 began to establish the concept of alcoholism as a disease. This notion began to be accepted by the medical community in the 1950s and 1960s.

Today alcoholism is understood to be not simply a symptom of an underlying condition but rather a primary illness. It is a chronic illness that cannot be cured but can be treated through education, counseling, and social support. Because of the chronic nature of this illness, alcoholics who have stopped drinking generally consider themselves to be recovering from this illness rather than being totally recovered. Given that alcoholism is an illness, alcoholics do not consider themselves personally responsible for being an alcoholic, but—as with any chronic illness—they consider themselves responsible for securing the proper treatment and support that can help in their recovery.

The illness of alcoholism is characterized primarily by a loss of control of one's drinking behavior and a continued use of alcohol despite negative consequences. Alcoholism is also generally characterized by a denial of the problem on the part of the alcoholic.

The alcoholic's denial of the problem is frequently "supported" by family members, friends, and/or coworkers and supervisors at work. These people in the alcoholic's life often inadvertently enable the alcoholic to avoid the negative consequences of his/her own behavior and thus enable the alcoholic to continue drinking. Enabling frequently takes the form of covering or making excuses for the alcoholic when things go wrong. Family members who are enablers are often considered to be codependent; their lives have become as rigid, distorted, and stuck in their relationship with the chemically-dependent family member as is the chemically dependent person's own life. When alcoholics are surrounded by enablers—as is usually the case—helping the alcoholic to enter treatment frequently requires helping the enablers to stop their enabling behaviors.

The disease concept of alcoholism also applies to other drugs of abuse (see Table 16-5). In fact many alcoholics and other drug abusers are addicted to a variety of prescription and/or nonprescription drugs. Given this wide spectrum of addictions, the term "chemical dependency" has come to be used to refer to any and all addictions formerly referred to as alcoholism or drug abuse.

As with any illness, the illness of chemical dependency may coexist with other illnesses. The term "dual diagnosis" is used to refer to chemically dependent patients who also have a psychiatric disorder (Thompson, 1990).

Table 16-5 The Disease Concept of Chemical Dependency

- A primary illness, rather than a symptom of an underlying condition
- Loss of control of one's chemical-using behavior
- Continued use of chemical(s) despite negative consequences
- Denial of problem

Substance abuse education is an important element of a comprehensive approach to substance abuse in the workplace. Education for employees on this topic should include not only information about substance abuse (e.g., the disease concept, substances of abuse, the progression of the illness, how the illness is treated) but also information regarding the company's policy concerning substance abuse at work and the availability of EAP services. Substance abuse education should also include family members.

In addition to the above, supervisors also need to be trained regarding their special role in situations involving employees who might be impaired due to substance abuse, job performance problems that might be related to substance abuse, and employees returning to work following substance abuse treatment. With respect to the impaired employee and the job performance problem, the supervisor training must emphasize that it is the supervisor's job to observe, document, and refer. It is not the supervisor's job to attempt to diagnose the nature of what might be an employee's personal problem. By focusing exclusively on work-related issues, the supervisor stays within his/her own area of expertise and does not run the risk of accusing someone of having a personal problem they may or may not actually have (Scanlon, 1991; Thompson, 1990).

Drug Testing and Fitness-for-Duty

In a time of intense cost-cutting, 98% of Fortune 200 corporations conduct drug testing on one or more categories of applicants and employees. Only three percent of this group did so in 1983 (DeLancey, 1994). This increase in testing reflects an overall increase in what is expected of the workforce. Employees are expected to perform a variety of work roles in a responsible, efficient, and trustworthy manner. As complex individuals, we perform numerous roles. In addition to being employees, we may also operate in the roles of parent, sibling, friend, or spouse. These demands outside the workplace have an influence on our job performance, causing fatigue, stress, psychological problems, substance use or abuse, illness, etc. Fitness-for-duty testing allows the EAP to do more early interventions.

A Drug-Free Workplace

Substance use in the workplace is not a modern phenomenon (Backer & O'Hara, 1991). Historically, employees had taken "grog breaks" and, later, the "three-martini lunch" during work hours. However, during the 1980s, the impact of workplace substance use on productivity, medical insurance costs, and safety became widely recognized. During the mid-1980s, several fatal train and subway accidents occurred which strongly increased support for drug testing in the workplace. In 1986, the problem was featured in a radio address by President Reagan. Shortly after, *Time* magazine devoted a cover story to the topic of workplace substance use (Backer & O'Hara, 1991). By the latter half of the decade, it became clear that actions needed to be taken to curb substance use on the job. A pervasive sense of a national drug crisis, as well as a shift to a more conservative political climate, made the time ripe for a national "War on Drugs." In September 1986, the "War on Drugs" was introduced by President Reagan. A key component of this effort was an executive order calling for a drug-free workplace. This order made random urine testing of federal employees mandatory (Gilliom, 1994).

The Drug-Free Workplace Act of 1988 requires that all federal contractors and grantees receiving payments of $25,000 implement a comprehensive Drug-Free Workplace Program. In 1989, the Federal Drug Control Strategy urged private employers to follow suit (Hanson, 1993). The U.S. Department of Transportation (DOT) issued new regulations in 1994 requiring all transportation workers in "safety-sensitive" positions to undergo alcohol and drug testing. In 1995, the rules became effective for public and private organizations with 50 or more DOT-covered transportation workers. The next year, these rules were expanded to include organizations with 50 or fewer DOT-covered workers (Buckley, 1995).

Random drug testing has increased 1,200% since 1987, and it is estimated that over 7.5 million workers will be tested for drugs annually (DeLancey, 1994). Because EAPs are a required component in federally mandated Drug-Free Workplace Programs, the demand for EAP services has grown substantially.

This demand will continue to grow because drug abuse is once again rising in the next generation of workers. Approximately 11% of employees between the ages of 18 and 34 used illegal drugs in 1992. Currently, it is estimated that about five million employed drug abusers and 18 million employed alcohol abusers need substance abuse treatment (DeLancey, 1994). The American Management Association found that 22% of the companies that have drug testing programs immediately terminate those who test positive. Twenty-one percent elected to suspend or put those employees on probation, while 70% referred them to treatment or counseling. Just over half of this sample had formal EAPs in place (Blum, Fields, Milne, & Spell, 1992).

Legal Issues

Drug and alcohol testing is a sensitive issue. Testing positive not only jeopardizes an employee's career but also carries with it a negative stigma. Although part of the rationale behind a drug testing program should be rehabilitation, employers are not required to offer treatment as an option to maintaining employment. Due to the sensitive nature of positive tests, it is extremely important that companies realize that the risk of litigation exists for the employer, the collection site, laboratories, and the Medical Review Officer (MRO) (Judge, 1993).

Thousands of employees have filed lawsuits based on charges that their Constitutional rights have been violated as a result of a mandatory drug test. The threat of litigation can be significantly reduced by seeking appropriate legal counsel and realizing the extent of responsibility employers assume for the welfare of their staff. Choosing to ignore or failing to take preventative measures regarding employee drug use can place an employer at risk of liability as well. If a drug- or alcohol-impaired employee working in a "safety-sensitive" position accidentally injures a fellow worker, there is a risk that the injured worker will file a lawsuit against the employer for negligence (Judge, 1993). Drug and alcohol prevention and awareness programs may be the best insurance for employers in guarding against accidents.

Despite the fact that the Drug-Free Workplace Act has been in effect since 1988, drug testing remains controversial. Most of the controversy stems from the fact that drug testing involves several fundamental yet conflicting interests: the individual's right to privacy, the employer's responsibility to maintain a safe working environment, and the public's right to safety. For the most part, the issue of safety and security has superseded an individual's right to privacy. This is especially true when the safety of the general public is at risk (Judge, 1993; Willette & Kadehjian, 1992).

Drug testing raises complex legal questions. An organization contemplating initiating a testing program must carefully review its particular needs as well as seek the advice of its legal counsel in order to gain a thorough understanding of the legal guidelines involved in drug testing programs (Hanson, 1990; Judge, 1993). If the intrusiveness of the testing process is kept to a minimum, the likelihood of the program withstanding legal scrutiny is maximized.

Drug Testing and the Americans with Disabilities Act (ADA)

The ADA considers addiction to be a disability. However, job protection for those disabled by substances applies only to those who have successfully completed a rehabilitation program and are not currently engaging in substance abuse. Under the ADA, drug testing and any disciplinary actions that are the result of a positive test do not fall under the protection of the ADA. An important component of ADA coverage that employers need to be aware of applies to preemployment drug testing. In accordance with the ADA, an employer may conduct a preemployment drug screen only after a conditional offer of employment has been made (Judge, 1995).

Policy Guidelines

Prior to implementing a drug testing program, employers should identify any federal or state laws with which they must comply. A formal drug testing policy should be drawn up and distributed to all employees.

At a minimum, the policy should include the following categories (Swotinsky, 1992):

- Who answers employee questions about policy
- How testing will differ by work category and the situation (i.e., after on-the-job accidents)
- Specific expectations for nonuse while on-call, at breaks, or for a specified period of time prior to reporting to work
- Other specifics about what type of conduct is prohibited
- The conditions in which a worker will be tested for alcohol or drugs
- Procedures for specimen analysis, accuracy, quality control, and quality assurance
- Explanation of what is considered a refusal to test and the consequences of such a refusal
- Return-to-work and aftercare procedures
- Consequences of violation of policies
- Substance cut-off levels according to the U.S. Department of Health and Human Services.
- Specific details of how confirmatory tests will be carried out

Refusal to take a drug test is regarded by most companies as a positive result. However, there are some exceptions. The 1995 Federal Aviation Association (FAA) regulations contain a loophole. While the FAA considers a refusal to test as a positive result, it does not count toward the two-strike permanent ban for working in any FAA covered job (Judge, 1995).

A positive test should mandate a referral to the EAP for an assessment. Those in safety-sensitive positions should be removed from service (unless company policies or union agreements state otherwise) while their test is verified for accuracy. Often random testing is required of employees working in such positions. As a method of protecting against "false positives," it is suggested that employees disclose all therapeutic drug use to the MRO prior to a drug test. However, release of such information by nonsafety-sensitive employees should not be mandated, as it could be considered a violation of the ADA (Judge, 1995). Employees should be aware that improper use of prescription drugs (i.e., taking a medication that

has not been prescribed to the user) could make the tester subject to the consequences of a positive test (Swotinsky, 1992).

Types of Drug Testing

Companies often post notices in their Human Resources Department that read: "Drug-free Workplace—We Test Applicants for Illegal Substances." Baxter Healthcare found that posting this sign alone has the power to significantly reduce the percentage of applicants who test positive (DeLancey, 1994). To be legal, alcohol testing is only allowed after a conditional offer of employment has been made (see Table 16-6). Drug tests are not considered medical examinations under the ADA so they may be conducted as a screening measure. Employers should not discriminate against candidates who are currently in the aftercare process of treatment, but employers are mandated (in workplaces with federal contracts) to verify that candidates have no record of substance abuse violations within the past six months (Judge, 1995). These are the only instances where discussions of a future employee's substance abuse history does not require a signed release specifically authorizing it; this is because employers with federal contracts are mandated to do this background check. *Preemployment tests* can greatly reduce costs associated with substance abuse. A 1993 analysis of the U.S. Postal Service's preemployment testing policy found the USPS

Table 16-6 Circumstances for Drug Testing

- Preemployment
- For-cause (when there is a reasonable suspicion of drug use based on observed behavior)
- As required by federal regulation
- Random testing for safety-sensitive jobs (i.e., jobs where impairment could pose a threat to public safety)
- Postaccident testing (to determine if drugs played a role in the accident)
- Following treatment for substance abuse (to ensure that the employee who is returning to work is drug free and remains drug free)
- As part of regularly scheduled physical exams for all employees

realized $162.48 in net savings per employee hired due to this type of screen. The costs considered in the analysis included collection and processing of the sample as well as those associated with recruiting and hiring employees to replace those who had not qualified for positions due to a positive result. The benefits were calculated in terms of accidents, injuries, turnovers, and absences avoided (DeLancey, 1994).

For-cause tests (also called reasonable suspicion) are controversial. It is important that drug testing policies detail under what conditions these sorts of tests will occur.

> "Tests should not be based solely on a series of absences or tardiness. Reasonable cause for testing exists when [a worker looks, acts, talks, or smells like someone withdrawing from substances]. The person who makes the determination that reasonable cause for alcohol testing exists should not perform the test. Also, it must be performed within eight hours of a for-cause decision" (Judge, 1995, p. 18).

Random testing has been found to be the most effective testing type in identifying substance abusers in the workplace. Federal mandates specify that 25% of the total random-testing pool of employees must be tested for alcohol annually. Half of the total random-testing pool should be tested for drugs annually. Company policy should clearly state what types of workers will be put in an additional random-testing pool for safety-sensitive employees, if any. Research has determined that "in general, pre-employment drug testing and testing 'for reasonable cause' continue to be much more prevalent in the workplace than random testing. The data indicate that this state of affairs is likely to continue," (Blum, Fields, Milne, & Spell, 1992, p. 318).

Postaccident testing has been found to be a consistently effective way to lower disability and worker's compensation costs over time. Clairson International (560 employees) experienced a 30–35% decrease in the number of industrial accidents reported after a postaccident testing program was implemented (DeLancey, 1994). Federally mandated workplaces often require employees to be substance-free up to eight hours after an accident or until a drug and alcohol test can be performed (Judge, 1995).

Determining Fitness-for-Duty

Fitness-for-duty is a condition of employment with adequate job performance being the minimum expectation. Employers have the right to insist that employees report to work in a condition conducive to performing their job to the utmost of their ability. A fitness-for-duty policy establishes a criterion for employee on-the-job fitness, methods for assessing fitness, and the company's response to employees deemed unfit. Often used in conjunction with a workplace's rules prohibiting substance use, possession, or sale on company premises, the policy provides fair and unified standards for employees and eliminates a myriad of problems for management confronted with unfit employees (Nye, 1990).

Although the issue of substance use lies at the core of a fitness-for-duty policy, there are numerous factors that could impede an employee's job performance that should not be overlooked. These factors include illness, lack of sleep, stress, family problems, and financial planning concerns. In dealing with the topic of fitness-for-duty, employers need to look at the overall picture of holistic health. In assisting employees with personal problems that inevitably spill over into the workplace, EAPs play a fundamental role in promoting greater workplace health and well-being.

Drug testing has been touted as an integral ingredient in workplace safety and employee fitness-for-duty. However, a major impediment of drug testing by means of urinalysis is its limited ability to determine whether or not a person is fit-for-duty at any particular time. Due to the fact that drugs and drug metabolites may appear in the urine for several days or weeks after the drug was last used, urine tests can only provide evidence of prior drug use. They cannot show job impairment, recency of use, level of intoxication, or pattern of use (Comer, 1995; Willette & Kadehjian, 1992).

Due to the limitations of drug testing by means of urinalysis, the development of indirect methods for assessing alcohol and other drug use has been rapidly growing. Indirect approaches typically involve measuring or observing behaviors or responses that are frequently associated with alcohol and other drug use and inferring such use from what is observed.

Indirect testing methods are certainly not a new phenomenon; they had been developed and utilized decades ago by the United States military. However, the mandatory drug testing element in the Drug-Free Workplace Act led to urinalysis replacing many alternative fitness-for-duty testing methods.

Since substance use may not be the only reason that an employee is not fit for duty on a particular day, performance tests have been developed to aid an employer in making this determination. Some of the more common indirect approaches are: Drug Abuse Scales (DAS), Drug Evaluation and Classification Programs (DEC), attitude prototype theory, and computerized performance-based fitness-for-duty testing (ACLU, 1996; Comer, 1995; Swotinsky, 1992).

Drug abuse scales were developed out of the theoretical framework of Zuckerman's theory of sensation seeking (National Research Council Institute of Medicine, 1994). According to Zuckerman, sensation seeking correlates with multidrug use. DAS are designed to measure the psychodynamic mechanisms that are posited to influence attitudes toward drug use. DEC programs identify illicit drug users by using observable behaviors and physiological signals. DEC programs allegedly determine whether a person is impaired at the time, whether the impairment is drug- or medically-related, and the broad category or combination of drugs likely to have caused the impairment. Based on the assessment, the DEC programs can provide probable cause for a urine sample, can assist laboratories in determining which drugs to test for, and can provide evidence of impairment that may not be available through chemical testing alone (ACLU, 1996).

EAPs Role in Fitness-for-Duty

Next to home, the workplace is probably the most influential environment in shaping substance-related behavior. According to the Drug-Free Workplace Act, assistance should be offered to any employee exhibiting possible substance-abuse-related behavior (Hanson, 1993). Thus, all employees testing positive or experiencing repeated fitness failures should be referred to the EAP for a substance abuse assessment.

In accordance with the Drug-Free Workplace Act, the EAP is an essential component in providing confidential problem assessment, counseling, referral to treatment, support, and guidance throughout the formal treatment program and the rehabilitation process and in continuing case management services for one to two years (Swotinsky, 1992).

As part of the recovery program, periodic drug testing may be implemented as a preventive measure. Often employees find this component helpful in staying sober or promptly seeking help should a relapse occur. Additionally, it is advisable that the EAP, along with the employee, develop an after-care program consisting of formal after-care support services and regular attendance of an informal support group such as Alcoholics Anonymous or Narcotics Anonymous.

After completion of a treatment program, the EAP partners with the MRO to determine whether or not the employee is fit to return to full duty. If it is determined that the employee is fit to return to duty, the MRO and EAP counselor may choose to draw up a "last-chance agreement." A last-chance agreement is a rehabilitation agreement in which an employer reinstates an employee who has violated workplace drug policies in exchange for a promise to follow an agreed upon after-care program. The employee agrees that violation of the terms of the agreement will result in disciplinary action, up to and including termination (Nye, 1990). Table 16-7 provides an overview of other relevant workplace legislation.

CRITICAL INCIDENT STRESS DEBRIEFING (CISD)

CISD was developed for use in managing stress among emergency service personnel (e.g., firefighters, paramedics, policemen, etc.) following exposure to traumatic events. The goal in developing CISD was to reduce the emotional strain of repeated exposure to trauma to prevent professional burnout and lower the incidence of more pronounced stress-related disorders among this population. CISD is a group process employing both crisis intervention and educational processes and is targeted towards mitigating or resolving the psychological distress associated with a critical incident or traumatic event (Mitchell & Everly, 1993).

Table 16-7 Overview of Other Relevant Workplace Legislation

The Americans with Disabilities Act, (ADA) 1991	• Disability under the ADA includes any individual who has a physical or mental impairment that substantially limits one or more major life activities. • An individual must have, have a record of, or be regarded as having a substantial impairment that limits a major life activity. • An individual must be qualified to perform the essential functions of the job with or without reasonable accommodations. • The ADA does not limit the employer's right to hire the best qualified employee nor does it impose any affirmative action. • The ADA prohibits the employer from discriminating against anyone due to disability. • Conditions specifically exempt from ADA coverage include homosexuality, bisexuality, transvestitism, compulsive gambling, kleptomania, pyromania, pedophilia, exhibitionism, voyeurism, gender identity disorders not resulting from physical impairments, and current illegal drug use. • Individuals who pose a direct threat to the health or safety of others are not considered qualified for protection under the ADA. For example, an HIV-infected health care professional who performs surgery may pose a direct threat to the patient and, therefore, would not be covered. An employer should consider the duration, nature, and likelihood and imminence of potential harm when determining a direct threat. • A reasonable accommodation is any change or modification to a job or work environment that permits an individual with a disability to perform the essential functions of a job, or to enjoy benefits and privileges granted to those who do not carry a disability. • Employers cannot ask an applicant questions that are likely to bring forth information or are closely related to making disclosures concerning a disability. In other words, one cannot ask if an individual has a disability at the preoffer stage but is allowed to ask if the individual is capable of fulfilling the functions of the position. Employers may request applicants to perform an examination to determine their ability but only if all applicants are asked to do so. • The ADA prohibits prejob-offer examinations. • Testing to determine use of illegal drugs is not considered a medical examination by the ADA and therefore can be administrated at any time. • Unlike illegal drugs, alcohol tests are considered by the Equal Employment Opportunity Commission (EEOC) to be a medical examination. One can only be questioned or examined concerning job-related matters, and it must serve a legitimate business purpose. • The ADA considers addiction to be a disability. However, job protection for those disabled by substances apply only to those who have successfully completed a rehabilitation program and are not currently engaging in substance abuse.
The Civil Rights Act 1964 and 1991	• The Civil Rights Act prohibits discrimination in the workplace based on gender. • Sexual harassment is considered by Title VII as a form of sexual discrimination and is prohibited. • Gender-based actions that cause a hostile environment are also considered to be a form of sexual harassment. A hostile work environment is one in which a person feels hassled or degraded because of constant unwelcome obscene joking, suggestive comments, or flirtation.

Racial discrimination	• Title VII of the Civil Rights Act of 1991 prohibits discrimination based on race or color. Federal courts have defined race discrimination as discrimination based on ancestry or ethnic characteristics.
	• Ethnic groups are those not classified as racial groups.
National origin discrimination	• Discrimination based on national origin includes physical, cultural, and language characteristics, and any activities or surname associated with an ethnic group.
	• Employers have the right to require English communication skills if it is considered a business necessity and is applied to all applicants and employees equally.
	• Requiring English to be spoken at all times in the workplace is considered a form of discrimination by the Equal Employment Opportunity Commission.
	• Employers cannot discriminate based on an individual's accent unless it is deemed a business necessity.
Religious discrimination	• Any earnest religious, moral, or ethical belief held with or without membership in a collective group is protected.
	• While some religions require specific dress and appearance, employers do not have to accommodate employees when paramount conditions exist.
	• Employers do not have to deny privileges to others to accommodate religious needs.
	• A preferred religious accommodation does not have to be made when other more reasonable alternatives exist. When participation in religious activities conflicts with work schedules, employers have the right to grant paid or unpaid leave, reschedule work hours, or deny leave when a hardship is created.
The Family and Medical Leave Act (FMLA) 1993	• FMLA allows employees to take a limited amount of unpaid leave for certain family needs, and FMLA protects the employer from abuse and excessive hardship and the employee from discrimination for tending to family and medical needs.
	• Covered employees are eligible for no more than 12 workweeks of unpaid leave in a 12-month period of time. Protected FMLA leave is for the care of an employee's child, immediate family member, or spouse.
	• Leave is granted for prenatal care, birth of a child or an adoption, or foster care placement. With the onset of a serious health condition, employees are entitled to unpaid medical leave. Serious health conditions must involve an illness, injury, impairment, or physical/mental condition that involves hospital, hospice, or residential medical care facility inpatient care or continuing health care of a health care provider.
	• FMLA extends to both male and female employees. In the event that a spouse, employed by the same employer, wishes to take FMLA leave, the total leave time cannot exceed 12 weeks.
	• Upon returning from approved FMLA leave, employees must be restored to their original jobs at the same site or a site that is not a significant increase in time or miles. If the original position is not available, the employees must be offered an "equivalent position," which means virtually identical in terms of pay, benefits, and other employment terms and conditions.
	• An employer can refuse job restoration to "key" employees whose employment will cause a "substantial and grievous economic injury" to the company's operation. Key employees are those whose salaries are within the top 10% for the company site.

The effectiveness of CISD is derived from several aspects. Early intervention within one to three days after the trauma is the best prevention against developing delayed stress reactions that are more difficult to cope with. While a strong emotional response to a trauma is not considered pathological, people's instinctive reactions (closing down, shock, intrusive thoughts) due to the intensity of the impact may inhibit the essential need for catharsis. CISD provides a safe, supportive structured environment wherein individuals can vent emotions. Disclosure of the traumatic event subsequently reduces stress arousal. Importantly, CISD provides the opportunity to verbally reconstruct and express specific traumas, fears, and questions. Successful recovery from a trauma is based not only on the ability to express feelings but also on the ability to reconstruct and integrate the trauma using verbal expression (Mitchell & Everly, 1993).

The CISD Process

CISD is a group meeting for recently traumatized individuals to help alleviate initial acute stress responses and accelerate the healing process. CISD ideally occurs within one to three days of the incident.

CISDs are usually conducted by employee assistance professionals, peer counselors, or a trained community- or organization-based team (hospital or family service agency). Debriefing leaders should include at least one mental health professional who serves as the lead facilitator. The trained "peer" plays a key role in CISD, especially in debriefings with emergency personnel and, more recently, in occupational settings. "Peers" add credibility in that they know the work culture and can lend strategic insight since they are a part of that culture.

Goals of Debriefings

Debriefing groups typically have the following goals:

- Reduce the emotional impact of the trauma by providing supportive counseling, an opportunity for cathartic ventilation of emotional reactions and a chance to review the event to "make sense" of it in the context of a supportive group.

- Provide education about the emotional, physical, and interpersonal impact of traumatic events. This occurs through didactic teaching by the leaders, as well as (and perhaps more powerfully) by group members discussing their reactions to the event with one another, and learning that many are experiencing similar reactions. The realization that, for most individuals, their reactions are normal, is a source of tremendous relief and is one of the most important objectives in providing a group (Plaggemars, in press).

Mitchell and Everly (1993) also outline several secondary goals for CISD. These are:

- Normalization of reaction to an abnormal event
- Reassurance that the stress response is controllable and that recovery is likely
- Reduction of the fallacy of uniqueness
- Reduction of the fallacy of abnormality
- Forewarning about possible signs and symptoms in the future
- Enhancement of group uniqueness
- Assessment of those who may need follow-up or individual counseling

Additional secondary goals in this process are the appropriate framing of anger and guilt responses and the clarification of misconceptions or distortions of the event itself.

Critical-incident stress management through the debriefing process provides structured early intervention at a time when the "window of opportunity" for providing assistance remains the greatest. Since post-traumatic stress reaction may occur regardless of the premorbid personality, it is important to provide crisis response services to all those who are affected by the tragedy as a preventative measure. This remains the ideal strategy for managing the risk of individuals from developing prolonged, hurtful stress reactions.

The debriefing process consists of seven phases:

1. The **introduction phase** sets the stage for the subsequent phases of the debriefing. It defines an actual beginning. The mental health professional introduces himself/herself and the team members.

The purpose, context, and the process of the meeting are explained. Guidelines are explained, including attention to confidentiality. Furthermore, the process is carefully disassociated from a critical analysis of the event. A supportive nonjudgmental tone is established to reduce resistance and anxiety and to encourage mutual help from the participants.

2. In the **fact phase,** participants are asked to introduce themselves and their role during the incident. Responses may range from where they were when they first became aware of the incident to what happened from their point of view and what their first reactions were. Since the facts are objective in nature, they are the easiest to discuss. Through a discussion of the facts, a collective, realistic picture of the event is created. It is crucial that, for a timely, healthy recovery to occur, the witnesses' memories and subsequent recollections be based on as accurate an account as possible.

3. In the **thought phase,** group members are asked to state their first thoughts about the incident. The thought phase represents a transition from the cognitive domain to the affective domain, thus setting the stage for more personalized responses from the participants.

4. The **reaction phase** is perhaps the most intense phase in that participants are asked to recall the worst part of the event. Responses are invited, and no particular structure is followed. The facilitator may rephrase what has been said or suggest what some people typically feel in response to a traumatic event. This allows group members a moment to sort out their emotions. The group culture influences the ease with which emotions are expressed. Often the thought and reaction phases blend together. By gradually putting words to what was most difficult for them, individuals begin to expose content that, if not dealt with, in all likelihood would prove most troublesome in the future.

5. The **symptom phase** redirects the participants from the reaction phase toward a more cognitive consideration of the physical, emotional, or behavioral symptoms they experienced during the event. The facilitator may stimulate the process by mentioning a few common symptoms then asking for a show of hands or a nod. The team will ask what it was like for the participants following the incident. Typically, the discussion turns to the symptoms of stress that were experienced over the next few days. The CISD team then asks the group if they are currently experiencing any stress symptoms. These symptoms are "normalized" and hopefully diffused in the process.

6. The **teaching phase** relays clear information on normative stress responses (what is considered a normal response to a trauma) and describes behaviors that assist individual recovery. Such timely clarification provides a calming effect by minimizing cognitive confusion and disorienting fears. This allows the victim to better focus on healthy self-care for the moment, such as the need to minimize alcohol consumption and to focus on remaining open to the support of others during the time of acute crisis. Also helpful as part of the education offered is identification of the phases through which people progress in the aftermath of a trauma or loss. This information helps those involved to orient their emotions, engenders a sense of self-control, and encourages ongoing self-assessment during recovery.

7. The **re-entry phase** offers the opportunity to summarize, clarify particular issues, reemphasize key points, and respond to remaining questions. It is also the time for facilitators to state any feelings that seem apparent but have not been expressed. At this point additional handouts are distributed, suggesting sources for further assistance. At the close of the debriefing the facilitators remain available for questions or may initiate debriefings with tangential groups (i.e., dispatchers, spouses, or families) as deemed appropriate. Peers may be deployed strategically or assigned to connect with certain distraught workers. Follow-up activities must be considered and applied depending on the circumstances unique to the event and those affected. Gaining postdebriefing feedback from those who invited the facilitators is desirable. Managers may in turn be given specific recommendations based on the feedback received. Other types of follow-up may include telephone calls to the managers, chaplain visits, an educational session, individual consultation, or referrals for therapy.

In summary, the CISD process facilitates the formation of a group support process led by training mental health professionals and possibly peers wherein the presentation of factual data prepares the way for the expression of more emotionally charged content. Through the group process, participants are encouraged to share their feelings and concerns and to listen to the others as they become educated about posttraumatic stress reactions. Through the direction of the facilitators, participants learn that their situation is not unique and that, with some care and attention, they can rebuild the sense of safety and security that they experienced prior to the crisis.

Given the dramatic increase in workplace violence, CISD has become an expected skill of EAP professionals. While some worksettings, due to the nature of the work, are viewed as higher risk for a trauma to occur, one cannot predict when a critical incident may occur. Consequently, the EAP must be prepared to provide assistance on very short notice to help workers cope with a range of trauma-producing events, such industrial accidents resulting in significant injury or death, violence, robberies, and natural disasters.

MANAGED BEHAVIORAL HEALTH CARE AND EAPS

Managed care is defined as any form of health care plan that initiates selective contracting as a means of channeling patients to a limited or set number of providers. It refers to a variety of market-driven systems and strategies to control costs by monitoring and controlling the utilization of health-related services. Managed behavioral care (MBC) refers to a system that generates and uses a plan to organize and quantify the delivery of behavioral care through specific providers in order to minimize the costs of care. Organizations purchasing MBC contracts expect to pay smaller plan premiums to cover their employees as a result of MBC vendors being able to control mental health costs.

Winegar (1996) proposes that three distinct historical events helped shape the face of MBC today. The first was the gradual development of prepaid health care coverage. During the late 1930s and early 1940s, industrialist Henry J. Kaiser and physician Sydney Garfield established the first HMOs in Oregon and California. The most prominent feature of this model was that the consumer paid one monthly fee and then received all health care services from selected providers at little or no cost. The success of these first organizations, designed specifically to serve the health care needs of Kaiser's employees, was the basis for the nation's largest group model HMO, Kaiser-Permanente HMO. Nevertheless, opposition from physician and hospital groups stunted the development of HMOs in the country until President Nixon signed the HMO Act of 1973. The law required employers of 25 or more people to offer an HMO option if an HMO is in operation in their locale and if requested by the HMO to do so. Though there was a large increase in enrollment and continued growth, rising health care costs made the entire industry struggle financially during the 1980s. The 1990s brought a financial turnaround in the industry, and the success of HMOs has spurred the development of other managed care systems such as preferred provider organizations (PPOs). Currently HMOs make up nearly 22% of all employee health benefits across the nation (Tolnai, 1996).

In 1975 the Diagnostic Related Group system (DRG) was developed at Yale University (Winegar, 1996). The federal government began using the DRG system for Medicare patients in order to contain costs and share financial risk with hospitals. Hospitals received maximum amounts based upon the DRG diagnosis given to the patient, no matter what the length of stay required. Though DRGs were used for medical hospital care, they were not applied to psychiatric diagnoses due to lack of professional consensus on treatment. Reduced profits in medical care motivated hospital management to shift expansion into specialty areas of mental health and substance abuse in the 1970s through the 1980s. The magnitude of this shift became overwhelming. Winegar (1996) reports that the incidence of teenage hospitalization went up 350% between 1982 and 1986, but the total adolescent population declined. Inpatient substance abuse and teenage treatment units proliferated, providing intensive and costly behavioral care. Hospital personnel aggressively marketed their inpatient units to EAP staff and psychiatrists who could make direct referrals to them.

Another development that influenced managed behavioral care was the expansion and divergence of the counseling professions (Masi, 1994). Before the 1960s, most insurance carriers reimbursed services provided only by psychiatrists. As the public's attitude toward therapy for emotional and substance abuse changed, the number of counseling professions and professionals expanded. The American Psychological Association (APA) and the National Association of Social Workers (NASW) successfully lobbied for legal recognition as providers of treatment services. Currently psychologists have achieved regulatory status in all 50 states and social work is regulated in 48 states. Other professions have statutory recognition as mental health providers in fewer numbers of states. Consumers flocked to the newer counseling professions, resulting in increased service utilization and increased mental health care costs. Insurance companies passed on these cost increases and their associated risks to the employers.

Struggling to contain the rising cost of health care on their profits, most of the nation's largest employers followed IBM's lead in the early 1980s (Winegar, 1996). They either developed or expanded their EAPs in the search for ways to provide appropriate, cost-effective care for employees' mental health and substance abuse treatments. Many of these employers already had managed health care in the form of HMOs and PPOs. These organizations gratefully resolved employers' questions on how to provide adequate mental health and substance abuse care while containing escalating costs by bringing the managed care to the forefront.

Managed Behavioral Care (MBC) Components

Four common components are present in MBC today, along with a range of secondary functions (Winegar, 1996). Any or all of the components can be delivered to HMO or purchasers' employees by "carve-out," specialty MBC firms or EAPs. The core components are precertification, provider network development, clinical case management, and utilization management.

Precertification

The precertification function is responsible for assessment and treatment planning. After assessing a client's presenting problem, a diagnostic impression is reached and matched to a service provider and the type, level, and intensity of treatment required. Precertification requires clinical assessment before hospitalization, thereby eliminating or reducing the client's option to select inpatient treatment without conferring with affiliated clinicians.

Provider Network Development

MBC systems utilize provider networks to provide service to clients. Clinicians are recruited who agree to reduced reimbursement rates for service, have recognized credentials, congruent values, and a willingness to comply with utilization review requirements. Credentialing and screening ensure quality service provision to clients. Agreed-upon rate structuring maximizes cost containment for the MBC.

Clinical Case Management

This component refers to the coordination and monitoring of client services throughout the treatment process. Clinical case managers may be treatment providers or other MBC staff who consult with providers and conduct periodic, concurrent reviews. Primary functions of the case manager include coordination of care with treatment providers, referral to outside community resources, and benefit interpretation.

Utilization Management

Utilization management or utilization review is the use of several techniques and procedures to monitor and evaluate the necessity or appropriateness of care for insurance coverage or provider reimbursement. Service decisions are based on objective information such as symptoms, diagnostic impressions, response to treatment, and treatment outcomes. Utilization management limits risk to the MBC and ensures that services delivered are appropriate, necessary, and authorized for advanced reimbursement.

Integrating Employee Assistance and Managed Care

EAPs promote easy access to care for troubled employees and early identification of and intervention into job performance problems (Robbins, Gerson, & Moore, 1992). Effective EAPs provide alternatives to termination, along with short-term counseling and educational and prevention components to reduce hospitalization as the first option for mental health and substance abuse problems. Conversely, EAPs have done little else in the way of controlling actual behavioral health care costs. Companies have responded by contracting with MBC vendors to check the rising cost of care. Managed behavioral care programs aggressively oversee mental health care in order to contain costs, while continuing to coordinate all facets of client treatment. Unfortunately, clients often have not been satisfied with restrictions to higher levels of care. Huge profits realized by MBCs over the last decade are suspect and may occur at the expense of effective treatment of the employee. The amicable solution would be for the EAP and MBC to cooperate and perform those functions in which they have the greatest expertise. This integrated partnership would enhance the qualities of both programs, while ultimately benefiting all areas of the work organization.

Winegar (1996) proposes three models for creation of enhanced EAPs with different managed care components. All three models also provide indirect services in the areas of policy development, consultation and statistical reporting, training, and awareness activities. The models are listed with direct client services as follows:

1. A managed care EAP with a network
   a. Self/supervisor/others identify client.
   b. EAP staff verify eligibility.
   c. EAP staff assess client.
   d. EAP staff educate client about benefits.
   e. EAP staff refer client to a participating network provider (formal arrangement may include acceptance of discounted fees).
   f. Benefit design provides a financial incentive for clients to use the network provider. Selection of out-of-network-providers is still a cov-

ered benefit. Incentives to the client to use in-network-providers may include: lower or no copayment, no claim forms to complete, richer benefits with in-network-providers, and broader selection of providers.
   g. EAP staff provide follow-up, monitoring, and coordination with supervisor (if needed).

2. A managed care EAP with an extended treatment component, plus a network
   a. Self/Supervisor/Others identify client.
   b. EAP staff verify eligibility.
   c. EAP staff assess client.
   d. EAP staff educate client about benefits.
   e. EAP staff clinicians provide direct treatment services to an eight-visit limit. If the need exists for further services after the eighth visit, the client is referred into the Network.
   f. Benefit design encourages the client to use the EAP clinician (i.e., there is no cost to the employee as these services have been prepaid by the employer).

3. A managed care EAP with concurrent review functions
   a. Self/Supervisor/Others identify client.
   b. EAP staff verify eligibility.
   c. EAP staff assess client.
   d. All clients must be assessed by EAP staff in order to access benefits.
   e. EAP staff educate client about benefits.
   f. EAP staff refer client to in-network-provider network (client may opt for out-of-network-provider with inherent disincentives).
   g. EAP staff authorize treatment, forward authorization to provider, and perform claims payment function.
   h. EAP staff precertify admissions on a 24-hour basis.
   i. EAP staff provide concurrent review of hospital admissions and of outpatient care.
   j. Benefit design encourages the client to use the EAP network provider.
   k. Claims function pays providers based on EAP authorization (out-of-network benefits/claims payment may be made through this operation as well).
   l. EAP staff monitor treatment, provide follow-up, coordinate with supervisor (if needed).

EAPs are valued elements in the workplace today. Their effectiveness has repeatedly been proven in reducing absenteeism, detecting substance abuse, and dealing with employee problems that can impact job performance. The EAP field continues to evolve and an enormous opportunity exists to increase its utility to organizations. Since EAPs have expertise about employee mental health problems that affect the workplace, the addition of an MBC component to the EAP will further ensure appropriate treatment and referral to maintain a healthy workforce.

Employee assistance practitioners have lost touch with the task of serving multiple clients. Because they are focused on providing the best treatment available to employees, EAPs have willingly relinquished mental health cost containment functions to separate managed behavioral care vendors. Now MBCs are absorbing EAPs at a record pace, much like they did with not-for-profit hospitals in the past, in order to eliminate other competitors from the market. The challenge for EAPs will be to incorporate managed care elements into their practice or face extinction. Employees, who have retained their jobs because of EAP interventions, hope their futures do not rely solely on the decisions of megamerger MBCs. EAPs should not abdicate their responsibility to provide the highest quality of workplace services and, therefore, should actively seek ways to include the MBC component into their programs.

EAPs and Employee Stress

Employee stress and stress management are addressed in detail elsewhere in this book. Responsibility for stress management activities may be given to any of a variety of workplace professionals in the areas of EAP, health promotion, medical services, organizational development, or employee relations. For this chapter, the specific question is: What is the unique contribution EAPs can make to stress management?

As part of the process of EAP counseling, EAP counselors learn about specific sources of stress in the workplace and the impact of these stressors on employees. For example, the EAP counselor may talk to a number of employees in the same department who describe stressful supervisory or personnel practices. The EAP may also learn that certain work practices (e.g., self-directed work teams), work technology (e.g., monitoring quantity of data entry keystrokes), or organizational changes (e.g., department restructuring, layoffs) are particularly stressful. By sharing this information with management (while maintaining the confidentiality of the EAP clients), the EAP can go beyond its usual role of intervening at the individual level by affecting organizational-level sources of stress.

Finally the EAP counselor can develop—in cooperation with health promotion, medical, or employee relations functions—education and support activities regarding sources of stress that are encountered frequently by EAP clients. Frequent topics of such education and support include family issues (e.g., single parenting, coping with teenagers), health issues (e.g., coping with chronic illness), and mental health issues (e.g., adult children of alcoholics).

INTEGRATING EAPs, HEALTH PROMOTION, AND EMPLOYEE WELL-BEING

Like all fields of study, the fields of employee assistance and health promotion have created boundaries for their respective disciplines. EAPs are designed to help employees resolve personal problems such as chemical dependency, emotional problems, or family conflicts that may affect the workplace. Health promotion programs in the workplace are designed to help employees adopt healthy lifestyles, such as regular exercise, prudent diet, and stress management coping skills. These help reduce the risk for disease and enhance the ability to achieve at work and at home. While such boundaries facilitate the development of a discipline, these same boundaries can also interfere with or distort the delivery of services to clients who experience their well-being in a holistic rather than a segmented fashion.

For example, employees who are abusing alcohol and having family problems may be the same employees who are smoking and are overweight. When EAP and health promotion activities are separate programs, these employees need to decide which program to enter if they want to improve their well-being. (Employees who are taking their first steps toward enhancing their health rarely enter both programs at the same time). If they choose to start with losing weight and/or stopping smoking, they are unlikely to be successful. Their alcohol abuse will interfere with dietary changes, and their family problems will continue to generate stress, which makes smoking cessation more difficult. On the other hand, if the employees decide that they want to enter the EAP first, they have to overcome the stigma that is frequently associated with EAPs (especially with those EAPs that are perceived by employees as "the alcohol and drug program" rather than as a broadbrush EAP) but not with health promotion. Given the fact that the vast majority of employees who are struggling with serious personal problems never go to the EAP, this stigma apparently creates a hurdle that many employees cannot surmount.

Thus the boundaries that separate EAP and health promotion, and that serve the needs of each area as a professional discipline, can interfere with the clients of each discipline getting the help they actually need. It should be further pointed out that these boundaries also exclude the large portion of employees who fall into the middle ground between these two disciplines—those employees who are fatigued, moderately anxious or depressed, moderately overweight, drinking more alcohol than they should, etc., who do not have personal problems "serious" enough for EAP or health problems that fit the traditional categories of health promotion. When these employees want to improve their well-being, neither EAP nor health promotion seem to fit the bill.

How can we make sure that the boundaries between disciplines do not get in the way of employees receiving the proper health service? One way is to make sure that EAP and health promotion practitioners know enough about each other's fields in order to assess, educate, and refer employees who could benefit by receiving services from the other provider. For example, nutrition and weight-loss programs should include education and assessment regarding eating disorders. The instructor should be able to confidently refer to EAP any participants affected by these disorders. Similarly, smoking cessation programs should address other addictive behav-

iors (e.g., alcohol and drug addiction, gambling addiction, work addiction); stress management programs should address alcohol and drug use as attempts to cope with stress; and hypertension screening programs should address the role of alcohol use in hypertension (Carey, 1987).

Just as health promotion professionals can and should refer employees to EAP, referrals should also go in the other direction. For example, when employees are recovering from chemical dependency, it is important to replace old behaviors that were associated with the addiction (e.g., drinking in the bar; hanging out with drug-using friends) with new behaviors that support healthy living. While attending a chemical dependency support group is the primary avenue for filling this need, participating in fitness, nutrition, stress management, or smoking cessation activities can provide additional opportunities for joining with others in a health-oriented setting. Behavior change activities can, of course, be stressful. Thus the EAP counselor must use good judgment before recommending such activities for employees who are early in recovery (Metz, Miller, & Winchester, 1991).

The boundaries of EAP and health promotion (see Table 16-8) have traditionally focused EAP upon the treatment of mental health and substance abuse problems and health promotion upon the prevention of physical problems. These categories do not include the prevention of mental health and substance abuse problems nor the treatment of physical problems. The latter category fits into the area of medical services. Just as with EAP and health promotion, providers of medical services should be able to confidently assess, educate, and refer employees to EAP and health promotion as appropriate and vice versa. Again it is the responsibility of the health professionals, not the client, to have an integrated understanding of the various providers of health services so that

Table 16-8 The Boundaries of Health Services

	Prevention	Treatment
Physical well-being:	health promotion	medical
Mental well-being:	??	EAP

the client will receive the proper services regardless of which service he/she initially contacts.

The prevention of mental health and substance abuse problems currently falls in between traditional EAP and health promotion. One example of such a service is stress management—a preventive mental health issue that affects physical well-being. Other activities that fall into this category include substance abuse education, education regarding depression, and coping with change and loss. The whole area of work-family issues (e.g., child care, parenting, elderly parents), while becoming a discipline in its own right, can also be seen as a mental health prevention activity. Both EAP and health promotion professionals are starting to address these issues, and both bring their own strengths and limitations to the endeavor. EAP professionals often have content expertise in these areas but little experience in implementing primary prevention activities. Health promotion professionals are experienced in primary prevention but may have minimal content expertise.

While having EAP and health promotion programs refer to each other is one approach to overcoming the problem of discipline boundaries, another approach is to have the EAP and health promotion activities integrated into a single program. The advantages of such integration would include ensuring that employees receive proper service throughout the entire course of their health activities, destigmatizing the EAP service, increasing the likelihood of addressing those employees and those concerns that fall in between EAP and health promotion, enhancing crossover program promotion, and addressing workplace environmental and cultural issues in a more effective fashion (Shain, Suurvali, & Boutilier, 1986).

Ford Motor Company's Total Health Program is an example of a program that has taken a step in this direction. In the Total Health Program the EAP counselors are "Total Health Counselors" and are positioned to respond to any personal, health, or lifestyle concern. In this way, employees do not need to decide ahead of time whether their concern should go to EAP or health promotion (Vaccaro, 1991).

The potential integration of EAP and health promotion brings into focus a basic difference in approaches between these two disciplines. EAP is gen-

erally prescriptive in its approach (i.e., assessing a problem and prescribing a course of action). Health promotion has generally avoided this medical model, favoring instead a "public health" approach that encourages education and self-responsibility. One example of combining these approaches in the areas of smoking cessation and weight loss offered a broad array of public health (e.g., wellness screening, health information, and health education classes) and medical model (e.g., personalized one-on-one counseling) interventions. This study found that offering this wide array of interventions greatly increased employee participation rates (Erfurt, Foote, Heirich, & Gregg, 1990).

Just as integrating EAP and health promotion can create a beneficial synergy, integrating EAP and health promotion into the traditional corporate occupational health and safety arena (e.g., medical, industrial hygiene, safety)—as has been done with the Live for Life Program® at Johnson & Johnson (Desmond, 1987)—can have a similar effect. In this program, the EAP is part of the fleet accident review board, nurses are trained to identify and refer to EAP mental health and substance abuse problems, and all areas participate together in health fairs, employee orientations, and management training programs.

A different approach to integrating EAP and health promotion under a broader umbrella is what has been called employee assistance services. In this conceptual model, EAP and health promotion would be joined with medical services, family and child activities, legal/financial activities, and job counseling/career development. By recognizing that each of these disciplines is independent yet connected under a broad umbrella, no single discipline is overwhelmed by taking on activities outside of its area of expertise, yet opportunities for integration and synergy can also be pursued (Lanier, 1991).

CONCLUSION

Employee assistance programs have made significant inroads into the American workforce. They are now considered an essential component of the human resources management function by most larger employers in the private and public sectors alike. However, there is still considerable room for growth both in service delivery and outcomes measures.

The EAP field continues to expand. In keeping with the trend toward downsizing and outsourcing, many larger employers who once had internal programs have now shifted to an external program. Employee assistance programs are also being promoted to the small employer in the form of EAP consortiums in which employers in similar industries or close geographic proximity to each other pool their resources and contract with an EAP vendor for services. The Small Business Administration has also recently made funds available to promote drug-free workplaces and to educate employers on how to best manage this problem through education, drug testing, and implementation of EAPs.

EAPs now offer a range of "value added" services that extend well beyond the essential core components. Those discussed here include integrated managed behavioral health care and critical incident stress debriefing. Growth areas are in disability management, services to expatriates, organizational change, and corporate coaching. Many EAPs have also been integrated with employee health and safety programs. While giving the EAP a wider berth to deliver a broader range of services, concerns remain in their ability to continue to show value at the bottom line. Quantitative studies to date are lacking, and qualitative studies are practically non-existent.

While EAPs have matured in their development of workplace service delivery, they still appear to be in their infancy in demonstrating their significance and impact for change from a statistical perspective. This will continue to be their challenge in the foreseeable future.

References

Albelda, R. (1999). What welfare reform has wrought. In *Dollars and Sense.* January/February.

American Civil Liberties Union. (1996). *Briefing paper number 5: Drug testing in the workplace.* [On-line]. Available: http://www.aclu.org/library/pbr5.num.

Backer, T., & O'Hara, K. (1991). *Organizational change and drug-free workplaces: Templates for success.* New York: Quorum Books.

Bengen-Seltzer, B. (1995, June). Assessing cost and quality in behavioral health care. *Medicine and Health.*

Blair, B. (1995, March). Serving multiple clients. *Employee Assistance,* 16–18.

Blair, B. R.. 1987a. Internal & external models. In *The EAP Solution: Current Trends and Future Issues,* edited by J. Spicer. Center City, MN: Hazelden Foundation.

_____. 1987b. *Supervisors and managers as enablers.* Rev. ed. Minneapolis, MN: Johnson Institute.

_____. 1991. The *supervisors role in early recovery.* Rev. ed. Minneapolis, MN: Johnson Institute.

Blum, T. C., and P. M. Roman. 1987. Internal vs. external EAPs. in *Employee Assistance Programs: Benefits, Problems and Prospects* Washington, DC: Bureau of National Affairs.

Blum, T., Fields, D., Milne, S., & Spell, C. (1992). Workplace drug testing programs: A review of research and a survey of worksites. *Employee Assistance Research,* 1(2), 315–319.

Bruhnsen, K., and L. DuBuc. 1988. A first-year cost-benefit analysis of the University of Michigan Medical Center EAP. *The ALMACAN* 18:28–30.

Bureau of National Affairs, Inc. 1987. *Employee Assistance Programs: Benefits, problems and prospects.* Washington, DC.

Buckley, R. (1995). Trucks, buses, and DOT: New markets for EAPs. *EAPA Exchange,* 25(9), 32–35.

Carey, P. 1987. Views of the experts. In *Employee Assistance Programs: Benefits, Problems and Prospects.* Washington, DC: Bureau of National Affairs.

Comer, D. (1995, August 15). *An evaluation of fitness for duty testing.* Paper presented at the 103rd Annual Convention of the American Psychological Association, New York, NY. [On-line]. Available: http://www.lindesmith.org/ tlcomer.html.

Contin, D., & Burton, W. (1995, July/August). The cost of depression in the workplace. *Behavioral Health Care Tomorrow.*

DeLancey, M. (1994). *Does drug testing work?* (2nd ed.). Washington, DC: Institute for a Drug-Free Workplace.

Desmond, T. C. 1987. An internal broadbrush program: Johnson & Johnson's Live for Life® assistance program. In *the EAP Solution: Current Trends and Future Issues,* edited by J. Spicer. Center City, MN.: Hazelden Foundation.

Durkin, W. G. 1985. Evaluation of EAP programming. In *The Human Resource*

Management Handbook. Edited by S. H. Klarreich, J. L. Francek, & C. E. Moore. New York: Praeger.

Employee Assistance Professionals Association, Inc. 1992. *EAPA standards for employee assistance programs, Part II: Professional guidelines.* Arlington, VA.

Erfurt, J. C. A. Foote, M. A. Heirich, and W. Gregg. 1990. Improving participation in worksite wellness programs: Comparing health education classes, a menu approach, and follow-up counseling. *American Journal of Health Promotion,* 4:270–78.

Gilliom, J. (1994). *Surveillance, privacy, and the law: Employee drug testing and the politics of social control.* Ann Arbor, MI: The University of Michigan Press.

Googins, B. 1989. Revisiting the role of the supervisor in Employee Assistance Programs. In *Drugs in the Workplace: Research and Evaluation Data,* edited by S. W. Gust and J. M. Walsh. Rockville, MD: National Institute on Drug Abuse.

Grinstein, G., & Oliver, W. (1994, January/February). EAPs and drug testing. *Employee Assistance, 91,* 32–36.

Gust, S. W., and J. M. Walsh. (1989). Research on the prevalence, impact, and treatment of drug abuse in the workplace. In *Drugs in the Workplace: Research and Evaluation Data,* edited by S. W. Gust, and J. M. Walsh. Rockville, MD: National Institute on Drug Abuse.

Hanson, A. (1990). What employees say about drug testing. *Personnel, 67*(7), 32–36.

Hanson, M. (1993). Serving the substance abuser in the workplace. In P. Kurzman, & S. Akabas (Eds.), *Work and well being* (pp. 218–232). Washington, DC: NASW Press.

Hooks, J. M. and S. Weinstein, eds. 1991. *An emerging paradigm: EAPs and the new American workforce.* Arlington, VA: Employee Assistance Professionals Association, Inc.

The impact of behavioral healthcare on productivity: A look at employer and employee attitudes. (1995, July 30) *Medical Benefits,* newsletter.

Institute for a Drug Free Workplace. (Washington, DC, 1994). Does drug testing work? (2nd ed.).

Jones, D. 1987. Evaluation. In *The EAP Solution Current Trends and Future Issues,* edited by J. Spicer. Center City, MN: Hazelden Foundation.

Judge, W. (1993). Drug testing: The legal framework. In R. Wright, & D. Wright (Eds.), *Creating and maintaining the drug-free workforce.* Westminster, MD: Recovery Communications.

Judge, W. (1995). Testing policy for labor officials. *Employee Assistance, 8*(1), 16–23.

Kouzis, A. (1994, August). Emotional disability days: Prevalence predictors. *American Journal of Public Health.*

Kurtz, N. R., B. Googins, and W. C. Howard. 1984. Measuring the success of occupational alcoholism programs. *Journal of Studies on alcohol,* 45:33–45.

Lanier, D. 1991. Work/family programming rests comfortably under the employee assistance services (EAS) umbrella. *Exchange* 6:20–21.

Lechnyr, R. (1993). The cost savings of mental health services. *EAP Digest, 14*(1), 22–26, 43.

Maiden, R. P. (1999). Welfare to work: New opportunities for EAPs —Increased risk for employers. Paper presented at the annual national conference of the Employee Assistance Professionals Association, Orlando, FL.

Masi, D. A. (1994). *Evaluating your employee assistance and managed behavioral care program.* Troy, MI: Performance Resource Press, newsletter.

Masi, D. A., Jacobson, J. M., & Cooper, A. R. (2000). Quantifying quality: Findings from clinical reviews. *Employee Assistance Quarterly.* 15(4) 1–17.

Mastrich, J., and B. Beidel. 1987. Employee Assistance Programs cost-impact. *The ALMACAN,* 17:34–47.

Maynard, J. 1990. The Q.A. audit. *Exchange,* 20: 44–47.

Mesaro, E. (1995, October). Skies overcast, therapies variable. *Managed Healthcare.*

Metz, G. J., R. E. Miller, and K. Winchester. 1991. Relapse and 'the missing sound of birds.' *EAP Digest,* 5:21–24.

Mitchell, J., & Everly, G. (1993). *Critical Incident Stress Debriefing (CISD).* Ellicot City, MD: Chevron Publishing.

Molloy, D. J. 1985. Peer referral: A programmatic and administrative review. In *The Human Resources Management Handbook,* edited by S. H. Klarreich, J. L. Francek, and C. E. Moore. New York: Praeger.

Nadolski, J. N. and C. E. Sandonato. 1987. Evaluation of an Employee Assistance Program. *Journal of Occupational Medicine,* 29:32–37.

National Institute on Alcoholism and Alcohol Abuse. (1995, March 17). Press release.

National Institute on Drug Abuse. (1995). *National household survey on drug abuse: 1993 population estimates.* Washington, DC: Government Printing Office.

Nye, S. (1990). *Employee assistance law answer book.* New York: Panel Publishers.

Plaggemars, D. (in press). Critical incident stress debriefing applications: A look ahead, *Employee Assistance Quarterly.*

Plant, T. 1987. Managing EAP services. In *The EAP Solution: Current Trends and Future Issues,* edited by J. Spicer. Center City, MN: Hazelden Foundation.

Rathus, S., Nevid, J., & Fichner-Rathus, L. (1997). *Human sexuality in a world of diversity* (3rd ed). New York: Allyn-Bacon.

Rivard, J. M. 1990. Operation RedBlock. *EAP Digest,* 10:60–62.

Robbins, R., Gerson, S., & Moore, N. (1992, August). The cooperation of EA and managed care programs. *Employee Assistance,* 13–16, 37.

Roman, P. M., & Blum, T. C. (1988, August). The core technology of employee assistance programs: A reaffirmation. *The ALMACAN,* 17–22.

Scanlon, W. F. 1991. *Alcoholism and drug abuse in the workplace: Managing care and cost through employee assistance programs.* 2nd ed. New York: Praeger Publishers.

Selvik, R. 1987. Selecting and monitoring referents. In *The EAP Solution: Current Trends and Future Issues,* edited by J. Spicer. Center City, MN: Hazelden Foundation.

Shain, M., H. Suurvali, and M. Boutilier. 1986. *Healthier workers: Health promotion and Employee Assistance Programs,* Lexington, MA: Lexington Books.

Shirley, C. E. 1985. TOPEX study: Hitting bottom in high places. In *The Human Resources Management Handbook,* edited by S. H. Klarreich, J. L. Francek, and C. E. Moore. New York: Praeger.

Smits, S. J., & Pace, L. A. (1992). *The investment approach to employee assistance programs.* Westport, CT: Quorum Books.

Smollen, E. 1991. Facing the facts: Dealing with cultural diversity in the workplace. *Employee Assistance* 4:8–13.

Sonnenstuhl, W. J., and H. M. Trice. 1988. Peers in the tunnels: A union's solution to problem drinking. *The ALMACAN* 8:13–16.

Spicer, J., P. Owen, and M. Gjerdingen. 1990. Practical evaluation methods. *Exchange* 20:25–28.

Swotinsky, R. (1992). *The medical review officer's guide to drug testing.* New York: Van Nostrand Reinhold.

Thompson, R., Jr. 1990. *Substance abuse and employee rehabilitation.* Washington, DC: Bureau of National Affairs, Inc.

Tolnai, E. A. (1996). Navigating health care reform: Prevention in managed care. *Prevention Forum,* 16(2), 6–10.

Tompkins, C. P. (1991). Drug abuse among workers and Employee Assistance Programs. In *Background Papers on Drug Abuse Financing and Services Research.* Rockville, MD: National Institute on Drug Abuse.

Trice, H. M., and W. J. Sonnenstuhl. 1986. *Strategies for employee assistance programs: The crucial balance.* Ithaca, NY: ILR Press.

Turner, S. 1985. Assessment/referral. In *The Human Resources Management Handbook,* edited by S. H. Klarreich, J. L. Francek, and C. E. Moore. New York: Praeger.

Unscheduled absence survey. (1995, August 28). *Human Resources Management Ideas and Trends in Personnel,* 354–56.

U.S. Department of Health and Human Services. (1995). National household survey on drug abuse. Washington, DC: USOHHS-SUMSHA.

Vaccaro, V. A. 1991. *Depression: Corporate experiences and innovations.* Washington, DC: Washington Business Group on Health.

Walker, P. L. 1991. The glass ceiling: Breaking through the invisible barrier holding back many women. *Employee Assistance* 4:14–26.

Walsh, D. C., R. W. Hingson, D. M. Merrigan, S. M. Levenson, L. A. Rupples, T. H. Eccren, G. A. Coffman, C. A. Becker, T. A. Barker, and S. K. Hamilton. 1991. A randomized trial of treatment options for alcohol-abusing workers. *New England Journal of Medicine* 325:775–82.

Willette, R., & Kadehjian, L. (1992). Drug testing in the workplace. In R. Swotinsky (Ed.), *The medical review officer's guide to drug testing.* New York: Van Nostrand Reinhold.

Winegar, N. (1996). *The clinician's guide to managed behavioral care* (2nd ed.). New York: The Haworth Press.

Worker absence posts fourth annual rise. (1995, August 30) *Medical Benefits* newsletter.

Yandrick, R. M. 1992. Taking inventory. *EAPA Exchange* 22:22–29.

Young, N. K., & Gardner, S. L. (1997). *Implementing welfare reform: Solutions to the substance abuse problem.* Washington, DC: Drug Strategies.

CHAPTER

17

Social Health in the Workplace

Kenneth R. McLeroy, Nell H. Gottlieb,
and Catherine A. Heaney

INTRODUCTION

Social well-being was included along with physical and mental well-being in the definition of health in the constitution of the World Health Organization (1947). Early definitions of social health focused on the integration of the individual into the community, including participation in community activities, conformity to social norms or standards, and adequate performance of social roles (such as parent or employee). More recent definitions of social health, and definitions that will be used throughout this chapter, have included three key aspects of social relationships as they affect health status (House, Umberson, & Landis, 1988):

1. **Social integration or involvement**—refers to the existence or quantity of social relationships individuals have with others, such as the number of social contacts or the presence of specific types of relationships (including marriage, friendships, or organizational membership)

2. **Social support**—refers to the functional content of social relationships, such as emotional or affective support received from others

3. **Social networks**—refers to the structure of the relationships and ties that exist between individuals and others in their social environment.

When referring to all three aspects of social health, we will use the term **social participation.**

The importance of social participation in health promotion programming is that social relationships provide modeling for lifestyle health behavior. They also provide constraints or controls on behavior that may be direct (e.g., prescription or proscription of behavior) or indirect (e.g., conformity with social norms). For example, religious involvement may preclude use of alcohol or tobacco or may prescribe dietary patterns; marriage and parenthood may induce an individual to reduce risk-taking behavior through a sense of responsibility to the family. Social relationships are an important source of information and regulation related to health care seeking. They provide a sense of meaning and purpose to life and provide much of our sense of social identity—who we are and what we are about (Antonovsky, 1984).

Social relationships may provide important resources for changing behavior and dealing with life crises, such as coping with illnesses, job loss, or geographical relocation.

Membership in formal and informal organizations is part of individuals' participation in the larger society and may serve an important mediating role by linking individuals to the broader communities in which they reside. Thus church attendance, close affective relationships, and norms for marriage, family, and friendship provide a cognitive map for behavior, a sense of belonging in the world, and a means of participating in the larger society (House, Umberson, 1988; Putnam, 2000; Umberson, 1992).

In this chapter we cover four major social health topics. First, we briefly review some of the research evidence for the effects of social participation on the health of individuals, including research studies on the effects of social participation on mental and physical health, the importance of social support, and the use of social health as an outcome of health-related interventions. Second, we address the context within which social support occurs. Specifically, we relate the types of support individuals receive from others to the relationships that most individuals have with family, neighbors, coworkers, friends, confidants, and others. Moreover we associate types of relationships to the organizations to which individuals belong, including worksites, churches, voluntary organizations, and other informal and formal social groups. Third, we describe the previous uses of social relationships for health promotion program planning, strategies, and evaluation. Finally, we discuss ethical and policy issues in using social relationships for worksite health promotion.

The promotion of social health has not been an integral part of worksite health promotion, and social health was not included in the first edition of this book. However, we believe that the worksite offers unique, largely untapped opportunities to enhance the social health of employees and their networks. To date, worksite health promotion programs have typically concentrated on social support in the context of behavior change. For example, self-help groups for smoking cessation and weight management focus first on initial behavior change and then on maintenance. Contracts are made between "buddies" for program participation and the achievement of specific behavioral goals. Teams participate in competitions to provide motivation and incentives for exercise, weight loss, and smoking outcomes (e.g., Brownell & Felix, 1987; Ewart, 1991; Gottlieb & Nelson, 1990). In general the focus has been on social ties as a mechanism for behavioral risk reduction, acting as a direct impact on physical health for the individual. Little, if any, attention has been placed on the enhancement of social health as an end in itself or as a buffer to environmental stressors.

However, there are often other activities within the organization that address, overtly or indirectly, social health. With increasing numbers of women (including single parents) in the labor force, family concerns have become a business issue (Carlson & Perrewe, 1999; Rodgers & Rodgers, 1989). Education, resources, and referral for care for dependants (both children and aging parents) are provided by many companies. Preretirement planning and relocation services offer assistance to employees to cope with disrupted social networks (Behrens, 1990; Starker, 1990). Education on the importance of social support and strategies for developing new relationships and adapting existing ties to the new situation is crucial but often overlooked, with the emphasis remaining on changes in benefits and work routines. Total quality management, an important force in United States industry today, includes an emphasis on functioning teams, improved communications, and empowered employees who are active participants in their work community (Juran, 1988; Lawler, 1986; Lawler, Mohrman, & Ledford, 1992). It is the challenge of a comprehensive worksite health promotion program to link together these efforts conducted within a variety of departments and to redirect and enhance them as necessary in order to have a coherent and synergistic intervention to improve employee social health.

SOCIAL PARTICIPATION, SOCIAL RELATIONSHIPS, AND HEALTH

Social participation can have both direct and indirect effects on physical and mental health and may serve as an indicator of quality of life in studying the effects of health-related interventions. The direct effects of social participation on health include studies linking the nature and extent of individuals' social relationships at one period of time to the risk of dying in subsequent years. Indirect effects of social participation on health include the effects of social support in moderating the effects of life changes or life strains on physical and mental health, so that individuals with strong social relationships do not experience as many stress-induced illnesses as those with weaker social relationships. As a critical component of quality of life, social participation is important in and of itself and may be used as a measure of the effectiveness of health-related interventions.

Direct Effects of Social Participation on Health

Several longitudinal studies have examined the direct effects of social participation on mortality and longevity (Berkman, 1995). Longitudinal studies are particularly important since they are better than cross-sectional studies or other designs in establishing causal direction and may elucidate the processes through which social participation affects health. These studies typically use measures of social participation as independent variables and study their potential effects over time on measures of health status. The following section will briefly review the findings from four of these studies.

In Alameda County, California, marriage, contacts with extended family and friends, church membership, and other group affiliations measured among 2,229 men and 2,496 women in 1965 predicted mortality in the following nine years. The independent effects of marriage and contact with family and friends were stronger than were those of church and other group membership. Independent of their physical health, socioeconomic status, lifestyle health behavior, race, life satisfaction, and use of preventive health services (all self-reported in 1965), men and women with few social ties were over twice as likely to die during the following nine years. This increase in risk was found for death from ischemic heart disease, cancer, stroke, circulatory diseases, and all other causes of death, as well as for mortality from all causes (Berkman & Syme, 1979).

Similar findings were obtained in the Tecumseh, Michigan, Community Health Study. Intimate social relationships, formal organizational involvements outside of work, and active leisure pursuits involving social contact were measured in 1,322 men and 1,432 women as part of an initial interview and physical examination in 1967–1969. An index of these social relationships was inversely related to mortality through 1979, independent of age and biomedically-assessed and self-reported risk factors of mortality. The effect of social relationships on mortality was stronger for men than for women (House, Robbins, & Metzner, 1982).

During a 30-month follow-up period of a study of 331 older adults in Durham, North Carolina, researchers found—after adjusting for baseline risk factors—an increase in mortality among those with a low frequency of interaction with friends and relatives. Persons with low perceived social support, including loneliness and lack of someone in whom to trust and confide, were over three times as likely to die in the long-term follow-up period as their peers with high perceived support (Blazer, 1982). These findings were replicated in a long-term (10-to 12-year) follow-up of older adults in Georgia (Schoenbach, Kaplan, Fredman, & Kleinbaum, 1986).

In a recent study of 726 African-American elderly women, severe social isolation (i.e., living alone and not having had contact with family or friends during the last two weeks) was related to a three-fold increase in the likelihood of dying within five years of the initial interview. In addition, the use of community-based senior support services (such as assistance with meal preparation and bathing) was not related to subsequent mortality (LaVeist, Sellers, Elliott Brown, & Nickerson, 1997). The authors suggested that such services could buffer against the effects of extreme isolation on mortality, but they could not empirically test this hypothesis. Thus, the extent to which formal services can replace informal support systems for this vulnerable population remains unknown.

In addition to the longitudinal studies, a substantial number of cross-sectional and retrospective studies of social participation, social support, and health have been conducted. For example, the Medline bibliographic database lists 3600 articles published from 1997 to 2000 on social support and social networks.

Since many of these studies have been previously reviewed by other authors (Berkman, 1995; Heaney & Israel, 1997; House, et al., 1988; Israel, 1982; Suls, 1982), no attempt will be made to provide an in-depth review of specific studies. Several generalizations may be drawn from the recent reviews (Berkman, 1995; Israel & Rounds, 1987; House, et al., 1988; Shumaker & Hill, 1991). First, the impact of social relationships on physical health is nonspecific and is related to all-cause mortality rather than to certain specific causes of death. Second, risk of dying is increased with very low levels of social relationships (social isolation); levels of social support above a moderate threshold make little difference. Third, the impact of social interaction on health varies with community size and with gender. The relationship between social interaction and mortality is stronger in urban than in rural areas, where social relationships may be more pervasive. In general, the risk ratios are stronger for men than for women.

Indirect Effects of Social Participation on Health

Not only may social participation affect health directly, but specific aspects of social participation—such as social support—may affect health only under specific conditions, such as exposure to life changes or other potentially stressful events. In studies of the indirect effects of social participation on health, researchers typically use measures of stress or exposure to specific stressors as independent measures, social support is treated as an effect modifier, and health outcomes are the dependent variables. For example, psychosocial resources—including ego strength, qualities of marriage, relationships with extended family members, friendship patterns, and feelings about the pregnancy—were found to be related to complications of pregnancy in 26 of 170 army wives experiencing high life stress prior to delivering at a military hospital. Stressed women with strong psychosocial resources were less likely to experience complications than those with weak resources. Psychosocial assets, however, had no effect on the pregnancy outcomes of those women who had not experienced a high degree of life stress (Nuckolls, Cassel, & Kaplan 1972).

When studying the indirect effects of social participation on health, researchers typically use measures of social support. Social support refers to the types of support individuals receive, or perceive as having available to them, from the interpersonal relationships in which they are involved. Israel (1982), for example, has included five types of support that may be received through interpersonal relationships: affective support, instrumental support, cognitive support, maintenance of social identity, and social outreach. Affective or emotional support provides comfort to a person, including the feeling that he or she is cared for, loved, valued, and respected. Instrumental aid or material support refers to goods and services, such as a loan of money, food, or child care assistance, that help solve practical problems. Cognitive support includes information and advice that help a person develop an understanding for his or her world and adjust to changes in it. Maintenance of social identity includes validation of a shared worldview through feedback about behavior. Social outreach is access to social contacts and roles (Israel, 1982; Jacobson, 1986).

A considerable number of studies have examined the role of social support in mitigating the effects of both specific and global stresses and strains on physical and mental health and in adaptation to physical illnesses (Cohen & Wills, 1985). For example, social support has been found to buffer the effects of job-related stress (Holt, 1982), to assist in coping with widowhood and divorce (Minkler, 1985), and to reduce the psychological and physical effects of job loss (Kasl & Wells, 1985). In addition, social support has been associated with successful coping with chronic and acute life-threatening illness (Singer & Lord, 1984) and may mitigate the effects of life's routine stresses and strains (Lazarus & Folkman, 1984). Many of these studies have been previously reviewed (Brownell & Shumaker, 1984, 1985; Cohen & Syme, 1985; House, et al., 1988), with some of the reviews suggesting that the evidence for the buffering effect of social support is too inconsistent to be conclusive (Beehr, 1995; Kahn & Byosiere, 1992). However, a few of the studies will be presented for illustrative purposes.

In a study of the process of coping with job loss, Gore (1978) followed 100 employees of two plants that were closed down—one plant in a large city and one plant in a small rural town. During the five interview periods—six weeks before plant closings, one month after the closing, six months after the plant closings, and at one and two years after the closing—she collected information on social support, including support from wife, friends, and relatives; frequency of activity outside the home; and opportunities to talk about their problems. In addition she collected information on depression, self-blame, illness symptoms, and serum cholesterol. In general the results of her study were consistent with an indirect, stress-buffering model of social support. Among those who were promptly able to secure employment, social support had little effect. However, among those with longer, more severe unemployment, social support had a positive effect on anxiety, tension, and economic insecurity. Moreover, serum cholesterol levels dropped over the two-year period for all of the sample except those who remained unemployed and reported low levels of social support.

While they did not measure social support directly, similar results were obtained in a study of General Motors plant closings in Michigan between 1986 and 1990. Hamilton, Broman, Hoffman, and Renner (1990) interviewed 1,597 workers at four plants to be closed and 12 comparison plants expected to remain open. In general, distress was higher among women and unmarried workers. More important, among workers laid off or anticipating layoff, those with fewer social

resources—lower social class, lower income, and lower education—reported more depression and anxiety.

In an Israeli prospective study of ischemic heart disease with approximately 10,000 adult males, individuals with psychosocial problems were at increased risk of developing angina pectoris during a five-year period (Medalie et al., 1973). Moreover, during the five-year follow-up, when anxiety was low, perceptions of wife's love and support were not associated with angina. However, when anxiety was high, those who reported not having their wive's love and support were almost twice as likely to develop angina than men with their wife's love and support.

Social support interventions have also been used to increase individuals' ability to deal with life crises (Gottlieb, 1988). In a study in Guatemala City, Guatemala, for example, 40 pregnant women at a hospital for delivery were randomly assigned to treatment and control groups. The treatment group received constant support from lay women from admission to delivery in the hospital. Since hospital routines called for pregnant women to deliver alone, the control group went through the normal delivery process without supportive partners. The length of delivery in the treatment group was 8.7 hours, compared to 19.3 hours for women in the control group (Sosa, Kennel, & Klaus, 1980).

Figure 17-1, adapted from the work of Lazarus and Folkman (1984) and Gore (1985), provides a conceptual overview of the processes through which social

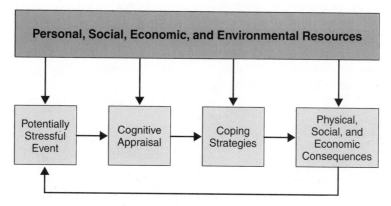

Figure 17-1 This coping-process model provides a conceptual overview of the processes through which social support may mitigate the effects of life stress.

support may mitigate the effects of life stress. In the model, individuals are exposed to potentially stressful events. An individual's cognitive appraisal of the nature and extent of the threat is a key element in determining which coping strategies are adopted. The specific coping strategies that are adopted and the nature of the threat may have physical, social, or economic consequences. The physical, social, and economic consequences of a potentially stressful event and subsequent coping strategies that are used may in turn also be stressful.

Social support may mitigate the effects of potentially stressful life events or circumstances through the following mechanisms. At the psychological level, social support may affect an individual's perceptions of the meaning and extent of threat from potentially stressful life events. Whether an individual appraises a stressful situation as being personally harmful and whether that person believes he/she has the resources available to master the situation are influenced by observing the reactions of others who are exposed to the stressor. The latter appraisal is also a function of the availability and accessibility of personal resources and resources available through an individual's social relationships. An individual's ability to deal with his/her emotional reactions to potentially stressful events and the ability to maintain emotional balance in order to effectively deal with a threat are also affected by social support (Gottlieb, 1983).

Different types of support are needed depending on the nature of the threat. For example, the personal, social, and environmental resources needed to cope with job loss may be different from the resources needed to deal with geographic relocation. Moreover, different resources may be required at different stages in the coping process, such as in the anticipation, experience, and aftermath of a stressful event. In general, affective support is needed immediately following a stressful event, while cognitive support and social outreach become important as the individual adapts to the changed situation.

Even relatively successful coping with stressful life events may have important consequences for the individual and his or her intimate social relationships. For example, coping with job loss or divorce fre-

quently requires an individual to mobilize or call on important social contacts and social relationships for various forms of support, including emotional support, information, concrete assistance in dealing with problems, access to persons outside of the individual's immediate social relationships, and affirmation of the individual's social identity. Attempting to mobilize social resources may strain social ties, or the individual may learn that support is not available from specific relationships. These consequences in turn may be stressful and require further adaptation and coping.

As an intervening variable, then, social relationships and social ties—in addition to personal, economic, and environmental resources—may affect each stage in the process of coping with environmental demands or potential stressors. Social relationships may reduce individuals' exposure to potentially stressful events; they may affect how stressful events are appraised, the coping strategies that are employed, and the immediate and long-term consequences of the coping process.

In addition to the psychological processes described above, the physiological mechanisms through which social support affects health and buffers stress are being investigated. A growing area of research, psychoneuroimmunology, is elucidating the links between the availability of supportive relationships and physiological processes such as endocrine function, immune function, and cardiovascular reactivity to stressors (see Uchino, Cacioppo, & Kiecolt-Glaser, 1996, for a review). The effects of social participation on these basic physiological processes have been shown to translate into health outcomes. For example, in one experiment individuals with supportive social ties were less likely to develop a cold after being exposed to the cold virus than were people with fewer, weaker social relationships (Cohen et al., 1997).

Social Health as an Outcome of Health-Related Interventions

Social health may also be used as a dependent measure in studies of health interventions. As an important component of health in the 1947 WHO definition, social health—primarily measured in terms of social participation—is frequently included in studies of the impact of disease and health-related interventions and measures of well-being (Kaplan, 1985; Lohr & Ware, 1987). For example, social health was included in a study of variations in health insurance coverage ad payment systems on health status in the RAND Health Insurance Study (Donald, Ware, Brook, & Davies-Avery, 1978), studies on the impact of dental conditions (Reisine, 1988), studies of aging (Duke University Center for the Study of Aging and Human Development, 1978), and a study of the effects of cataract surgery (Legro, 1992).

Increasingly, social health is being recognized as an important goal and outcome of health promotion efforts. Green and Raeburn (1990), for example, have suggested that **enabling communities**—including families and neighborhoods—should be the central focus of health promotion strategies. The WHO-sponsored healthy cities projects have considered using measures of citizen participation and the interconnectedness of social networks as indicators of community capacity building (Duhl & Hancock, 1988). Wallerstein (1992) and Wallerstein and Bernstein (1988) have suggested community competence and empowerment as an important research outcome of social network and community interventions in health promotion. Minkler (1989) has argued for a broad approach to health promotion based on social system and structural changes in order to create healthy communities. She has contrasted this vision of health promotion with the more narrow behavioral risk reduction focus of health promotion that is the dominant paradigm in the United States today.

Recently, the concept of **social capital** is being applied to studies of health status and health promotion interventions. Robert Putnam, an oft-quoted scholar of social capital, states that "the core idea of social capital theory is that social networks have value" (Putnam, 2000, p. 19). The critical components of social capital are social trust, relationships characterized by reciprocity, cooperation for mutual benefit, and civic engagement. Because of the documented linkages between social capital and health status (e.g., Kawachi, Kennedy, & Glass, 1999), the effects of public health policies and health interventions on social capital should be monitored.

SOCIAL NETWORKS AND SOCIAL SUPPORT

Social health does not occur in a vacuum. As will be described, social health is a function of the extent and types of relationships individuals have with others; the extent of individuals' participation in social activities and social organizations is partially determined by the social environment; and the types and extent of social support that individuals perceive as available, requested, and/or receive is partly a function of the strength and nature of the relationships they have with others. For example, social change—such as industrialization, geographic mobility, and bureaucratization—can disrupt or change the nature of social relationships and weaken individuals' sense of community (Wellman, 1979; Wellman & Leighton, 1979). Participation in social relationships and community organizations is influenced by the communities and neighborhoods in which people live. Specific forms of social support, such as affective or emotional support, are more likely to occur within close interpersonal relationships such as marriage, families, and long-term friendships. Access to new social contacts (social outreach), on the other hand, may under some circumstances occur more often through loose friendships than more intimate relationships. Intensive, long-term instrumental assistance—such as long-term assistance for the disabled elderly—is more likely to be provided by close family members than by friends or neighbors. Short-term, less-intense instrumental assistance is more likely to be provided by friends and neighbors (Fisher, 1982; Gottlieb, 1988; Heinemann, 1985; Pearlin, 1982; Wellman & Leighton, 1979).

Of particular importance to this discussion of social health is the interpersonal context within which social support occurs. Since social support—including affective support, instrumental support, cognitive support, maintenance of social identity, and social outreach—can be thought of as social resources obtained through personal relationships, it is important to understand how these relationships affect and are affected by social support. Social networks provide a useful framework for understanding the interpersonal facts that affect the receipt and provision of social support.

A social network consists of a set of **nodes** (individuals, groups, organizations) joined by **ties** (specific types of relationships among them) (Hall & Wellman, 1985; Wellman, 1983). For example, employees of an organization may be conceived of as a social network. Each individual, work group, or organizational unit would represent a node in the network. The connections that exist among the individuals or groups (such as friendship, acquaintanceship, or communication flow) would represent the ties among the network members. Social networks have both structural and relationship properties among the network members (ties). Structural properties of social networks include the nine listed here (Hall & Wellman, 1985; Israel, 1982):

- Range—the number of network members.
- Density—the extent to which a network is connected. Density is measured by the proportion of direct ties that exist among network members out of all possible ties that could exist among them.
- Degree—the extent to which a network member has direct ties with other network members.
- Boundedness—the proportion of all ties of network members that stay within the networks' boundaries.
- Reach ability—the average number of ties required to link any two network members.
- Homogeneity—the extent to which network members have similar characteristics (age, race, sex, gender, economic status, etc.).
- Cliques—portions of networks in which all network members are tied directly.
- Clusters—portions of networks with high density but in which all members do not have direct ties.
- Components—portion of networks in which all members are tied directly or indirectly.

The relationship properties of social networks refers to the nature of the ties that exist among network members. Specific characteristics of the ties include the six listed here (Hall & Wellman, 1985; Israel, 1982):

- Strength—the quantity of resources between two network members.

- Frequency—the quantity of contact between two network members.
- Multiplexity—the number of different types of social support exchanged between two network members.
- Duration—the length of time a tie or relationship has existed.
- Symmetry—the extent to which social support is both given and received between two network members.
- Intimacy—the perceived emotional closeness among two network members.

Role properties of networks refer to the roles individuals within the network play. The three major role categories are group member, linking agent, and isolate with few ties to other network members (Fulk & Boyd, 1991). Linking agents are network members who are also members of other networks and serve a crucial role in communications across networks.

Positional characteristics of networks refer to individuals' positions within the network structure. Among positional characteristics, perhaps the most important is centrality. Centrality refers to the relative effect of an actor on other actors in the network, the speed with which an actor's effects are realized, and the extent to which a particular actor transmits to other network members the effects of other actors (Friedkin, 1991). Measures of centrality have been widely used in studies of communication processes in organizations, where centrality measures are used to identify actors who are centrally connected to other network actors and who may serve essential functions in communications within networks.

Content properties of networks refer to whether networks are primarily friendship, task-oriented organizational networks, kinship networks, or communication networks. Networks can also be characterized by the mechanisms through which network members interact, including face-to-face, telephone, or computer communications.

There are essentially two approaches to studying social network structure and ties. The **whole network** approach starts with a defined group of people, such as members of an organization, worksite, or neighborhood, and identifies the relationships that exist among them. For example, Figure 17-2 is a friendship map of a nine member work group. As depicted in the figure, there are three friendship cliques within the work group: ABC, DGF, and DEF. These three represent cliques since the members all have ties with each other. The nine members of the network represent a component, since each member is connected to other members directly or indirectly (through other members).

To create the diagram in Figure 17-2, each member of the work group would be asked about his or her relationships with all other members of the group. Thus studies of whole networks require specifying the boundaries of the network (Laumann, Marsden, & Prensky, 1983) and collecting information from each network member. By contrast, **egocentric network** approaches usually start with individuals and collect information on the persons with whom the individual has close personal ties or from whom they have received specific types of support (Bernard, Johnson, Killworth, & Robinson, 1991).

Each of these approaches has advantages and limitations. Whole network approaches allow the discovery of indirect relationships among individuals. For example, individual D in Figure 17-2 is connected to A through B and C. Since information and other forms of support flow through network ties, individual D may indirectly receive information from A through either B or C. Thus whole networks are useful in studying the flow of resources, including communication patterns, within a defined group. Whole

network approaches are also useful in identifying individuals who are members of multiple cliques or clusters. Such individuals may serve important roles, such as boundary spanners, by conveying information or other resources across cliques or components. Finally, the study of whole networks may be used to identify individuals with equivalent positions in the network for studies of organizational power and decision making (Wellman, 1983).

Egocentric network approaches, on the other hand, are particularly useful in studying who provides social support to whom and under what conditions. Since individuals typically belong to multiple networks—kinship, work, voluntary organizations, and friendship—they may receive different forms of social support from their ties in different networks. For example, they may receive affective support primarily from family members, information and a sense of social identity primarily from work and voluntary organizations, and information through their work and friendship networks. Thus whole network analysis is useful in studying the relationships among a defined group of actors, while egocentric approaches emphasize individuals' connections to multiple networks and the broader community.

It has been suggested that communities be considered networks of networks (Wellman, 1983). That is, individuals, groups, and organizations in communities are linked through a series of network ties (Mitchell, 1969). A network conceptualization of communities has several implications. First, the nature of

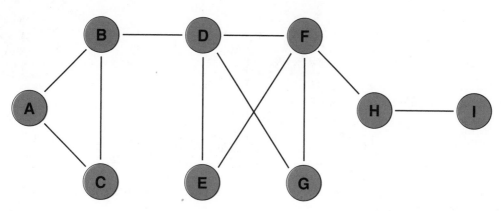

Figure 17-2 Sample friendship network in a work group.

the ties that exist in a community affects the ability of a community to meet the needs of its members. Second, the norms and expectations governing individuals' behaviors will be governed by the positions they occupy in specific networks and the nature and extent of their social ties. Finally, as will be described, access to social goods, such as social support, is affected by membership in social networks.

Figure 17-3 diagrammatically portrays the relationships among characteristics of individuals, environmental or situational factors, network structure and ties, and the provision of social support to network members. As suggested in the figure, individual characteristics affect the networks to which individuals belong and the subsequent support they receive from their networks. For example, individuals choose the networks to which they wish to belong based on individual aspirations and goals (Ellemers, Van Knippenberg, & Wilke, 1990). Moreover, individuals tend to choose networks consisting of individuals with similar social class, behaviors, and norms. The social support received by individuals is determined not only by the structure of the networks to which they belong and the ties that they have within the network, but by their willingness to seek support from network members. Some psychologists go so far as to conceptualize social support as a personality construct (driven by an individual's preferences, motivations, and skills) rather than as a characteristic of the social environment (Pierce et al., 1997).

Environmental factors also influence the social networks to which individuals belong (Fleming, Baum, & Singer, 1985; Pearlin, 1982). Access to social networks, particularly those requiring face-to-face interactions, may be constrained or enhanced by the neighborhoods in which individuals choose to live, the organizations in which they work, other organizations to which they belong, and family structure. It is difficult to overemphasize the effects of environmental factors on the networks to which people belong. In his study of East York, Toronto, Canada, for example, Wellman and Leighton (1979) found that 81% of respondents' interpersonal ties were part of mutual ties to larger groups and organizations, such as family, churches, and worksites (Hall & Wellman, 1985; Perl & Trickett, 1988; Wellman, 1979).

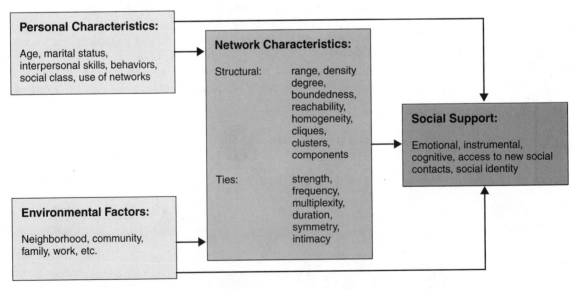

Figure 17-3 Conceptual framework for relationships among personal characteristics, environmental factors, network characteristics and network ties, and social support.

Source: Adapted from B. A. Israel, *Patient Counseling and Health Education*, 1982.

Some research suggests that social contexts that are strongly hierarchical and marked by inequality in the distribution of resources and power inhibit the building and maintaining of strong social networks. Wilkinson (1999) posits that social inequality is incompatible with friendships characterized by mutuality and reciprocity. Rather, relationships in such contexts are likely to be characterized by feelings of insecurity and inadequacy. Thus, organizations with strong vertical structures may make it difficult for employees to build social networks that span the status gradient and that can provide needed support.

Social networks may also choose their members. Membership in specific networks may be restricted by social class, occupation, residence, age, sex, gender, marital and family status, physical or intellectual prowess, or interpersonal skills, among others. Network norms concerning the behavior of members—such as use of tobacco, drugs, and alcohol—may also affect who chooses to belong, who is allowed to belong to the network, and subsequent behaviors of network members.

Network characteristics, including structure and characteristics of ties, influence the nature and extent of social support received by individuals. Affective, instrumental, and cognitive support, maintenance of social identity, and social outreach are more likely to be exchanged between individuals who have strong, intimate, multiplex relationships of long duration. Such individuals are more likely to receive emotional support, help in dealing with daily problems or extraordinary events, and a sense of belonging and social identity. Moreover with regard to network structure, there is evidence to suggest that individuals who belong to a relatively small (low range), single network (highly bounded) of friends similar to themselves (high homogeneity), with strong ties, will be more influenced by group norms and behaviors than individuals who belong to larger, less-homogeneous, less-bounded groups (Agnew, 1991).

It would be tempting to conclude that dense, reachable, homogeneous networks with strong, intense, multiplex ties among members are ideal for providing and receiving social support and for their effects on health. However, such a conclusion would be misguided. Dense, homogeneous networks may limit an individual's access to information. Granovetter (1973, 1983) has argued that individuals' acquaintanceships are more likely to be loosely organized (less dense) than their friendships. Since acquaintanceships would also have close friends not tied to an individual, individuals with few acquaintanceships would be deprived of diverse information from sources outside of their network. It has been found, for example, that low-income pregnant women with stronger family ties and less-dispersed friendship networks were less likely to utilize prenatal care than women with weaker family ties and more disperse friendship networks (St. Clair, Smeriglio, Alexander, & Celentano, 1989). In a study of awareness of services by older persons, Ward, LaGory, and Sherman (1984) found that friends and neighbors (weak ties) were a greater source of information than strong ties and that the elderly with greater access to strong ties (children, confidants, and instrumental helpers) had the least knowledge about available services.

Dense networks with strong ties among the members may also be a source of strains and demands on individuals. Not all relationships are supportive. Individuals may be involved in mentally or physically abusive relationships. More common than abuse would be the daily hassles of relationships, advice when it is not wanted, and dominance rather than caring (House, et al., 1988; Israel, 1982).

Social networks and social relationships impose behavioral norms on their members through informational feedback from network members. Social regulation or control may be either positively or negatively associated with health, depending on the specific content of the norms and the behaviors that are regulated. For example, subgroups may have norms about the use of alcohol and other drugs, breast-feeding, use of health and social services, work performance, or other health-related behaviors. The extent to which individuals perform behavioral norms in large part will be dependent on the information they receive from their networks and the strength of the network ties. In addition, individuals with weak ties and individuals belonging to diverse networks will be less influenced by the norms within a single network.

While social support is generally considered to have only positive consequences, it should be obvious that not all social support is helpful and that the timing and sources of social support may be critical. McLeroy, De Vellis, De Vellis, Kaplan, and Toole (1984), for example, reported that the magnitude of support received from family and friends had negative effects on recovery from stroke for up to one year following the stroke. Pearlin and Schooler (1978) found that self-reliance was more effective in coping with strains from work, finances, parenting, and marriage than was seeking help and advice from others. In a study of social support and adaptation to widowhood, Bankoff (1983) found that the overall support from network members had no effect during the crisis stage of coping with widowhood and only modest effect during the transition phrase. In addition, support from family and married friends had no effect on the widows' sense of well-being, while support from widowed friends did. In interpreting results from similar studies, Walker, MacBridi, and Vachon (1977) suggest that the stage of the crisis, the timing of social support, and characteristics of widowers' social networks may be critical in coping with bereavement. For example, during the initial grief of widowhood, emotional support is more likely to be provided by dense networks with strong ties, such as extended family. In making the later transition from being part of a marital dyad to being single, access to new social contacts through weaker friendship ties may be more important. In addition, the transition from married to widowed may disrupt previous strong ties due to changes in role responsibilities and social definitions (Lopata, 1986).

Communities composed primarily of networks with strong ties would have restricted information flow among the networks and would be composed of insular subgroups. It has been suggested, for example, that low-income groups rely more on strong ties than other economic groups (Granovetter, 1983; McKinlay, 1980). Among economically marginal individuals, networks with strong reciprocal ties may be necessary for providing a minimum of economic security to their members. The absence of weak ties, however, limits the access of group members to the larger community (Oliver, 1988).

A useful framework for understanding the importance of social networks in improving social health is provided by Steuart (Eng, Hatch, & Callan, 1985; Steckler, Dawson, Israel, & Eng, 1992). Steuart suggests that most health problems—including those of concern to health promotion, such as diet, exercise, stress, smoking, drug use, and risk of injuries—occur within a specific social and cultural context. The social groups to which individuals belong and from which they draw their social identity (families, neighborhoods, communities, informal social networks, formal and informal organizations) may have enormous influence on the behavior of individuals. Not only do individuals draw much of their sense of social identity from the social groups and organizations to which they belong, but these social groups and organizations frequently meet many of their participants' individual and collective needs.

Steuart suggests that interventions should target the social units, including families, social networks, and organizations, within which individuals participate as members, maintain their social identity, and within which they already meet many of their individual and social needs. Thus the purpose of interventions is to strengthen the ability of social units to more effectively meet the needs of their members. As noted by Eng, Hatch, and Callan (1985, p. 83),

> The general thrust of these programs is to place behavior change strategies in the hands of people who can motivate and assist one another to adopt healthier life-styles. The assumption is that affiliations with family, friends, neighbor, co-workers, or people with a common problem like alcoholism can provide the necessary intimacy of association and warmth of mutual support for bringing about behavior change. The expectation is that through their social networks, members will not only be able to persuade one another to effect change but will also be able to offer social support for sustaining change.

Partly as a result of his emphasis on strengthening existing social units, Steuart emphasized the role of professionals as consultants to the true practitioners, the individuals and social units with whom they work. Appropriate models of professional practice, then, include process consultation (Schein, 1969), community organization strategies (Cox, Erlich,

Rothman, & Tropman, 1979), and participatory action research (Whyte, 1991), among others.

AN ECOLOGICAL FRAMEWORK FOR ENHANCING SOCIAL HEALTH AT THE WORKSITE

To effectively intervene for the promotion of social health, it is essential to use an ecological approach (McLeroy, Bibeau, Steckler, & Glanz, 1988). As seen in Figure 17-4, individuals are embedded within networks (e.g., families, workgroups), which are embedded within organizations (e.g., worksites, schools, churches). Similarly, organizations are subsystems of communities, which in turn are subsystems of society. Each system forms the context for those at more microlevels. For example, the corporation provides the context for employee networks within it. However, the causal influences are reciprocal: the employee network can act to change the corporation. Thus in considering worksite health promotion approaches to social health, one ecological level or system may be targeted for change, but interventions can be directed across levels to effect that change. For example, the establishment of flexible work schedules can enable families to provide more continuous care for young children (Winett, King, & Altman, 1988).

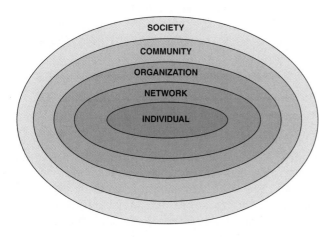

Figure 17-4 Ecological systems for health promotion planning.

Table 17-1, adapted from the work of McLeroy, Steckler, Goodman, and Burdine (1992), illustrates five levels of intervention to support the improvement of social health through worksite health promotion: intrapersonal, interpersonal, organizational, community, and public policy. Strategies appropriate for each level are also suggested. Worksite programming is most often direct to the individual, the work group, or the organization. However, for change interventions to be successful, it is important that each level be supportive of change. For example, if a program objective is for an individual to share feelings with a coworker buddy and the worksite culture proscribes any interaction beyond that required to carry out one's job or the normative culture for blue-collar workers does not encourage affective exchange, it is unlikely that the program will be successful.

Strategies for Enhancing Social Health at the Worksite

Full consideration of worksite social health interventions requires that we examine social health at each ecological level, both as the primary target of health promotion intervention and as the secondary target to support a primary target at another level. After a brief discussion of social health programming at the intrapersonal, interpersonal, organizational, community, and public-policy levels within the context of worksite health promotion, we will apply an ecological approach to planning programs directed to the social health, first of the family unit and then of the work group. Since the focus is on worksite health promotion, we will limit our discussion of interventions directed to the community and policy levels to those within the purview of worksite programming. At each level the outcome desired is a) that the system be able to function effectively to meet the needs of its members, and b) that its members be linked to larger systems.

Intrapersonal

The objective of intrapersonal interventions is to provide the motivation, values, knowledge, and skills individuals need for relationship enhancement

Table 17-1 A Social Ecology Framework for Interventions Aimed at Social Networks and Social Support at the Worksite

Ecological Level	Target of Change	Strategies
Intrapersonal	Knowledge Attitudes Values Skills Behavior Self-concept	Information/Discussion Sessions Micromedia Newsletters Posters Skill-building sessions
Interpersonal	Social networks Social support Families Workgroup Peers Neighbors Small group norms	Mutual help support groups Interactive health Promotion program Changing group norms Enhancing social network
Organizational	Organizational norms Incentives/Policies Organizational culture Management styles Organizational structure Communication network	Organizational development Incentives programs Changes in structure Employee involvement Programs Linking agents Family-friendly policies Services to strengthen networks
Community	Community resources Neighborhood organizations Community competencies Social and health services Organizational relationships	Coalition development Support community services Conduct social health community campaigns Support community political and social institutions
Public Policy	Legislation Policy	Support employees' political activity Lobby of family-friendly policies Conduct media campaigns to support values related to social health

and for using social support to cope with problems, crises, and other stressful situations. This can be accomplished through educational and skill-building programs and through media communications for primary prevention or, for those with problems requiring a clinical approach, through counseling or therapy in Employee Assistance Programs. Intrapersonal health promotion interventions for social support are usually conducted in support of a target at the interpersonal or organizational level; for example, they may be utilized to enhance family, workgroup, or worksite functioning. Many of the chapters in this book address this level of intervention.

Interpersonal

At the interpersonal level the objective is to enable the target network (e.g., the family or the work group) to function effectively to meet the needs of its members and to link its members with other networks, the organization, neighborhood, and community. Interventions focus on strengthening social networks, changing group norms, and building social support groups. Contracting for program participation and goal attainment, team competitions, and self-help groups for behavior change and maintenance are common examples of programming at this level. However, the potential for intervention in interpersonal interaction goes far beyond supporting lifestyle behavior change. Increasing the quality and reliability of support available from existing social networks can impact both the physical and mental health of network members. Group norms to share feelings and experiences and to access one's network when needed may require shaping. Family-oriented programs for lifestyle change and recreation have the potential to improve the functioning of the family system and provide for more satisfying parent-child and marital relationships.

Israel and Rounds (1987) list four categories of network interventions to increase social health:

1. To strengthen already existing network ties.
2. To develop and enhance new network linkages.
3. To enhance the total network through natural helpers.
4. To bring together overlapping networks to meet identified needs.

Conceptualized within a person-centered social network paradigm, interventions to strengthen existing ties and develop new linkages have been targeted primarily to individuals and small groups. However, organization-level activities such as establishing quality circles, changing the organizational structure, or strengthening formal and informal communication systems are also important. These activities flow from the social network perspective, with groups of dense relationships seen as nodes or clusters. In the worksite context, intervention with natural helpers also occurs at the level of the network when these persons located throughout the organization are given additional knowledge, skills, and consultation to assist in social health enhancement of members of their networks and their organization. Bringing networks together occurs at a macrolevel and may involve networks within or outside the organization. The latter may be linkage with a neighborhood or professional association or a support group. (Chapter 8 discusses norms and norm change in more detail.)

Organizational

As with network interventions, the objective of this level is to enable the organization to better meet the needs of its departments, workgroups, and employees and to link them with each other and through the organization to the community and society. Organizational-level change to improve social health is directed toward organizational norms, culture, and policies. Workers' perceptions of involvement and commitment to their jobs, peer supportiveness and cohesion, and management's supportiveness of employees and encouragement of employees to be supportive of each other are important parts of the work environment related to relationships (Moos, 1986). Total quality management, which companies are adopting to maintain their global competitiveness, is based on participatory work teams and employee involvement (e.g., Juran, 1988; Lawler, Mohrman, & Ledford, 1992). Company benefits or services for childcare, eldercare referral, maternity/paternity leave, and flexible role scheduling are policies that enhance the family network (Behrens, 1990).

The social health of the corporation is an important focus of management, often viewed outside the purview of the health promotion unit. However, the organization's structure, culture, and norms related to communication flow, employee involvement, morale and well-being, and cultural diversity have direct influences on individual and family health. We will discuss multilevel programming to strengthen employee work relationships in the next section.

Community

Because our focus is on worksite health promotion, we will examine how the community affects the ability of the organization to meet the needs of its members and how organizations can influence the community system. Corporations can provide leadership and work in coalitions to improve the accessibility and quality of community services needed to foster social health. These might include the mounting of community campaigns to provide information about family and interpersonal relationships, increasing mental health services aimed at strengthening family systems and social networks, encouraging employees and their families outside of work. Examples of such supportive activities include the Adopt-a-School program, executive loan programs, and community-wide fitness events.

Support for community social health at the interpersonal level would include employees' planning or participating in community activities as a group. At the intrapersonal level, programming to increase the motivation and participation of employees in community activities would be key. This could be done through newsletter feature stories on the benefits of community involvement, announcements of community activities, and incentives for participation in community activities.

Public Policy

The legal, regulatory, and policy environment provides the structure for social health at the level of society and reflects our cultural understandings of social health. From the vantage of worksite health promotion, public policy acts as a support for programming at the community, organizational, and the intrapersonal levels. Examples of the policy context supporting social health include daycare services regulation and funding, support for community mental health services, laws related to divorce and child support, and the tax benefit structure. Organizations should have a social health agenda to influence public policy through their own advocacy activities and those of the community and industry-wide membership groups (e.g., a chamber of commerce, a Welcoa business coalition, and the Business Roundtable). Industry campaigns to promote values supportive of social health (e.g., a public service advertising campaign reinforcing the value of family)

help create support for broad-scale policy. Within the organization, management should keep employees informed of social health issues and encourage employee voting and participation in organizations that influence public policy. Objectives of interpersonal and intrapersonal activities would include increased discussion of local and national policy issues, increased knowledge among employees of how to influence social health policy, and increased motivation and behavior to act in the political arena.

Multilevel Strategies to Strengthen the Family and the Workgroup

We will now take two interpersonal targets to increase network effectiveness—families and workgroups—and outline a multilevel approach organized through the worksite to increase the abilities of these networks to meet the needs of their members. The strategies suggested are by no means inclusive or appropriate for all worksites; they were chosen for illustrative purposes only. The best strategies to select depend on the specific issues faced by families or workgroups and the context of the organization, community, and policy environment. As discussed in the following section, an ecological diagnosis with assessment of needs and resources at each level is necessary for program planning.

Many of these strategies have been used previously in worksite health promotion programming. We will cite examples in our discussion. It is rare, however, to find them linked systematically to form a comprehensive multilevel approach. A number of these strategies to improve social health are not conducted within the health promotion program. The health promotion coordinator must coordinate with his or her counterparts in human resources, training, employee assistance, quality management, public relations, and occupational safety and health to design and provide this type of programming.

Social Health Strategies to Strengthen the Family

Figure 17-5 displays intervention strategies designed to increase the effectiveness of the family at meeting members' needs and linking them to other families and the community. The importance of this type of programming has been expressed by the Manager of Work/Life Issues Strategy at IBM.

"IBM has a number of programs that respond to the needs of a changing work force. Over half of our employees are part of a dual-income couple, others are single parents and about 30% have elder care responsibilities. I'm proud to say that as the demographics have changed, IBM has changed to help employees balance the demands of career and family" (Joan Sourenian, quoted in Behrens, 1990).

Public Policy
- Strong laws and regulations related to family (e.g., divorce, child care, tax deductions)
- Health and social services available for families
- Strong cultural values related to family

Community
- Child and eldercare resources
- Family and community events and programs
- Coalitions of organizations to promote family life in community

Worksite
- Family-friendly policies (maternity/paternity leave, flextime, relocation, child care benefits, mental health benefits)
- In-house child and family services (daycare, employee assistance counseling)
- Family values reinforced through newsletter feature stories
- Training for supervisors on family issues
- System of natural helpers to assist with family issues
- Family picnics and other events
- Health promotion program open to family members
- Programs to encourage families to volunteer for community service

Interpersonal
- Mutual help support groups on family issues (new parents, parenting teens, sandwich generation, marital enrichment)
- Interactive family-centered health promotion activities
- Interactive groups on family communication skills
- Discussion of family issues related to work by employees in work groups

Intrapersonal
- Information/discussion seminars on marriage and family topics
- Skill-building sessions to build relationship skills
- Information on community services provided in newsletters
- Sessions on values clarification related to family/work
- Participation in family health promotion programs promoted through role model stories in newsletter
- Counseling services as needed

Figure 17-5 Intervention strategies to strengthen the family network.

Intrapersonal Level

At the intrapersonal level, the focus is on values clarification, information, and skill-building for communication and relationship skills. Various formats can be used. Newsletters delivered to the home—such as "Pipeline to Health" produced by Tenneco Gas for its remote-site employees or the commercially produced magazine and memo used by DuPont—can motivate families to participate in the worksite health promotion program and provide role models and information for family issues (W. B. Baun, personal communication, 1992; Behrens, 1990). Winett has recommended videotapes, based on behavioral modeling and behavior change theory, for teaching individual skills in time management, handling stressful family situations, the division of labor for child- and home care, choosing childcare, and giving and receiving support (Winett, King, & Altman, 1988). These could be used in worksite discussion groups and for home viewing. A video library can reach employees who are not fitness center members or who work at remote sites and use the service by mail (W. B. Baun, personal communication, 1992). IBM has offered a series of work and family seminars covering such topics as parenting (with tracks for different aged children), the conflicting demands of responsible parenting and working, negotiating rules with time, time management, and child development (Behrens, 1990).

The importance of family issues to employees is exemplified by a needs assessment that indicated that 25% of couples were experiencing serious marriage and family problems (Larson, Wilson, & Beyley, 1988). The most-requested service was a monthly family newsletter, followed by a marriage enrichment program and a family enrichment program. In the area of treatment, assessment, counseling, and referral services for marital and family problems are available in some companies through employee assistance programs to both employees and their families.

Interpersonal Level

At the interpersonal level, support groups and interactive health promotion activities may build strong ties among participants as they share experiences and provide cognitive and instrumental support for strengthening the family system. For example, Tenneco sponsors Alcoholics Anonymous, Co-dependents Anonymous, Overeaters Anonymous, and Weight Watchers groups. These groups are open to employees of other companies as well, providing network linkages outside the work environment (W. B. Baun, personal communication, 1992). As part of a relocation of 500 families from Pennsylvania to Florida, Westinghouse sponsored a weekend workshop for adolescent children of both newly transferred and long-time Florida employees. The focus was on increasing self-confidence, trusting others, problem solving, and adjusting to change. The format helped the recently arrived youth make friends with the current residents (Behrens, 1990). Support groups can be particularly effective strategies for participants who cannot mobilize needed social support in their other social relationships (Helgeson, Cohen, Schulz, & Yasko, 2000).

Worksite Level

At the worksite level, policies and programs have been directed toward strengthening the family. Behrens (1990) cites the findings of a Department of Labor survey of child-related policies of over 10,000 businesses. About 40% reported they had flexible hours; 40% had extended maternal or paternal leaves or other short-term leaves for handling childcare responsibilities; 33% had temporary shifts to fewer hours; 10% had special benefits or services for assistance in childcare arrangements; 3% had financial assistance designated specifically for childcare; and 2% had work-sponsored daycare centers. Childcare and eldercare referral services are offered by IBM and other companies, often using independent citywide services (Behrens, 1990).

Dual-career families are especially affected by recruitment techniques, nepotism policies, and relocation policies. Newman (1985) points out that employers have traditionally dealt with the problems of the dual-career family on a case-by-case basis. She suggests inclusion of both spouses in the preselection recruitment process, revising nepotism policies that prevent supervision or evaluation by a relative, and reducing transfers by finding other ways of advancing employees within the company. Spouse placement assistance programs support families when one spouse is transferred.

Insurance benefits are also of key importance for support of families. IBM offers a special care for children benefit of up to $50,000 in medical benefits per child for care of a mentally, emotionally, or physically disabled child. Mental health coverage of marriage and family counseling and counseling for family members is offered by many companies. Managed-care programs being implemented in increasing numbers offer the opportunity to provide these prevention services on a population-wide basis and should be integrated with health promotion programming. Company adoption of these policies and benefits requires confronting issues of basic values regarding family life; potential differential benefits to married/single, parents/nonparents, and males/females; and economic barriers (Behrens, 1990).

Opening the organization's health promotion program to families provides the opportunity for family ties to be strengthened through common activities, such as physical activity or other lifestyle change experiences. Tenneco has several programs designed to encourage parents to become involved in health promotion with their children. The health and fitness program sponsors a Kid's Club for six- to ten-year-olds that in 1992 had about 150 families enrolled. On a bimonthly basis the families are sent a newsletter and activity sheet; the kids are sent a commercially available coloring book. Topics have included self-esteem, nutrition, safety, personal hygiene, and fitness. The activity sheet includes an art or games activity and other ideas for the parents(s) and child(ren) to do together. Families are encouraged to return the completed activity sheet; these, along with information about the Kid's Club, are placed on a bulletin board prominently placed near the fitness center. In the summer, the company runs a one-day summer Adventure Camp for employee children at their off-site recreation center. The 1992 Great American Smoke Out used the innovative activity of having parents talk with their children about the importance of not smoking and encouraging their children to sign a pledge not to smoke. A cold turkey coloring sheet was included. Children who completed the coloring sheet and pledge re-ceived an "It's cool not to smoke" T-shirt and had their art work displayed at Tenneco (W. B. Baun, personal communication, 1992).

Special events involving families include picnics, walks or runs, "Bring the Kids to Work" day, and holiday parties. Recognizing holidays special to specific ethnic groups, such as El Cinco de Mayo, Hannukah, and Martin Luther King Day, can strengthen ties within and between families of different ethnic groups. Aguirre-Molina and Molina (1990) offer other examples of health promotion activities for a culturally diverse population. Adopt-a-School program links employees to schools through tutoring, counseling, special programs linked to the work of the company, and equipment and monetary donations. Motorola, Inc., allows two hours paid time per month for all employees to work at a school of their choice (P. Bossert, personal communication, 1992). Incentives and recognition programs and internal newsletter coverage of activities would reinforce employee family participation in community activities.

Enhancing the networks of natural helpers has been used in community programming but has not been applied systematically to the workplace. In this intervention laypersons to whom others turn for advice, emotional support, and material aid are selected from the population and are given training or process consultation aimed at strengthening the network for all members. The focus can be both on developing the natural helpers' existing skills and providing new skills. Called by such terms as health facilitators, natural neighbors, lay health advisors, and promoters, these individuals continue to provide support to their networks in their communities, housing projects, churches, and other settings (Eng, et al., 1985; Israel, 1985).

Community Level

Worksites exist within communities, and community resources, policies, and events provide the environment for worksite interventions to strengthen family life. Companies can assist in the organization of services needed by employees, such as child- and eldercare services and referral. In Houston, companies encouraged a local hospital to offer a sick-child daycare program. The companies offer copayment for childcare to employees who use the service so they can come to work. Companies can also encourage their employees to volunteer in their community. Tenneco sponsors an annual Community Service Fair at which employees may sign up to work as a group on such activities as housing improvement for the elderly (W. B. Baun, personal communication, 1992).

Organizations can influence local policies through business coalition activities and by encouraging employees to support local issues influencing families and to participate in the governance of their communities. In Austin, Texas, Motorola, Inc., employs an education liaison to work with local school boards and the city council on educational issues (P. Bossert, personal communication, 1992). Executive loan programs of many corporations provide volunteer leadership to the United Way and voluntary health and social service agencies, which provide important services to community residents. Fund-raising efforts within the worksite for these organizations allow employees to assist others in their communities.

Community-wide family events sponsored by organizations offer opportunities for recreation. Companies in Houston sponsored a Tunnel Walk in the underground system linking the downtown area. Different companies along the route provided refreshments and activities, such as an obstacle course for kids to complete. Following one of these events, the Tenneco fitness center sponsored on-site games and tricycle races, with blood pressure and cholesterol screenings for adults, for their employee families who had participated in the Tunnel Walk (W. B. Baun, personal communication, 1992).

A company, either individually or as part of a coalition, can also sponsor community campaigns that reach all residents. Examples of this have been in the areas of substance abuse prevention and nutrition education (Behrens, 1990). A community campaign "Good Friends Make Good Medicine", directed explicitly toward improving social health, was conducted in California in 1982 under the auspices of a local steering committee with representatives from county health and mental health departments, hospitals, school systems, and civic organizations and with technical assistance from the state Department of Mental Health. Its aim was to inform people about the influence of social support on health and to encourage people to nurture relationships. Both media and interpersonal discussion groups were used as communication channels.

The knowledge and beliefs the campaign was designed to foster were:

1. Social support influences physical health.
2. Lifestyle influences health.
3. Social support is especially important in times of stress.
4. Friendship takes attention and commitment.
5. There is no secret prescription for making friends (you are capable).
6. It is OK for you to share feelings.

These in turn were expected to increase two attitudes and values: increased importance of friendship and self-confidence about making friends. The behavioral outcomes included talking to a friend on the phone, getting together with friends, trading favors with friends, sharing feelings with friends, going someplace to meet someone new, calling a relative, getting together with family or relatives, trading favors with a relative, and sharing feelings with family (Hersey, Klibanoff, Lam, & Taylor, 1984).

Public Policy Level

Public policy shapes the environment within which organizations and networks act to strengthen family functioning. Policies determine the kind and amount of resources devoted to community mental health services, daycare programs for children and older adults, and homelessness; regulations relating to families in public aid programs, tax deductions for childcare, and legal issues with regard to divorce, including child support. As discussed earlier, organizations may be affected by public policy. They should advocate policies supportive of families themselves and advocacy groups to which they, as organizations, belong. Organizations should also encourage employees to act through their membership organizations, including their professional associations, and as individual citizens to influence policy.

Social Health Strategies to Strengthen Workgroups

Figure 17-6 lists, by ecological levels, intervention strategies to strengthen workgroups. Workgroups have not usually been considered as part of the health promotion strategy at a worksite; however, they are fundamental to the social health of the organization as a whole and of participating individuals. Workgroups, when structured with union and management involvement to link across functional and

Public Policy
- Services and policies related to increasing labor-management relations
- Tax policies and legislation to promote organization training and social services
- Labor-management cooperation for global competitiveness
- Cultural value on cooperation as opposed to radical individualism

Community
- Training and support for employee involvement and total quality programming by Chambers of Commerce and other interorganizational groups
- Unionwide training and support for employee involvement and total quality programs

Worksite
- Employee involvement and total quality programs
- Union/management development of work group systems
- Workgroups structured across hierarchical lines
- Flatten hierarchy to improve communication
- Incentives for teamwork
- Informal communication systems across employee groups and between employees and management
- Boundary spanners to link groups together

Interpersonal
- Interactive training to improve team functioning
- Interactive training in small group participation
- Boundary spanning across employee groups to improve communication
- Work group teams participate in health promotion competitions and contracting for behavior changes
- Interactive discussion to foster workgroup norms and values

Intrapersonal
- Skill-building sessions to improve relationships at work
- Role model stories about workgroup friendships and interaction to motivate closer relationships within groups
- Values clarification exercises on cooperation and competition
- Training in listening skills and communication

Figure 17-6 Intervention strategies to strengthen work groups.

hierarchical lines, empower employees and groups to participate in organization functioning and to control their work environment. For example, Pretty and McCarthy (1991) found that job involvement, peer cohesion, and supervisor support were positively associated with a psychological sense of community among workers at a larger public utilities corporation. In addition, the skills in communication and teamwork learned through workgroup experiences may transfer to family and friendship network interactions. Thus workgroups are an important focus for social health interventions at the worksite.

We will not discuss intervention strategies for strengthening work groups in the same detail we did for families. Most major companies use natural teams that link across broad processes, such as quality or engineering. In addition to technical training for their team tasks, interpersonal skill training is provided in the areas of communication, decision-making, and cultural diversity. Motorola University and Motorola Training and Development offer such short courses as Effective Interactions with Employees, Listening Skills Workshop, Teamwork Skills, Dealing with Difficult People, and Working with Diversity. Some of the classes are open to all employees; others are designed specifically for intact teams. The high-technology electronic manufacturing companies in Austin, Texas, cooperate to offer Boot Camp, one-week courses in facilitating and leading teams (Bossert, personal communication, 1992).

At Tenneco, fitness programming has been used to foster work group relationships. Product personnel and buyers outside the company participated together in Team-bound, a Project Adventure-type ropes course to strengthen their relationships. Fitness center activities serve a similar function in-house. Department wallyball teams play each other and learn about the skills and potential within their team. For example, one executive noted that he had worked with his secretary for 20 years and got a whole different perspective on her abilities and strengths by playing on a team with her. The fitness center also serves a linking function. For example, accountants on different floors who had never met before joining center activities began to communicate and exchange information. Individual sports and fitness activities enable employees to share experiences not possible through work and to build stronger relationships with each other (W. B. Baun, personal communication, 1992).

In addition to health promotion-related activities, employee involvement programs have been implemented in 82% of Fortune 1000 companies (1987), with 72% of the implementing companies indicating that employee involvement programs were designed to improve quality and 70% to improve productivity (Lawler et al., 1992). A follow-up survey examined companies' training programs, reward systems, and power-sharing practices. Over half of the companies reported that more than 20% of their employees had been trained in the following areas during the three years prior to the survey: job skills training (84%), team-building skills (56%), group decision-making and problem-solving skills (55%), and leadership skills (54%).

Individual employee incentives were offered more frequently than team incentives, even though team incentives may be more supportive of employee involvement. Specifically almost one-half of the companies (44%) reported that at least one-fifth of their employees were covered by individual incentives, while 21% of companies reported the use of team incentives.

Over one-half (51%) of the companies reported power-sharing approaches other than quality circles covering at least one-fifth of their employees; 30% of companies reported using quality circles; 15% reported combined union-management quality-of-working-life committees; 52% reported job enrichment or redesign; 10% reported self-managing work teams; and 5% of companies reported using minienterprise units.

Partly as a result of these employee involvement programs, over one-half of the companies reported some change to a more participatory management style (78%), improved organizational processes and procedures (75%), increased employee trust in management (66%), improved implementation of technology (69%), and elimination of management or supervision (50%) (Lawler et al., 1992).

To achieve the benefits of high employee involvement, Lawler (1986) has argued that pay and incentive systems, personnel and selection policies, and training orientation must reflect a management philosophy and core values congruent with employee involvement. He also notes that egalitarian physical surroundings (without special parking, dining facilities, furniture, and dress for management) encourage team identity and support employee involvement.

Planning for Social Health

An ecological perspective on social health at the worksite suggests that planning should occur at multiple levels of analysis, including the individual, network, organization, community, and the linkages among them. By using multiple levels of analysis, the organization is viewed as a social system with a climate and culture supported and maintained by a particular pattern of intra- and interorganizational relationships. While a detailed presentation of planning techniques and methods is beyond the scope of this chapter, the following sections briefly identify selected issues in planning for social health for individuals, social networks, the organization, and the community.

Intrapersonal Needs Assessment

The purpose of a social health needs assessment of individual members of an organization is to determine:

1. the nature and extent of stresses and strains in employees' daily lives, including those primarily due to job demands;
2. employee perceptions of the supportiveness of the organization and organizational units, including work groups and organizational units, as well as specific relationships (such as relationships with peers, supervisors, administrators, and support units);
3. the nature of support needs among individual employees and their families and the extent to which these needs are being met through both formal and informal services and programs within the organization and the community.

There are a variety of techniques for conducting individual needs assessments, ranging from in-depth, unstructured or semistructured interviews with em-

ployees at different levels of the organization to more formal techniques, such as focus groups, group discussions with formal organizational units, and sample surveys (Bailey, 1978; Miller, 1991; Price, 1972). In addition there are numerous scales and instruments available for assessing work- and nonwork-related stresses and strains (Hurrell, Nelson, & Simmons, 1998), perceptions of organizational climate and culture (Basen-Engquist, Hudmon, Tripp, & Chamberlain, 1998; Moos, 1986; Taylor & Bowers, 1972), social support (House & Kahn, 1985; Payne & Jones, 1995), and service and program needs (Moroney, 1977).

Regardless of the individual needs assessment technique employed, an essential element in planning for social health is the ability to link individual needs to organizational structure. That is, the needs of the individual within an organization and the extent to which needs are perceived as addressed by the organization will vary, depending upon the individual's specific work group, organizational unit, and position. For example, in a recent study of organizational climate within 20 school districts, there were significant differences between teachers and administrators and across school buildings in the extent to which the social environment of the school districts was perceived as supportive and participatory (McLeroy, Steckler, McCormick, et al., 1992). By linking individuals' perceptions to their positions within the organization, it may be possible to identify dysfunctional organizational units and to develop appropriate interventions.

Network Assessment

Network analysis is designed to provide information on the structure, role, content, and relational and positional properties of social networks. It can be used to identify

1. key individuals to participate in the planning and implementation of worksite health promotion activities;
2. informal communication systems for disseminating information about health promotion programs;
3. network norms or characteristics that may affect participation in health promotion activities;

4. work groups or organizational units with low group cohesiveness and weak ties among the members and units with weak connections or ties to other units;
5. the potential for intergroup conflict.

Key Individuals

Of particular importance in the planning of health promotion programs is identifying key individuals within the organization who should be involved. The network concept of centrality would suggest that individuals within the organization who are perceived by others as influential decision makers should be involved. Parham (1990), for example, used a network survey of teachers and administrators in 22 school districts to identify key administrators to include in an intervention designed to encourage school districts to adopt tobacco use prevention curricula. Other techniques for identifying key decision makers would include key informants (Burt, 1983a) or archival records (Burt, 1983b).

Communication Systems

Individuals' access to information within organizations is a function of their participation in both formal and informal communication systems. In order to effectively disseminate information about health promotion programs, it is important to use both channels (Heirich, Cameron, & Erfurt, 1989). However, accessing informal communication channels can be difficult. A network approach to identifying informal communication networks would focus on communication patterns within and across organizational networks. For example, if each organizational unit or work group within a company or worksite were defined as a network, then a communications network analysis would focus on the structure and ties within each unit and the connections among units. A network analysis would identify individuals within networks with a high degree of connectedness to other network members and individuals who serve boundary spanning roles by being members of two or more networks. Such individuals could be recruited to provide information on program activities. As noted by Heirich and colleagues (1989 p. 113),

Even in a plant that operates primarily by assembly line there are a series of work roles that regularly involve travel around the plant, much like bees going from flower to flower. Additionally, people in some other work roles are regularly contacted by a wide group of people, even though they stay in a single location. If a few of these people become personally interested in a health venture, word about it can pass rapidly throughout the plant in a context that endorses the health message as it is being circulated.

Norms

Workgroups and informal friendship networks will vary in norms and expectations about members' participation in health promotion activities. In worksites characterized by management and labor conflict, for example, selected workgroups may be suspicious of organization-sponsored health promotion programs and discourage member participation. Work and friendship groups will also vary in norms concerning alcohol consumption and dietary, exercise, and fitness behaviors. Allen and Allen (1986) have developed a scale that can be used to identify workgroup norms concerning health-related activities.

Weak Ties

Workgroups may differ in the value placed on friendship ties, with some workgroups being primarily task-oriented and some emphasizing personal relationships. Some workgroups and friendship groups may be relatively insular and well-bounded with weak ties to other organizational units. Some work groups may have numerous isolates within the unit with strong ties among a few of the work group members (Bollen & Hoyle, 1990). By linking individuals' perceptions of work group norms and interaction patterns to their position within the organization and organizational unit, it may be possible to identify dysfunctional organizational units and to develop appropriate interventions.

Intergroup Conflict

Network information may also be used to identify the potential for intergroup conflict. For example, the extent of conflict within organizations has been linked to the types of ties across organizational units. In his study of 20 organizations, Nelson (1989) found that low-conflict organizations were characterized by consistent, if not homogeneous, groups bound together by strong ties, such as intergroup relations managed by a dominant group or linking hierarchy.

As with intrapersonal needs assessment, network analysis techniques include both formal and informal techniques. Sample surveys may be used to identify key opinion leaders, individuals with a high degree of connectedness, boundary spanners, and the nature of ties among network members. Key informant interviews and participant observation may be used to identify boundary spanners and individuals with a high degree of connectedness by studying who talks to whom within the organization and which key positions require considerable interaction with other members (Cairns, Kindermann, & Gariepy, 1987; Fisher, 1982; House & Kahn, 1985). Moreover there are microcomputer programs, such as NEGOPY (Richards & Rice, 1981), for analyzing network information.

Organizational Needs Assessment

The purpose of an organizational needs assessment is to identify how organizational mission and goals, climate, leadership, culture, structures, services, and programs are related to the social health of organizational members and the functioning of organizational units and informal networks. Each of these organizational factors is the context within which social health, including the structure and function of social networks, is developed and maintained in the worksite. Since each of these factors may affect the social health of organizational members, a comprehensive worksite needs assessment should incorporate each of these elements. Moreover, each of the organizational factors may be the target of worksite interventions to improve the health of employees. For example, an important objective of social health interventions is to institutionalize the importance of employee health, including social health, in the mission and goals statements of the organization. Organizational climate, leadership, culture, and structure should incorporate social health as an important organiza-

tional value. Organizational services and programs should be tailored to meet the social health needs of employees and their families.

There are a variety of techniques and measures available for assessing organizational factors related to social health in the worksite. (These are discussed in more detail in Chapters 3, 4, 5, and 8.)

Community Needs Assessment

While social health in the worksite is the principle focus of this chapter, it should be recognized that communities are the context within which organizations function. An important purpose of organizational needs assessment, then, is identifying local community organizations and services, developing ways of linking organizational members and their families to local programs and services, and assessing the community political and social climate in order to influence the availability of community services for organization members.

For discussions of community needs assessment techniques see Green and Kreuter (1991), McKillip (1987), and Warheit, Bell, and Schwab (1977).

Evaluation

Evaluation is a key stage of the program cycle, enabling health promotion programmers to evaluate whether a program is being carried out as planned and whether project goals have been reached. In addition program evaluations can contribute to health education and health promotion theory through identifying mechanisms by which change is produced, developing more comprehensive program models, identifying limitations to existing theories, and identifying new issues to be studied (McLeroy, Steckler, Goodman, & Burdine, 1992).

In order to accomplish these goals, it is important to understand the causal relationships among health promotion interventions and expected outcomes. Figure 17-7 is an adaptation of the Health Promotion Research Agenda Model published in the *American Journal of Health Promotion*. The original model serves as a conceptual framework of hypothesized crucial relationships among health promotion inputs,

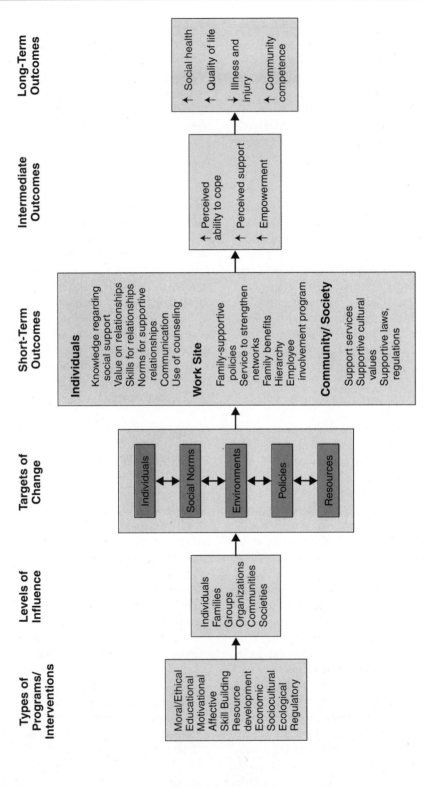

Figure 17-7 Evaluation research model for social health.
Source: Adapted from L. W. Green, *American Journal of Health Promotion*, 1992.

processes of change, and outcomes that require documenting through research and evaluation (Green, 1992a). While the model has primarily been used descriptively to characterize research and evaluation reports and articles, the model can also be used proscriptively. That is, consistent with an ecological perspective, evaluation plans within this framework would include strategies and outcomes at multiple ecological levels.

Specifically, we know relatively little about how health promotion programs targeted at individuals and individual behaviors within the worksite may influence workgroup norms, the social environment of the organization, or organizational policies and resources. Conversely there is relatively little research information on the reciprocal effects of organizational policies, social environment, and workgroup norms on the development and implementation of worksite health promotion strategies. Moreover there is relatively little information on the synergistic effects of combining interventions at multiple levels (e.g., combining family support and individual education programs to enhance social support). Thus there is a need for worksite programs to begin evaluating program effects at multiple levels, including effects on individuals, social groups, the organization, and the community. Moreover there is a need to develop and appropriately evaluate multi-level interventions.

By placing program evaluation within an ecological perspective, we may begin to develop appropriate theories of how worksite programs achieve desired effects and what works, with whom, and under what conditions. An ecological perspective on program evaluation, then, can contribute to health education and health promotion theory building by identifying how interventions at one ecological level may have reciprocal influences at other levels of the model (Burdine & McLeroy, 1992; McLeroy, Steckler, Goodman, & Burdine, 1992).

As seen in Figure 17-7, long-term outcomes include the primary goal of increased social health at each ecological level and the secondary goals of decreased morbidity, increased quality of life, and increased community competence. The secondary goals flow from the intermediate outcomes in the causal path toward social health and from improved social health itself (Green, 1992a). Intermediate outcomes include perceptions of ability to cope with life stresses and perceived support from one's network (House & Kahn, 1985). The outcomes of increased empowerment and sense of community occur at both the individual level and higher order levels.

The short-term outcomes of this model are those that flow most immediately from the strategies we suggested in Figures 17-5 and 17-6. At the individual level and the network level, they include increased knowledge of the relationship of social, physical, and mental health; increased value on relationships; increased skills for interaction; more supportive norms for relationships; increased communication between family, friends, and coworkers; and increased used of counseling where needed. At the worksite level, the variables are increased family-supportive policies and benefits, increased services to strengthen networks, decreased levels of hierarchy, and increased employee involvement programs; for community and society levels, the variables are increased supportive services, cultural values, and laws and regulations. The types of programs and interventions listed in generic terms in Figure 17-7 are outlined with more specificity in Table 17-1 and Figures 17-5 and 17-6.

In studying these linkages in program evaluations, it is important to remain alert to unexpected negative consequences of interventions to strengthen social networks. For example, employees forming an exercise group at work may develop new ties and, as a consequence, weaken family ties. Also health promotion interventions may carry negative social health consequences. Gottlieb and Nelson (1990) and Gottlieb, Lovato, Weinstein, Green, & Eriksen, (1992), for example, found that a restrictive smoking policy in some instances disrupted worksite social activities and strengthened the bonds among smokers as an isolated group. The formation of lifestyle enclaves within larger social groups as a result of market segmentation for health promotion may lead to isolation and division within communities and society (Green, 1992b).

CONCLUSION

In this chapter we have discussed the importance of social relationships in promoting and maintaining health. The research evidence for the effects of social participation on the health of individuals was reviewed. Five different types of social support (affective, cognitive, and instrumental support, maintenance of social identity, and social outreach) were seen to flow through interpersonal relationships. The structural basis for social support through social networks was described and properties of social networks defined.

We then applied this information to the promotion of social health at the worksite using an ecological model, with emphasis on supporting the family and workgroup networks. It was suggested that an ecological perspective provides an innovative approach for organizing programs that link contextual and environmental supports to the target for change (e.g., behavior, group norms, organization culture, etc.). An ecological perspective provides a multilevel heuristic for program design, rather than a new intervention technique. As such, we recommend an ecological approach by health promotion specialists to ensure the comprehensiveness of interventions. An overview of planning and evaluation of social health interventions concluded the section on the promotion of social health at the worksite.

In closing the chapter, we considered broad policy and ethical issues related to social health. The discussion and recommendations in this chapter on improving social health in the worksite occur within a political, social, and scientific context. Politically, strengthening families and communities has become the clarion call of both the Democratic and Republican parties, with renewed emphasis on traditional community and family values, including mutual and self-help. Volunteer community coalitions to address AIDS, alcohol and other drug problems, community violence, and adolescent pregnancy have sprung up in communities across the country, many of them partially supported by federal, state, or local funds.

Within the social, behavioral, and health sciences, there appears to be a reemergence of interest in community and families and working with communities, families, networks, and organizations to address community and social problems. Research on community-based approaches to health promotion has burgeoned (Israel, Schulz, Parker, & Becker, 1998), and volumes have begun to appear on working with communities for health promotion (e.g., Bracht, 1990). Research on the role of families, social support, social networks, and self-help continues to expand. Professional treatises have been produced discussing the importance of community in American life (Bellah, Madsen, Sullivan, Swidler, & Tipton, 1985, 1991; Putnam, 2000; Reynolds & Norman, 1988). Professional organizations have begun to focus attention on the importance of community in American life.

As we embrace this rediscovery of community, social networks, and interpersonal relationships, however, we must be cautious in our interventions to improve social health. In this chapter we have emphasized the importance of the social environment as the context of change. As pointed out by Pilisuk and Parks (1986), there must be resources for caring, such as child- and eldercare programs, social security, and mental and physical health care services, or else an emphasis on interpersonal social support becomes an exercise in victim blaming.

Another issue of concern is cooptation of natural sources of support by professionals. The informal, spontaneous helping processes offered by mutual support groups and natural helpers are different from those provided by professionals. Professional dominance and control, which flows from the assumption of expert power, can coopt the natural system and destroy its potency. Also the network assessments and training can isolate natural helpers from their networks. Gottlieb (1988) has discussed the appropriate roles for professionals working with natural helping systems, emphasizing the more indirect roles of consultant, referral agent, and advocate. Group members and natural helpers can also act as consultants to professionals regarding the nature of informal helping behaviors and the improvement of professional services and delivery system organization. Where assessment and research activities interfere with the effectiveness of the interventions, they should be curtailed.

Although there is strong evidence relating social support both directly and indirectly to physical and mental health outcomes, we do not understand completely how social support works and how this varies with culture and personality. We must allow the natural processes of helping to work and, as noted before, should emphasize environmental interventions to provide a supportive context for natural helping. Health promotion practitioners must be aware of the potentially coercive nature of social network interventions; these involve changing organization and group norms and the expectations of one person for another. In the interventions we have suggested for increasing the knowledge, attitudes, and behaviors of individuals and the norms and incentives for network interaction, the voluntariness of individuals' participation is key.

Finally, while we have discussed in detail the measurement of social health of individuals and networks, the conceptualization of social health at the levels of organization, community, and society has not been fully developed. While we use the terms "healthy organizations" and "healthy communities," health at each of these levels is usually viewed as the aggregate health of the respective members. Perhaps it is time for us to begin to identify and define the structural meaning of healthy communities, organizations, networks, and families—that is, to extend the concepts of health beyond the health of individuals. While the health promotion goals of decreased illness and injury and increased quality of life have been included in evaluation studies (e.g., Abelin, 1986; Woodruff & Conway, 1992), the systematic conceptualization and measurement of healthy communities, healthy families, and healthy organizations are lacking, as are related concepts such as community competence and empowerment (Goodman et al., 1998; Green, 1992a; Wallerstein, 1992).

References

Abelin, T. (1986). Positive indicators in health promotion and protection. *WHO Statistical Quarterly, 39,* 353–374.

Agnew, R. (1991). The interactive effects of peer variables on delinquency. *Criminology, 29* (1), 47–72.

Aguirre-Molina, M., & Molina, C. W. (1990). Ethnic-racial populations and worksite health problems. In M. E. Scofield (Ed.), *Medicine: State-of-the-art reviews. 5* (4), 789–806.

Allen, Jr., & Allen, R. F. (1986). From short term compliance to long term freedom; Culture-based health promotion by health professionals. *American Journal of Health Promotion, 1*(2), 39–47.

Antonovsky, A. (1984). The sense of coherence as a determinant of health. In J. D. Matarazzo, S. M. Weiss, J. A. Herd, N. E. Miller, & S. M. Weiss (Eds.), *Behavioral health: A handbook of health enhancement and disease prevention.* New York: John Wiley & Sons.

Bailey, K. D. (1978). *Methods of social research.* New York: Free Press.

Bankoff, E. A. (1983). Social support and adaptation to widowhood. *Journal of Marriage and the Family, 45,* 827–839.

Basen-Engquist, K., Hudmon, K., Tripp, M., & Chamberlain, R. (1998). Worksite health and safety climate: Scale development and effects of a health promotion intervention. *Preventive Medicine, 27,* 111–119.

Beehr, T. (1995). *Psychological stress in the workplace.* London: Routledge.

Behrens, R. (1990). *Reaching families through work-site and community health promotion programs.* (Available from the Washington Business Group on Health, 777 North Capitol Street, NE, Suite 800, Washington, DC 20002.)

Bellah, R. N., Madsen, R., Sullivan, W. M., Swidler, A., & Tipton, S. M. (1985). *Habits of the Heart.* Berkeley: University of California Press.

_____. (1991). *The good society.* New York: Knopf.

Berkman, L. F. (1995). The role of social relations in health promotion. *Psychosomatic Medicine, 57,* 245–254.

Berkman, L., & S. L. Syme. (1979). Social networks, host resistance, and mortality. A nine-year follow-up study of Alameda County residents. *American Journal of Epidemiology, 109,* 186–204.

Bernard, H. R., Johnson, E. C., Killworth, P. D., & Robinson, S. (1991). Estimating the size of an average personal network and of an event subpopulation: Some empirical results. *Social Science Research, 20,* 109–121.

Blazer, D. (1982). Social support and mortality in an elderly community population. *American Journal of Epidemiology, 115,* 684–621.

Bollen, K. A., & Hoyle, R. H. (1990). Perceived cohesion: A conceptual and empirical examination. *Social Forces, 69,*(2), 479–504.

Bracht, N. (Ed.) (1990). *Health promotion at the community level.* Newbury Park, CA: Sage.

_____. (1985). *Social support: New perspectives in theory, research, and intervention. Part II. Interventions and policy.*

Brownell, K. D., & Felix, M. R. J. (1987). Competitions to facilitate health promotion: Review and conceptual analysis. *American Journal of Health Promotion, 2,* 28–36.

Brownell, A., & Shumaker, S. A. (Eds.). (1984). Social support: New perspectives in theory, research, and intervention. Part 1. Theory and research. *Journal of Social Issues,* 40(4).

Burdine, J. N., & McLeroy, K. R. (1992). Practitioners' use of theory: Examples from a workgroup. *Health Education Quarterly, 19* (3), 331–340.

Burt, R. S. (1983a). Network data from archival records. In R. S. Burt & M. J. Minor (Eds.), *Applied network analysis: A methodological introduction,* Beverly Hills, CA: Sage.

_____. (1983b). Network data from informant interviews. In R. S. Burt & M. J. Minor, (Eds.), *Applied network analysis:* A methodological introduction, Beverly Hills, CA: Sage.

Cairns, R. B., Kindermann, T., & Gariepy, L. (1987). *Cognitive sociometry: How to identify peer clusters through composite social maps.* Unpublished manuscript, University of North Carolina at Chapel Hill.

Carlson, D. S., & Perrewe, P. L. (1999). The role of social support in the stressor-strain relationship: An examination of work-family conflict. *Journal of Management, 25,* 513–540.

Cohen, S., Doyle, W. J., & Skoner, D. P. (1997). Social ties and susceptibility to the common cold. *Journal of the American Medical Association, 277,* 1940–1944.

Cohen, S., & Syme, S. L. (Eds.). (1985). *Social support and health.* New York: Academic Press.

Cohen, S., & Wills, T. A. (1985). Stress, social support, and the buffering hypothesis. *Psychological Bulletin, 98,* 310–357.

Cox, F. M., Erlich, J. L., Rothman, J., & J. E. Tropman, (Eds.). (1979). *Strategies of community organization.* Itasca, IL: F. E. Peacock.

Donald, C. A., Ware, J. E., Jr., Brook, R. H., & Davies-Avery, A. (1978). *Conceptualization and measurement of health for adults in the health insurance study: Vol. 4. Social health.* Santa Monica, CA: The Rand Corporation.

Duhl, L., & Hancock, T. (1988). *The healthy cities papers: No. 3 Community self-evaluation, A guide to assessing healthy cities.* Denmark: WHO Regional Office for Europe.

Duke University Center for Study of Aging and Human Development. (1978). *Multidimensional functional assessment: The OARS methodology.* Durham, NC: Duke University.

Ellemers, N., Van Knippenberg, A., & Wilke, H. (1990). The influence of permeability of group boundaries and stability of group status on strategies of individual mobility and social change. *British Journal of Social Psychology, 29,* 233–246.

Eng, E., Hatch, J., & Callan, A. (1985). Institutionalizing social support through the church and into the community. *Health Education Quarterly, 12*(1), 81–92.

Ewart, C. K. (1991). Social action theory for a public health psychology. *American Psychologist, 48,* 931–946.

Fisher, C. S. (1982). *To dwell among friends: Personal networks in town and city.* Chicago: University of Chicago Press.

Fleming, R., Baum, A., & Singer, J. E. (1985). Social support and the physical environment. In S. Cohen & S. L. Syme (Eds.), *Social support and health.* New York: Academic Press.

Friedkin, N. E. (1991). Theoretical foundations for centrality measures. *American Journal of Sociology, 96*(6), 1478–1504.

Fulk, J., & Boyd, B. (1991). Emerging theories of communication in organizations. *Journal of Management, 17*(2), 407–446.

Goodman, R. M., Speers, M. A., McLeroy, K., (1998). Identifying and defining the dimensions of community capacity to provide a basis for measurement. *Health Education & Behavior, 25,* 258–278.

Gore, S. (1978). The effect of social support in moderating the health consequences of unemployment. *Journal of Health and Social Behavior, 19*(2), 157–165.

_____. (1985). Social support and style of coping with stress. In S. Cohen & S. Syme (Eds.), *Social support and health* (pp. 263–280). New York: Academic Press.

Gottlieb, B. H. (1983). Social support as a focus for integrative research in psychology. *American Psychologist, 38,* 278–287.

Gottlieb, B. H. (1988). Marshalling social support: The state of the art in research practice. In B. H. Gottlieb (Ed.), *Marshalling social support: Formats, processes, and effects,* Newbury Park: Sage.

Gottlieb, N. H., Lovato, C. Y., Weinstein, R. P., Green, L. W., & Eriksen, M. P. (1992). The implementation of a restrictive smoking policy in a large decentralized organization. *Health Education Quarterly, 19*(1), 77–100.

Gottlieb, N. H., & Nelson, A. (1990). A systematic effort to reduce smoking at the work-site. *Health Education Quarterly, 17,* 99–118.

Granovetter, M. (1973). The strength of weak ties. *American Journal of Sociology, 78*(6), 1360–1380.

Granovetter, M. (1983). The strength of weak ties: A network theory revisited. In R. Collins (Ed.), *Sociological theory,* San Francisco: Jossey-Bass.

Green, L. W. (1992a). The health promotion research agenda revised. *American Journal of Health Promotion, 6,* 411–413.

_____. (1992b, June 18). *Public policy and health education practice.* Paper presented at the Society for Public Health Education Mid-Year Scientific Conference, Austin, TX.

Green, L., & Kreuter, M. (1991). *Health education planning: An educational and environmental approach* (2nd ed.). Mountain View, CA: Mayfield.

Green, L. W., & Raeburn, J. (1990). Contemporary developments in health promotion: Definitions and challenges. In N. Bracht (Ed.), *Health promotion at the community level,* Newbury Park, CA: Sage.

Hall, A., & Wellman, B. (1985). Social networks and social support. In S. Cohen & L. Syme (Eds.), *Social support and health* (pp. 000). New York: Academic Press.

Hamilton, V. L., Broman, C. L., Hoffman, W. S., & Renner, D. S. (1990). Hard times and vulnerable people: Initial effects of plant closing on auto-workers' mental health. *Journal of Health and Social Behavior, 31*(2), 123–140.

Heaney, C. A. & Israel, B. A. (1997). In K. Glanz, F. M. Lewis, & B. K. Rimer (Eds.), *Health behavior and health education* (2nd ed., pp. 179–205). San Francisco: Jossey-Bass, 179–205.

Heinemann, G. D. (1985). Interdependence in informal support systems: The case of elderly, urban widows. In W. A. Peterson & J. Quadagno (Eds.), *Social bonds in later life: Aging and interdependence,* Beverly Hills: Sage.

Heirich, M. A., Cameron, V., & Erfurt, J. C. (1989). Establishing communication networks for health promotion in industrial settings. *American Journal of Health Promotion, 4* (2), 108–117.

Helgeson, V. S., Cohen, S., Schulz, R., & Yasko, J. (2000). Group support interventions for women with breast cancer: Who benefits from what? *Health Psychology, 19,* 107–114.

Hersey, J. C., Klibanoff, L. S., Lam, D. J., & Taylor, R. L. (1984). Promoting social support: The impact of California's "Friends Can be Good Medicine" campaign. *Health Education Quarterly, 11,* 293–311.

Holt, R. R. (1982). Occupational stress. In L. Goldberger & S. Breznitz (Eds.), *Handbook of stress: Theoretical and clinical aspects,* New York: Free Press.

House, J. S., & Kahn, R. L. (1985). Measures and concepts of social support. In S. Cohen & S. L. Syme (Eds.), *Social support and health,* New York: Academic Press.

House, J., Robbins, C., & Metzner, H. (1982). The association of social relationships and activities with mortality: Prospective evidence from the Tecumseh Community Health Study. *American Journal of Epidemiology, 116,* 123–140.

House, J. S., Umberson, D., & Landis, K. R. (1988). Structures and processes of social support. *Annual Review of Sociology, 14,* 293–318.

Hurrell, J. J., Nelson, D. L., & Simmons, B. L. (1998). Measuring job stressors and strain: Where we have been, where we are, and where we need to go. *Journal of Occupational Health Psychology, 3,* 368–389.

Israel, B. A. (1982). Social networks and health status: Linking theory, research, and practice. *Patient Counseling and Health Education, 4,* 65–79.

_____. (1985). Social networks and social support: Implications for natural helper and community level interventions. *Health Education Quarterly, 12,* 65–80.

Israel, B. A., & Rounds, K. (1987). Social networks and social support: A synthesis for health educators. *Advances in Health Education and Promotion, 2,* 311–351.

Israel, B. A., Schulz, A. J., Parker, E. A., & Becker, A. B. (1998). Review of community-based research: Assessing partnership approaches to improve public health. *Annual Review of Public Health, 19,* 173–202.

Jacobson, D. E. (1986). Types and timing of social support. *Journal of Health and Social Behavior, 27,* 250–264.

Juran, J. M. (1988). *Juran on planning for quality.* New York: Free Press.

Kahn, R. L., & Byosiere, P. (1992). Stress in organizations. In M. D. Dunnette & L. M. Hough (Eds.), *Handbook of Industrial and Organizational Psychology* (2nd ed., pp. 571–650). Palo Alto, CA: Consulting Psychologists Press.

Kaplan, R. M. (1985). Quality of life measurement. In P. Karoly (Ed.), *Measurement Strategies in Health Psychology,* New York: Wiley & Sons.

Kasl, S. V., & Wells, J. A. (1985). Social support and health in the middle years: Work and the family. In S. Cohen & S. L. Syme (Eds.), *Social support and health,* New York: Academic Press.

Kawachi, I., Kennedy, B. P., & Glass, R. (1999). Social capital and self-rated health: A contextual analysis. *American Journal of Public Health, 89,* 1187–1193.

Larson, J. H., Wilson, S. M., & Beyley, R. (1988). The assessment of family wellness in a university employee wellness program. *American Journal of Health Promotion, 2* (3), 20–30.

Laumann, E. O., Marsden, P. V., & Prensky, D. (1983). The boundary specification problem in network analysis. In R. S. Burt & M. J. Minor (Eds.), *Applied network analysis: A pethodological introduction,* Beverly Hills, CA: Sage.

LaVeist, T. A., Sellers, R. M., Elliott Brown, K. A., & Nickerson, K. J. (1997). Extreme social isolation, use of community-based senior support services, and mortality among African American elderly women. *American Journal of Community Psychology, 25,* 721–732.

Lawler, E. E. (1986). *High-involvement management.* San Francisco: Jossey-Bass.

Lawler, E. E., Mohrman, S. A., & Ledford, G. E., Jr. (1992). Employee involvement and total quality management: *Practices and Results in Fortune 1000 Companies.* San Francisco: Jossey-Bass.

Lazarus, R. S., & Folkman, S. (1984). *Stress, appraisal, and coping.* New York: Springer.

Legro, M. (1992, July). The paradox of quality of life outcomes: The case of cataract surgery. *SPSSI Newsletter, 188,* 20–21.

Lohr, K. N., & Ware, J. E. (Eds.). (1987). *Proceedings of the Advances in Health Assessment Conference, 40* (Suppl. 1), 1s–193s.

Lopata, H. Z. (1986). Becoming and being a widow: Reconstruction of the self and support system. *Journal of Geriatric Psychiatry, 2,* 203–214.

McKillip, J. (1987). *Needs analysis: Tools for the Human Services and Education.* Newbury Park, CA: Sage.

McKinlay, J. B. (1980). Social network influences on morbid episodes and the career of help seeking. In L. Eisenberg & A. Kleinman (Eds.), *The relevance of social science for medicine,* Boston: D. Reidel.

McLeroy, K. R., Bibeau, D., Steckler, A., & Glanz, K. (1988). An ecological perspective on health promotion programs. *Health Education Quarterly, 15,* 351–378.

McLeroy, K. R., De Vellis, R., De Vellis, B., Kaplan, B., & Toole, J. T. (1984). Social support and physical recovery in a stroke population. *Journal of Social and Personal Relationships, 1,* 395–413.

McLeroy, K. R., Steckler, A. B., Goodman, R. M., & Burdine, J. N. (1992). Health education research: Theory and practice-future directions. *Health Education Research: Theory and Practice, 7,* 1–8.

McCormick, L., Steckler, A., and McLeroy, K. (1994). Adoption and implementation of health curricula: A study of diffusion and organizational change processes. *American Journal of Health Promotion, 9*(3), 210–219. University of North Carolina at Greensboro.

Medalie, J., Snyder, M., Groen, J. J., Neufeld, H. N., Goldbourt, Y., & Riss, E. (1973). Angina pectoris among 10,000 men: 5 year incidence and univariate analysis. *American Journal of Medicine, 55,* 583–594.

Miller, D. C. (1991). *Handbook of research design and social measurement.* Newbury Park, CA: Sage.

Minkler, M. (1985). Social support and health of the elderly. In S. Cohen & S. L. Syme (Eds.), *Social support and health,* New York: Academic Press.

_____. (1989). Health education, health promotion, and the open society: An historical perspective. *Health Education Quarterly, 16*(1), 17–30.

Mitchell, J. C. (1969). *Social networks in urban situations.* Manchester, UK: The University of Manchester Press.

Moos, R. H. (1986). *Work environment scale manual* (2nd ed.). Palo Alto: Consulting Psychologists Press.

Moroney, R. (1977). Needs assessment for human services. In *Management human services,* International Cities Managers Association.

Nelson, R. E. (1989). The strength of strong ties: Social networks and intergroup conflict in organizations. *Academy of Management Journal, 32,* 377–401.

Newman, E. C. (1985). Health promotion for the working couple: A health promotion program for dual-career couples. In G. S. Everly, Jr. & R. H. L. Feldman (Eds.), *Occupational health promotion: Health behavior in the workplace,* New York: John Wiley & Sons.

Nuckolls, K. B., Cassel, J. C., & Kaplan, B. H. (1972). Psycho-social assets, life crisis, and prognosis of pregnancy. *American Journal of Epidemiology, 95,* 431–441.

Oliver, M. L. (1988). The urban black community as network: Toward a social network perspective. *The Sociological Quarterly, 29*(4), 623–645.

Parham, D. L. (1990). *Organization innovation: A study of adoption of a health education/tobacco prevention curriculum in North Carolina school districts.* Unpublished doctoral dissertation, University of North Carolina at Chapel Hill.

Payne, R. L., & Jones, G. (1995). Measurement and methodological issues in social support. In S. V. Kasl & C. L. Cooper (Eds.), *Stress and health: Issues in research methodology* (pp. 167–205). New York: Wiley & Sons.

Pearlin, L. I. (1982). Social structure and processes of support. In G. S. Sanders & J. Suls (Eds.), *Social psychology of health and illness,* Hillsdale, NJ: Lawrence Erlbaum Associates.

Perl, H. I., & Trickett, E. J. (1988). Social network formation of college freshmen: Personal and environmental determinants. *American Journal of Community Psychology, 16*(2), 207–224.

Pierce, G. R., Lakey, B., & Sarason, I. G. (1997). Personality and social support processes: A conceptual overview. In G. R. Pierce, B. Lakey, I. G. Sarason, & B. R. Sarason (Eds.), *Sourcebook of social support and personality* (pp. 3–18). New York: Plenum Press.

Pilisuk, M., & Parks, S. H. (1986). *The healing web: Social networks and survival.* Hanover, NH: University Press of New England.

Pretty, G. M. H., & McCarthy, M. (1991). Exploring psychological sense of community among men and women of the corporation. *Journal of Community Psychology, 19,* 351–361.

Price, J. L. (1972). *Handbook of organizational measurement.* Lexington, MA: DC Heath.

Putnam, R. D. (2000). *Bowling alone: The collapse and revival of American community.* New York: Simon & Schuster.

Reisine, S. T. (1988). The impact of dental conditions on social functioning and the quality of life. In L. Breslow, J. E. Fielding, & L. B. Lave (Eds.), *Annual review of public health,* Palo Alto: Annual Reviews.

Reynolds, C. H., & Norman, R. V. (1988). *Community in America.* Berkeley: University of California Press.

Richards, W. D., & Rice, R. E. (1981). The NEGOPY network analysis program. *Social Networks, 3,* 215–223.

Rodgers, F. S., & Rodgers, C. (1989). Business and the facts of family life. *Harvard Business Review, 67,* 121–129.

St. Clair, P. A., Smeriglio, V. L., Alexander, C. S., & Celentano, D. D. (1989). Social network structure and prenatal care utilization. *Medical Care, 27*(8), 823–832.

Schein, E. H. (1969). *Process consultation: Its role in organization development.* Reading, MA: Addison-Wesley.

Schoenbach, V. I., Kaplan, B. H., Fredman, L., & Kleinbaum, D. B. (1986). Social ties and mortality in Evans County, Georgia. *American Journal of Epidemiology, 123,* 577–591.

Shumaker, S. A., & Hill, D. R. (1991). Gender differences in social support and physical health. *Health Psychology, 10*(2), 102–111.

Singer, J. E., & Lord, D. (1984). The role of social support in coping with chronic or life-threatening illness. In A. Baum, S. E. Taylor, & J. E. Singer (Eds.), *Handbook of Psychology and Health,* Hillsdale, NJ: Lawrence Erlbaum Associates.

Sosa, R., Kennel, J., & Klaus, M. (1980). The effect of a supportive companion on perinatal problems, length of labor, and mother-infant interactions. *New England Journal of Medicine, 305,* 597–600.

Starker, J. E. (1990). Psycho-social aspects of geographic relocation: The development of a new social network. *American Journal of Health Promotion, 5,* 52–57.

Steckler, A., Dawson, L., Israel, B., & Eng, G. (1992). Unpublished manuscript, University of North Carolina at Chapel Hill.

Suls, J. (1982). Social support, interpersonal relations, and health: Benefits and liabilities. In G. S. Sanders & J. Suls (Eds.), *Social psychology of health and illness,* Hillsdale, NJ: Lawrence Erlbaum Associates.

Taylor, J., & Bowers, D. (1972). *Survey of organizations: A machine-scored standardized questionnaires.* Ann Arbor, MI: Institute for Social Research, University of Michigan.

Uchino, B. N., Cacioppo, J. T., & Kiecolt-Glaser, J. K. (1996). The relationship between social support and physiological processes: A review with emphasis on underlying mechanisms and implications for health. *Psychological Bulletin, 119,* 488–531.

Umberson, D. (1992). Gender, marital status, and the social control of health behavior. *Social Science and Medicine, 34,* 907–918.

Walker, K. N., MacBridi, A., & Vachon, M. L. S. (1977). Social support networks and the crisis of bereavement. *Social Science and Medicine, 11,* 35–41.

Wallerstein, N. (1992). Powerlessness, empowerment, and health: Implications for health promotion programs. *American Journal of Health Promotion, 6*(3), 197–205.

Wallerstein, N., & Bernstein, E. (1988). Empowerment education: Freire's ideas adapted to health education. *Health Education Quarterly, 15*(4), 379–394.

Ward, R. A., LaGory, M., & Sherman, S. R. (1984). Informal networks and knowledge of services for older persons. *Journal of Gerontology, 39,* 216–223.

Warheit, G. J., Bell, R. A., & Schwab, J. J. (1977). *Needs assessment approaches: Concepts and methods.* Washington, DC: NIMH (ADM 79-472).

Wellman, B. (1979). The community question: The intimate networks of East Yorkers. *American Journal of Sociology, 84,* 1201–1231.

Wellman, B. (1983). Network analysis: Some principles. In R. Collins (Ed.), *Sociological theory 1983,* San Francisco: Jossey-Bass.

Wellman, B., & Leighton, B. (1979). Networks, neighborhoods, and communities. *Urban Affairs Quarterly, 14,* 363–390.

Whyte, W. F. (1991). *Participatory action research.* Newbury Park, CA: Sage.

Wilkinson, R. G. (1999). Putting the picture together: prosperity, redistribution, health, and welfare. In M. Marmot & R. G. Wilkinson (Eds.), *Social determinants of health* (pp. 256–274). Oxford, UK: Oxford University Press.

Winett, R. A., King, A. C., & Altman, D. G. (1988). *Health psychology and public health.* New York: Pergamon Press.

Woodruff, S. I., & Conway, T. L. (1992). Impact of health and fitness-related behavior on quality of life. *Social Indicators Research, 25,* 391–405.

World Health Organization. (1947). Constitution of the world health organization. *Chronicle of WHO, 1,* 1.

CHAPTER
18

Workplace Health Promotion in Small Businesses

Daniel Stokols, Shari McMahan, and Kimari Phillips

INTRODUCTION

The present chapter addresses one of the most understudied yet potentially influential contexts for workplace health promotion: small business organizations. Small businesses are defined as firms employing between 2–500 employees (Muchnick-Baku & Orrick, 1992; U.S. Small Business Administration [USSBA], 2000a). According to the 1996 data compiled by the U.S. Small Business Administration (USSBA), small firms represented 99% of all employers in the U.S. in 1995 (USSBA, 1998b), employed approximately 53% of U.S. private sector nonfarm workers (USSBA, 2000a), and accounted for virtually all of the net new jobs created in the U.S. between 1990–1995 (USSBA, 2000a; Wellness Councils of America [WELCOA], 1998) (see Table 18-1). Yet, very little empirical research has been conducted previously concerning the particular stressors and health problems faced by small business workers, let alone the prevalence and effectiveness of health promotion programs in small firms.

Table 18-1 Profile of U.S. Small Businesses

- 24.8 million U.S. businesses have between 2–500 employees
- Nearly 80% of U.S. private firms have fewer than 10 employees
- U.S. small businesses represent 99% of all employers in the U.S.
- U.S. small businesses employ 53% of U.S. private sector nonfarm workers
- U.S. small businesses accounted for 76% of the net new jobs between 1990–1995
- Nearly 57% of U.S. small businesses occupy home-based worksites
- U.S. small businesses provide 67% of workers with their first-time job and initial on-the-job training
- U.S. small businesses employ higher proportions of younger (under age 25), older (age 65 and over), female, minority, less educated, and part-time workers
- U.S. small businesses produce 39% of the gross national product
- U.S. small businesses invent more than half the nation's technological innovations
- A growing number of U.S. small businesses are owned and managed by women and minorities

Sources: USSBA, 1998; USSBA, 2000a; USSBA, 2000b; WELCOA, 1998.

The major purposes of this chapter are to describe the unique needs of small businesses relative to health promotion and to outline a conceptual model for meeting those needs. The proposed model offers a programmatic framework that identifies several health promotion strategies for small businesses, including those directed at changing employees' health behaviors, improving conditions of the physical environment and corporate culture at work, and facilitating greater collaboration among small businesses, nonprofit organizations, and government agencies. The suggested model is applicable to companies of all sizes, but the level of priority and financial investment assigned to each of the strategies included in the model will vary between small and large firms.

Before presenting a conceptual model for promoting employee wellness in small businesses, it is important first to characterize the unique attributes and health promotion needs of small firms. The next section of the chapter describes these attributes and needs of small firms, and highlights the special opportunities and challenges associated with workplace health promotion in small companies.

OPPORTUNITIES AND CHALLENGES FOR WORKSITE HEALTH PROMOTION IN SMALL BUSINESSES

Earlier studies to evaluate the health and cost effectiveness of workplace health promotion (WHP) programs in the U.S. have focused primarily on very large companies employing thousands of workers rather than on small businesses (Everly & Feldman, 1985; Fielding, 1984; O'Donnell & Ainsworth, 1984; Pelletier, 1996). Three national surveys of WHP activities in the U.S., for example, omitted companies with fewer than 50 employees despite the fact that nearly 80% of the country's private firms have fewer than 10 workers (Fielding & Piserchia, 1989; USSBA, 2000a; U.S. Department of Health and Human Services [US-DHHS], 1993; Association for Worksite Health Promotion [AWHP], Mercer, & USDHHS, 1999). Similarly, the 1994 National Health Interview Survey (NHIS), a household-based probability survey conducted by the National Center for Health Statistics, examined the availability and use of WHP programs by U.S. workers but included only individuals work-

ing at a location with 50 or more employees (Grosch, Alterman, Petersen, & Murphy, 1998). The sampling restrictions imposed by these earlier surveys of WHP activities suggest that individuals working in small organizations—especially those employed by firms with fewer than 50 employees—comprise an *understudied* and *underrepresented population* in the research literature on health promotion.

Small business organizations constitute an exciting yet challenging target of opportunity for workplace health promotion in the coming decades. Because small firms employ the majority of American private sector workers, they represent a strategic, high-leverage context for improving the health of the U.S. population. Small businesses provide a highly advantageous context for promoting employee health in view of their unique social, organizational, and environmental attributes (AWHP et al., 1999; Chenoweth, 1998; Muchnick-Baku & Orrick, 1992; WELCOA, 1998) (see Table 18-2). For example, small businesses have fewer people to accommodate, fewer administrative costs, and less space to manage; therefore, less time and money are required for communicating with employees about health and safety issues. Also, small busi-

Table 18-2 Small Business *Advantages* in Workplace Health Promotion

- Visible, accessible, and approachable top management
- Fewer people to accommodate
- Fewer administrative costs
- Less space to manage
- Less time and money required for communicating with employees about health and safety issues
- Easier to integrate and link health promotion objectives with business outcomes
- Interdependency among employees
- Supportive environment conducive to group participation
- Higher rates of employee participation
- More visible employee health improvements
- Simpler, less expensive data gathering for program evaluation
- Large and locally accessible marketplace for community health agencies and organizations to direct their free and low-cost services

nesses report significantly higher rates of employee participation in workplace health promotion activities than do larger firms (AWHP et al., 1999). The sense of community among employees that typifies small business settings affords a supportive environment conducive to group participation in WHP programs; and among certain types of small businesses, such as rapidly expanding high-technology firms that have relatively low overhead costs, the requisite financial resources and organizational innovation can be directed toward the development of truly outstanding WHP programs.

Another factor within small companies conducive to their members' participation in WHP programs is that employee health improvements tend to be more visible to coworkers in smaller versus larger firms. The more visible health improvements are, the less resources a company needs to invest in promoting and formally evaluating program efforts. Because one of the keys to successful worksite health promotion is management involvement, small businesses also have the distinct advantage of having visible, accessible, and approachable top management. Thus, there are fewer layers in the decision-making process and less organizational bureaucracy to go through in order to get a supportive health policy formulated or a WHP program implemented quickly. In addition, the approachability of top management in small firms makes it easier to integrate and link health promotion objectives with business outcomes, thereby enabling the program to become established as an integral part of the organization's culture. Finally, small businesses constitute a large and locally accessible sector of the workforce toward which community health agencies and organizations can direct their free and low-cost services.

Despite the above-mentioned advantages and opportunities for health promotion in the context of small businesses, future efforts to implement effective workplace health programs for small business workers must confront certain complexities and challenges inherent in the economic organization of small firms, the variety of physical facilities used by small companies, and the greater vulnerability of employees in small firms to health problems as compared to workers in large corporations (see Table 18-3). Economic and organizational factors that have constrained the development of health promotion programs in small businesses include the lower profit margins of many small firms as compared to larger ones, which make it more difficult for small companies to invest in and sustain workplace wellness programs. Moreover, small businesses rarely include an owner or other individual who is expert in the design and implementation of health promotion programs. Small companies often feel overburdened by regulatory requirements and are hesitant to offer health programs that are not mandated by law (Chenoweth, 1995). And, although some health maintenance organizations (HMOs) and preferred provider organizations (PPOs) offer subsidies to support worksite health promotion programs, many of these health plan-sponsored programs require a minimum group size of 50 or more employees (Donaldson, Gooler, & Weiss, 1998).

Table 18-3 Small Business *Challenges* in Workplace Health Promotion (WHP)

- Lack of time—WHP is often a low priority for management, as productivity and cost issues take precedence
- Overburdened by safety and health regulations/legislation
- Poor financial support—lower profit margins limit funding for WHP
- Rising employer health costs
- Downsizing and shifts toward part-time, temporary, or "contingency" workforce
- Employee turnover
- Lack of formal departments and in-house experts responsible for WHP
- Constrained by the group-size requirement (usually 50+ employees) of many health-plan-sponsored WHP programs
- Diversity and geographic dispersion of physical work settings (e.g., offices, factories, warehouses, restaurants, schools, retail shops, vehicles, residences, satellite locations)
- Large percentage of workers with low socioeconomic status (SES)
- Large percentage of employees without health insurance and employee benefits
- Aging and ethnic diversification of the U.S. workforce

The great diversity of physical facilities used by small businesses also has made it difficult for health professionals and researchers to implement standardized health promotion programs tailored to the unique worksites of small firms. **Worksites** are those settings in which one or more individuals engage in work-related tasks, including the offices, factories, warehouses, and other facilities controlled by organizations, vehicles operated by employees (e.g., trucks, buses, taxis), and residential offices of home workers. Comprehensive approaches to workplace health promotion combine behavioral and lifestyle change strategies with those focusing on environmental restructuring and enhancement (Stokols, 1992; Stokols, Pelletier, & Fielding, 1996). Examples of environmental enhancement strategies include interventions aimed at improving the ergonomic features and social climate of work settings and reducing levels of noise, air pollution, and hazardous substances in those environments. Yet, because the majority of small businesses (firms with 200 or fewer workers) occupy home-based worksites (56.5% of all small firms in the U.S. were home-based in 1992 according to the USSBA, 1998), it is difficult to catalog the unique environmental and family circumstances faced by individuals working in these multipurpose (occupational/residential) settings. Moreover, the diversity of small business facilities makes it difficult to implement environmentally-based WHP programs in a systematic and replicable fashion.

Finally, the demographic composition of the small business workforce poses another set of challenges for the future development of health promotion programs in small firms. Whereas some small companies (such as law firms, medical offices, accounting firms, and internet-based companies) are quite profitable and their employees are very well-off, small firms as a group employ larger percentages of workers with low socioeconomic status than larger firms do (USSBA, 1998). Thus, although not all small firms and their employees are financially constrained, small businesses generally employ larger percentages of vulnerable employees (i.e., low-income and minority workers who lack health insurance) than do larger companies (Rubio & Arteaga, 2000). In view of the well-documented correlation between socioeconomic status and health status (Adler et al., 1994; Yen & Syme, 1999), the small business workforce constitutes not only an understudied and underrepresented group in the health promotion literature but also a highly vulnerable population in view of their greater susceptibility to illness and their relative lack of health insurance and employee health benefits.

The vulnerability of small business workers is likely to be exacerbated by contemporary societal trends (including the aging and ethnic diversification of the U.S. workforce, and rising employer health costs) and corresponding shifts toward corporate down-sizing and part-time "contingency" work, reduced employee health benefits, and managed health care plans (HMOs, PPOs) that offer greater financial support for worksite wellness programs to large, high-volume employers as compared to smaller firms (Donaldson et al., 1998; Dooley, Fielding, & Levi, 1996; Green & Cargo, 1994; Hudson Institute, 1987; U.S. Bureau of the Census, 1992, 1993). Moreover, the shift from manufacturing to office-based work, society's growing reliance on digital communications technologies, and the increasing demand for workers skilled in information technology will create greater competition for jobs and heightened levels of job insecurity among older, very young, and less-educated minority workers (Freeman & Aspray, 1999; Kochar, 1994; Special report: Rethinking work, 1994; Stokols, 1999; U.S. Department of Commerce, 1995, 1998). The greater prevalence of these vulnerable groups in small firms suggests that the small business workforce is increasingly becoming a strategic target for future workplace wellness programming efforts.

In the remaining sections of the chapter, we examine in greater detail the unique circumstances of small businesses and the special challenges they face in their efforts to promote employee health. We begin by taking a closer look at the substantial impact of small businesses on the U.S. economy and the unique financial, demographic, facilities design, and health challenges faced by small versus large firms. We also examine the prevalence of WHP programs within small businesses and certain areas of WHP programming that have been relatively neglected by small firms. Particular attention is given to the challenge of providing more extensive health insurance coverage and family health benefits to workers in small companies. This issue is discussed in light of recent national and regional surveys regarding the availability of health insurance benefits to employees of companies with fewer than 50 workers (McMahan, Stokols, Clitheroe, Wells, & Phillips, 1997; Rubio & Arteaga, 2000; USDHHS, 1997; Wilson, DeJoy, Jorgensen, & Crump, 1999). Finally, in later sections of the chapter, we discuss several promising directions for future research and practice in the field of small business health promotion based on the findings from recent demonstration studies that have implemented and are evaluating the efficacy of workplace wellness programs in small firms (Chenoweth, 1998; Donaldson & Klein, 1997; Erfurt & Holtyn, 1991; Stokols, Clitheroe, McMahan, & Wells, 1995; Torres, 1999; Wells, Stokols, McMahan, & Clitheroe, 1997).

UNIQUE CHARACTERISTICS AND NEEDS OF SMALL BUSINESSES RELATIVE TO HEALTH PROMOTION

As a basis for understanding the unique characteristics and special needs of small businesses relative to health promotion, this section of the chapter examines four key issues: (a) the impact of small businesses on the U.S. economy; (b) the typical foci of worksite health promotion activities in small companies as reflected in the data from recent national surveys; (c) the extent to which small businesses provide health insurance plans for their workers relative to larger companies; and (d) the plight of ethnic minority and low-income employees in small firms.

Impact of Small Businesses on the U.S. Economy

There were approximately 24.8 million small businesses in the U.S. in 1998 (with fewer than 500 employees). These include corporations, partnerships, and sole proprietorships (USSBA, 2000a). The cumulative impact of these firms on the U.S. economy is substantial. For instance, small businesses produce 39% of the gross national product and invent more than half the nation's technological innovations. They also provide 67% of U.S. workers with their first-time jobs and initial on-the-job training (USSBA, 2000b). As well, small businesses offer employment and man-

agerial opportunities to a broader array of age and socioeconomic groups than larger companies. Specifically, they employ larger percentages of workers under age 25 and over age 65, and those with lower educational levels, than larger firms do. At the same time, a growing number of women and minority group members are taking advantage of opportunities to own and manage small firms. Women-owned small businesses, for example, increased 89% from 1987–1997. Between 1987–1997, the number of African-American-owned firms increased 108%, and the number of Hispanic-owned firms rose 232%. There also has been a marked increase in the number of businesses owned by Asian and Pacific Islanders, American Indians, and Alaskan Natives during the same period (USSBA, 2000a).

Whereas small businesses offer a broad range of employment opportunities to diverse subgroups of the population, employees of small firms tend to be more vulnerable to financial and health difficulties than those working in large companies. The fact that small business workers, as a group, tend to be less educated and have lower incomes than their counterparts in large corporations makes them more vulnerable to many acute and chronic illnesses. Furthermore, part-time employment is more prevalent in smaller companies (20.5%) as compared to larger firms (17.4%). In fact, very small firms (fewer than 10 employees) hire part-time employees at a rate almost twice that of large firms (USSBA, 1998). Part-time workers and their dependents are much less likely to be covered by health insurance at work than are full-time employees (18% coverage for part-time vs. 82% for full-time workers, reported in USDHHS, 1997; see also Wilson et al., 1999). The greater vulnerability of small business workers to illness and injury also is reflected in the disproportionately higher number of work-related fatalities that occur in establishments with fewer than 10 employees. In addition, these individuals account for approximately 33% of all workplace fatalities and for about one million employer-related injuries each year (Twardowski, 1998).

The increased vulnerability of small business workers to various illnesses, relative to those working in large companies, suggests that worksite health programs aimed at preventing and reducing medical problems would be especially beneficial to the employees of small firms (Chenoweth, 1995; Stokols, Pelletier, & Fielding, 1995). Yet several international, national, and regional occupational health surveys have found that smaller companies offer significantly fewer worksite health and safety programs to their employees than larger firms. The findings from these surveys are outlined below.

Health Promotion Activities of Small Businesses

The Office of Disease Prevention and Health Promotion (ODPHP) of the U.S. Public Health Services conducted the 1985 National Survey of Worksite Health Promotion Activities (National Survey) to assess health promotion activities in private worksites with 50 or more employees (Fielding & Piserchia, 1989). In 1992, ODPHP commissioned the second National Survey to elaborate on the substance and prevalence of WHP programs in U.S. companies (USDHHS, 1993), and, in 1999, the findings of the third National Worksite Health Promotion Survey were published (AWHP et al., 1999). These surveys provided a basis for tracking changes in WHP activities between 1985–1999 and differences in the prevalence of WHP activities related to company size and industry type. The 1985, 1992, and 1999 surveys also compared the actual levels of WHP activities in U.S. companies with the goals and objectives outlined in *Healthy People 2000: National Health Promotion and Disease Prevention Objectives* (USDHHS, 1991) and, more recently, in *Healthy People 2010* (USDHHS, 1999). As noted earlier, all three National Surveys omitted companies with fewer than 50 employees.

The 1985 National Survey indicated that two-thirds of the participating companies offered at least one health promotion activity (Fielding & Piserchia, 1989). Smoking cessation, health risk appraisal, back care, stress management, and physical fitness programs were the most frequently cited health promotion activities at these worksites. Also, spouses and dependents of workers, as well as retirees, were found to have less access to corporate health programs than employees do themselves. Specifically, all permanent employees were eligible to participate in health promotion activities at 85.4% of the worksites, whereas spouses and dependents were eligible for these programs at only 30.1% and retirees at 30.4% of the participating companies.

The second National Survey found that by 1992, 81% of the worksites sampled offered at least one health promotion activity (USDHHS, 1993). The activities mentioned most frequently in the 1992 survey included injury prevention, physical fitness, smoking control, and stress management, with the prevalence of worksite smoking policies increasing by 118% between 1985–92. Both the 1985 and 1992 surveys indicated that larger companies sponsor a broader array of health promotion activities than smaller ones. In 1992, for example, worksites with 750 or more employees were nine times as likely to offer cancer screening programs than companies with fewer than 100 workers and about three times as likely to provide blood pressure control, physical fitness, and weight management programs.

The third National Survey found that by 1999, 90% of all worksites reported offering at least one health promotion activity, an increase of 9% from 1992 (AWHP et al., 1999). Among the WHP programs showing the greatest gains in prevalence were back injury prevention programs, which rose from 29% in 1985 and 32% in 1992 to 53% in 1999. As documented in the 1985 and 1992 surveys, the 1999 survey also found that worksites with large numbers of employees offer more health promotion services than smaller worksites. Yet, for most categories of WHP programs (including health screenings, health risk assessments, awareness information, and lifestyle change programs), smaller worksites reported higher rates of employee participation in worksite health programs than larger ones. According to the 1999 survey data, the availability of health promotion services to employees increases substantially within both small and large firms if access to such services is offered through a corporate health plan. Moreover, worksites of all sizes reporting that employee wellness was an important corporate goal offered more health promotion services, stronger evaluation efforts, and had higher utilization rates than those that did not identify employee health improvement as an explicit part of the company's mission.

The significant positive relationship between company size and availability of WHP activities, as documented in the 1985, 1992, and 1999 surveys, has been found in other international, national, and regional WHP surveys as well. In 1996, a postal survey of Scottish workplaces was carried out to assess the current state of health promotion activity in the workplace and to establish the context for the evaluation of Scotland's Health at Work (SHAW) award scheme, which recognizes and encourages Scottish workplaces seeking to improve the health of their workforce (Docherty, Fraser, & Hardin, 1999). The results of the Scottish survey echo the findings of other surveys in that small- and medium-sized workplaces tend to have the lowest levels of health promotion activity. Based on national probability survey data gathered by the U.S. Centers for Disease Control and Prevention as part of the Business Responds to AIDS Program, Wilson et al. (1999) also found a significant positive correlation between company size and the availability of corporate WHP programs. Specifically, companies employing 100 or more workers were more likely to offer a variety of health promotion programs (e.g., physical activity, smoking cessation) than firms with fewer than 100 employees. An important aspect of the survey sample used by Wilson et al. (1999) is that it included companies with 15 or more employees, thereby representing a major segment of small businesses—those with 15–49 workers—that had been ignored by the earlier National Surveys.

The positive association between company size and availability of health promotion programs at the worksite was replicated in a regional survey of nearly 2000 small businesses based in Orange County, California (McMahan et al., 1997; Stokols et al., 1995). The sampling frame for this telephone survey, conducted by Interviewing Services of America on behalf of the University of California, Irvine Health Promotion Center (UCIHPC), included the phone numbers of all Orange County, California, businesses employing between 2–500 workers. The companies participating in the UCIHPC Small Business Workplace Wellness Survey (Small Business Survey) consisted of 2000 companies drawn randomly from the initial sampling frame. A unique feature of the Small Business Survey sample is that it included companies employing as few as 2–14 employees—"microfirms" that had been excluded from the earlier national probability surveys. The exclusion of microfirms from earlier surveys of small business worksite health promotion is striking, considering the fact that 75–80% of U.S. companies employ fewer than 10 workers (Chenoweth, 1995; USSBA, 1998).

The results of the Small Business Survey not only corroborate the previously reported positive link between company size and the availability of WHP programs, but also reveal the markedly lower levels of WHP programs, activities, policies, and benefits available within microfirms as compared to companies with either 15–99 or 100–500 workers (see Table 18-4). For example, 9% of the firms employing 2–14 employees provided smoking cessation programs at the worksite, whereas 13.4% of the firms with 15–99 workers and 18.5% of the companies with 100–500 employees offered such programs at work. The corresponding percentages for stress management programs at the workplace, across the three company-size groups (from lowest to highest), were 9.2%, 13.6%, and 29.4%, respectively. Similarly, the percentages of firms providing workplace violence prevention programs at work were 11.1%, 20.3%, and 34.5%, respectively. This positive linear relationship between company size and WHP programs/activities is evident for most of the program categories listed in Table 18-4.

The generalizability of the Small Business Survey data is limited to Orange County, California. The findings from this regional survey, however, are provocative as they strongly indicate that WHP programs and activities are even more unavailable to workers in very small firms (i.e., microfirms employing between 2–14 workers) than to those employed by companies with 15–99 and 100–500 workers. Moreover, these data underscore the need for more extensive research at state and national levels and for WHP intervention studies focusing on the needs of individuals working in very small firms—a highly underrepresented population in the field of WHP research and practice.

The Small Business Survey findings summarized in Table 18-4 also indicate that the reduced availability of disease prevention and health promotion

Table 18-4 UCIHPC Small Business Workplace Wellness Survey (1996): Programs, Activities, Facilities, Policies, and Benefits Reported by Size of Company

Program, Activity, Facility, Policy, or Benefit	2–14 Employees (n = 637)	15–99 Employees (n = 936)	100–500 Employees (n = 250)	Total Number of Employees (n = 1823)
Adjustable furniture	56.0%	59.3%	73.3%	60.1%
Americans with disabilities compliance	62.4%	79.4%	89.3%	74.9%
Cholesterol or blood pressure	8.7%	8.9%	20.6%	10.5%
Diet/Nutrition	6.5%	7.0%	16.2%	8.1%
Disease screening programs	5.2%	9.0%	14.3%	8.4%
Drug-free policy	76.5%	85.8%	92.5%	83.5%
Emergency & disaster training	36.4%	57.4%	69.7%	51.8%
Employee safety	24.8%	51.9%	77.8%	46.0%
Ergonomics	30.0%	46.6%	64.3%	43.3%
First aid	32.0%	50.1%	68.1%	46.3%
Fitness	7.5%	9.2%	20.2%	10.0%
Hazardous materials	34.0%	52.7%	67.5%	48.2%
Health benefits available to dependents	58.0%	95.7%	97.9%	95.1%
Health insurance	64.2%	83.7%	93.3%	78.2%
Healthy food	15.6%	26.7%	50.6%	26.2%
Immunizations	9.4%	16.5%	33.9%	16.5%
Lockers	15.5%	28.6%	43.4%	26.1%
Lounge	36.5%	55.0%	70.8%	50.8%
No-smoking policy	78.6%	84.8%	86.9%	82.9%
Personal/Mental health	12.7%	19.0%	36.7%	19.9%
Safe work practices	52.4%	71.5%	84.1%	66.6%
Safety policy	81.0%	93.3%	97.2%	89.9%
Sexual harassment policy	66.3%	84.3%	94.8%	79.5%
Showers	7.2%	14.3%	24.5%	13.3%
Smoking cessation	9.0%	13.4%	18.5%	12.5%
Social activities	29.7%	44.8%	64.0%	42.2%
Stress management	9.2%	13.6%	29.4%	14.2%
Substance abuse	12.7%	21.1%	33.9%	19.9%
Suggestion box	25.0%	43.4%	67.1%	40.3%
Violence prevention policy	38.1%	46.4%	63.1%	45.8%
Weight management	7.2%	6.7%	14.4%	8.0%
Workplace violence	11.1%	20.3%	34.5%	18.4%

Note. UCIHPC = University of California, Irvine Health Promotion Center.

programs in the workplace among employees of very small companies is compounded by the lower capacity of these microfirms to provide health insurance benefits to their employees. Specifically, 64.2% of the Small Business Survey firms employing 2–14 workers offered health insurance to their employees, whereas 83.8% of the firms with 15–99 workers and 93.3% of those with 100–500 workers provided health insurance coverage to their employees. These differences in health insurance coverage across the three company-size groups are significant according to chi-square analyses computed on the dichotomous (yes/no) data on which the percentages listed in Table 18-4 are based ($\chi^2 = 124.51$, df = 2, $p < 0.001$).

Furthermore, health insurance benefits were made available to workers' dependents in 58% of the companies with 2–14 employees, whereas health benefits were provided to workers' dependents in 95.7% of the companies with 15–99 employees and in 97.9% of those firms with 100–500 workers (χ^2 = 11.09, df = 2, $p < 0.004$). Thus, the employees of very small firms not only have the most limited access to disease prevention and health promotion programs at work but also sustain the lowest rates of company-based health insurance coverage. The low rates of health insurance coverage for workers in very small firms is a major problem in view of the higher per capita medical costs paid by the owners of these firms (Kathawala & Elmuti, 1994). We turn now to a more detailed discussion of these economic and worksite wellness challenges currently facing the owners and managers of small businesses.

Health Insurance and Small Businesses

Small business employers have been hardest hit by medical care costs. Expenditures for health care plans totaled $145.7 billion in 1992 for businesses with fewer than 500 employees. Of that, $92.2 billion was spent on health care for those establishments with fewer than 100 employees. Health insurance premiums for small businesses are 20–50% higher than premiums for larger businesses (National Governor's Association, 1991).

In a report investigating insurance coverage and firm size, Berger, Black, and Scott (1994) found that the number of uninsured in the United States increased from 31.0 million to 35.5 million people between 1988–92. In 1992, almost 21 million (about 60%) of the uninsured were working. Most of the 35.5 million people who lacked health insurance coverage in 1992 were small business employees or their dependents (Wilcox, 1992). Estimated rates of health insurance coverage among small business workers vary across earlier studies. In a nationwide survey of 1500 small businesses, Kathawala and Elmuti (1994) observed that 79% of the participating firms offered some sort of health insurance coverage to their employees, but only 49% of those employing fewer than 25 employees provided any such coverage. Among companies employing 301–500 workers, however,

94% of the firms provided health insurance benefits to their employees.

The more restricted access to health insurance benefits among workers in very small firms also was observed in a national survey conducted by the USDHHS (1997), indicating that 33% of small businesses with fewer than 10 employees offer health insurance coverage as compared with 96% of firms with 100 or more employees. The national Business Responds to AIDS Program (BRAP) survey conducted by Wilson et al. (1999) reported health insurance rates of 91.9% and 98% in companies with 15–99 and 100+ workers, respectively; but, as noted earlier, the BRAP survey sample omitted firms with only 2–14 employees, which are less likely to offer health insurance coverage to their members than larger employers.

In considering the issue of health plans relative to small companies, it is important to recognize that not all businesses can afford to provide health insurance for their workers. Providing a health promotion program may typically cost $5, $10, $50, $100, or $200 per employee per year, depending on the type of program (e.g., awareness level program, behavior change program, or comprehensive supportive environment program). (O'Donnell & Harris, 1994). Providing health insurance, on the other hand, costs approximately $2000 to $6000 per employee per year. The greater cost of providing employee health insurance suggests that small business managers will be more likely to try implementing a WHP program than investing resources simultaneously to establish both WHP programs and employee health insurance plans. Furthermore, to the extent that employees can access medical coverage through spouses or Medicaid or that the employer is able to supplement employees' salaries so they can purchase insurance on their own, it may not make sense for the employer to provide medical insurance. Finally, reducing medical care costs through WHP programs may not be as great a motivator for employers who do not provide medical insurance as compared to those firms that do provide employee health plans. The medical insurance payment dynamics are quite different for small versus large businesses. Unlike large corporations, small firms can lose their coverage if their claims are high, but cost savings resulting from low utilization rates generally are not passed along to small businesses.

While acknowledging the above-noted barriers to employee health insurance coverage in small firms, it is also important to recognize that the findings from several earlier studies strongly suggest that the employees of very small companies are uniquely disadvantaged by their restricted access to medical benefits as compared to workers in larger firms. This is especially true for small businesses within the wholesale/retail, services, and manufacturing industries as compared to professional offices (e.g., legal and medical firms), finance firms, and rapidly expanding high-technology companies (California HealthCare Foundation & Mercer, Inc., 1999; Torres, 1999). Moreover, among employees working in very small firms in those industries, certain groups appear to be especially vulnerable to medical problems and financial hardships—namely, ethnic minority and low socioeconomic status workers.

The relative lack of health insurance coverage among small versus large business workers is an issue that is highly relevant to the development of future health promotion strategies in small business settings. Clearly, not all small businesses can afford to offer health insurance. Nonetheless, the absence of such coverage may create anxiety, insecurity, and greater financial and illness-related vulnerabilities among substantial segments of the small business workforce—all of which can seriously compromise the physical and emotional well-being of these individuals and their dependents and thereby undermine the effectiveness of WHP programming efforts in some small companies. The following section examines the particular needs of these vulnerable groups, namely, ethnic minority and low-income employees of small firms.

The Plight of Ethnic Minority and Low Socioeconomic Status Workers in Small Businesses

Members of ethnic minority groups, especially those characterized by low household incomes and socioeconomic status (SES), face enormous financial and health challenges in the U.S. These persons are much more likely to be unemployed or underemployed (Dooley et al., 1996) and to lack family health insurance and worksite health benefits than are more affluent, high-SES individuals (Berger et al., 1994; Donaldson et al., 1998; Schauffler, Brown, & Rice, 1997; USDHHS, 1991). The disproportionate lack of access to adequate employment and health insurance coverage leaves low-income, uneducated, and minority group members particularly vulnerable to financial hardship and premature morbidity/mortality, owing to the pervasive and strongly positive correlation between SES and favorable health status (Adler et al., 1994; Yen & Syme, 1999).

Another source of vulnerability among low-income minority group members is the growing "digital divide" between them and more affluent, nonminority workers (U.S. Department of Commerce, 1995). Although the rate of computer ownership among U.S. citizens has risen in recent years (to about 33% of the population in 1998), the gap between computer "haves" and "have-nots" continues to grow. About half as many Black and Hispanic people own computers as do non-Hispanic Whites, and White households are three times as likely as Black households to have Internet access. In 1997, the difference in computer ownership rates between Whites and Blacks was 21.5 percentage points; and the difference between Whites and Hispanics was 21.4 percentage points (U.S. Department of Commerce, 1998). Moreover, computer ownership is positively correlated with educational attainment. About 63% of people with some college education own computers—a level of ownership that is about 10 times greater than for those who never attended high school.

The relative lack of access to computer training and ownership among low-SES minority group members will create even greater economic difficulties for them, as the demand for workers skilled in information technology continues to expand in the coming decade (Freeman & Aspray, 1999). For example, Kochar (1994), analyzing data from the 1991 Current Population Survey of 50,000 U.S. households (compiled by the Bureau of the Census), found that small businesses were hiring college educated workers and creating jobs at the top end of the wage spectrum in greater proportions than in earlier years. The highest premium for computer users over nonusers was found in rapidly growing small firms, where a premium of nearly 24.8% in wages was observed. Thus, although the proportions of low-SES minority persons entering the small business workforce has grown in recent years, it is precisely those individuals who lack the requisite training to compete for higher paying computer-based jobs in small high-technology firms.

Finally, low-SES minority individuals are disadvantaged not only by restricted financial resources, but also by starkly unequal incomes relative to other groups in society. Income inequality has been found to exert a negative impact on health status, above and beyond the effects of low SES and low levels of household income (Yen & Syme, 1999). Some researchers (Kawachi, Kennedy, Lochner, & Prothrow-Stith, 1997) have hypothesized that the deleterious effects of income inequality on health are mediated by the social isolation and relative deprivation experienced by disadvantaged individuals, which in turn, lead to a decline of "social capital"—those "features of social organization such as networks, norms, and social trust that facilitate coordination and cooperation for mutual benefit" (Putnam, 1995, p. 67). Thus, income inequality, social isolation, and loss of social capital, along with restricted access to health insurance, technology training, and full-time employment, are among the factors that place low-SES minority workers at highest risk for illness, injury, and financial hardship.

The National Health Interview Survey data reported by Grosch et al. (1998) clearly indicate that the availability of WHP programs is highest for employees who are well-educated, White, and between the ages of 25–54, and lowest for less educated and Black workers—groups that may have the most to gain from access to worksite health programs. Thus, one challenge facing the WHP field is to develop disease prevention and health promotion programs that reach these disadvantaged and underserved groups (Stokols, Allen, & Bellingham, 1996). Simply making more WHP programs available to underrepresented groups of workers, however, will not necessarily result in health improvement for those individuals. To be effective, future worksite health programs for small businesses must address the specific needs of low-SES minority persons, as well as those of other underserved groups, such as older workers, highly mobile employees (e.g., those whose jobs are vehicle-based), employees in rural locations, and blue-collar workers in injury-prone occupations (such as farming, mining, construction, and transportation) (McMahan, 1999; Scharf, Kidd, Cole, & Wiehagen, 1999; Stokols, Clitheroe et al., 1995).

Earlier WHP research strongly suggests that the most effective worksite health programs include multiple components (e.g., encompassing lifestyle modification, changes in the work environment, personalized risk appraisal, and counseling) that identify the employees in an organization who are most at risk for illness and injury, then provide programs that are tailored to their specialized needs (DeJoy & Southern, 1993; Erfurt, Foote, Heirich, & Brock, 1995; Erfurt & Holtyn, 1991; Foote & Erfurt, 1991; Fries, Harrington, Edwards, Kent, & Richardson, 1994; Harvey, Whitmer, Hilyer, & Brown, 1993; Heaney & Goetzel, 1997). For low-SES minority workers, small business owners first and foremost must develop cost-effective strategies for providing health insurance to their employees—for example, by partnering with other small firms to establish health insurance purchasing cooperatives (Chenoweth, 1995; Schauffler et al., 1997; UCIHPC, 1998). Future WHP programs also should be designed to enhance social support and encourage a stronger sense of community among minority workers by incorporating culturally appropriate language and programming options that are consistent with the health beliefs and needs of a culturally diverse workforce (Edmunson, 1995; Ramirez, 1994; Rubio & Arteaga, 2000; Torres, 1999).

Finally, greater efforts should be made by small business managers to offer on-the-job computer training to their lower SES and entry-level employees (Donaldson et al., 1998; Freeman & Aspray, 1999). Several lines of research suggest that a major risk factor for illness is job insecurity and that such insecurity is widespread among large segments of the small business workforce due to the greater volatility of small firms and the fact that a large proportion of low-income workers in small companies lack the requisite technological skills to compete for stable and high-paying jobs. Thus, computer skills training should be considered as an important facet of future WHP programs targeted toward small business employees.

TOWARD MORE COMPREHENSIVE WORKSITE HEALTH PROMOTION PROGRAMS FOR SMALL BUSINESSES

The preceding discussion of small firms and their specialized needs relative to health promotion suggests the value of developing a conceptual model that can be used to identify: (a) important directions for WHP practice and research in small companies, and (b) a set of programmatic strategies that are uniquely tailored to meet the worksite health goals of small businesses (see Table 18-5). We next outline a conceptual model for organizing WHP activities in small firms and then discuss some recent case studies in which certain of the strategies outlined in the model are being implemented and evaluated for their efficacy within small business settings.

A Model for Meeting the Health Promotion Needs of Small Businesses

The proposed model of worksite health promotion reflects certain core assumptions. The first assumption is that comprehensive, multicomponent WHP programs are generally preferable to single-component and more narrowly targeted programs. We recognize that efforts to implement single-component WHP programs are sometimes more affordable than those involving multicomponent programs and that establishing even a limited WHP program in a company is preferable to neglecting health promotion activities altogether. Nonetheless, multicomponent WHP programs have some distinct advantages over narrowly gauged programs and often can be implemented in a cost-effective manner within both small and large firms.

The emphasis on comprehensive WHP programs in the proposed model is consistent with recent developments in the health promotion field. During the 1990s, the conceptualization of WHP programs expanded to include not only informational or awareness-raising strategies and behavioral/lifestyle change programs to foster improved employee health, but also facilities design and organizational changes to create a more healthful work environment (DeJoy & Wilson, 1995; O'Donnell, 1989; O'Donnell & Harris, 1994; World Health Organization [WHO], 1994). This trend toward developing comprehensive worksite health programs reflects an increasing emphasis on the value of broad-gauged, integrated worksite health improvement strategies that encompass: (a) individually-focused lifestyle change, self-care, clinical preventive

---

Table 18-5 High-Leverage Strategies for Workplace Health Promotion in Small Businesses

Management Training Strategies:	Community Partnering Strategies:
Provide small business managers with educational training and resources to cultivate: 1. Sensitivity to cultural, gender-based, and age-related needs of employees 2. Awareness of multicomponent, comprehensive health promotion programs 3. Core competencies for designing, implementing, and evaluating comprehensive workplace health promotion programs • Manager training programs in the area of workplace health promotion. • Practical, "how-to" programming guides and educational resources. • Consultation services provided by knowledgeable workplace health promotion experts.	Provide small business managers with outside technical assistance and economic support to enhance worksite wellness using new community-based delivery systems to provide: • Small business health insurance purchasing cooperatives • Government-sponsored grants-in-aid for small business health promotion • Corporate-community consortia for delivering medical and EAP services to small business workers • Small business partnerships to facilitate collaborative workplace health promotion efforts (e.g., informal worksite wellness coalitions, support networks).

services, mental health management, and health awareness programs (Docherty et al., 1999; Fries et al., 1993; Green, 1984; Maccoby & Alexander, 1980; U.S. Preventive Service Task Force, 1989; Vickery & Fries, 1996); as well as (b) organizational culture, policies, and benefits, (c) environmental change, facilities planning, and management strategies, and (d) collaborative efforts with other businesses, nonprofit agencies, and government organizations in the community for purposes of promoting employee wellness and a healthy workplace (Allen & Allen, 1986; McLeroy, Bibeau, Steckler, & Glanz, 1988; McMahan & Kuang, 1999; Stokols, 1996; Wandersman et al., 1996). Comprehensive programs that integrate activities and policies spanning these four levels of analysis and intervention exemplify **social ecological models** of health promotion (Breslow, 1996; Green, Richard, & Potvin, 1996; Levi, 1992; Richard, Potvin, Kishchuk, Prlic, & Green, 1996; Stokols, 1992; Stokols et al., 1996; UCIHPC, 1998).[1]

A second key assumption underlying the proposed model of health promotion is that the model is applicable to companies of all sizes, but the *relative priority and effectiveness of the WHP strategies included in the model varies between small and large firms.* Specifically, we suggest that certain combinations of WHP strategies are likely to afford greater *leverage* for achieving the worksite health goals of small companies than others. For instance, because small businesses typically lack formal departments and in-house experts responsible for wellness programming, the owners and managers of small firms must play a more active and central role in promoting worksite health than their counterparts in large companies. Thus, one promising strategy for small business health promotion is to place greater emphasis on developing educational resources and training programs designed to

cultivate certain core competencies for small business managers—especially those skills that appear to be essential for effective delivery and maintenance of wellness programs in small firms.

In subsequent sections of the chapter, we give particular attention to four managerial skills that are becoming increasingly important as a basis for promoting employee health in small companies: (a) sensitivity to cultural, gender-based, and age-related needs of employees, (b) an awareness of multicomponent, comprehensive health promotion programs, (c) the knowledge to design, implement, and evaluate comprehensive workplace health promotion programs, and (d) the ability to incorporate low-cost community resources into workplace health promotion programs. Examples of recently published training resources designed to enhance these core competencies of small business managers are the *Health Promotion: Sourcebook for Small Businesses* (WELCOA, 1998) and the *Manager's Guide to Workplace Wellness* (UCIHPC, 1998). Similarly, *Design of Workplace Health Promotion Programs* (O'Donnell, 1995) and *Well Now: A Manager's Guide to Worksite Health Promotion* (Eddy & Kahler, 1992) provide business managers with extensive hands-on information about the design and implementation of worksite wellness programs. An important direction for future research on WHP programs in small business settings is to evaluate the extent to which the managers of small firms are using these new educational resources and the extent to which these efforts are effective in enabling small business managers to cultivate new WHP competencies and skills.

The findings from recent studies also suggest that to be maximally effective, health promotion training programs aimed at small business managers should be supplemented by community-based interventions

---

[1]The integration of these multiple levels of worksite health promotion provides the basis for establishing corporate health programs that go beyond individual behavior change to improve the collective health of all employees working in a particular location. Using the issues of smoking cessation as an example, the employees working at a particular company will be more likely, as a group, to refrain from or quit smoking if their employer offers not only a smoking cessation program targeted at high-risk workers (individual strategy), but also implements a "no-smoking" policy (organizational strategy), removes all ashtrays from the building (environmental strategy), and arranges for a local nonprofit agency (community strategy) to provide information to workers about the health and financial costs associated with smoking and the availability of local support groups to facilitate smoking cessation (Sorensen, Glasgow, Corbett, & Topor, 1992, Sorensen, Lando, & Pechacek, 1993).

designed to establish informal worksite wellness coalitions, support networks, and public/private sector consortia as a basis for promoting cost-effective, cooperative health promotion ventures spanning multiple employers, nonprofit organizations, philanthropic foundations, universities, and government agencies (Chenoweth, 1998; Donaldson & Klein, 1997; Pelletier, Klehr, & McPhee, 1988; Torres, 1999; UCIHPC, 1998; USDHHS, 1987; Wandersman et al., 1996). These organizational networking strategies, which create linkages between multiple businesses, community settings, and intervention targets (Richard et al., 1996), appear to be especially crucial for effective health promotion in small firms, owing to the special needs and more limited resources of small versus large companies. In the following sections of the chapter, we review recent efforts to cultivate core WHP competencies among small business managers and to establish community consortia for small business health promotion. We also examine the implications of these recent efforts for future practice and research in the field of health promotion.

Cultivating Core Competencies for Worksite Health Promotion Among Small Business Managers

Our earlier discussion of small businesses and their specialized needs relative to health promotion highlights a crucial core competency for small business managers, which can help promote more effective WHP programs in the 21st Century—namely, the *development of cultural sensitivity and the ability to recognize and serve the needs of an increasingly diverse workforce.* A business manager sensitive to the cultural, gender-based, and age-related needs of his or her employees will make concerted efforts to communicate directly with them about their health and family concerns in a linguistically appropriate and supportive manner; provide personalized health risk appraisals and counseling (e.g., with the assistance of outside consultants) to encourage health-promotive lifestyle change; take the necessary steps to ensure a healthy and safe work environment; and, very importantly, offer company-sponsored health insurance and access to low-cost preventive services and medical care for employees and their dependents.

The previously noted findings that WHP programs tend to be most influential and effective when they incorporate multiple components tailored to the specialized needs of vulnerable workers (DeJoy & Southern, 1993; Erfurt et al., 1995; Fries et al., 1994; Harvey et al., 1993; Heaney & Goetzel, 1997) underscore the value of cultivating at least two additional core competencies among small business managers for WHP: namely, an *awareness and understanding of comprehensive, integrated WHP programs,* and the *ability to design, implement, and evaluate integrated multicomponent WHP programs.* We turn now to a more detailed discussion of these issues.

Because small businesses typically lack in-house expertise and formal departments in the areas of human resources, medical services, and occupational safety and health, they face the complex challenges of (a) compiling/integrating research and regulatory information pertinent to these concerns and (b) designing and delivering effective worksite health programs based on that information. Typically, these tasks fall by the wayside in small businesses since their managers are confronted by more stringent time and resource constraints than those working in larger firms. Given these constraints, new training resources and consultation services must be developed to assist small business managers in their efforts to become more knowledgeable about worksite health and more capable of designing and implementing cost-effective worksite health promotion programs. As noted earlier, several resource books and hands-on programming guides have been developed in recent years to assist the owners and managers of small firms in these efforts (Eddy & Kahler, 1992; O'Donnell, 1995; UCIHPC, 1998; USDHHS, 1987; WELCOA, 1998).

The task of compiling and integrating information pertinent to the development of effective worksite health promotion programs is a daunting one because worksite health encompasses a wide array of research and practice areas, including occupational safety and health (OSH), employee assistance programs (EAP), employee wellness or worksite health promotion (WHP) programs, and employee benefits/relations (DeJoy & Southern, 1993). According to DeJoy and Southern (1993), the first step in developing effective worksite health programs is the creation of a comprehensive health policy or mission statement by the company. The importance of this strategy is borne out by recent findings from the 1999 National Worksite Health Promotion Survey (AWHP et al., 1999), indicating that companies (of all sizes) identifying employee health improvement as an explicit part of their corporate mission undertake more extensive WHP efforts and report higher rates of employee participation in their WHP programs as compared to businesses lacking clear worksite health goals.

A prerequisite for establishing comprehensive and effective corporate health policies is a basic awareness and understanding among business managers of the many facets of worksite wellness (e.g., OSH, EAP, WHP, state and federal regulations, and human resources and benefits programs). In an effort to increase managers' awareness and understanding of these issues, several worksite health training programs and resource guides have been developed in recent years and tested for their effectiveness. For example, researchers at the UCI Health Promotion Center (UCIHPC) developed the *REACH OUT for Safety* training program for small business managers to improve corporate awareness of, and compliance with, California's worksite Injury and Illness Prevention Program (IIPP) legislation (Injury and Illness Prevention Program 198, 1989; Wells et al., 1997).[2] In this train-the-trainer program, the REACH OUT acronym represents the various worksite health requirements stipulated by California's IIPP law and was created to better communicate the relevant aspects of the legislation to business managers and to enhance managers' comprehension and memory of key regulatory requirements. Components of the REACH OUT training program include:

Responsibility assignment, Evaluation procedure, Accident investigation, Corrective action, Hazard prevention training, Obeying the law, Understanding through communication, and Tracking and Record-Keeping.

Wells et al. (1997) conducted a two-year field-experimental study of 100 firms in Orange and Los Angeles Counties, California. The results demonstrated that those companies randomly assigned to the REACH OUT training sessions during the first year of the study demonstrated greater managerial awareness of the IIPP regulatory requirements and achieved higher levels of corporate compliance with the law than the nonintervention firms that received the REACH OUT training at the conclusion of the study.[3]

The UCIHPC team subsequently developed a more comprehensive training program, the Small Business Workplace Wellness Project (SBWWP), which not only addresses occupational safety and health regulations but also encompasses individually oriented strategies of lifestyle/health behavior change, organizational policies and programs, facilities planning and management interventions, and collaboration among business organizations and other community groups, all aimed at achieving higher levels of worksite wellness, quality of working life, employee productivity, corporate cost containment and profitability (McMahan et al., 1997; McMahan, Stokols, & Phillips, 2000; Stokols, Clitheroe et al., 1995). To achieve these goals, UCIHPC administered a Worksite Wellness Telephone Appraisal (Small Business Survey) to 2000 small businesses in southern California and developed several informational resources for managers and employees, including the

---

[2]In 1989, the state of California passed Senate Bill 198, which requires businesses not only to report and evaluate accidents, but also to actively promote health and disease prevention. The legislation specifically requires California employers to establish, implement, and maintain a worksite Injury and Illness Prevention Program (IIPP). An effective IIPP includes several key elements: (a) identification of the person responsible for implementing the program, (b) identification and evaluation of workplace hazards, (c) investigation of occupational injuries and illnesses, (d) correction of unsafe conditions and work practices, (e) a training program to instruct employees in both general and job-specific safe work practices, (f) procedures for ensuring that employees comply with safe work practices, (g) communication between employers and employees on health and safety matters, and (h) IIPP-related record keeping.

[3]Levels of corporate compliance were measured from multiple perspectives, using a 16-item checklist administered to (1) business managers, (2) employees in participating firms who did not hold managerial positions, and (3) researchers who made onsite visits to the participating companies both before and after the REACH OUT sessions occurred.

Workplace Health Promotion Information & Resource Kit, an interactive internet site (http://www.healthpro-motioncenter.uci.edu) that provides detailed information about worksite health promotion (WHP) and numerous links to related internet sites, and a comprehensive WHP programming guide—the *Manager's Guide to Workplace Wellness* (UCIHPC, 1998).

The *Manager's Guide to Workplace Wellness* is organized into seven modules that provide information about the multiple components of comprehensive programs and policies (including the individual/behavioral, organizational, environmental, and community levels of WHP) and introduce managers to strategies for identifying employee health concerns and company health needs, planning and presenting workplace wellness programs (including lifestyle improvement, environment and safety, and workplace relations programs), and monitoring and evaluating these programs. The *Manager's Guide* also provides several practical tools for WHP, including copy-ready, self-scorable forms for surveying managers and employees about their health concerns, checklists for conducting environmental health audits, descriptions of community resources that can be used by business managers to promote workplace wellness, and a program planner for planning, presenting, and monitoring WHP programs.

The effectiveness of the SBWWP in promoting higher levels of worksite wellness is being evaluated in a longitudinal (1996–1999) field-experimental study in which 80 small businesses are randomly assigned to four different training levels. Managers in the nonintervention (comparison) group received no WHP training or resources at the outset of the study; the second group received the *Manager's Guide to Workplace Wellness* at the outset of the study; the third group received the *Manager's Guide* and a follow-up

WHP coaching visit by a member of the research team; and the fourth group received the training components provided to Group 3 and also participated in a partnering group with other business managers in an effort to facilitate community collaboration toward worksite health improvement.

Analyses conducted on the Small Business Survey data, gathered from nearly 2000 Orange County businesses during the first year of the SBWWP, indicated that the comprehensiveness (or multicomponent/integrative quality) of WHP programs is associated with higher levels of organizational health as reported by the managers of participating firms. The integrative quality of WHP programs was measured using multiple survey items that assessed the breadth, existence, and availability of multiple worksite health policies and activities within each of the participating firms (e.g., health risk appraisal and lifestyle change programs, physical environmental strategies, organizational policies and employee health benefits, use of community resources for WHP).[4] Preliminary findings suggest the potential value of comprehensive WHP programs is greater than those that are narrower in scope (e.g., implementing behavior change programs without implementing related policies).

The relative effectiveness of the SBWWP intervention components in promoting higher levels of worksite health in small businesses is being examined through a series of pre/postanalyses of employee wellness and related organizational outcomes associated with (a) use of the *Manager's Guide to Workplace Wellness,* (b) WHP coaching visits involving project staff and small business managers, and (c) participation in a small business partnering group aimed at fostering greater collaboration between businesses, nonprofit agencies, and government organizations in

---

[4]A median split was performed on the comprehensive factor scores to identify companies with relatively narrow, nonintegrated WHP programs and those with broader-gauged, more integrated programs. Two five-point Likert scales were combined to measure managers' appraisals of organizational health in their companies: "How would you rate the general health of your company's employees during the last year?" (from excellent to poor), and "How would you describe employee morale at your company?" (from excellent to poor). An analysis of variance indicated that the managers of small businesses with more comprehensive WHP programs reported higher levels of organizational health than those representing firms with less comprehensive and integrated programs ($F = 10.77$, df = 1, $p < 0.001$). These data are from a cross-sectional survey and must be viewed as preliminary in view of the methodological limitations inherent in retrospective, self-report surveys.

the development of WHP activities. Examples of outcomes to be measured include intervention group differences in employee health status and morale, quantity and types of WHP programs/activities offered by the company, and manager awareness about (a) the kinds of programs/activities that can be included in a WHP program, (b) the kinds of health risks their employees may be exposed to, and (c) the kinds of benefits their company might experience by implementing WHP programs. Although training resources such as the *Manager's Guide* appear to be useful in enabling small business managers to develop more effective WHP programs, it is also likely that the value of these informational tools will be augmented substantially by the availability of community resources, such as outside WHP consultants and business-community coalitions, who can assist managers in their efforts to promote health in the workplace.

For instance, the processes of planning, presenting, and monitoring WHP programs entail several sequential steps: raising corporate awareness of worksite health concerns, conducting a WHP needs assessment, developing a broad-ranging corporate health policy or mission statement, selecting and implementing key program components in an integrated fashion, monitoring their effectiveness, and revising program components to enhance their effectiveness. Training resources such as the *Manager's Guide to Workplace Wellness* provide a useful means for managers to learn about and implement these sequential phases of WHP programming. At the same time, however, the assistance of outside health promotion experts and business-community partnerships may prove invaluable to those managers of small firms who lack sufficient time and organizational resources to establish comprehensive, effective WHP programs on their own.

A broad array of community resources for WHP is potentially available to small business managers, however the managers themselves may not know how to locate and make use of the WHP expertise and assistance within their local communities and at state and national levels. An additional and critical core competency for effective WHP programming among small business managers is the *capacity to identify and*

incorporate low-cost community resources into corporate health promotion programs. We turn now to a discussion of community-partnering strategies to link managers with these critical resources.

Enhancing Worksite Wellness through Community Partnering Strategies

An exciting new frontier for small business health promotion is the development of community coalitions and partnering groups, which can substantially augment managers' efforts to develop comprehensive and effective worksite health promotion programs. An extensive research literature on the formation of community coalitions for health promotion presently exists (Bracht & Gleason, 1990; Butterfoss, Goodman, & Wandersman, 1993; Conner, Tanjasiri, Davidson, Dempsey, & Robles, 1999; McLeroy, Kegler, Steckler, Burdine, & Wisotzky, 1994; Pelletier et al., 1988; USDHHS, 1995, Wandersman et al., 1996); yet, prior studies have given sparse attention to the development of small business-community coalitions whose goal is to foster greater collaboration among small firms and community groups for worksite health improvement.

Nonetheless, several demonstration projects involving small businesses partnering with each other and various community groups to enhance worksite health have been spawned in recent years. These projects, which include corporate health insurance purchasing cooperatives (Chenoweth, 1995), government-sponsored grants to small businesses for developing worksite health promotion programs (Cyzman & Lafkas, 1991), mentoring initiatives matching interested business managers with managers from other local employers who are experienced in developing health promotion programs (Joint Venture: Silicon Valley Network, 1998), and community collaboration to provide low-cost employee assistance programs and medical services to low-SES workers (Donaldson & Klein, 1997; Torres, 1999), offer a provocative and informative glimpse into the field of small business health promotion during the 21st century. In the following section, we summarize some of these innovative community-partnering strategies for worksite health improvement.

Small Business Health Insurance Purchasing Cooperatives

We noted earlier that very small businesses are at a distinct disadvantage in working with HMOs and PPOs due to their more limited resources and purchasing power relative to large corporations. For example, many worksite health promotion subsidies provided to companies by HMOs are restricted to firms with 50 or more employees (Donaldson et al., 1998). Thus, small businesses increasingly are joining health insurance purchasing "cooperatives" to enhance their ability to provide high-quality medical benefits for their workers.

In Cleveland, Ohio, a group of small businesses formed a large purchasing pool, the Council of Smaller Enterprises (COSE). "The council consists of 9,000 firms representing 54,000 employees and 120,000 dependents. All COSE members can purchase affordable health insurance coverage because the council has persuaded large insurers to offer their coalition the same advantages given to larger companies. The most important of these advantages is the clout to pressure doctors and hospitals to keep costs down. The COSE arrangement has been a successful cost-control strategy for its members, whose annual premiums typically rise only about one-fourth as much as they do for non-COSE businesses" (Chenoweth, 1998, pp. 129–130). Small business purchasing cooperatives similar to COSE are likely to arise in many other regions of the country, as managers confront the pressing demand for cost-effective health insurance coverage among their employees—especially low-SES minority workers (Schauffler et al., 1997).

Government-Sponsored Grants-in-Aid for Small Business Health Promotion

The Worksite and Community Health Promotion Program (WCHPP) was established by the Michigan Department of Public Health to provide small grants to companies with fewer than 500 employees, with the goal of assisting underserved firms in their efforts to develop and maintain cost-effective WHP programs (Chenoweth, 1995; Cyzman & Lafkas, 1991). Created in 1987, this state-sponsored program provides one-year WHP grants of up to $9,000 to small businesses. The grants are awarded on a quarterly basis. The WCHPP requires that WHP vendors be trained and certified by the state before working directly with the grant-funded firms. Also, the program requires that evaluative measures be gathered at each of the participating worksites to assess WHP processes and outcomes. A particularly valuable feature of this innovative program is its assignment of highest priority to small firms employing large percentages of low-SES and minority workers in the grant-making process. This Michigan-based program stands as an exemplar of government-sponsored support for small business health promotion which, hopefully, will expand to additional states in the coming years.

Corporate-Community Consortia for Delivering Medical and Employee Assistance Program Services to Small Business Workers

As noted earlier, one of the most pressing challenges facing the managers of small businesses is finding cost-effective ways of offering their employees clinical preventive services, employee assistance programs, and medical care for injury and illness. In southern California, two innovative coalitions involving small businesses, nonprofit agencies, and medical providers have been established to promote employee wellness: the Los Angeles Worksite Wellness Project (Torres, 1999) and The Pasadena Consortium (Donaldson & Klein, 1997).

The Los Angeles Worksite Wellness Project (LAWWP) is a three-year demonstration project that brings wellness education and basic health care to the worksites of medically underserved and uninsured low-wage workers in Los Angeles. The Project aims to increase health awareness and improve the health status of low-income workers by facilitating their use of existing health education and medical resources. The LAWWP links these traditionally underserved workers to community health resources by distributing information at the worksite that encourages healthy lifestyle choices, self-care, and timely utilization of medical services.

The LAWWP targets workers in the food processing, furniture manufacturing, and apparel/textile industries, all of which employ large percentages of low-income workers and typically do not offer health benefits or health education programs to their employees. During its first two years, the LAWWP established worksite wellness programs at 10 small firms employing a total of 400 predominantly low-wage, Latino workers. Key components of the LAWWP include clinical preventive services, risk factor screening programs, and health care utilization and referral. To deliver worksite health services in a cost-effective manner, the LAWWP has established a community network of nonprofit health providers who offer health education and screening programs to participating worksites. Also, to better achieve the health education goals identified by participating companies, the health awareness materials distributed at the worksite are culturally sensitive and linguistically appropriate.

An especially valuable feature of the LAWWP is that employees at each worksite receive personalized counseling on how to access community medical services in an efficient and timely manner. As part of this counseling process, uninsured workers are informed about the availability of free or low-cost services, while those workers with medical benefits receive assistance in contacting their designated medical providers. The LAWWP serves as a model program for delivering cost-effective health education and medical services to underserved small business workers in California and beyond.

The Pasadena Consortium (Consortium) was established as a low-cost delivery system for providing WHP and EAP services to small business workers (Donaldson & Klein, 1997). The Consortium, established in 1993 with funding support from The California Wellness Foundation, has provided community health services to more than 4000 small business workers. The Consortium was created to promote collaboration among businesses, nonprofit agencies, university researchers, and medical providers for purposes of enhancing worksite health among traditionally underserved employee populations. Like the WCHPP in Michigan and the LAWWP in California, the Pasadena Consortium targets ethnically diverse employees working in small companies, especially those that are owned by women and/or minorities. The Consortium's network of providers includes behavioral health specialists from both the public and private sectors. Participating vendors agree to pro-

vide health services and wellness education to managers, employees, and their families on a *pro bono* basis. Several intervention components that are being delivered as part of the Consortium (e.g., EAP services, wellness education and lifestyle change programs, and managerial training in WHP strategies) are currently being evaluated for their health and cost effectiveness. The number of small businesses participating in the Consortium has increased dramatically in recent years. The Pasadena Consortium, like the WCHPP and LAWWP described earlier, has established itself as an innovative model for future community-business partnerships that are intended to promote more collaborative and effective worksite health programs.

Establishing Small Business Partnerships to Facilitate Collaborative Worksite Health Promotion Efforts

At the University of California, Irvine, small business managers participating in the highest intervention group within the Small Business Workplace Wellness Project (SBWWP) were assigned to a small (8–10 person) WHP partnering group. The purpose of this group was to help managers of multiple companies identify common worksite health concerns and help them share resources and expertise. Ideally, these identified concerns would then be addressed through the development of joint WHP programs. This approach differs from the WCHPP, the LAWWP, and the Pasadena Consortium described earlier in that it entails a series of task-oriented discussion sessions and programming meetings where representatives from several small companies actively collaborate in the formulation of new WHP initiatives. Initial indications are that these small business partnering groups can serve as a powerful tool for promoting improved levels of worksite health within the participating firms. In effect, these partnering groups provide small business managers with interpersonal support and information exchange as they work together to design innovative and cost-effective WHP programs. By pooling their financial and personnel resources and sharing programming ideas, the managers of these firms may improve their capacity for identifying low-cost strategies for promoting

Table 18-6 Community Resources for Workplace Health Promotion

- **Government agencies** (e.g., the U.S. Small Business Administration, city and county health departments, state Occupational Safety and Health Administration [OSHA] consultation services) will provide free information about workplace health and safety and may be available to visit a workplace to offer suggestions.

- **Local health agencies and educational institutions** (e.g., chapters of national organizations such as the American Heart Association and American Cancer Society, hospitals/health clinics and HMOs, colleges and universities, and county libraries) offer a variety of free services, including informational brochures and pamphlets, speakers, training sessions, health education seminars, meeting space, health fairs, and health services.

- **Professional, industry, and service organizations** (e.g., chambers of commerce; service clubs like Rotary, Kiwanis, Lions; industry or professional associations appropriate for different companies) can provide free information, speakers, and assistance.

- **Community involvement opportunities** are available, which can help a company expand its health promotion efforts. For example, they can research the availability of local health-related services for employees, such as childcare and eldercare; they can post information about free local health services that might interest employees; they can help sponsor a health-related event for a local charity, such as a 5K walk/run; and they can encourage and reward employees for volunteering their own time within the community.

- **Networking and partnering with other businesses** (e.g., similar size, industry, or geographic region) can be a very powerful strategy for small business managers to increase the effectiveness and success of their health promotion efforts. For example, they may be able to identify other companies similar to theirs through their property management company, the local chamber of commerce, or professional and industry associations; they can pool financial and personnel resources with similar companies to provide shared workplace health promotion programs that might not otherwise be feasible, such as expanded health insurance coverage or a health fair; and they can establish an ongoing group of small business owners and managers who meet regularly to talk about the health of their businesses, including the health of their employees and the relative effectiveness of alternative health promotion strategies.

wellness in their respective companies. An evaluation of the processes and outcomes associated with SBWWP's business-partnering intervention is currently being conducted (Stokols, Clitheroe, McMahan , & Wells, 1995). The results of this evaluation will provide detailed information about the effectiveness of the program and guide future efforts to establish corporate partnering groups for enhancing worksite health in small companies.

In sum, the development of business-community coalitions and partnering groups to promote more effective and comprehensive worksite health programs has emerged in recent years as a new and exciting frontier for future WHP practice and research. A variety of community resources are currently available to small business managers to assist them in their efforts to establish effective WHP programs, as outlined in Table 18-6. The WHP field is likely to witness more extensive utilization of these community strategies and resources by the managers of small firms during the 21st Century.

CONCLUSION: THE FUTURE OF HEALTH PROMOTION IN SMALL BUSINESSES

The small business sector constitutes an extremely important part of the American economy. Roughly 80% of the nation's workers are employed by companies with fewer than 500 employees. Small businesses are a tremendous source of innovation and account for most of the net job growth in the U.S. They also provide most first-time workers with the opportunity to enter the job market in America. At the same time, small firms face enormous financial and organizational challenges since they operate on tighter profit margins and employ higher percentages of low-SES, minority, and technologically-untrained individuals than do large firms. They also lack the in-house expertise and corporate infrastructure (e.g., occupational safety and health specialists, human resource departments) to facilitate the establishment and maintenance of comprehensive worksite health programs. It is not surprising, then, that over the past two decades, the most extensive WHP programs and research studies have been implemented in companies with 500 or more workers.

Appendix: Online Resources for Small Businesses

- **AllBusiness.com—Solutions for Growing Businesses**
  www.allbusiness.com

- **BenefitMall.com—Employee Benefits for Small Business**
  www.benefitmall.com

- **Biztalk—Small Business Community**
  www.biztalk.com

- **Business Resource Center**
  www.morebusiness.com

- **BusinessWeek Online**
  www.businessweek.com/smallbiz/index.html

- **ChamberBiz—The Ultimate Small Business Resource**
  www.chamberbiz.com/

- **Convey.com—Communication and Web Resources for Small Businesses**
  www.convey.com

- **Department of Social and Preventive Medicine, University of Queensland**
  www.spmed.uq.edu.au

- **Health On the Net Foundation**
  www.hon.ch

- **Health Canada Online—Small Business Health Model**
  www.hcsc.gc.ca/hppb/ahi/workplace/pube/smallbusiness/healthmodel.htm

- **Heartland Healthcare Coalition**
  www.hhco.org

- **Idea Café—The Small Business Channel**
  www.ideacafe.com

- **National Health Information Center**
  http://nhic-nt.health.org

- **OneCore.com—Financial Expertise for Small Businesses**
  www.onecore.com

- **Partnership for Prevention**
  www.prevent.org

- **SmallOffice.com—Big Ideas for Small Business**
  www.smalloffice.com

- **Small Business Development Center, New York State**
  www.smallbiz.suny.edu

- **Small Business Resources**
  http://smallbusinessresources.com

- **SmallBizSavings—The Online Purchasing Alliance for Small Business Buyers**
  www.smallbizsavings.com

- **SmartAge.com—Smart Commerce for Small Business**
  www.smartage.com

- **University of California, Irvine Health Promotion Center**
  www.healthpromotioncenter.uci.edu

- **U.S. Business Advisor**
  www.business.gov

- **U.S. Chamber of Commerce**
  www.uschamber.org

- **U.S. Small Business Administration**
  www.sba.gov

- **Wellness Councils of America**
  www.welcoa.org/prod_and_srvcs/sourcebooks/sourcebooks.htm

- **WomenConnect.com—Connecting Women in Business**
  www.womenconnect.com

- **Workz.com—Helping Small Businesses Grow and Prosper Online**
  www.workz.com

To better meet the challenge of improving worksite health in the 21st Century, small business managers will need to find innovative ways of addressing the health needs of their workers and providing cost-effective preventive services, EAP programs, and basic medical care to both high-risk and less vulnerable employees. Accomplishing these tasks in the context of constrained budgets and a tight job market will not be easy and will require small business managers to acquire certain critical core competencies. These competencies include: (a) *cultural sensitivity and the ability to recognize and serve the needs of an increasingly diverse workforce*; (b) *a basic awareness and understanding of comprehensive, integrated WHP programs*; (c) *the ability to design, implement, and evaluate integrated, multicomponent WHP programs*; and (d) *the capacity to identify low-cost community resources and integrate them into corporate health promotion programs.*

The present chapter outlined a two-pronged approach for providing small business managers the wherewithal to cultivate these core competencies. First, new educational resources, including WHP training programs and hands-on programming guides, have been developed (e.g., UCIHPC, 1998; WELCOA, 1998). These resources are being delivered to small business managers and tested for their effectiveness in several demonstration projects throughout the country. Second, new community-based delivery systems are being established to provide outside technical assistance and economic support to small business managers and to champion their efforts to address worksite health concerns in their companies. These new delivery systems include: (a) *small business health insurance purchasing cooperatives* (Chenoweth, 1995; Schauffler et al., 1997); (b) *government-sponsored grants-in-aid programs for small business WHP activities* (Chenoweth, 1995; Cyzman & Lafkas, 1991); (c) *corporate-community consortia for delivering medical and EAP services to small business workers* (Donaldson & Klein, 1997; Torres, 1999); and (d) *small business partnerships to facilitate greater WHP collaboration among managers from multiple firms* (e.g. matched pairs of businesses with and without WHP programming experience and businesses in a similar geographic area or industry) (Joint Venture: Silicon Valley Network, 1998; UCIHPC, 1998).

During the 21st Century, new WHP training resources for small business managers will be developed and refined, and community-based support networks for small business WHP will continue to expand and undergo rigorous evaluation for their health benefits and cost-effectiveness. A key issue that can be expected to receive greater attention in the coming years, from both WHP researchers and practitioners, is the challenge of achieving comprehensive worksite health programs that not only are beneficial to employees' well-being, but also sustainable by small companies over extended periods (Altman, 1995; Warner, Wickizer, Wolfe, Schildroth, & Samuelson, 1988). It is at the expanding frontier of small business health promotion that these challenges of creating comprehensive, cost-effective, and sustainable worksite health promotion programs will be met.

References

Adler, N. E., Boyce, T., Chesney, M. A., Cohen, S., Folkman, S., Kahn, R. L., & Syme, S. L. (1994). Socioeconomic status and health: The challenge of the gradient. *American Psychologist, 49*, 15–24.

Allen, J., & Allen, R. F. (1986). Achieving health promotion objectives through cultural change systems. *American Journal of Health Promotion, 1*, 42–49.

Altman, D. G. (1995). Sustaining interventions in community systems: On the relationship between researchers and communities. *Health Psychology, 14*, 526–536.

Association for Worksite Health Promotion, Mercer, W. M., Inc., & U.S. Department of Health and Human Services. (1999). *1999 National worksite health promotion survey: Report of survey findings.* Northbrook, IL: Author.

Berger, M. C., Black, D. A., & Scott, F. A. (1994). *Measuring the uninsured by firm size and employment status: Variation in health insurance coverage rates (Part I).* Springfield, VA: National Technical Information Service. (NTIS No. PB 94-195153).

Bracht, N., & Gleason, J. (1990). Strategies and structures for citizen partnerships. In N. Bracht (Ed.), *Health promotion at the community level* (pp. 109–124). Newbury Park, CA: Sage Publications.

Breslow, L. (1996). Social ecological strategies for promoting healthy lifestyles. *American Journal of Health Promotion, 10*(4), 253–257.

Butterfoss, F. D., Goodman, R. M., & Wandersman, A. (1993). Community coalitions for prevention and health promotion. *Health Education Research: Theory & Practice, 8,* 315–330.

California HealthCare Foundation, & Mercer, W. M., Inc. (1999). *Employer-sponsored health insurance: A survey of small employers in California.* Oakland, CA: Author.

Chenoweth, D. H. (1995). Health promotion in small businesses. In D. M DeJoy & M. G. Wilson (Eds.), *Critical issues in worksite health promotion* (pp. 275–294). Boston: Allyn & Bacon.

Chenoweth, D. H. (1998). *Worksite health promotion.* Champaign, IL: Human Kinetics.

Conner, R. F., Tanjasiri, S. P., Davidson, M., Dempsey, C., & Robles, G. (1999). *Executive summary—The first steps toward healthier communities: Outcomes from the planning phase of the Colorado Healthy Communities Initiative.* Denver, CO: The Colorado Trust.

Cyzman, D., & Lafkas, G. (1991, Winter/Spring). Wellness dollars for Michigan worksites. *Wellness Management,* pp. 1–2.

DeJoy, D. M., & Southern, D. J. (1993). An integrative perspective on work-site health promotion. *Journal of Occupational Medicine, 35,* 1221–1230.

DeJoy, D. M., & Wilson, M. G. (1995). *Critical issues in worksite health promotion.* Boston: Allyn & Bacon.

Docherty, G., Fraser, E., & Hardin, J. (1999). Health promotion in the Scottish workplace: A case for moving the goalposts. *Health Education Research: Theory & Practice, 14*(4), 565–573.

Donaldson, S. I., Gooler, L. E., & Weiss, R. (1998). Promoting health and well-being through work: Science and practice. In X. B. Arriaga & S. Oskamp (Eds.), *Addressing community problems: Psychological research and intervention* (pp. 160–194). Thousand Oaks, CA: Sage Publications.

Donaldson, S. I., & Klein, D. (1997). Creating healthful work environments for ethnically diverse employees working in small and medium-size businesses: A non-profit industry/community/university collaboration model. *Employee Assistance Quarterly, 13,* 17–32.

Dooley, D., Fielding, J., & Levi, L. (1996). Health and unemployment. *Annual Review of Public Health, 17,* 449–465.

Eddy, J. M., & Kahler, H. S., Jr. (1992). *Well now: A manager's guide to worksite health promotion.* Omaha, NE: Wellness Councils of America.

Edmunson, J. M. (1995). Special populations in worksite health promotion: Focusing on underserved employees. In D. M DeJoy & M. G. Wilson (Eds.), *Critical issues in worksite health promotion* (pp. 221–250). Boston: Allyn & Bacon.

Erfurt, J. C., Foote, A., Heirich, M. A., & Brock, B. M. (1995). *The wellness outreach at work program: A step-by-step guide* (NIH Publication No. 95-3043). Washington, DC: National Institutes of Health.

Erfurt, J. C., & Holtyn, K. (1991). Health promotion in small business: What works and what doesn't work. *Journal of Occupational Medicine, 33*(1), 66–73.

Everly, G. S., Jr., & Feldman, R. H. L. (Eds.). (1985). *Occupational health promotion: Health behavior in the workplace.* New York: John Wiley & Sons.

Fielding, J. E. (1984). *Corporate health management.* Reading, MA: Addison-Wesley.

Fielding, J. E., & Piserchia, P. V. (1989). Frequency of worksite health promotion activities. *American Journal of Public Health, 73,* 538–542.

Foote, A., & Erfurt, J. C. (1991). The benefit to cost ratio of worksite blood pressure control programs. *Journal of the American Medical Association, 265,* 1283–1286.

Freeman, P., & Aspray, W. (1999). *The supply of information technology workers available in the United States.* Washington, DC: Computing Research Association.

Fries, J. F., Harrington, H., Edwards, R., Kent, L. A., & Richardson, N. (1994). Randomized controlled trial of cost reductions from a health education program: The California Public Employees' Retirement System (PERS) Study. *American Journal of Health Promotion, 8,* 216–223.

Fries, J. F., Koop, C. E., Beadle, C. E., Cooper, P. P., England, M. J., Greaves, R. F., Sokolov, J. J., & Wright, D. (1993). Reducing health care costs by reducing the need and demand for medical services. *New England Journal of Medicine, 329*(5), 321–325.

Green, L. W. (1984). Modifying and developing health behavior. *Annual Review of Public Health, 5,* 215–236.

Green, L. W., & Cargo, M. D. (1994). The changing context of health promotion in the workplace. In M. P. O'Donnell & J. S. Harris (Eds.), *Health promotion in the workplace* (2nd ed., pp. 497–524). Albany, NY: Delmar Publishers.

Green, L. W., Richard, L., & Potvin, L. (1996). Ecological foundations of health promotion. *American Journal of Health Promotion, 10*(4), 270–281.

Grosch, J. W., Alterman, T., Petersen, M. R., & Murphy, L. (1998). Worksite health promotion programs in the U.S.: Factors associated with availability and participation. *American Journal of Health Promotion, 13*, 36–45.

Harvey, M. R., Whitmer, R. W., Hilyer, J. C., & Brown, K. C. (1993). The impact of a comprehensive medical benefit cost management program for the city of Birmingham: Results at five years. *American Journal of Health Promotion, 7*, 296–303.

Heaney, C., & Goetzel, R. (1997). A review of health-related outcomes of multi-component worksite health promotion programs. *American Journal of Health Promotion, 11*(4), 290–308.

Hudson Institute. (1987). *Workforce 2000: Work and workers for the 21st Century.* Indianapolis, IN: Author.

Injury and Illness Prevention Program, Labor Code, Section 142.3 and C401.7(401.) (1989).

Joint Venture: Silicon Valley Network. (1998). *Healthy workforce mentor program evaluation (1995-1997).* San Jose, CA: Author.

Kathawala, Y., & Elmuti, D. (1994). An empirical investigation of health care coverage and costs in U.S. small businesses. *Journal of Small Business Management, 32*(4), 61–72.

Kawachi, I., Kennedy, B. P., Lochner, K., & Prothrow-Stith, D. (1997). Social capital, income inequality, and mortality. *American Journal of Public Health, 87*, 1491–1498.

Kochar, R. (1994). *The effect of computer use on the earnings of workers by firm size.* [On-line]. Available: http://www.sba.gov/advo/research/rs156.html.

Levi, L. (1992). Psychosocial, occupational, environmental, and health concepts; research results; and applications. In G. P. Keita & S. L. Sauter (Eds.), *Work and well-being: An agenda for the 1990s* (pp. 199–210). Washington, DC: American Psychological Association.

Maccoby, N., & Alexander, J. (1980). Use of media in lifestyle programs. In P. O. Davidson & S. M. Davidson (Eds.), *Behavioral medicine: Changing health lifestyles* (pp. 351–370). New York: Brunner/Mazel.

McLeroy, K. R., Bibeau, D., Steckler, A., & Glanz, K. (1988). An ecological perspective on health promotion programs. *Health Education Quarterly, 15*, 351–377.

McLeroy, K. R., Kegler, M., Steckler, A., Burdine, J. M., & Wisotzky, M. (1994). Community coalitions for health promotion: Summary and further reflections. *Health Education Research: Theory & Practice, 9*, 1–11.

McMahan, S. (1999, March 10). *Enhancing health in the mature worker: A social ecological approach for small businesses.* Paper presented at APA/NIOSH Work, Stress, and Health Conference '99. Baltimore, MD.

McMahan, S., & Kuang, J. (1999, July). Merging health promotion and health protection: A unified philosophy toward employee health. *Professional Safety, 44*(7), 38–39.

McMahan, S., Stokols, D., Clitheroe, H. C., Jr., Wells, M., & Phillips, K. (1997). *Do small businesses differ from larger ones? A small business workplace wellness appraisal.* Research report session at the *American Journal of Health Promotion's* 8th Annual Art and Science of Health Promotion Conference, Hilton Head Island, SC.

McMahan, S., Stokols, D., & Phillips, K. (2000). *Strategic planning for workplace health promotion in small business.* Research report session at the *American Journal of Health Promotion's* 11th Annual Art and Science of Health Promotion Conference, Colorado Springs, CO.

Muchnick-Baku, S., & Orrick, S. (1992). *Working for good health: Health promotion and small businesses.* Washington, DC: The National Resource Center on Worksite Health Promotion, a cooperative between the Washington Business Group on Health and the U.S. Department of Health and Human Services.

National Governor's Association. (1991). *A healthy America: The challenge for states.* Washington, DC: Author.

O'Donnell, M. P. (1989). Definition of health promotion: Part III: Expanding the definition. *American Journal of Health Promotion, 3*, 5.

O'Donnell, M. P. (1995). *Design of workplace health promotion programs* (4th ed.). Rochester Hills, MI: American Journal of Health Promotion.

O'Donnell, M. P., & Ainsworth, T. (Eds.). (1984). *Health promotion in the workplace.* New York: John Wiley & Sons.

O'Donnell, M. P., & Harris, J. S. (Eds.). (1994). *Health promotion in the workplace* (2nd Ed.) Albany, NY: Delmar Publishers.

Pelletier, K. R. (1996). A review and analysis of the health and cost-effective outcome studies of comprehensive health promotion and disease prevention programs at the worksite: 1993-1995 update. *American Journal of Health Promotion, 10*(5), 380–388.

Pelletier, K. R., Klehr, N. L., & McPhee, S. J. (1988). Developing workplace health promotion programs through university and corporate collaboration: A review of the Corporate Health Promotion Research Program. *American Journal of Health Promotion, 2,* 75–81.

Putnam, P. D. (1995). Bowling alone: America's declining social capital. *Journal of Democracy, 6,* 65–78.

Ramirez, S. (1994). *Health promotion for all: Strategies for reaching diverse populations at the workplace.* Omaha, NE: Wellness Councils of America.

Richard, L., Potvin, L., Kishchuk, N., Prlic, H., & Green, L. W. (1996). Assessment of the integration of the ecological approach in health promotion programs. *American Journal of Health Promotion, 10*(4), 318–328.

Rubio, M., & Arteaga, L. M. (2000). *A new bottom line: Health insurance and minority owned small businesses in California.* San Francisco: Latino Issues Forum.

Scharf, T., Kidd, P., Cole, H. P., & Wiehagen, W. (1999, March 10). *Workload, stress, and risks for injury in hazardous work environments.* Symposium presented at APA/NIOSH Work, Stress, and Health Conference '99. Baltimore, MD.

Schauffler, H. H., Brown, E. R., & Rice, T. (1997). *The state of health insurance in California, 1996.* Los Angeles, CA: UCLA Center for Health Policy Research.

Sorensen, G., Glasgow, R. E., Corbett, K., & Topor, M. (1992). Compliance with worksite nonsmoking policies: Baseline results from the COMMIT study of worksites. *American Journal of Health Promotion, 7*(2), 103–109.

Sorensen, G., Lando, H., & Pechacek, T. F. (1993). Promoting smoking cessation at the workplace: Results of a randomized controlled intervention study. *Journal of Occupational Medicine, 35*(2), 121–126.

Special report: Rethinking work. (1994, October 17). *Business Week,* pp. 74–93.

Stokols, D. (1992). Establishing and maintaining healthy environments: Toward a social ecology of health promotion. *American Psychologist, 47, 6*–22.

Stokols, D. (1996). Translating social ecological theory into guidelines for community health promotion. *American Journal of Health Promotion, 10,* 282–298.

Stokols, D. (1999). Human development in the age of the internet: Conceptual and methodological horizons. In S. L. Friedman & T. D. Wachs (Eds.), *Measuring environment across the lifespan: Emerging methods and concepts* (pp. 327–356). Washington, DC: American Psychological Association.

Stokols, D., Allen, J., & Bellingham, R. L. (1996). The social ecology of health promotion: Implications for research and practice. *American Journal of Health Promotion, 10*(4), 247–251.

Stokols, D., Clitheroe, C., McMahan, S., & Wells, M. (1995). *Developing and delivering workplace wellness programs for small and medium-sized California businesses.* Grant #96-31, funded by The California Wellness Foundation, 1995–1999.

Stokols, D., Pelletier, K. R., & Fielding, J. E. (1995). Integration of medical care and worksite health promotion. *Journal of the American Medical Association, 273,* 1136–1142.

Stokols, D., Pelletier, K., & Fielding, J. E. (1996). The ecology of work and health—Research and policy directions for the promotion of employee health. *Health Education Quarterly, 23,* 137–158.

Twardowski, T. (1998, Fall/Winter). OSHA asks small businesses for input on safety and health program proposal. *Job Safety and Health Quarterly,* pp. 31–35.

Torres, L. A. (1999, March 10). *Worksite Wellness Project: Delivering culturally appropriate health promotion to small manufacturing businesses.* Paper presented at APA/NIOSH Work, Stress, and Health Conference '99. Baltimore, MD.

United States Bureau of the Census. (1992). *Statistical abstract of the United States,* 1992, The National Data Book (ISBN 0-16-060935-6), Washington, DC: Government Printing Office.

United States Bureau of the Census. (1993). *Current population reports: Hispanic Americans today* (pp. 23–183). Washington, DC: Government Printing Office.

United States Department of Commerce. (1995). *Falling through the net: A survey of the "have nots" in rural and urban America.* [On-line]. Available: http://www.ntia.doc.gov/ntiahome/fallingthru.html.

United States Department of Commerce. (1998). *Falling through the net II: New data on the digital divide.* [On-line]. Available: http://www.ntia.doc.gov/ntiahome/net2/.

United States Department of Health and Human Services. (1987). *Small business basics: Guidelines for heart and lung health at the workplace.* Washington, DC: U.S. Government Printing Office.

United States Department of Health and Human Services. (1991). *Healthy people 2000: National health promotion and disease prevention objectives* (DHHS Publication No. PHS 91-50212). Washington, DC: U.S. Government Printing Office.

United States Department of Health and Human Services. (1993). 1992 National survey of worksite health promotion activities: Summary. *American Journal of Health Promotion, 7,* 452–464.

United States Department of Health and Human Services. (1995). *The prevention marketing initiative: Coalitions & public health.* Washington, DC: Centers for Disease Control and Prevention.

United States Department of Health and Human Services. (1997). *Employer-sponsored health insurance: State and national estimates* (DHHS Publication No. PHS 98-1017). Hyattsville, MD: Author.

United States Department of Health and Human Services. (1999). *Healthy people 2010: National health promotion and disease prevention objectives.* [On-line]. Available: http://www.health.gov/healthypeople.

United States Preventive Service Task Force. (1989). *Guide to clinical preventive services: An assessment of the effectiveness of 169 interventions.* Baltimore: Williams & Wilkins.

United States Small Business Administration. (2000, August). *The facts about small business, 1999.* [On-line]. Available: http://www.sba.gov/advo/stats/fact1.html.

United States Small Business Administration. (1998a, January). *Characteristics of small business employees and owners, 1997.* [On-line]. Available: http://www.sba.gov/advo/stats/ch_emp_o.html#1.

United States Small Business Administration. (2000b, September). *Learn about SBA.* [On-line]. Available: http://www.sba.gov/aboutsba.

University of California, Irvine Health Promotion Center. (1998). *Manager's guide to workplace wellness.* Irvine, CA: Regents of the University of California.

Vickery, D. M., & Fries, J. F. (1996). *Take care of yourself* (6th ed.). Reading, MA: Addison-Wesley.

Wandersman, A., Valois, R., Ochs, L., de la Cruz, D. S., Adkins, E., & Goodman, R. M. (1996). Toward a social ecology of community coalitions. *American Journal of Health Promotion, 10*(4), 299–307.

Warner, K. E., Wickizer, T. M., Wolfe, R. A., Schildroth, J. E., & Samuelson, M. H. (1988). Economic implications of workplace health promotion programs: Review of the literature. *Journal of Occupational Medicine, 30*(2), 106–112.

Wellness Councils of America. (1998). *Health promotion: Sourcebook for small businesses.* Omaha, NE: Author.

Wells, M., Stokols, D., McMahan, S., & Clitheroe, C. (1997). Evaluation of a worksite injury and illness prevention program: Do the effects of the REACH OUT Training Program reach the employees? *Journal of Occupational Health Psychology, 2,* 25–34.

Wilcox, M. (1992, February). Health insurance, help for small business. *Kiplinger's Personal Finance Magazine,* p. 73.

Wilson, M. G., DeJoy, D. M., Jorgensen, C. M., & Crump, C. J. (1999). Health promotion programs in small worksites: Results of a national survey. *American Journal of Health Promotion, 13*(6), 358–365.

World Health Organization. (1994). Health promotion: A discussion document on the concept and principles. *Health Promotion, 1,* 73–76.

Yen, I. H., & Syme, S. L. (1999). The social environment and health: A discussion of the epidemiologic literature. *Annual Review of Public Health, 20,* 287–308.

CHAPTER

19

Aging and Worksite Health Promotion

David Gobble

INTRODUCTION

The American workforce is rapidly aging. The median age of workers in 1994 was 38 years, but by 2005 it will be 41 (Poulos & Nightingale, 1999). The labor force as a whole will continue to age until about 2015.

In 1995, there were about 41 million workers aged 45 and older, representing approximately 31% of the labor force. By 2005, 55 million workers will be 45 and older, making up 37% of the labor force. Much of this increase occurs in the 50–60-year age group. After 2005, there will also be an increase in the 60–70-year-old category until the early baby boomers (born 1946–1964) begin retiring in large numbers after 2015. In essence, we have a rapidly aging workforce, and the work environment will be altered in response to the needs and abilities of this large work cohort.

One of the most consistent findings from the study of older workers and retirees is the presence of chronic disease conditions. In 1995, over one-third (37.2%) of older persons (55+) reported they were limited by chronic conditions. Among all elderly (65+), 10.5% were unable to carry on a major life activity. In con-

trast, only 13.9% of the total population were limited in their activities, and only 4.3% had a major activity restriction (American Association of Retired Persons [AARP], 1998). In general, older workers below the age of 65 experience more absenteeism and higher health care costs than younger workers (Shephard, 1997). The basic demographics of this age wave are not going to change. The only unknown is our response to this development.

This chapter addresses the potential for and rationale behind worksite health promotion and wellness programs for older workers (45 or older) and retirees. The principle goals of the chapter are:

1. To describe the demographics of our aging workforce within the context of worldwide aging
2. To review the epidemiology of older workers and retirees
3. To describe the unique needs of the older worker
4. To describe worksite modifications that enable the older worker to remain productive
5. To review the variables involved in decision-making regarding continuation of work or entering retirement
6. To describe theories of aging relevant for older workers and retirees

7. To describe the potential for worksite health promotion to impact the health and productivity of older workers and retirees

These goals are approached through a summary of a wide range of information that captures the dynamic forces of economics, culture, and health. Successful worksite programs for older workers and retirees require a broad perspective on the many forces impacting the health of older individuals, corporations, and the economy.

This chapter introduces the context of an aging world and its impact in the changing work place. The impact of an aging work force on disability patterns and health benefits is the context used to underscore the need for modifications in worksite health promotion programming. Finally, theories of aging and specific recommendations are presented for inclusion in planning and management of health promotion in the workplace. The chapter concludes with a comment on the bottom-line question of "Is program modification worth the effort for older workers and retirees?"

THE DRIVING FORCES BEHIND THE AGING WORKFORCE

Several factors are driving the trend of an aging workforce, including the baby boom cohort (70 million individuals), the current reduced fertility rate, and the success of health promotion and disease management, including secondary and tertiary prevention. The boomers were born into families having 3 or more children and created smaller families of their own (having 1 or more children). Therefore, the emerging labor force will not be sufficient to meet the demands of a growing economy. Examples abound in today's economy, with very low unemployment rates and many jobs going unfilled. If the boomer cohort retires in numbers similar to previous generations, large economic and social stresses will emerge that challenge all our assumptions about work, retirement, and related benefits.

Medical technology, including secondary and tertiary prevention, also helped create an aging population that either continues to work or to draw retirement benefits from employers and government. A prominent example is the decline of heart disease death rates by over 50% from 1968 to the present (National Heart, Lung, and Blood Institute, 1999). Through improved screening for risk factors and successful cardiac surgery and treatment, prognosis for those with this disease is very good. Fries (1980) also argued that the compression of morbidity resulting from positive lifestyle would result in a rectangularization of Survival Cures for aging cohorts. According to Fries (1980), as people adopt good health practices and have access to appropriate medical care, they live more of their lives in a healthy state, minimizing the impact of chronic debilitating conditions until the end of life. The evidence (Fries, Koop, Sokolov, Beadle, & Wright, 1998) is now showing support for this hypothesis and provides support for prevention and early intervention programs in the workplace and in society.

DEMOGRAPHICS OF AGING

In 1997, there were 20.1 million older women and 14 million older men over age 65. Since 1900, the percentage of Americans who are 65+ has more than tripled (4.1% in 1900 to 12.7% in 1997), and the number has increased 11 times (from 3.1 million to 34.1 million). Since 1990, the number of older Americans increased by 2.8 million (9.1%) while those under 65 increased only by 7.0%. The only thing that has slowed growth in percent of older people is the relatively small birth cohort of the Great Depression (1929–1940). From this point in time until 2030, the over-65 group will grow rapidly. The United States will have 34 million people over 65 in 2000, rising to approximately 70 million in 2030—representing 13% of the population in 1997 and 20% of the population in 2030, respectively.

Minority individuals currently make up 13% of the over-65 population but will comprise 25% of the 65+ population by 2030. Table 19-1, presents specific information about the explosive growth of minorities in the over-65 age group.

Between 1999 and 2030, the white non-Hispanic population is projected to increase by 79%, compared with 238% for other minorities.

Table 19-1 Percent Increase in Minority Populations Over Age 65

Minority Population	% by 2030
White non-Hispanic	79
Hispanic	368
Non-Hispanic Blacks	134
Non-Hispanic American Indians, Inuit, Aleuts	159
Non-Hispanic Asians and Pacific Islanders	354

Source: Adapted from Administration on Aging *Profile of Older Americans,* 1998.

Table 19-2 Comparison of the Years in which the Aging Populations of Selected Countries will Reach the Current Level (18.5%) of the Florida Population in the Over 65 Years of Age Group

Country	Year Population Is Predicted to Have the Same Age Distribution as Florida
Florida	1999
Italy	2003
Japan	2005
Germany	2006
U.K.	2016
France	2016
Canada	2021
U.S.	2023

Source: Adapted from Longman, P. How Global Aging will Challenge the World's Economic Well-being. *U.S. News & World Report,* pp. 30–59. March 1, 1999.

Most Americans know our population is aging, and much has been written concerning the impact of aging on society. The focus of concern has been the emergence of the baby boomers into middle age and the impact this development has on work, the economy, and retirement. We can project what this will mean for the United States, but we can also learn from other countries that are currently several decades ahead of us in their aging profiles. This brief review places the development of our aging population within the context of the worldwide aging demographics.

Aging Patterns from an International Perspective

Globally, the average life span has increased from 49 years in 1972 to 63 years in 1999. According to the United Nations (Longman, 1999), for the first time in history, people over 60 were to outnumber children under 14 by the year 2000. These numbers are somewhat abstract; but, by comparison with data from Florida, our most senior-dominated state, these data can be brought into perspective. Table 19-2 compares other countries' aging experience to that in Florida, which has 18.5% of its population over age 65. As can be seen from this brief comparison, we are a young nation compared to other developed countries. Italy will have 18.5% of its population over 65 by 2003, and the United States will not reach that percentage until 2023.

We must keep this aging trend in perspective in the United States, as we are the youngest developed soci-

ety. We won't have the same age structure as Europe does today until 2015 (Marmor & Okma, 1998). Northern and western European countries have made modest adjustments to their entitlement programs and continue to prosper. We can learn from these societies as they have already responded to what we must face as our largest population ages. Finally, by 2050, one in every five people in the world will be over 60 years old.

With world fertility rates declining (women average 1/2 the number of children birthed in 1972), fewer people will be entering the workforce to support the large number of older individuals in each culture. Workers also have been retiring earlier, which compounds the problem of a shrinking work force combined with an expanding retiree population. For example, in 1960, the typical retirement age in the developed world was approximately 65 years old. Today, in the developed world, the low is 59 in France and the high is 66 in Japan; the median retirement age in the developed world is approximately 62 years old. Only time will determine if this trend can continue or even be reversed. This issue will be covered in more detail in the discussion of the current benefit packages offered to older workers in the United States.

Challenges to the Current Economic System

Using current projections, within 20 years the workforce in developed countries will start decreasing by approximately one percent per year. This will be caused by the joint contributions of fewer new workers entering the workforce and more workers retiring, resulting in an increase of 70 million people over 65, eligible for pensions. At the same time, the working-age population increases by only 5 million (Poulos & Nightingale, 1999). For example, in 1999, working taxpayers outnumbered retirees by over 3-to-1. By 2030, that ratio will be 1.5-to-1. This contracting workforce will have significant economic impact for the developed world economies. But, since many of the developed countries are ahead of the United States in the aging of their populations, we can look to them for guidance regarding this demographic shift. Governments, businesses, and individuals will need to work together to address these changing demographics and workforce trends.

Developing Countries

The developing world is also faced with similar problems. Even in Africa, the youngest continent demographically, aging is evident, with the only exception being the Muslim countries of North Africa. Data on Aging are compounded in the developing world by communicable disease and emigration of the younger generation. These countries are becoming old before becoming rich, so they will be challenged when responding to increasing numbers of older individuals requesting comprehensive retirement benefit programs. The imbalance created by an aging population and a decreasing birth rate in these countries will cause severe readjustments in role expectations for generations of citizens. Resources for basic public health services and infectious disease management will compete for resources that older citizens need for a quality old age. Resolving this conflict will be one of the most difficult social and health issues facing the developing world. The prospect for retirement in these countries is not great. Most people able to work will be required to contribute to their own and society's economic and health-related needs.

Complexity of Workforce Populations

Population shifts described previously, and their projected impacts, are based upon a model of three living generations: young dependents, working adults, and the elderly (defined as over 65 years old). However, this division has largely disappeared in the U.S. and other developed societies. We now have large numbers of individuals over 65 who are healthy and continue to work. We have young workers earning money for discretionary spending. And, we have people in the middle who move into and out of the work force, both by choice and because of the realignment of our economy from traditional production to a service- and technology-driven economy. According to Borst-Eilers & Okam, as cited in Marmor & Okmal (1998), it is possible to distinguish six or seven specific population groups with their own unique circumstances and potential for work and well-being. Table 19-3 presents a summary of these population groups.

Each group presents challenges and opportunities; but, if we use the traditional public health model of intervention (high-risk targets), most of our programming resources will be expended upon groups 2, 6, and 7. For example, if we use the traditional health promotion method of needs assessment, health risk appraisal, we would focus on those individuals or, more likely, clusters of individuals possessing risk factors for disease and disability. This approach eliminates consideration of large numbers who might benefit and, at best, points to interventions that only postpone costs of disease and illness. Our real challenge with workers and retirees representing each of these groups is to think in a more comprehensive manner that addresses individual, work, and community options for illness, health promotion, and wellness for each segment of the population. Each worksite must make its own evaluation of need and plan for appropriate intervention. Later in this chapter, more information will be provided on program design and decision making for health promotion programming.

The Baby Boom Effect on Work and Society

In America, after World War II, the baby boom set the stage for the current focus of workforce planning and

Table 19-3 Population Targets for Worksite Health Promotion

1. **Young adults**—often with multiple incomes, accumulating savings, investments, and pension benefits
2. **Young unemployed**—usually lower education levels and probably the future poor elderly
3. **Middle-aged adult working**—high accumulated savings and benefits, financially secure and looking forward to a healthy active retirement
4. **Young retired (50–70 years old)**—healthy, with resources to enjoy early retirement. This is the new image of the elderly portrayed in commercials
5. **Elderly healthy retired**—vast majority of those over 65 and retired are healthy, but there are large differences in income and functional levels
6. **Frail but independent elderly**—most frail elderly still manage their health, with nonofficial assistance, and consider themselves independent, even though they may need temporary home care, or short-term hospital or nursing home care
7. **Frail and dependent very old**—highly dependent on professional permanent interventions from various health care resources; in the 75–85-year-old group, 6% are institutionalized and 26% are institutionalized in the over-85-year-old group

Source: Adapted from Borst-Eilers, Okma, & Kieke, 1996. Marmor, T. R., & Okma, K. (1998), Societal interventions affecting elderly citizens: A comparative approach. *Annual Review of Gerontology and Geriatrics,* pp. 321–338.

program development. From 1946–1964, the birth rate remained elevated, compared to past cohorts. This large birth cohort influenced almost all segments of our culture as it aged. For example, when this cohort reached school age, we had to rapidly build schools to meet the demand for classroom space. As this cohort entered their teenage years, they fueled the growth of a new popular culture. They also caused the university system in the U.S. to grow faster than at any time in its history. Now, we are facing the aging boomers as they enter their fifties and change the face of the workplace and retirement. One thing is clear: this cohort changed everything as it moved through our culture and will change the meaning of work and retirement in the next 20 years. The key now is that the boomers are such a large cohort that the workplace

and society at large must modify programs to meet the needs of this group.

The boomers are reaching the later stages of their worklife and considering the options of staying in the workforce or adopting some sort of retirement. Boomers don't usually decide in an either/or fashion, and the retirement decision appears no different. At this time, 80% of the boomers intend to work at some level during retirement (AARP/Roper Baby Boomer Study, 1998). What is very interesting about this cohort is their view of work and its influence on deciding to retire. For those with incomes over $70,000, 52% plan to work after retirement because "it's fun," while 24% of those with incomes below $30,000, plan to work because "it's fun." So, the traditional view of the life cycle of education, work, and retirement does not fit this cohort.

Extending Worklife and Balancing Health-Related Costs

It may be possible to extend the worklife of most workers by improving the work environment; decreasing productivity demands, flexibility of amount, and timing of work; provision of rehabilitative services; and changing financial incentives. As we extend the worklife of older workers though, we open the door to managing the health care costs that are associated with more mature workers. In a recent study completed at Ball State University (McCarthy, Gobble, Fitzgerald, & Treloar, 1999), medical claims data for employees increased in each decade from a median value of $1,496 for the 20–29 year age group to a high of $3,738 for the 60–69 year age group. Figure 19-1 presents a graphic picture of the accelerating costs of older workers in a University setting. These workers (3000+ employees) represented all employment categories, including service personnel, professional staff, and faculty. Job descriptions included classic blue-collar through white-collar and resemble the modern workplace across America in age distribution, ethnicity, and variety of job description.

This pattern is typical of most work settings, and with aging workers, the cost of health insurance continues to accelerate. Absenteeism and other productivity issues need to be managed with sensitivity for

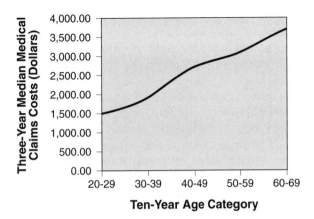

Figure 19-1 Three-year median medical claims cost among all employees at Ball State University by 10-year age categories.

Source: T. H. McCarthy, D. C. Gobble, J. Fitzgerald, & J. Treloar, *The Best Predictors of Medical Claims Costs at Ball State University,* unpublished manuscript, 1999.

this mature work-group. The challenge for business will be to find the balance between productivity and health claims cost of this category of employee.

The Changing Workplace: Challenges for the Older Worker

The nature of work has evolved rapidly from being dominated by physical work to being dominated by cognitive/intellectual tasks. Currently, approximately 25% of work requires high physical capability (Shephard, 1991). Most work being created in the new technological economy requires knowledge-based skills or services. This is both very good and very bad for the mature worker. Most mature workers lose some ability to do hard physical work and would be forced to either retire or work reduced hours to maintain employment, so the movement toward work that emphasizes knowledge-based productivity removes the barrier of declining physical ability of the older worker. However, new knowledge-based jobs require high levels of technical skills, and most older workers were trained for work in a pretechnological era. Older workers need retraining to successfully perform the new work. It is well-documented that older workers'

performance in high-skill tasks declines over time. But, according to Sterns (1998), little evidence exists to indicate that age alone predicts lower job performance (Sterns & Doverspike, 1998). It appears that older workers can learn appropriate compensatory skills that support job functions. What we don't fully understand at this time is how successful older workers manage to overcome declines in cognitive and physical ability. It is possible that the wealth of knowledge that older workers possess about work-specific tasks allows them to work "smarter" rather than harder to meet demands in the workplace. In general, older workers who have demonstrated good work performance during their work careers generally continue to perform at acceptable productivity levels, given appropriate modifications in the work environment. Training for the older worker is discussed in more detail later in the chapter.

Work environment modifications are an essential part of the process of keeping the mature worker both productive and in the workplace. Sensitivity to ergonomic needs of the mature worker involves seating options, computer screen size, lighting, and noise management. Simple but consistent attention to the work environment enables the mature worker to manage work demands more productively. If the mature worker is to continue to assist in physical work tasks, work hardening activities are essential to minimize injury and illness.

The changing nature of supervision in the modern workplace is also a challenge for mature workers. Most mature workers experienced work that was directed through a management hierarchy and required little decision making. The typical job entailed doing a repetitive task over an 8-hour day. Today, work is organized around teams, with shared decision making throughout the organization. The productivity of the worker is measured through team accomplishment and is dependent on continuous learning and quality improvement. Social interaction skills form the basis for work success in the new workplace. The mature worker might find this work environment requires a set of communication skills that have not been well-developed during the past 30 years of work. And finally, the issue of a career path nurtured at one workplace with one work culture building seniority is now not the workplace reality. The older worker is in a skills-driven economy, not a seniority-driven one, so acquiring new skills is required to remain in the work place.

Patterns of Work and Age

During the 1930s, 51% of men over 65 continued working. By 1950, workforce participation rates for men between ages 45–54 were approximately 96%, 87% for men 55–64, and 46% for those over 65. But a significant decline in participation emerged by 1995 with only 91% of men aged 45–54 working, 64% of men aged 55–64 working, and only 13% of those over 65 remaining in the workplace. This significant decline was offset by the increasing participation of women in the workplace over the past 60 years (U.S. Bureau of Labor Statistics, 1995). However, at this point in time, we are approaching a balance between men and women participating in work outside the home, so a continuing trend toward early retirement creates special problems for both the specific employer and the national economy. When unemployment rates are high, the need to keep older workers in the workforce accelerates. Employers are willing to spend more in employee benefits for the older worker for several reasons. First, based upon birth rates for the past 20 years, younger workers will not be available to fill all the positions vacated through early retirement. And second, with increased training costs for new workers and the amount invested in current employees, the motivation to protect employer investment in the current workforce is greater.

Many mature workers are approaching retirement facing two developments that may force longer work careers. According to many financial analysts, most people nearing retirement have not saved enough money for retirement. Many mature workers will need to stay in the workforce in some capacity to supplement income needs. Currently, over 70% of boomers plan to work, either full or part-time after retirement age (65–67, depending on present age) (AARP, *Roper Baby Boomers Study*, 1998). Others will opt for a flexible work arrangement. Baby boomers have already shown a tendency to use flexible employment arrangements throughout their careers

(AARP/*Roper Baby Boomers Study*, 1998), so this pattern should accelerate as boomers approach retirement decision making. Boomers currently make up one-third of contingent workers (flexible or short-term). As the economic needs for retirement become clearer for boomers, and as the pool of qualified workers available to enter the job market shrinks, employers will be challenged to create a workplace that allows a wide range of relationships with older employees. Evidence already supports the willingness of employers to offer flexible staffing patterns because it allows management to respond to changing needs in a rapidly changing marketplace (Lenz, 1996).

Older workers are also looking forward to a longer life expectancy. The worker who retires at 65 without any major chronic disease can expect to live for 30 or more years. This extended life challenges the economic resources of most people, and the fear of outliving retirement savings is very real. And, how much golf, bridge, and other activities can anyone play? Boredom is a very real issue for retirees. These factors will influence the decision to stay in the workforce. It appears that, as boomers move toward their middle 60s, retirement at 65 may be a distant memory of another generation.

Disability and the Aging Employee and Retiree

The good news is that disability in the United States is trending downward. People are moving through the life span with fewer health problems than previous generations. Data on disability has focused upon the ability to carry out specific roles, usually measured by activities of daily living (ADLs) (including bathing, eating, and other basic personal maintenance behaviors) and instrumental activities of daily living (IADLs) (including outside activities such as shopping and laundry) (Freedman & Martin, 1998). These measures have shown a slight declining trend, but these data may be influenced by older people's expectations. For example, as people stop working, they might not place the same demands upon themselves and under-report limits in function. Whereas, if they had to work or perform other required social roles daily, they might indicate functionally higher activity limitations.

Another measure reported by Freedman and Martin (1998) measures functional limitations such as seeing, walking, lifting, and climbing more closely reflect activities required to continue working outside the home (Freedman & Martin, 1998). Based upon U.S. Bureau of Census data (1998) gathered from 1984 through 1993, projections indicate declines in these disabilities among age groups for all functional categories. Declines in chronic disability ranged from a low of 0.9% to a high of 2.3%, depending on functional category. In the 50–64-year-old group, seeing disabilities declined from 11.1% in 1984 to 7.8% in 1993. Walking disability declined from 15.2% to 13.7% over the same period. Even though these declines appear small, they have a large effect in health claims and productivity in the workplace. When the aging population is growing so rapidly, these small percentage declines indicate many people are not losing function at the same rate as a decade earlier. This is a remarkable reversal in a short time. Table 19-4 provides more detail covering this rapid reversal of disability.

One of the contributing factors to this decline could be the increasing education level of the "young" old (age 65–74). Education is one of the strongest predictors of a successful life experience in our culture. In 1984, 43% of the over-50 group had not finished high school, and in 1993, 31% had not completed high school. Only 25% of the over-50 group had completed some education after high school, compared to 33% in 1993. This trend will continue since the baby boom generation is the highest educated generation in history.

The second contributing factor to the decline in disability might be the increased availability and use of various assertive devices, including vision, hearing, and mobility aids. According to Freedman and Martin (1998), after controlling for use of these items, a significant decline in disability still existed. Apparently, we are remaining fully functional for longer periods of time, providing support for Fries' (1980) compression of morbidity hypothesis. Therefore, many people who in the past had to stop working because of physical limitations now can continue to do productive work.

So, what does the older worker and retiree bring to each day? In general, they are better off than previous

Table 19-4 Adjusted Rates[a] of Functional Limitations by Age Group (Percent of Population Reporting Disability)

Age	Year 1984	Year 1993	Percent Change
50–64			
Seeing	10.1	6.8	3.3
Lifting	15.3	11.8	3.5
Climbing	16.1	13.6	2.4
Walking	16.4	13.8	2.6
65–79			
Seeing	17.6	13.6	4.1
Lifting	28.8	22.3	6.5
Climbing	30.5	27.2	3.2
Walking	32.7	26.6	6.1
80+			
Seeing	38.9	35.2	9.6
Lifting	54.6	43.1	11.5
Climbing	53.7	27.2	8.4
Walking	58.0	50.1	7.9

[a]Adjusted for age, sex, marital status, race, ethnicity, education, ownership of liquid assets, and region of residence.
Source: Adapted from L. G. Martin, & V. A. Freedman. *American Journal of Public Health,* 1998.

older workers and retirees, but some significant disability issues remain. Mobility is the classic example of the magnitude of the disability challenge. Approximately 5 million people use canes, 1.8 million use walkers, and 1.6 million use wheelchairs (Russell, Hendershot, LeCleere, Howie, & Alder, 1997). The problem accelerates in the over-70 age group. For example, 18% have visual impairments, 33% are hearing impaired, 8.6% are both visually and hearing impaired, 30% fall at least once per year, and 20% use psychotropic drugs (which double the risk of falls). And finally, looking at the old over 75, a pattern emerges that is characterized by severe gait disorders, arthritis, dementia, cardiovascular disease, podiatric and orthopedic problems, severe visual impairment, and incontinence. As the sheer number of people continue to age, we can look forward to assisting large numbers of individuals with multiple disabilities. Our success with meeting these needs will determine the final number of older workers and retirees who are able to fulfill both work and other productive societal roles.

In summary, disability increases with age. Work performance and daily activity limitation may result if appropriate interventions are not tailored to individual needs. Based upon the increasing education level of the work force and improved access to health care and assistive devices, the rate of disability appears to be declining compared to earlier age-related cohorts. With appropriate interventions, we can anticipate a larger percentage of older workers being able to both remain in the work force and continue to lead active, productive lives. The challenge for health promotion and wellness professionals is to integrate what we know about programming in general to a target audience with great physical diversity, that learns differently, and has different motivations for their behavior.

CURRENT HEALTH BENEFITS MIX AFFECTING HEALTH PROMOTION FOR OLDER WORKERS AND RETIREES

A significant percentage of workers leave the labor force before becoming eligible for Medicare at age 65, and many do not have health insurance. In 1992, approximately 40% of the labor force between the ages of 51–61 were not working, compared to 24% between ages 41–50 (Loprest & Zedlewski, 1998). Over 15% of these individuals not in the workforce were without health insurance. Their health and economic security were at risk. Some of these individuals may have been uninsured while working, but others lost insurance coverage upon retirement. The current trend for business is to aggressively manage health insurance costs of retirees. New federal accounting rules require corporations to report future costs of promised health benefits to retirees against the current "bottom line," and this has made business very aware of health insurance costs of an aging workforce and retiree group. Under the 1985 Consolidated Budget Reconciliation Act (COBRA), workers are eligible for continued health benefits from their employer for 18 months after retirement but may be forced to pay the entire premium. Many workers struggle to remain in the workforce until they are within 18 months of qualifying for Medicare

benefits so they will have access to health care until Medicare eligibility is reached. Other workers who cannot afford to pay the health insurance premiums remain in the workforce until 65, working at a reduced functional capacity, just to qualify for Medicare. However, persons in poor health cannot choose to continue to work, and persons with lower skills may be forced out of jobs and lose benefits (Dulitzky, 1999).

Employment-based health insurance coverage has been the primary source of insurance for early retirees. About 70% of workers who retire before 65 were covered by group health insurance plans (Dulitzky, 1999), but the trend is to reduce this benefit, with mid-sized and large employers reducing this benefit from 75% in 1985 to 52% in 1994 (Holahan & Winterbottom, 1995)—and, for those who have access to this benefit, premiums are being increased almost across the board (Higgins, 1995).

The aging worker and retiree typically deals with a higher number of health problems and uses health care services more than do younger populations. Work-related benefits and government entitlement programs provide critical support for continuing a lifestyle of productivity and quality. One of the greatest fears of older workers and retirees is the cost of health care. An appropriate mix of both work-related and government benefits is ideal for the retiree. For the aging employee, health care coverage is one of the most important variables in the decision to continue working or to retire.

From the employer standpoint, a decision to offer early retirees health benefits increases early retirement rates. A decision to withdraw this benefit increases the retirement age of the workforce. If an employer has a high payroll cost associated with long-term workers, expanding health benefits for early retirees makes good economic sense. If the employer needs to retain workers because of labor supply problems, reducing health care coverage for early retirees increases the likelihood of keeping older workers in the workforce. A basic understanding of current benefits provided through the workplace and government provides insight into the challenge of balancing the needs of the older worker and retiree with the needs of the employer.

Employee Benefits and the Retirement Decision

Many things will influence the decisions made by this large cohort, but one of the most central is the availability of health benefits after full-time work. At this time, health insurance benefits provided through work are the primary source of insurance coverage for the near-retired, aged 55–64. Of these 21.5 million people, approximately 86% are receiving health insurance and other benefits at work, but it is important to note that 2.3 million of this group are already not working because of illness or disability and that their benefits coverage is spotty at best (Fronstin, 1998). According to the Health Confidence Survey cosponsored by the Employee Benefit Research Institute and Mathew Greenwald & Associates (as cited by Fronstin, 1997), 74% of workers indicated that they would not retire early if they could not get their worksite to extend health insurance benefits until Medicare eligibility. With the tight job market, many employers are looking for ways to keep workers in the workplace. Reducing benefits for early retirees is one strategy that meets the needs of the employer at the expense of those wishing to retire early.

In general, for the past 50 years the trend has been for workers, especially men, to retire at an earlier age in each decade. However, this trend appears to be stalled in the United States and may be reversing. In 1996, there were 1.5 million more men between the ages of 60–69 working than would be expected based upon projections of past retirement rates (Smith, 1997). As baby boomers age, this trend should accelerate because boomers are more educated, and higher-educated workers continue working longer. The general trend is that with each year of education, workers continue in the labor force four more years. It appears that the cost of securing education and training increases the motivation to reap the economic benefits of continued employment (Besl & Kale, 1996).

Finally, changes in Social Security benefits may have influenced this new trend. For example, those born in 1949–1959 will not qualify for full benefits until age 66. With those born in 1960 or later, they will not qualify for full benefits until age 67. Also, by 2005, persons delaying retirement to age 70 will receive an 8% increase in the monthly pension payment. It seems logical these trends will work to keep more people in the workplace, producing an older workforce. This will place interesting financial and organizational demands upon the workplace to meet the needs of the aging worker.

Government Programs

Older Americans are eligible for both Social Security and Medicare at age 65. Reduced Social Security benefits (20% reduction of benefits) are available as early as 62. Social Security benefits were designed to replace up to 40% of lost income upon retirement. However, for wage earners making over $45,000 per year, replacement would be below 30% of previous income. A general rule for retirement is that persons should have various income sources that replace approximately 70–80% of preretirement income. For workers retiring in the year 2000, Social Security is the major source of income, replacing (on average) 40% of preretirement income. So, many new retirees face the retirement transition with limited economic resources for basic living expenses.

Assuming a worker retires at 65, Medicare is the federal government health insurance program available to all citizens. Organized in two parts, A, Hospital Insurance, and B, Medical Insurance, it has been available since 1966 as a core entitlement program for older Americans. It is truly a national health insurance program, with benefits primarily limited to those 65 and over. Part A is a benefit purchased through payroll taxes of the worker or spouse. Part B requires the retired person to pay a monthly premium so is very similar to other types of health insurance. In general, both Parts A and B have significant copayment requirements and limitations on maximum payment for hospital, physician, and nursing-home care (Health Care Financing Administration, 1999). Prescription drugs are not covered under the Medicare program and result in significant out-of-pocket monthly expense for most retirees. Significant medical costs are so routine for this population that a subindustry has evolved (Medigap insurance) to help the cost-strapped retiree.

THE CONTEXT OF HEALTH PROMOTION FOR OLDER WORKERS AND RETIREES

Theories of Aging

When considering the biological and psychological theories of aging, a clear distinction exists between normal, optimal, and pathological processes of aging. Variability between individuals becomes greater with life experiences so that a random group of 5-year-old children will have much more in common with each other than a random group of 75-year-old elders. Unfortunately, most of our knowledge about aging has come from cross-sectional studies that show patterns of decline. These studies mask the subgroups within the aging population that are aging very well. Comparing younger aged cohorts to older cohorts exaggerates the true physical losses and psychological differences between generations. Each generation has unique life experiences that affect aging, and younger workers today have had more opportunities for health care, education, nutrition, and financial well-being than their grandparents. Therefore, much of the current research on aging focuses on the pathological aspects of aging and provides little information on normal or successful aging (Rowe & Kahn, 1997).

The best information on normal aging processes comes from a few longitudinal studies that have followed people through time to determine individual patterns of aging. The Baltimore Longitudinal Study of Aging, begun in 1959 and focusing on physical aging, and the Alameda Study of lifestyle and social relationships, begun in 1965 (Breslow & Beckman, 1983), are providing some very important data to build accurate theories of aging. To date, there is sparse research on optimal aging processes that might be possible with health promotion programs over the lifespan of individuals (Fries, Koop, Sokolov, Beadle, & Wright, 1998).

Out of these cross-sectional and longitudinal studies of aging, a number of theories of aging have emerged. Theories about physical and biological processes of aging provide the basis for most of the nutritional and exercise programs for older adults and can be found in many resources (O'Brien Cousins, 1998; Shephard, 1997). Since much of health promotion and wellness management depends on motivating people to change, the theories of late life development will be reviewed.

Few psychologists have been interested in old age and the study of human development and behavior. Freud and other psychoanalytic theorists believed that childhood experiences shaped behavior in adulthood and that unconscious motivations were the underlying cause of a person's actions. The subconscious controlled conscious behavior and was difficult to change. The psychoanalysts believed that personality was fixed by young adulthood and that older people were incapable of significant change in behavior and personality. As a consequence of such psychological views, many of the stereotypes of old age in our society have led us to believe in the intractable rigidity of thought and behavior in later life. *"You can't teach an old dog new tricks!" "Old people are set in their ways." "Old soldiers never die, they just fade away." "Older people should act their age!"* Some of the earliest gerontological theories of aging focused on "disengagement" (Cumming & Henery, 1961) and "age-based roles" (Neugarten & Associates, 1964). These theories left little room for change in later life and, thus, little hope to correct negative health habits and attitudes. Only a few decades ago, the common view was that longevity had more to do with genetic programming than with lifestyle choices. Even though the debate continues concerning the balance of genetics and lifestyle, it is clear that individual behavioral choices are important components of long-term health.

As the study of human behavior became more popular, the theories of behavioral psychologists took a mechanical view of human actions and did not consider age to be much of a factor. The theories asserted that a human organism responds and reacts the same to stimuli, no matter what the age. Researchers professed that environment and/or cognition reinforced behavior and that change occurred by modifying the antecedents, consequences, or thoughts that were associated with the behavior. So, no matter the age of the person, behaviors could be changed by contextual and educational interventions. Likewise, in the mid 1960's, some gerontologists began to promote an "activity" theory of aging. They believed that, rather than "disengage," older people should be encouraged and motivated to become or to stay active after retirement, and that would greatly improve the quality of life, as well as the quantity of years. Active aging became the basis for much of the program planning for older adults. Long-term care facilities were evaluated on their "activity" programs and their abilities to get residents to participate in bingo, music, art, and other activities. Senior centers developed educational, exercise, and recreational activities. Travel excursions and volunteer opportunities were promoted for retirees. Adages like *"Use it or lose it!"* or, *"You're only as old as you feel"* became popular. Activity and involvement programs, once the domain of the young, were now "pushed" onto the older worker and retirees.

Yet, neither of these theories, disengagement nor activity, has proven to be applicable to all older adults. Much of the research on human development of behavior and personality finds there is truth in both theories. In summary, activity theory supports the programming philosophy that the individual must "use it or lose it." A continuing variety of programming should be provided as people move through the life span. Little worth is given to quiet contemplation or relaxation. Conversely, the theory of disengagement promotes the gradual withdrawal from the time commitments and tasks of work and a complex lifestyle. So, as people age, they should be allowed to peacefully "pontificate" and reflect on life and be a spectator. This is the reward for a well-lived life. Neither of these theories has proven to capture the experience of individuals as they move through the life span. A more accurate pattern of life experience is that personality and behavior appear to become relatively stabilized in adulthood (Costa & McCrae, 1988). It is more difficult to change after a behavior or attitude has been practiced over time.

A third theoretical view emerged, called the "continuity theory of aging" (Atchley, 1989). This theory recognized that people do not typically make dramatic or drastic changes in their behaviors or attitudes; however, it leaves room for adaptation, growth, and change as interests and needs change with life experiences. Individuals continue much the same in old age as they were at younger ages, so if they were active as young people they will probably prefer to be active in old age. On the other hand, if they were disengaged from relationships, work roles, etc. in early life, they will probably become even more disengaged with age. Continuity theories of aging are consistent with those of the developmental psychological theories of Erik Erikson (1963) and Carl Jung (Mattoon, 1981). Erikson and Jung both believed that old age was a time of continued growth and development. Not only can people change in old age, but they can find wisdom, integrity, and maturity impossible at younger ages. These theories suggest that not all people are able to achieve maturity in later life, but those who have stayed open to learning new things and deepening their understanding of life will find old age filled with wonder and richness.

Health professionals, from physicians and nurses to psychologists and social workers, health educators, exercise specialists, and caregivers, are all concerned with physical and mental health of older adults. Cardiac rehabilitation and physical therapy for stroke victims are examples of the typical treatment plans for most older patients who have been hospitalized. Residents of long-term health facilities or retirement communities are offered physical exercise programs and a variety of social activities to prevent decline and social isolation. Most communities have some kind of senior services that provide information, travel opportunities, support groups, and even some meals to promote health. However, these programs are typically designed from a "behavioral" or "activity" theory and have not taken the wide variability of older adults nor the "continuity" theory of aging into account.

According to the continuity theory of aging, older workers are going to continue to respond to health promotion program offerings as they have in the past. So, the history of local health promotion efforts will be very predictive of how successful any intervention will be as the workforce ages.

Prevention Programs: Examples/Benchmarks

The primary questions for health promotion professionals concerning programs for older workers and retirees are "What modifications must be made to traditional health promotion programs?" "What programs are needed for this population?" and, "Are the modifications worth the effort?"

The good news is that many of the traditional risk factor reduction programs are appropriate for the aging worker. For example, most chronic conditions that are targets of health risk appraisal instruments (high blood pressure, heart disease, diabetes, cancer, etc.) are common problems for the aging worker. Our challenge is in recruitment and retention of participants into our health promotion efforts. Specific recommendations are made later in the chapter that should improve the chances of impacting behaviors in this population that influence health and well-being.

In general, as workers age, they experience a higher rate of chronic disease and generate more health claims than younger workers. However, risk factor change and relative risk of disease are not perfectly correlated with increasing age. In a thorough review of changing risk factors with increasing age published in the Annual Review of Public Health (Kaplan, Haan, & Wallace, 1999), common risks and chronic conditions are shown to vary across age groups. These data indicate that, depending on how the data are collected (either from longitudinal or cross-sectional data sets), general support exists for a strong relationship of age risk factors and morbidity. It appears that evidence from both longitudinal and cross-sectional data show a relationship of age and chronic disease, but the precise contributions of age and lifestyle are not clear. Many variables, including access to health care, ethnicity, and economic status, need to be controlled to clearly see the strength of this relationship.

In general, the relative risk of most major detectable chronic conditions is higher for older individuals than for those under 45. The potential for identifying high-risk older workers is great; and, according to Chapman (1999), this risk factor approach results in significant potential reduction in risk and increased cost savings for business and improved quality of life for the worker and retiree.

PLANNING AND DESIGN ISSUES: OLDER WORKERS AND RETIREES

Health risks, or health problems identified in the older worker, are imbedded in a rich matrix of family, social supports, and health behavior history. Workers and retirees have had many experiences managing health

and health care within the context of their culture and have developed unique coping and management strategies, both positive and negative. Patterns of under- or over-utilization of health care are well established, and general beliefs about personal responsibility for health management are in place. Openness to traditional and alternative strategies for managing health are based upon personal and cultural experiences. For example, an increasing number of aging workers and retirees are no longer committed to standard medical care. Forty-two percent were regularly using alternative care sources (Eisenberg, Kessler, Foster, Norlock, Calkins, and Delbanco 1998). They spent $21 billion over the past decade outside the traditional health care system, so they are very interested in being involved with their health, but they are also skeptical of much of what traditional health authority groups, including worksite sponsored programs, offer.

Systems Model of Health Promotion and Wellness

We know that older workers and seniors are more dissimilar in their ability to do physical work and in their health status than a typical group of younger workers. We also know that older workers and retirees have literally invested a lifetime in becoming who they are within their cultural context. Individuals developing a worksite health promotion program for older workers need to understand who they are, how they see themselves meeting their life needs through work and retirement, and how they view the role of work as partner or adversary. This is a very tall order—and one that promotes a comprehensive approach. The systems model proposed in 1991 by Nicholas and Gobble and applied to women and aging by Crose, Nicholas, Gobble, & Frank (1992) and Gobble & Crose (1998) is one way to conceptualize the organizational structure needed to be successful in planning programs for older workers and retirees. The premise of systems thinking is that nothing happens out of context. Individuals respond to work- and health-related issues based upon their social, emotional, intellectual, spiritual, physical, and environmental histories. This ecological approach is becoming the foundation for successful programs in organizations and communities. This rich context can be the basis of successful health promotion and wellness programs for the older worker and retiree.

The older worker and retiree has needs that are defined by their special life stage and driven by the ever present reality of physical and mental decline. Programs that enable the older worker to fulfill a workrole more efficiently while reducing the physical demands or the mental strain have the potential to be well-supported. These programs need to be viewed by the worker as a partnership between the worker and the employer, where each has responsibility for the well-being of the other. An ecological systems approach (Green Richard, & Potvin et al., 1998) that shares the responsibility between all parties and proposes solutions that are shared by all parties has the best chance of getting and keeping the attention of the older worker and retiree.

Motivation for Change

As people age, the variation among participants increases. In any program requiring movement or skill, more personal teaching and support are needed. According to Caserta and Gillett (1998), retirees with diminished function were more likely to continue to participate in an exercise program if they did it at home rather than in a group setting. Apparently, as individuals become more disabled, they are self-conscious about their lack of functional ability and prefer to do their workouts in the privacy of their homes.

For the older worker, a combination of knowledge, skill, and "determination" are predictive of motivation for change (Straka, 1998). Of the three, will seems to be the most critical for understanding participation and sustained change in the older worker and retiree. Determination is a very abstract construct, but it points toward the issues raised earlier in the chapter concerning the deeper motivations of older workers and retirees compared to younger workers. The older population is not generally interested in experimenting with something new just for the experience. They are primarily interested in problem-solving behavior, so programs must be clearly tied to expressed needs. They are motivated when they see something that meets their own needs, not by a professed organizational or government need.

Planning and Program Design

The planning and program design process for older workers and retirees includes similar issues and concerns involved in all program development, but unique aspects of design and planning involve the stability of lifestyle behaviors, the diversity of the aged population, and the impact of culture on health-related behavior change. Table 19-5 presents a summary of specific issues for planning and designing programs for older workers and retirees.

Many items are discussed in Table 19-5, but the key issues involve: (a) developing trust so accurate assessments can be made; (b) focusing on the appropriate target of remedial rehabilitation, prevention, or life quality; (c) incorporating social supports; (d) increasing self-efficacy; (e) providing high amounts of personal attention, and (f) providing staff trained in the unique needs and learning styles of the older learner.

Programming for the Older Worker, Young-Old, and Old-Old: An Example

In many ways, appropriate program planning and design for the older worker (aged 50–64), the young-old, (65–74), and the old-old (75+) requires each group to be considered as a separate audience. Functional ability and disability varies significantly both within and across these three populations, but a strong trend toward greater functional disability with age is supported by the data.

Physical activity, a very common health promotion program, may serve to illustrate the need for individual targeting in these three (older worker, young-old, and old-old) populations. For the older worker (50–64), physical response to exercise of any type is fairly predictable, based upon a preliminary screening for underlying risks and current exercise capability. Programs can be carried out in the workplace focused upon the specific work task needed, or a general fitness program can be offered to all workers. Assessment needs to be sensitive to emerging physical health problems, including chronic diseases and loss of physical strength through nonuse. This group, while different from the young worker, still has the potential to make fairly rapid adjustment to increased

Table 19-5 Planning and Designing Programs for Older Workers and Retirees (Special Factors)

1. Needs Assessment
   a. **Trust:** What cooperative work experiences support partnerships? Know the local programming history and the management and labor relationships.
   b. **Self-management concepts:** How does this population view personal health and illness? Identify the level of interest/commitment to lifestyle modification.
   c. **Diversity assessment:** Market segmentation is critical (see Table 19-3 concerning different populations). Assume significant diversity exists.
   d. **Program target:** Remedial/rehabilitative, prevention and lifestyle enhancement (see Table 19-6) problems and program opportunities represent primary targets for programming.
2. Program Design
   a. **Staffing:** Age-sensitive or age-appropriate staff are critical for success. Most individuals trained in health promotion and wellness have very little sensitivity/training about unique needs of older adults. Visual, hearing, mobility, pain management, communication, and learning style all need special attention in program design.
   b. **Physical modifications:** If activity programs are planned, accessibility to space must be considered for those with disability, and equipment modification may be necessary to allow participation for all ability levels. The older the target audience, the more individualized the assessment.
   c. **Individual support:** Older workers and retirees require more supervision and individual support to complete activity programs. Self-esteem is generally lower in the older worker and retiree, and more feedback is needed to keep motivation levels high (Noe & Wilk, 1993).
   d. **Family and group support:** Programs must be sensitive to family values and local cultural mores and incorporate these values into program materials.
   e. **Learning styles:** Self-efficacy is usually low in this population (Farr & Middlebrooks, 1990),

particularly when new skills must be learned. Constant reinforcement and early rewards are needed to insure continued participation. Determine which theory of aging is represented in the target population: activity, disengagement, or continuity? Most individuals will continue similar patterns over time, so develop programs reflecting past history.

3. Program Delivery
   a. **Physical modifications:** Disability rates are significant, and mobility issues are always a concern. Variability in functional capacity is very large, and individual assessments are required. Pain management is essential for continued participation. As population disability increases with age, so does the need for personal attention and program variation.
   b. **Social interaction:** A primary motivation for participation among nondisabled workers and retirees is the quality of group interaction. Time must be allotted for group affiliations as a core part of programs.
   c. **Personal feedback:** Older workers and retirees require more personal contact when starting programs. Any program must begin with very small increments of change that allow early success and formal recognition of each participant's successes.
   d. **Personnel training:** Exposure of current staff to special training programs on needs of the older worker are highly recommended. Training should include social, cognitive, physical, and other unique needs of this population.
4. Program Evaluation
   a. **Participant satisfaction:** Monitoring individual acceptance of program processes is critical for continued participation. This group is very tolerant when they perceive their opinions are heard and incorporated into programs.
   b. **Outcome measures:** Such tremendous variability in subjects requires assessing individual successes instead of basing success on group scores. What is successful for one group will be inappropriate for another that is either younger or older.

Source: Adapted from J. L. Farr, P. E. Tesluk, & S. R. Klein (1998). Organizational structure of the workplace and the older worker. *Impact of Work on Older Adults*, pp. 143–185.

physical loads. However, the motivation to exercise is very low in this population (O'Brien Cousins, 1998), and most programs that demonstrate any success have a very high degree of individual attention. The successful exercise program for this population is usually aimed at improving specific work performance. Work-hardening programs requiring employee attendance have had success because they mandate participation in order to return to work after injury or to continue in a particular position (Cady, Biscoff, O'Connell, Thomas, & Allan, 1979). Finally, in the 50–64-year-old work force, chronic diseases (including hypertension, diabetes, arthritis, and other cardiovascular diseases) affect the level of performance of physical tasks and require individualized attention for successful exercise program participation.

For the young-old (65–74), either still in the workforce or retired, the variability of physical performance is more pronounced. A significant percentage of workers and new retirees will be able to perform a wide range of both physical and mental tasks at a level comparable to the 50–64-year-old work population. In many ways, this population represents the "golden age." The ability to do work and the energy to live fully are still intact. Physical activity programs for this group need to emphasize both maintenance and development of specific strength and skill levels to continue to work or to perform specific life tasks. Most young-old are interested in working but not necessarily full-time.

When planning physical activity programs for the old-old (75+), each individual is truly a unique participant. Health and medical history are critical, along with a thorough assessment of current flexibility and strength. The oldest people in our culture have had the longest time to express their genetic potential within a particular environment, so they represent a true uniqueness that can only be appreciated by taking more time to conduct individual interviews and testing and basing intervention upon a person's complete history. Once this information is obtained, appropriate individual physical activity programs can significantly improve physical performance of the old-old (Evens & Rosenberg, 1991). This increased functional ability accrues to the individual and to society at large but not usually to an employer, as these individuals are typically retired.

General fitness programs have not worked well for the older worker and retiree. According to Shephard (1997), O'Brien Cousins (1998), and others, the better educated the workforce, the greater the chance to get exercise participation. So, depending upon the mix of employees (white- and blue-collar) and the level of physical activity specified, participation varied from a low of 6% to a high of 40% of workers (Wilson, Holman, & Hammock, 1996). The boomer, now approaching midfifties, however, has had more exposure to the general fitness movement and may be open to adopt an active lifestyle change in later life.

Health Promotion Program Targets for Older Workers and Retirees

Depending on worksite rationale and goals, health promotion programs for older adults and retirees may target one of three areas: remedial/rehabilitative, prevention, or life quality. With older workers and retirees, significant health problems exist that must be addressed (remediated) to both maintain current job functions and limit losses in productivity. A commitment to this phase of worksite health should enable many workers to remain in the workforce. Prevention programming based upon risk factor identification should minimize the impact of problems associated with both lifestyle and age. By promoting positive lifestyles and instituting secondary prevention programs, significant impact on the workforce is possible. Finally, life satisfaction program targets demonstrate concern for the whole person and promote employee participation by demonstrating strong interest in employee well-being. Table 19-6 identifies programming targets that are appropriate for health promotion and wellness providers.

If programs are designed for those needing rehabilitative/remedial assistance, clear analysis based upon the individual disability should be the basis for action. If programs are designed for prevention, high-risk populations should be identified and targeted. However, all individuals benefit from this category of programming. If programs are designed for lifestyle and well-being, local mores and values need to be the basis of programming.

Table 19-6 Program Targets for Worksite Health Promotion

1. **Remedial and rehabilitative programs:** People who have suffered disability and illness must be individually evaluated to determine appropriate interventions. Work-hardening programs that focus on a specific skill or function have great value to both the individual and employer.
2. **Prevention programs:** Keeping people active and functioning independently by supporting positive lifestyle programming improves day-to-day functioning and reduces the risk of many chronic diseases.
3. **Life-enhancing and growth producing programs:** Programs that encourage people to reach new levels of well-being in late life demonstrate a caring and concerned employer.

Recruitment Strategies

Blanket interventions aimed at the total workplace will miss most older workers. Prochaska's stages of change model (Prochaska & Velicer, 1997) is an example of the level of analysis needed when thinking about interventions within this population. It would be critical to know which older workers and retirees are in the preparation and action stages as a basis for program planning. However, the stage model is only the beginning of understanding the motivation to participate in worksite health programs. The use of focus groups and in-depth interviews of intended work groups is necessary to fine-tune recruitment and marketing efforts. Knowing where the population falls in terms of needs and interest in the three program target areas of remedial/rehabilitative, prevention, or life-enhancing programs will assist in tailoring attractive program interventions.

In general, what excites the younger worker will not usually attract older workers and retirees. These individuals have been purchasers and consumers for many years and are "wise" to the world of marketing and promotion. It is difficult to create a need through marketing for these individuals. But, they have real health and wellness needs and recognize opportunities to efficiently and effectively meet these needs. For example, a beautiful body is not as high a priority for

a 58-year-old as is dealing with chronic pain or financing retirement, so a fitness program that emphasizes getting ready for swimsuit season may not sell well. Nonetheless, the same program may be marketed successfully if it reduces pain and increases a grandparent's ability to play with grandchildren.

It is always dangerous making generalizations; but, as workers age, it appears they have deeper motivations for either changing a behavior or not (Shalomi-Schachter & Miller, 1995). They also have a great deal of experience evaluating the quality and sincerity of the programs offered, so successful worksite health promotion programs must tap into these deeper emotional bases for health-related behavior change. In summary, according to Cross (1981), participation is influenced by: (a) self-evaluation, (b) attitudes toward a program, (c) importance of goals and expectations that goals will be met, (d) life transitions, (e) opportunities and barriers, and (f) information about availability of program offerings.

Changing health behavior has proven to be very difficult in these populations (Dzewaltowski, 1989); and, in older populations, positive health behaviors may not be clustered as they are in younger populations (Misra, Quandt, & Aguillon, 1999). When working with younger groups, we could usually infer that when either new positive behaviors were established or supported, other positive behaviors followed. This has not proven to be the case with older workers or retirees. Other social factors, including poverty, social support, or lack thereof, may moderate the crossover effect of positive lifestyle. As a result, a strong case can be made to focus on those behaviors and basic health conditions that are directly related to morbidity, mortality, and quality of late life.

Program Content

Based upon frequency in the population, the most promising targets for health-related intervention and control are blood pressure detection and management, serum glucose, not smoking, and obesity (Reed et al., 1998). Other programs of high interest for the older worker and retiree include financial health, relationship skill-building, spiritual wellness, and retirement transition planning.

Table 19-7 Design of Content for Health Promotion Programs

1. **Fear Management:** Older learners fear failure and comparison to younger workers. Feedback on successful performance, either physical or cognitive, needs to be delivered early and often.
2. **Relevance:** Content needs to have obvious application to either job performance or a functional need in retirement.
3. **Skill Level:** Appropriate complexity is critical for success, and clear articulation of the old and new behavior need to be demonstrated.
4. **Program Support:** New behavior or knowledge needs to be in context of larger work or retirement culture.
5. **Completion Rates:** Older workers and retirees vary greatly in their abilities and may need more time to complete tasks or learn new skills. Independent learning is important for the older learner so content should be organized in units that allow self-study.

Source: Adapted from Straka, 1998. Commentary: Organization; self-directed learning and chronological age. In K. W. Schaie, & C. Schooler (Eds.), *Impactive Work on Older Adults*, pp. 186–194.

Successful programs need to be organized with the special learning needs of this population in mind. According to Sterns and Doverspike (1988), five basic issues need to be addressed in organizing content. Table 19-7 reviews core issues in organizing program materials. All learning materials need to be viewed by the learner as appropriate to specific needs and organized in a manner that supports current skill and knowledge levels.

Program interventions in worksite health have been extensively reviewed (Wilson, Holman & Hammock, 1996) in a series of articles that appeared in the *American Journal of Health Promotion* in 1996. Program areas included physical activity, weight control, cholesterol, nutrition, smoking control, high blood pressure, stress management, HIV, health risk appraisal, and seat belt use. These program areas represent the core of most worksite-based health promotion programs. Based upon these reviews, it is clear that the level of impact of most programs in the workplace have good success in producing short-term change but mixed to limited impact on long-term behavioral change. Older workers and retirees present some of

the most difficult challenges for worksite health promotion because behavior patterns are very well established, and population variability is great, therefore the patterns of success demonstrated in the field of worksite health will be amplified with the older worker and retiree.

Program Format

Individual attention and support will be necessary to achieve significant positive response from this population. This attention could come from programs that use high technology to tailor individual feedback. A computer-assisted intervention with algorithms that make follow-up health messages appropriate for each individual is being demonstrated by Victor Strecher at the University of Michigan (Strecher, 1999). Participants receive personal mail based upon their ongoing health-related data. Through this computerized contact system, individuals feel they are getting the personal attention they deserve. This technique has great potential for reaching the older worker and retiree.

Regardless of the specific methodology, older workers and retirees will participate in health promotion and wellness programs if they deem them as relevant to their needs and life stage. The challenge for health promotion and wellness programmers is to understand the complexity of the older worker and retiree health decision-making process.

Program Management

Programs must be organized and managed by available staff or outsourced through contracts. This decision should be based upon an assessment of an organization's philosophy of ownership of programs and experience with health promotion vendors and community resources. Specifically, working with older adults and retirees is going to be more expensive in terms of time and money than working with the general workforce population. It is essential that programs be guided by staff with experience working with this age group. Each organization must decide if they want to employ or retrain employees to provide these programs or contract for this expertise.

CONCLUSION

Planning and designing programs requires an awareness of the diversity of the older worker and retiree and how immersed they are in their culture. Programmers must be aware of the difficulty this population has with breaking old habits that are supported by a work and home culture. Those who are willing to move into this culture and build trust and develop a deep understanding of the history of the workplace, the community, and the individual have the greatest potential for success.

In general, most older workers would be very willing to continue to work if their current employer would make work hours more flexible and specific physical tasks less demanding (AARP, 1998). In a workplace dominated by cognitive tasks, older workers may hold the most important positions because of longevity in positions, and older workers may outperform younger workers by using accumulated on-the-job knowledge. Based upon quantitative measures of job performance, most cognitive tasks in the workplace appear to be performed equally well by older and younger workers (Clancy & Hoyer, 1994), so good planning and program design could result in significant older worker retention and productivity. In the retiree population, good design would result in improvement in functional health status and quality of life.

Finally, each organization must decide if these program modifications are worth the effort. If the only criterion is direct associated costs, then a net present value analysis should help in making the decision to either do, or not do, a particular program for older workers and retirees. However, most program decisions are based upon a complex set of variables that includes costs, benefits, local program history, staffing levels, and commitment of upper management. Based upon the large population shift taking place and the economic power of this well-educated cohort, it will be difficult to ignore their health and wellness needs. It appears that most workplaces will find it necessary to include planning and delivery of appropriate programs for this large population.

References

Administration on Aging. (1998). *Profile of older Americans: 1998.* [On-line]. Available: http://www.aoa.dhhs.gov/aoa/stats/profile/default.htm.

American Association of Retired Persons. (1998). *A profile of older Americans* [Brochure]. Washington, DC: Author.

American Association for World Health. (1999). *Healthy aging, healthy living: Start now.* Washington, DC: American Association for World Health.

Atchley, R. C. (1989). A continuity theory of normal aging. *The Gerontologist, 29,* 183–190.

Besl, J.R., & Kale, B.D. (1996). Older workers in the 21st century: Active and educated, a case study. *Monthly Labor Review 119(6):* 18-28.

Breslow, L., & Beckman, L. (1983). *Health and ways of living: The Alameda county studies.* New York: Oxford University Press.

Cady, L., Biscoff, D., O'Connell, E., Thomas, P., & Allan, J. (1979). Strength and fitness and subsequent back injury in firefighters. *Journal of Occupational Medicine, 4,* 269–272.

Caserta, M. S., & Gillett, P. A. (1998). Older women's feelings about exercise and their adherence to an aerobic regimen over time. *The Gerontologist, 38,* 602–609.

Chapman, L. S. (1999). Population health management. *The Art of Health Promotion, 3(2),* 1–10.

Clancy, S. M., & Hoyer, W. J. (1994). Age and skill in visual search. *Developmental Psychology, 30,* 545–552.

Costa, P. T., & McCrae, R. R. (1988). Personality in adulthood: A six-year longitudinal study of self-reports and spouse ratings on the NEO Personality Inventory. *Journal of Personality and Social Psychology, 54,* 853–863.

Crose, R., Nicholas, D. R., Gobble, D. C., & Frank, B. (1992). Gender and wellness: A multidimensional systems model for counseling. *Journal of Counseling and Development, 71,* 149–156.

Cross, P.L. (1981). *Adults as learners.* San Francisco: Jossey-Bass.

Cumming, E., & Henery, W. (1961). *Growing old.* New York: Basic Books.

Dulitzky, D. (1999). *Incentives for early retirement in private pension and health insurance plans.* Urban Institute: The Retirement Project. Brief Series No. 3, (March).

Dzewaltowski, D.A. (1989). *A social cognitive theory of older adult exercise motivation*. In A.C. Ostrow (Ed.), Aging and motor behavior. Indianapolis, IN: Benchmar, 257-81.

Frostin, P. (1997). *Employee benefits, retirement plans, and implications for increased worklife*. Employee Benefits Research Institute. EBRI Issue Brief No. 1984, Washington, D.C.

Eisenburg, D. M., Kessler, R. C., Foster, C., Norlock, F. E., Calkins, D. R., & Delbanco, D. L. (1998). Unconventional medicine in the United States: Prevalence, costs, and patterns of use. *New England Journal of Medicine, 328*, 246–252.

Employing a productive workforce. (Accessed 1999, July 27). [On-line]. Available: http://www.nsf.gov/sbe/sber/social/worksla.htm.

Erikson, E. H. (1963). *Childhood and society.* New York: Norton.

Etheridge, L. (1999). Three streams, one river: A coordinated approach to financing retirement. *Health Affairs, 18,* 80–85.

Evans, W., & Rosenberg, I. H. (1991). *Biomarkers: The 10 keys to prolonging vitality.* New York: Fireside.

Farr, J. L., & Middlebrooks, C. L. (1990). Enhancing motivation to participate in progressional development. In S. L. Willis & S. S. Durbin (Eds.), *Maintaining professional competence: Approaches to career enhancement, vitality, and success throughout a work life* (pp. 132–155). San Francisco: Jossey-Bass.

Farr, J. F., Tesluk, P. E., & Klien, S. R. (1998). Organizational structure of the workplace and the older adult. In K. W. Schaie & C. Schooler (Eds.), *Impact of work on older adults* (pp. 143–185). New York: Springer.

Fosu, G. B. (1995). Social support and compliance with hypertensive regimens among the elderly. *Journal of Mental Health and Aging, 1,* 7–20.

Freedman, V. A., & Martin, L. G. (1998). Understanding trends in functional limitations among older Americans. *American Journal of Public Health, 88,* 1458–1462.

Fries, J. F. (1980). Aging, natural death, and the compression of morbidity. *New England Journal of Medicine, 303,* 130–135.

Fries, J. F., Koop, C. E., Sokolov, J., Beadle, C. E., & Wright, D. (1998). Beyond health promotion: Reducing need and demand for medical care. *Health Affairs, 17,* 70–84.

Gobble, D., & Crose, R. (1998). *Living long and loving it: Ingredients for a good old age.* Preconference

workshop presented at the annual meeting of the American Journal of Health Promotion, Monterey, CA.

Glanz, K. (1999). Commentary: Participation, retention, and adherence: Implications for health promotion research and practice. *American Journal of Health Promotion, 13,* 276–277.

Goetzel, R. Z., Anderson, D. H., & Whitmer, R. W. (1998). The relationship between modifiable health risks and health care expenditures: An analysis of the multi-employer HERO health risk and cost database. *Journal of Environmental Medicine, 40,* 843–854.

Green, L., Richard, L., & Potvin, L. (1998). Ecological foundations of health promotion. *American Journal of Health Promotion, 10,* 270-81.

Health Care Financing Administration. (1999). *Medicare and you, 2000* (Publication No. 10050r) [Brochure]. Baltimore: Author.

Higgins, F. (1995). *Highlights: A monthly summary of benefits news.* Princeton, NJ: A. Foster Higgins Co.

Hoyer, W. J. (1998). The older individual in a rapidly changing work context: Developmental and cognitive issues. In K. W. Schaie & C. Schooler (Eds.), *Impact of work on older adults* (pp. 28–44). New York: Springer.

Kaplan, G. A., Haan, M. N, & Wallace R. B. (1999). Understanding changing risk factor associations with increasing age in adults. In J. E. Fielding, L. B. Lave, & B. Starfield (Eds.), *Annual review of public health* (20th ed., pp. 89–108). Palo Alto, California: Annual Reviews.

Kreuter, M. W., Lezin, N. A., & Green, L. W (1998). *Community health promotion ideas that work.* Boston: Jones & Bartlett.

Lenz, E. A. (1996). *Flexible employment: Positive work strategies for the 21st century: National Association of Temporary and Staffing Services.* (Accessed 1999, April 28). [On-line]. Available: http://natss.org/flx.txt.

Lewin-VHI, Inc. (1994). *Aging baby boomers: How secure is their economic future?* Washington, DC: American Association of Retired Persons.

Longino, C. F. (1994). *American demographics/marketing tools.* (Accessed 1998, November 6) [On-line]. Available: http://marketingtools.com/cgi-bin/tex.

Longman, P. (1999, March). How global aging will challenge the world's economic well-being. *U.S. News & World Report,* pp. 30–39.

Loprest, P. J., & Zedlewski, S. R. (1998). Health insurance coverage transitions of older Americans. [On-line]. Available: http://urban.org/health_older.html.

Marmor, T. R., & Okma, K. G. H. (1998). Societal interventions affecting elderly citizens: A comparative approach. In R. Schulz, G. Maddox, & M. P. Lawton (Eds.), *Annual review of gerontology and geriatrics* (18th ed., pp. 321–338). New York: Springer.

Mattoon, M. A. (1981). *Jungian psychology in perspective.* New York: Free Press.

Mazzeo, R. S., Cavanagh, P., Evans, W., Fiatarone, M., Hagberg, J., McAuley, E., & Statzell, J. (1998). Exercise and physical activity for older adults. *Medicine Science in Sports and Exercise, 30,* 992–1008.

McCarthy, T. H., Gobble, D. C., Fitzgerald, J., & Treloar, J. (1999). *The best predictors of medical claims costs at Ball State University.* Unpublished manuscript. Ball State University.

Minnesota Department of Human Services. (1999). *Project 2030: Workforce and economic vitality.* [On-line]. Available: http://www.dhs.state.mn.us/agingint./proj2030/report/workfrce.htm.

Misra, R., Quandt, S. A., & Aguillon, S. (1999). Differences in nutritional risk and nutrition related behaviors in exercising and nonexercising rural elders. *American Journal of Health Promotion, 13,* (3), 149–52.

Morgan, D. (1998). Facts and figures about the baby boom. *Generations, 22,* 5–33.

Morris, W. R., Conrad, K. M., Marcantonio, R. J., Marks, B. A., & Ribisl, K. M. (1999). Do blue-collar workers perceive the worksite health climate differently than white-collar workers? *American Journal of Health Promotion, 13,* 319–324.

National Heart, Lung, and Blood Institute. (1999). *Cardiovascular health for all: NHLBI sets new heart agenda* (Summer ed.) [Brochure]. Bethesda, MD: Heart Memo, National Institute of Health.

Neugarten, B. L., & Associates (Eds.). (1964). *Personality in middle and late life.* New York: Atherton.

Nicholas, D. R., & Gobble, D. C. (1991). World views, systems theory, and health promotion. *American Journal of Health Promotion, 6,* 30–35.

Noe, R. A., & Wilk, S. L. (1993). Investigation of the factors that influence employees' participation in development activities. *Journal of Applied Psychology, 78,* 291–302.

O'Brien Cousins, S. (1998). *Exercise, aging and health: Overcoming barriers to an active old age.* Philadelphia: Taylor & Francis.

Poulos, S., & Nightingale, D. S. (1999). The aging baby boom: Implications for employment and training programs. [On-line]. Available: http://www.urban.org/aging/abb/agingbaby.html.

Prochaska, J. O., & Velicer, W. F. (1997). The transtheoretical model of health behavior change. *American Journal of Health Promotion, 12,* 38–48.

Public Policy Institute. (1998). *Boomers approaching midlife: How secure a future?* Washington, DC: American Association of Retired Persons.

Reed, D. M, Foley D. J., White, L. R., Heimovitz, H., Burchfiel, C. M., & Masaki, K. (1998). Predictors of healthy aging in men with high life expectations. *American Journal of Public Health, 88,* 1463–68.

Reynolds, A. (1998). Quitting while they're ahead (but what about the rest of us?). [On-line]. Available: http://www.hudson.org/American_Outlook/fa98/reynolds.htm.

Rowe, J. W., & Kahn, R. L. (1997). Successful aging. *The Gerontologist, 37,* 433–440.

Russell, J.N., Hendershot, G.E., LeClere, F., Howie, L.J., & Alder, M. (1997). *Trends and differential use of assistance technology devices: United States, 1994.* Advace Data No. 292. National Center for Health Statistics, Hyattsville, MD.

Schneider, J. K. (1997). Self-regulation and exercise behavior in older women. *Journal of Gerontology, 52B,* 235–241.

Schooler, C., Caplan, L., & Oates, G. (1998). Aging and work: An overview. In K. W. Schaie & C. Schooler (Eds.), *Impact of work on older adults* (pp. 1–19). New York: Springer.

Shalomi-Schachter, Z., & Miller, R. (1995). *Age-ing to sage-ing: A profound new vision of growing older.* New York: Warner Books.

Shephard, R. (1991). Fitness and aging. In C. Blais (Ed.), *Aging into the twenty-first century* (pp. 12–35). North York, ON: Captus University Publications.

Shephard, R. J. (1997). The aging labor force. *Aging, physical activity and health* (pp. 327–349). Champaign, IL: Human Kinetics.

Smith, J.P. (1997). *The changing economic circumstances of the elderly: Income, wealth and social security.* Policy Brief No. 8, New York: Center for Policy Research, Syracuse University.

Sterns, H.L., & Doverspike, D. (1988). *Training and developing the older worker: Implications for human resource management.* In H. Dennis (Ed.), Fourteen steps in managing an aging worforce. Lexington Books: Lexington, KY, 97-110.

Sterns, H. L., Matheson, N. K., & Schwartz G. (1989). Aging and the training and learning process in organizations. In I. Goldstein & R. Katzel (Eds.), *Training and development in work organizations.* San Francisco: Jossey-Bass.

Stofan, Depietro, L., Davis, D., Kohl, H. W., & Blair, S. N. (1998). Physical activity patterns associated with cardiorespiratory fitness and reduced mortality: The aerobics center longitudinal study. *American Journal of Public Health, 88,* 1807–1813.

Straka, G. (1998). Commentary: Organization, self-directed learning, and chronological age. In K. W. Schaie & C. Schooler (Eds.), *Impact of work on older adults.* New York: Springer, 186-94.

Strecher, V. J. (1999). Computer-tailored smoking cessation materials: A review and discussion. *Patient Education Counseling, 36*(2), 107–17.

Vita, A. J., Terry, R. B., Hubet, H. B., & Fries, J. (1998). Aging, health risks, and cumulative disability. *The New England Journal of Medicine, 338,* 1035–41.

Wilson, M., Holman, P., & Hammock (1996). A comprehensive review of the effects of worksite health promotion on health-related outcomes. *American Journal of Health Promotion, 10,* 429-435.

CHAPTER

20

Global Perspectives in Workplace Health Promotion

Wolf Kirsten

INTRODUCTION TO INTERNATIONAL HEALTH PROMOTION

In line with the current globalization and the increasing interest of U.S. health promotion professionals in international trends and initiatives in the field, the following chapter has the purpose of providing an overview of health promotion in the workplace abroad. This will include an account of the new challenges in global health and the global emergence of health promotion, descriptions of health promotion programs implemented by multinational corporations, and introductions to initiatives in various selected countries. The chapter will conclude with an analysis of the differences between international and U.S. programs and an outlook into the future where the field of global workplace health promotion may be heading.

Much of the following content is drawn from the experience of the author, Wolf Kirsten, who has been heavily involved in international health promotion over the last six years. Many interviews were conducted specifically for the compilation of this chapter, in addition to previously gathered data from international conferences, seminars, meetings, and daily communications.

New Challenges in Global Health

The leading cause of mortality and morbidity worldwide is chronic disease (e.g., cardiovascular disease, cancer). Although developing countries still face major challenges in controlling infectious disease, an epidemiological transition is taking place due to the rapid increase in chronic disease incidence. Most chronic diseases can be attributed to unhealthy lifestyles and behaviors that are preventable. In line with economic growth, people in developing countries are acquiring the unhealthy lifestyles of the industrialized countries (e.g., smoking, high-fat diets, inactivity), resulting in a changing disease pattern. Mortality statistics follow similar patterns in regions with different socioeconomic conditions as demonstrated in Table 20-1.

Table 20-1 Leading Causes of Mortality and Disability-Adjusted Life Years (DALYs) in All Member States and Their Ranks in WHO Regions.

	All Member States		Africa		The Americas		Eastern Mediterranean		Europe		South-East Asia		Western Pacific	
	Rank	% of total	Rank	% of total	Rank	% of total	Rank	% of total	Rank	% of total	Rank	% of total	Rank	% of total
Deaths														
Ischemic heart disease	1	13.7	9	2.9	1	17.9	1	13.6	1	25.5	1	13.8	3	11.1
Cerebrovascular disease	2	9.5	7	4.7	2	10.3	5	5.3	2	13.7	4	6.5	1	14.3
Acute lower respiratory infections	3	6.4	3	8.2	3	4.2	2	9.1	4	3.6	2	9.3	4	4.0
HIV/AIDS	4	4.2	1	19.0	13	1.8	27	0.4	42	0.2	8	2.2	42	0.2
Chronic obstructive pulmonary disease	5	4.2	14	1.1	6	2.8	10	1.7	5	2.7	11	1.6	2	12.0
Diarrheal diseases	6	4.1	4	7.6	10	2.0	3	7.4	22	0.7	3	6.6	17	1.2
Perinatal conditions	7	4.0	5	5.5	7	2.6	4	7.3	13	1.2	5	6.0	10	2.2
Tuberculosis	8	2.8	11	2.2	19	1.0	7	3.7	23	0.6	6	5.1	9	2.9
Trachea/bronchus/lung	9	2.3	38	0.3	4	3.2	20	1.0	3	4.2	15	1.2	6	3.6
Road traffic accidents	10	2.2	12	1.8	5	3.1	9	1.9	8	1.9	7	2.5	12	2.0
DALYs														
Acute lower respiratory infections	1	6.0	4	7.0	9	2.9	2	8.1	8	2.5	1	8.1	4	3.9
Perinatal conditions	2	5.8	5	6.2	5	4.2	1	8.2	5	2.9	2	7.9	5	3.7
Diarrheal diseases	3	5.3	3	7.5	8	3.0	3	7.7	17	1.6	3	7.2	13	1.9
HIV/AIDS	4	5.1	1	16.6	13	2.0	7	2.8	46	0.4	12	2.2	36	0.6
Unipolar major depression	5	4.2	11	1.7	1	5.7	6	3.6	3	5.5	4	4.0	2	6.5
Ischemic heart disease	6	3.8	20	0.9	2	4.9	5	3.7	1	9.7	5	3.8	7	3.5
Cerebrovascular disease	7	3.0	13	1.5	6	3.5	12	1.8	2	5.6	13	2.1	3	5.1
Malaria	8	2.8	2	10.6	80	0.1	16	1.5	97	0.0	39	0.6	60	0.2
Road traffic accidents	9	2.8	9	1.9	4	4.7	11	2.1	4	3.7	8	2.9	9	2.8
Measles	10	2.2	6	5.3	92	0.0	8	2.7	67	0.2	11	2.2	48	0.3

Source: World Health Organization, *The World Health Report 1999*, 1999.

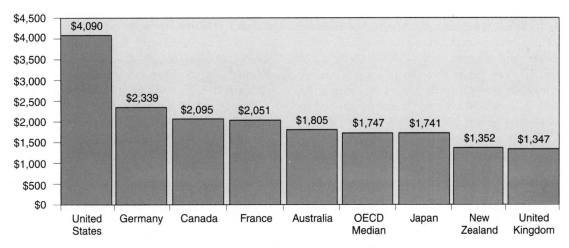

Figure 20-1 Health care expenditures per capita in 1997, Adjusted for cost-of-living differences (OECD-Organization for Economic Cooperation and Development)

Source: Gerard F. Anderson, Multinational Comparisons of Health Care: Expenditures, Coverage, and Outcomes, 1998.

This transition in lifestyles is enhanced by emerging global developments, such as population growth, urbanization, aging, and a changing family structure. Most countries will face a tremendous economic burden in the next century as health care costs are rising. Many countries, developed and emerging, authorize large and increasing health care budgets, with the United States allotting the highest percentage in the world of their annual budget to health care as shown in Figure 20-1.

Continuing to apply administrative cost-containment strategies will not alleviate the situation and, coupled with rapidly changing demographics, presents a number of fiscal and social challenges.

Reacting to these challenges, there has been a recent increased focus in the international community on the importance of maintaining or improving one's health status through the practice of health-enhancing activities. The rising popularity of the promotion of healthy lifestyles has been spurred by the participation of institutions from many different fields. Academic institutions, government authorities, private corporations, insurance companies, hospitals, medical groups, and community groups, as well as other significant individuals in health promotion, have

joined the universal effort to improve the quality of life. Specifically, a number of multinational corporations are taking a close look at the health status of their global workforce and are consequently designing and implementing health promotion programs. Numerous well-designed programs have shown an increase in productivity, reduction in health care costs, and improved morale among employees. These developments have generated a global desire for intense networking and international collaboration in the area of health promotion.

Major international organizations such as the World Health Organization and the World Bank have begun to incorporate health promotion components into their large-scale health-related initiatives. The World Health Organization articulated health promotion as a focal point of their overall strategy since the announcement of the Ottawa Charter in 1986, but a biomedical perspective still dominates throughout the ranks.

The Global Emergence of Health Promotion

Health promotion is on the verge of becoming a recognized science in the United States and a few other select countries, and many other countries are also displaying considerable momentum for advancement of the field. For example, Poland has demonstrated a remarkable turnaround in mortality rates from chronic disease since 1991. After rising since 1960, mortality rates from diseases of the circulatory system dropped by 40% in the 20–44 age group, by nearly 30% in the 45–64 age group, and by 12–14% in the over-65 age group between 1991 and 1996. A similar trend has been noted in the Czech Republic and Slovakia since the beginning of the 1990s and in Hungary since 1993 (Zatonski, 1996). This decrease in premature mortality in Poland is of a magnitude apparently without precedent in peacetime. The decline is largely attributed to the introduction of a market economy and corresponding dietary changes, specifically the decrease in animal fat consumption and increase in vegetable and fruit consumption. The fact that this change in lifestyle can have such a profound impact underlines the enormous potential of health promotion (e.g., advocating a decreased intake of animal fat). In addition, some of the most progressive tobacco control legislation was passed in Poland in 1999, including a total ban on tobacco advertising, promotion, and sponsorship.

In Brazil, a physical activity program called "Agita" was launched in the state of São Paulo in 1996 and, to date, has spread the message to an estimated 21 million people through the media. The program outcome with regard to health status has not been scientifically documented yet; however, as the program is now being expanded to other Brazilian cities and other Latin American countries, the number of people affected by this cleverly marketed program is large.

In the People's Republic of China, obesity is on the rise. According to the latest Nationwide Nutrition Survey, 14.9% of the urban Chinese population and 32.9% of Beijing residents are overweight. (Ge Ke You, 1992). This compares to 12% in 1989 and 9.7% in 1982 in urban areas. While the intake of grains and potatoes has decreased, intake of meats, eggs, and milk has significantly increased over the last 15 years. One has to keep in mind that still many Chinese peasants and rural workers are grossly undernourished. In addition to the increasing trend of obesity, more and more Chinese are becoming inactive; a recent investigation of 112,000 workers by the Department of Mass

Exercise of the Chinese Sports Committee (1998) showed 41.9% were sedentary individuals and 27% were occasionally active individuals. This is hard to believe if one frequents one of the city parks early in the morning to observe the many activities, ranging from tai chi to sword fighting and ballroom dancing.

The age of globalization also provides numerous opportunities for the improvement of quality of life, such as improved information flow through use of new technologies. But globalization is also a "double-edged sword." Take, for example, the case of tobacco consumption. Increased free trade has contributed to the doubling of the world's cigarette production over the last 30 years. In 1998, 5,609 billion cigarettes were produced, which amounts to 948 per person (U.S. Dept. of Agriculture, 1999). Many tobacco companies aggressively market their products in the developing world in a move to offset the legal challenges they face back home. At the same time, advocacy measures against tobacco consumption have multiplied and improved drastically worldwide as researchers, politicians, and advocates have been sharing facts as well as advocacy strategies. Furthermore, unhealthy dietary habits are being adopted worldwide with the increased exposure to "Western" foods due to globalization.

There are many fascinating and successful examples in different countries underlining the positive impact of health promotion worldwide. This chapter will introduce some of the more interesting programs implemented at the worksite.

CURRENT INTERNATIONAL DEVELOPMENTS IN WORKPLACE HEALTH PROMOTION

Much of the history of health promotion programs offered in and through the work environment has been linked to programs in North America. However, as you will read throughout this chapter, there are many very fine examples of well-developed workplace health promotion programs that have been and continue to be operating in many countries throughout the world.

Alfred Marshall, Cambridge's great economist at the turn of the century, was once quoted as saying "The most valuable of all capital is that invested in human beings." (Karch, 1999). The allocation of capital that is specifically committed to the development, implementation, and ongoing operation of high quality workplace health promotion is not only "the most valuable of all capital" but is "imperative capital" if a company, or for that matter a country, wants to be competitive in local, regional, or global marketplaces. Companies, first and foremost, accomplish their goals through people—their employees. Thus, strategies and programs that call for building, recruiting, and maintaining healthy and vital employees can be unequivocally linked to high performance.

As important as it is, the impetus for workplace health promotion is not tied exclusively to performance. Concurrent with the need to be competitive in the marketplace, companies throughout the world, to varying degrees, are faced with soaring health care costs, nationalization and privatization of health insurance plans, and an aging workforce. Companies have pursued a workplace health policy as long they have existed. However, with some major changes taking place, such as changes in the demography of the labor market, changes in the nature of economic activity, and changes in the nature of work, this area of human resource management has gained a new significance. Corporate activities have shifted from production to complex work operations requiring highly qualified employees. In most large companies, the ratio of blue- and white-collar workers reversed over the last 20 years (Pot & Gründemann, 1999). A growing number of high-technology companies are in need of "intellectual capital"—qualified, innovative, flexible, and motivated employees. To find these employees, employers must provide more than material benefits, such as personal freedom of action, possibilities of further development, respect and recognition by superiors, and healthy working conditions (Goth, 1999). This is where health promotion becomes an important business factor in a comprehensive human resource strategy.

Given these factors, companies around the globe are confronted with a critical strategic choice: invest additional capital to get and keep all employees (young and old) as healthy as possible or expect and plan to expend significant capital to pay for the associated medical and lost-production cost incurred as a result of the poor health of their workers. Fortunately, many insightful companies have already made the choice to be proactive in developing and promoting programs that are not only focused on issues of controlling health care costs and increasing productivity, but also on organizational issues such as the development of social, environmental, and educational policies. These programs are key elements to building and maintaining a truly healthy workplace and workforce.

Creating a Healthy Global Workforce

There are many different approaches to creating a healthy global workforce. The strategies employed by six multinational corporations are described below. Each of the six companies has taken a distinctly different approach in the development and operation of their respective workplace health promotion programs. This information was compiled through past discussions and interviews with the program managers and interactive sessions at seminars on this topic.

Case Study #1: Coca-Cola

The Coca-Cola Company is the world's leading beverage company, conducting business in more than 200 countries with nearly one million employees in a worldwide system. This includes a vast global distribution network of local bottling companies that employs more than 500,000 people. Coca-Cola is one of the few multinational corporations to have taken a global approach to health management. The headquarters in Atlanta have devised an integrated health management strategy combining health promotion, early detection of disease, occupational medicine, disease management, health plan design, and return to work/disability programs. The overriding goal is to increase employee satisfaction, productivity, and the value of health care dollars spent by linking health strategies to business strategies and integrating the components (Landgreen, 1999b).

Coca-Cola started its health management programs 15 years ago with a fragmented approach. The evolution towards integrating programs has come only recently, with the result that many worksites now have well-established, effective health promotion programs up and running. The challenge has been to transfer some of the successes and learnings across complex company structures and diverse country borders. Success stories can be found from the headquarters in Atlanta, where a 70% fitness center participation rate has been documented, to Drogheda in Ireland, Manaus in Brazil, and Cidra in Puerto Rico where 80% participation rates have been tracked for nearly a decade (Landgreen, 1999a). The programs have a distinct character according to country, culture, and environment. For example, in Bangkok, Thailand, all office staff members go to an adjacent park with a fitness leader on Thursday afternoons to exercise and play volleyball. In Japan, any employee absent from work with a physical disability must participate in the on-site rehabilitation program to ensure a speedy return to work. The production facility in Manaus, Brazil, is located in the Amazon River Basin and can be reached only by air or barge. Here it is especially important to provide a healthy environment because employees and dependents spend all their time in the area. All services ranging from medical care to recreational activities and healthy eating choices are provided on-site.

Coca-Cola's system of bottling partners represents a rich diversity reflecting the cultures served. These billion dollar bottling systems have major production and distribution processes, which require large numbers of employees. The overall business strategy takes a local approach, using marketing and advertising techniques that reflect local culture and therefore create local ownership. This multilocal approach, however, does present unique challenges in applying health management programs and practices. The sharing of best practices and pooling resources requires a concerted effort within an organization that does business throughout the world. It is a priority to raise awareness among the working populations by building communications capabilities through use of all types of communication channels (such as worldwide intranet and videoconferencing). Independent of the location, the goal is to create active participants who take responsibility for their health and lifestyles and, at the same time, to provide convenient on-site

health management services, which range from exercise facilities to primary medical care.

The challenge to implementing an integrated health management system worldwide is to achieve a single community mindset and bridge the gap between the corporate headquarters viewpoint of health management and the reality of the local culture and environment. This process can take years and can encounter formidable resistance. Coca-Cola follows a transformation process which includes seven stages: transition, connection, focus, activation, integration, sustainability, and rejuvenation. Due to the limited staff, Coca-Cola's corporate health management team decided to start system implementation in the Latin America division, which has 210,000 employees. Mexico, which has 80,000 employees, was selected as the charter country to test the concept because it is reasonably accessible from corporate headquarters in Atlanta and has capable occupational medicine staff. The initiative involves identifying key resources in Mexico, which includes the Mexico City division office, two major bottling partners, the Mexican community and government, consulting firms, and local and global health insurance carriers; assessing current health management best practices; and identifying viable partnership opportunities. The goals are to design and implement integrated programs and services, evaluate outcomes, share knowledge, and eventually expand the programs across Latin America. In spite of the time and effort involved to put the necessary communication structure in place and achieve a team-building effect, the stakeholders are committed to the process aimed at integration and sustainability.

Cola-Cola plans to extend the concept to worksites in Africa, Asia, and Europe if the outcomes of the Latin America charter program prove an added value to the business, working towards a globally integrated, cost effective health management system.

Case Study # 2: Dow Chemical

The Dow Chemical Company is a global science and technology-based company that develops and manufactures a portfolio of chemical, plastic, and agricultural products and services for customers in 168 countries around the world. With annual sales of more than $18 billion, Dow conducts its operations through 14 global businesses employing 39,000 people. The company has 123 manufacturing sites in 32 countries and supplies more than 3,500 products. Dow's vision is to "provide superior solutions for our customers and society through science and good thinking" (Dow Chemical website, 3/11/00).

Health promotion has a strong tradition at Dow Chemical. The Occupational Health Services function has been serving the employees for more than seven decades with health education and preventive health activities. A formal distinct health promotion program was started at the corporate headquarters in 1985. In 1988, this effort evolved to include the creation of a corporate expertise/resource center for health promotion to serve the global operations of Dow. The program received the C. Everett Koop Award for Health Promotion in 1994 and international recognition in 1996 when the Brazilian Association of Life Quality presented Dow with the award for outstanding performance in health promotion. Dow Chemical administers health promotion as part of the Health Services Expertise Center within the Environment, Health, and Safety function. It is a shared service, which is leveraged across the entire corporation and individual business units. Dow's health promotion management standard is a key factor for global standardization, effective focus, and future success. Health promotion at Dow has three objectives: to improve the health status of Dow people, to positively affect the health-related costs of Dow people, and to be perceived as a valued service by Dow people. Health promotion at Dow is part of a larger integrated health management effort designed to capitalize on Dow's human investment.

Dow's Global Health Promotion Resource Center coordinates services to international locations, develops and/or identifies core products and services, provides subject matter expertise, maintains best-practice technology, ensures standardization, eliminates redundancy, evaluates effectiveness, and monitors quality. The mission is to drive and leverage the most cost-effective and impactful health promotion programs, services, and resources across global sites for optimal health promotion delivery.

Dow has a truly global approach to its health services, including health promotion. For example, a global stress assessment tool exists to promote stress management, and monthly health awareness fliers are translated and distributed internationally. The programmatic issues for 2000 are life management and physical preparedness; in other words, being healthy to perform the job successfully. A more holistic approach to health promotion is envisioned for the future. A worldwide health campaign addressing total health (mind, body, and spirit) is planned, including issues such as depression, nutrition, stress, substance abuse, and workload. Improved integration with other health-related services, including health benefits, training and development, employee assistance programs (EAP), and occupational health services, is also a priority.

Health promotion site expertise leaders are accountable for site health promotion planning, delivery, administration, and evaluation within North America. Outside of North America, health promotion is implemented primarily by occupational health physicians, nurses, and/or contractors. Health promotion professionals with the proper credentials are recruited from a variety of health-related sources, primarily from either the health education or physical education field.

Comprehensive information systems are being looked at to integrate group health, worker's compensation, participation, and absenteeism data. Global participation data is not available. However, the global injury and illness rates have steadily dropped over the last decade. The best year so far in Dow's history was 1999, with an all-time low of 0.98 injuries and/or illnesses per 200,000 workhours. The health promotion programs are believed to be a major factor in this trend. Dow will continue to recognize the value of health promotion in improving health and employee productivity and therefore will continue to link health strategies with business strategies.

Case Study #3: Applied Materials

Applied Materials is the leading supplier of semiconductor wafer processing systems and services worldwide. Established in 1967, it now has approximately

15,000 employees in over 80 locations worldwide and revenues of over US$ 4 billion per year. Applied Materials employees have an average age of early thirties. The company mission is to be the leading supplier of semiconductor fabrication solutions worldwide through innovation and enhancement of customer productivity with systems, process modules, and service solutions. The wellness program was initiated in 1989 at the request of Chairman of the Board Jim Morgan, to help employees improve basic health and thereby increase productivity. Applied Materials strives to provide a variety of tools and resources to employees throughout the world to enable them to develop their own personal wellness program, a key to success at Applied Materials (Applied Materials, 2000).

All full-time employees worldwide are eligible to participate in the wellness programs. Applied Materials follows a decentralized approach with regionally specific programs. Multiple departments work together to create an integrated approach: Benefits, Safety, Occupational Health, Risk Management, Human Resources, Food Services, and Corporate Affairs. In addition, individual product divisions administer joint programs to maximize resources. The programs focus on lifestyles and self-care to maintain and improve basic health and maximize productivity. Depending on the location, the following areas are targeted: health appraisals, nutrition/weight control, physical activity/fitness, stress management/worklife balance (e.g., employee assistance programs, community events), special population programs, and online services. Specific risk factors targeted are stress, lack of physical activity, obesity, high blood pressure, and nutrition. While participation varies from program to program, an overall rate of 39% has been documented. Every two years a global employee survey is conducted, which includes questions on wellness and worklife programs. The U.S. operations also administer an employee satisfaction survey. Some international offices have their own employee wellness satisfaction surveys. A formal evaluation including the tracking of health care costs, worker's compensation, absenteeism, turnover rates, and disability data is performed in the United States. The annual report compares health claim costs and absenteeism rates between participants and nonparticipants.

The programs have corporate health promotion staff in Santa Clara, California, Austin, Texas, and Taiwan. All other sites often rely on individuals from nursing and human-performance-related fields, who volunteer to organize employee wellness activities. The programs have a different focus according to country and culture:

- China: the government sponsors group exercises in the office during work time. Other activities include such sports competitions as table tennis, jump rope, volleyball, and walking.
- Japan: the offices are smoke-free, health club memberships are subsidized in some locations, and other discounted sports and social activities are offered.
- Korea: the program is closely tied to occupational health services and features smoking cessation, fatigue management, and stress reduction.
- Taiwan: the office has an on-site fitness center with full-time staff which offers massage, hair salon, facials, relaxation lounge, and evening educational sessions.
- Singapore: the site offers employee sports days, family days, bowling, sports leagues, and lunch-and-learn sessions on basic health, fatigue management, travel health, and shift-work health.
- Israel: various on-site fitness centers exist. Other programs offer employee fitness events, healthy foods in cafeterias, recreation days, and stress management.
- Ireland: offerings include educational sessions, stress management weekends, and reimbursement for health and fitness activities.
- England: health and fitness club memberships are subsidized, cafeterias serve healthy foods, smoking cessation and exercise classes are offered on-site.
- Rest of Europe: various sites focus on family recreation activities, provide subsidized health club memberships, and offer stress management activities.

Challenges for the future include reaching remote employee groups and securing participation in fast-paced work environments, which allow little time for personal activities. Other critical issues Applied

Materials face abroad are finding qualified staff, complying with local and employee welfare legislation, and making programs culturally appropriate. A continuing need exists to convince the management of the value of health promotion for the employees and company.

Case Study #4: Caterpillar Inc.

Caterpillar began operations in 1925 with three facilities in the United States and has grown to more than 200 facilities and 66,000 employees worldwide, of which 28,500 are outside the U.S. Headquartered in Peoria, Illinois, Caterpillar Inc. is the world's largest manufacturer of construction and mining equipment, diesel and natural gas engines, and industrial gas turbines. Caterpillar is one of only a handful of U.S. companies that leads its industry while competing globally from a primarily domestic manufacturing base. A U.S.-based global competitor, more than half of Caterpillar's sales are to overseas customers. Caterpillar is committed to servicing a product throughout its life, monitoring its health and scheduling maintenance and repairs, and minimizing their customers' cost of doing their work. This same philosophy is extended to the way its employees are treated: the company invests in the health and well-being of employees throughout their worklife. (informal interview with Beverlee Gilmore on 2/28/00)

Caterpillar has encouraged facilities throughout the world to implement health promotion programs that fit the culture of their population. Until 1997, programming had no central focus but met the needs of each geographic location. In 1997, the Corporate Medical Department developed a core program to provide consistency, direction, and measurements to evaluate the effectiveness of interventions offered. The program was designed to improve the health of employees, reduce health care costs, and urge employees and their families to assume responsibility for their health. As a self-insured employer, health care has had a direct impact on the profitability of the company. Caterpillar spent over a million dollars a day in 1999 to pay for medical benefits for U.S.-based employees, retirees, and dependents. The U.S.-based programming is geared toward reducing health care costs. Outside of the U.S., it focuses on risk reduction, productivity, and quality of life. The core program uses health assessments to identify health risks then monitors and educates accordingly to fit the needs of the individual, workgroup, and families. Ninety-five percent of the U.S.-based employees and 76% of spouses participate in the Healthy Balance program. Health assessments are completed around the world. "Healthy Balance News," a health newsletter developed internally, is distributed to most English-speaking employees around the world. It is also translated into French and Portuguese where appropriate. The Healthy Balance program gets its direction from the corporate medical director located at corporate headquarters and is supported by a small staff, including a health promotion manager. All facilities are encouraged to enhance the core program with exercise programs, weight loss campaigns, smoking cessation techniques and other health initiatives provided in the community. Most of the larger facilities have medical departments staffed with physicians and registered nurses who provide screening exams and other occupational health initiatives. Other sites have coordinators whose job responsibilities are outside of health promotion but who volunteer to administer health promotion programs.

Some examples by location outside the U.S. are: Caterpillar Overseas S.A. in Geneva, Switzerland, offers an improved Quality of Life program through an on-site fitness center, support of sports activities, physical examinations, gym classes, healthy food in their employee restaurant, stress management programs, and exposure to health professionals to increase awareness of health risks and help employees balance work and private life responsibilities. This site works with other multinational institutions to develop active prevention programs and insurance coalitions.

Caterpillar Brasil S.A. in Piracicaba, Brazil, has a very comprehensive Quality of Life program, directed by a Caterpillar physician, that includes a medical clinic for employees and their families where health needs and lifestyle behaviors are addressed. Physicians may prescribe any number of behavioral classes at their Quality of Life Center, exercise regimes, etc. In addition, the Employee Center offers recreational facilities for the entire family. Their focus on quality and employee initiatives resulted in their receipt of the Brazilian National Quality Award in 1999.

Caterpillar's live satellite broadcasts often feature health initiatives at facilities from around the world. Recently, a group of employees from Skinningrove, England, were shown walking along the coast at lunch time and challenging other global facilities to do the same. Testimonials from employees are also featured; for example, an employee in Russia was encouraged and supported by his coworkers to quit smoking, and he succeeded. One Japanese employee and his wife have begun to walk five miles a day around the Imperial Palace in Tokyo, Japan, after being encouraged by Healthy Balance News. The facility in Australia offers blood pressure and other screenings along with health newsletters to support healthy lifestyle changes.

Caterpillar anticipates that, with the ability to measure the impact on productivity, the Healthy Balance program will be expanded throughout Europe and many other parts of the world. Where medical care is dictated by governmental agencies, there is no motivation to measure the incidence of disease. However, absenteeism and productivity issues are prevalent worldwide. Caterpillar's health promotion programs will also be expanded to retirees in the U.S. and Europe as appropriate. Some disease management modules, which show lots of promise in the area of diabetes and heart diseases as secondary prevention, are being piloted.

Case Study #5: Siemens

Siemens is a global electrical engineering and electronics company based in Germany with 436,000 employees in 190 countries. This multinational corporation has adopted a holistic approach to health management. It has been calculated that Siemens spends roughly 100 million Deutsch marks (DM), which amounts to approximately US $ 50 million, on employee health care every year. This includes 80 occupational physicians and their first-aid stations, occupational medical check-ups, spa facilities used by 2,100 employees every year, sports amenities, rehabilitation measures after serious illnesses, social

consultants, and other health-promotion activities (Goth, 1999). In order to stay competitive in the global marketplace, especially in the high-technology industry, Siemens has made it a priority to address the demands of the modern-day employee by creating a favorable working environment, motivation incentives, and a corporate culture with which everyone identifies. The human resources policy is an integral element of Siemens' business strategy. The policy is based on the following factors: leadership and cooperation, staff development, recruitment, pay systems, and workplace health management. Under health management, the company strives to create general conditions in which the employees enjoy working by advocating proactive health promotion. In 1996, the project "Top in Form" was initiated. This project started with a detailed analysis of absenteeism causes and obstacles to better performance. Crucial factors affecting health and performance were leadership style, work stress and personal behavior, poor working climate, information and communication, working conditions, job security, individual constitution, private life, corporate culture, self-motivation, and "unjust" pay. This analysis had far-reaching consequences for the managerial staff. Managers are now assessed on their efforts to promote cooperation within their team as well as the extent to which they support the personal development of their staff. The managers are also accountable for what they do to maintain their own personal physical and mental capacity. The system is aimed at establishing a culture of dialogue and trust. This culture is enhanced through interviews regarding development, promotion, and recognition of staff; "manager discussions" during which employees get the chance to evaluate their direct superior; and staff surveys, in which employees can provide comments anonymously on a variety of issues (e.g., how the customer benefits from their work).

Through the "Top in Form" program, Siemens was able to produce financial savings by reducing absenteeism rates from 4.4% to 3.3% in two years. However, Siemens' philosophy with regard to workplace health promotion may be best described by Günther Goth's (co-director of human resource management at Siemens) statement that "it is totally non-sensible to compare the income and expense of a health management system in purely economic terms" (Goth, 1999). Dr. Goth views the measurement of motivation, commitment, and performance in units of currency as impossible and underlines that investments in employees always pay dividends.

Case Study #6: American International Group (AIG)

American International Group, Inc. (AIG) is a multinational company that primarily focuses on keeping the workforce of its U.S.-based multinational clients (rather than its own workforce) healthy through the Global Wellness Initiative. AIG is a U.S.-based international insurance organization and the largest underwriter of commercial and industrial coverage in the United States. AIG is headquartered in New York and employs 40,000 people through a network of worldwide offices. AIG's Group Management Division has operations in 85 countries and provides group life, medical, and disability products to more than 22,000 firms and 3.5 million lives.

AIG's Group Management Division developed the Global Wellness Initiative in 1996 in response to the overwhelming support for health promotion programs indicated in the Louis-Harris survey of 400 U.S.-based and 20 Europe-based multinational companies. More than 90% of respondents believe that employee wellness programs would become a key component of international benefit packages within the next five years. However, the primary concern of benefit managers was how to implement this type of program in a variety of countries (Schmitz, 2000). The Global Wellness Initiative works with the clients interested in wellness activities to identify specific goals, which vary from country to country. These goals can be tied to corporate priorities, health or business needs recognized by local management, statistics on the country's morbidity and mortality, medical claims data, or in-country health initiatives. An in-country needs assessment is completed to determine such items as the site's existing communication resources; past experiences with site-wide programs; and particular cultural concerns and supportive program activities and policies at the site that affect implementation decisions. This could include information on the per-

centage of office versus field workers; current demographics; involvement of the unions; availability of eligibility list; reliability of addresses; preferred delivery sites; on-site health care providers; company smoking policy; fitness and nutrition resources available at the facility (Schmitz, 2000). The programmatic features offered include adapted and translated brochures on topics such as walking, stress, smoking cessation, and weight management, as well as customized newsletters, both licensed from the HOPE Heart Institute.

The first health assessment for employees of the Otis Elevator Company in Spain, which is one the AIG Global Wellness Initiative's clients, reached participation rates of more than 30%. Other wellness activities, such as brochures and health fairs, have been offered in Peru, Mexico, and Panama. Evaluation measures are based on the health assessments' examination of risk areas, readiness to change, physician visits, hospital stays, and absenteeism.

The Global Wellness Initiative is becoming more and more aware of the differences in motivation, environment, and values with regard to health promotion in the international market compared to the U.S. For example, employee retention and recruitment rather than decreasing health care costs may be the prime reason for implementing programs. In addition, organizational health often plays a bigger role in other countries (e.g., in Europe) than in the U.S., where individual health is the priority. Cultural norms have varying influences on the programs; for example, the high status of the physician in many countries or the significance of confidentiality play an essential role. Lack of access to modern technology (e.g., computers, internet) is also an important factor when designing a program.

The Flavor of Workplace Health Promotion Around the World

The following section introduces several innovative workplace health promotion initiatives from around the globe. Programs are featured from countries in different regions (Europe, North America, South America, East Asia, and Southern Africa). Some countries (e.g., Finland) can look back on a strong tradition of workplace health, while others (e.g., Taiwan) have shown more recent and progressive activity in the field. The objective of the section is to describe various approaches to health promotion by addressing different realities and cultures, but by no means does it provide a complete review of workplace health promotion in the world.

Brazil

Brazil is a large country of approximately 165 million inhabitants and stark contrasts. A small portion of the population has a good standard of living, whereas the vast majority is poor and has either no access or limited access to health care and education. Different sectors of the economy—chemistry, cosmetics, aviation, automobiles, services, communications, information technology, electronics, tourism, and commerce—employ the countries' active economic population (informal interview with Ricardo De Marchion 3/15/00). These companies range in size from 100 to 100,000 employees, with approximately equal gender representation and average ages of 30–50 years old.

The health promotion concept was introduced to Brazil in the early 1980s by occupational doctors. Preliminary programs, called Preventive Medicine and Life Quality programs, targeted risk factors and their relation to the health of employees. Their main objective was to decrease costs related to disease management. Over the last two decades, the concept has grown gradually with regard to awareness among the population and within the companies, overcoming large political, economic, and social obstacles. In the last five years a more steady growth has occurred, and companies have started to incorporate the vision of a more motivated employee with a better health and life quality in their goals. Over the last few years, motivations for initiating workplace programs have been increasing. Desired outcomes now include better relationships, social quality, work environment, natural environment, work enjoyment, and balance between professional and personal life. Globalization and instant communication have transformed the nature of competition and created the necessity for increased retention of employees, general satisfaction,

and employee identification with the organization. Today, programs have many forms, from small educational actions and health campaigns to more elaborate processes with long duration, larger budgets, and a focus on personal responsibility in health and lifestyles.

Depending on the interests and needs of the company, health promotion programs are sometimes implemented only at the main office and/or the administrative sector, rather than being offered in different locations to all the employees and dependents. Some companies develop programs without having the necessary facilities. Many use meeting rooms as places for workshops and conferences, open spaces for physical activities, and occupational health offices for the control of health risks. However, some companies have built specific centers for health promotion with well-equipped fitness centers, health nutrition centers, etc.

The Brazilian Association for Quality of Life (ABQV) was founded in the early 1990s as a small and informal group. It now has more than 500 members from a variety of industries and six branches in different states of the country. Several large U.S.-based companies are ABQV members, including Dupont, Ford, IBM, Xerox, Monsanto, 3M, BankBoston, Citibank, and General Motors. In 1997, ABQV developed the National Award for Life Quality, which recognizes companies that develop health promotion programs.

Professionals involved with health promotion in the corporate environment come from different fields, including medicine, fitness, physiology, nutrition, nursing, social services, business, communication, technology, and marketing. There is a great need for more skilled professionals, and courses in this area have only recently been incorporated in academic curricula. Frequently, professionals in charge of health promotion programs come from the human resources or the occupational health department.

Program planning has become more formal, resembling the process followed in U.S. companies. This usually includes needs analysis, health risk reports, targeted goal setting aligned with business objectives, tailored action plans, incentive programs, and evaluation. However, evaluation designs are still rudimentary and need more systematic data collection. Participation rates vary from program to program. Fitness center membership rates range from 10–30% while campaigns and workshops sometimes reach 70–80% participation rates. More and more programs offer the possibility for dependents to participate. The most commonly targeted risk factors are cardiovascular risk factors (physical inactivity, obesity, stress, hypertension, cholesterol, diabetes, smoking, etc.), and alcohol and drug use. However, social and environmental factors such as depression, socialization, work quality, ergonomics, nutrition, traffic, overtime, work on the weekends, time spent seated during the day, and adequate use of the medical system are also addressed.

In spite of the similarities to U.S. worksite programs, numerous differences exist, the most obvious being that the field in Brazil is much smaller and has a shorter history. The Brazilian concept of quality of life is broader than the U.S. health promotion concept; it incorporates more social factors. In addition, the occupational health area is more involved and the nursing profession less involved in Brazil. Finally, Brazil only offers a small quantity of training courses and motivational and educational products and strategies in the field compared to the U.S.

Considerable growth is expected in this field within the next few years. Increasing doubts about personal life quality, corporate need for competitive strategies, and increasing costs and less quality in the medical system will make the demand for products and services in the health promotion area increase substantially. A large number of corporations will include the employee life quality concept as part of their strategic actions. Decisions based on economics will replace decisions based purely on values. This process surely will have some cultural, economic, and political obstacles. The opportunities are there, but great challenges remain with regard to filling the equity gap by generating benefits for all through health promotion programs. The government, more private companies, and other big organizations need to be attracted to contribute to the strategy with various actions. The challenge will also be to create possibilities for medium-sized and small companies to participate in this process.

Canada

Canada has a long tradition of health promotion including hosting the release of their landmark declaration, the "Ottawa Charter," in 1986 (see the section on the World Health Organization and Appendix A for more details). Health promotion has also played a significant role at the worksite. The approach taken by Canadian companies is often different than in the United States. One of the underlying reasons is that the Canadian government pays for health insurance for all citizens while most U.S. companies pay health insurance for their employees. Emphasis has been placed on the work environment and organizational health rather than solely on individual risk factors. Ron Labonte of the Saskatchewan Population Health and Evaluation Research Unit describes this more recent approach in his criticism of traditional workplace promotion in 1997: " It has spent far too much time concentrating on making workers healthier rather than making healthier workplaces" (Health Canada, 1998a, p. 42). Often cited by Canadian health promotion professionals, Michael Peterson of the University of Delaware points out the need for organizational health: "For health promotion to improve in effectiveness, it is time for professionals to adopt a more balanced approach and direction to programming that includes individual responsibility and health behaviors, and addresses psychosocial and socio-ecological issues—namely the work people do and the cultural context in which it is done" (Health Canada, 1998a, p. 37).

Health Canada's Workplace Health System

Along these lines, Health Canada has taken a comprehensive approach to health promotion with the Workplace Health System. Workplace health determinants addressed by the Workplace Health System strategy are: individual factors (worker characteristics, personal resources), job factors (pace and value of work, level of worker participation in decision-making, management philosophy), organizational factors (terms of employment, work hours, commitments to health and safety), and external factors (globalization, economic competition, changing structure of business). Links between these factors and injury rates, lost time, productivity, and profits are clear, but links between these factors and health outcomes can only be correlated and rarely can causality be inferred (Health Canada, 1998b). With the increased awareness of these determinants, a new approach was required. Therefore, Health Canada developed the Workplace Health System (WHS), which addresses three major avenues of influence on health: physical and psychosocial environment, personal resources, and health practices. The Workplace Health System is implemented as a seven-step process: commitment, workplace health committee, needs assessment, workplace health profile, health plan, program action plan, and review of progress. Separate models have been developed for different settings: corporate health model, small business health model, and the farm business health model. The WHS stresses an integrated approach due to the limitations of three important areas of health promotion: workplace health promotion, occupational health and safety, and organizational change interventions.

An example of a workhealth approach, which gives much attention to the organizational design and culture, is the "Workplace Sanctuary" model that has been applied in numerous worksites in Montreal. This model uses focus groups and work enjoyment surveys to analyze needs in a given workplace. The needs assessment looks at the learning opportunities within the workplace, relationships between people at work, and the ability to meet the needs of both internal and external customers. The interventions involve individual and team coaching, workshops, integration of values into committees and departments, and educational tools (e.g., experiential learning, values-centered leadership assessment). The overriding goal is to create more meaningful work and relationships at work.

Workplace Active Living

The Fitness and Active Living Unit of Health Canada has made major efforts promoting active living at the workplace. In Health Canada's 1998 Workplace Active Living Survey (Adams, 1999), organizations that encourage and support active living programs at the workplace were classified. The analysis led to the identification of seven habits of highly successful programs: leadership commitment, employee involvement, clear purpose, integrated effort, support structure, cultural context, and measured outcomes. These factors are reflective of the above-mentioned Workplace Health System approach. The Fitness and Active Living Unit is currently developing the "Business Case for Active Living at Work." This initiative will highlight and summarize the available research in this area, provide information about what works and how a company can get started, provide a template for practitioners to use when developing the business case approach, and other practical, ready-to-use information. This product will be web-based and presented in modules so that end-users can pick and choose what information they need to combine with their own data to build their case. The product will be kept current and relevant to changing needs and information in this area.

Healthy Workplace Award Program

Another significant milestone in the Canadian evolution of workplace health promotion is the Healthy Workplace Award Program. Conceived by Health Canada and managed by the National Quality Institute, the Healthy Workplace Award Program is new and is designed to recognize employers that provide exemplary workplace health promotion programs to their employees. In addition to the recognition, a trophy and related recognition through media coverage, etc., the award's process provides interested organizations with tools and information about how to develop or improve health policies and promotions at work, including physical activity as an important health practice. The award is based on the Healthy Workplace Criteria, which outline a set of comprehensive building blocks for organizations to follow on developing a healthy work environment, both physically and socially. This framework is intended for human resource managers, health promotion professionals, and other individuals interested in changing business practices to allow greater organizational effectiveness. The building blocks cover leadership, planning, people-focus, process management, and outcomes. The first Healthy Workplace Award Program awards were given out last October.

Further proof of the growing interest in health promotion at the workplace is the recent founding of the Health, Work and Wellness Institute, which provides a national network in the field and hosts an annual conference. The Institute has been focusing on networking, developing alliances, advocacy, and promotion, acting as a central resource, and research. The Health, Work and Wellness Institute has forged alliances with the National Quality Institute and Health Canada for significant initiatives such as the Healthy Workplace Criteria, the National Workplace Health Consortium, and the Workplace Health System Training Centers.

European Union

Outside of North America, Europe probably has the most developed and established workplace health promotion programs in the world. Strong traditions of sports and occupational health services in Scandinavia and Germany have spurred various activities to create and maintain healthy workers. As European countries are growing together through the European Union (EU), a common approach to workplace health promotion has been formulated within a European network, which is discussed below. In general, the European Union model has a stronger focus on the quality of working life and the work environment than on individual risk factors. Health actions at the workplace have not only focused on health screenings and healthy behaviors, but also on organizational interventions (e.g., shift schedule, job design, flexibility), social welfare activities (e.g., counseling support, community and social programs), and safety and physical environment activities (e.g., noise reduction) (Pot & Gründemann, 1999). Another characteristic is the involvement of different cross-sections within a company: management, staff representatives, trade union representatives, health and safety representatives, occupational health staff. The reasons for implementing health promotion programs are varied and not as focused on cost savings as in the United States European companies have reacted to external pressures such as legislation, industrial rela-

tions, company public image, internal demands (such as personnel/welfare problems), and health problems in the workplace. Programs in some of the European countries, which have been at the forefront of the advancement of worksite health promotion, are discussed below.

Netherlands

The Netherlands has put a lot of emphasis on workplace health and specifically work stress. In line with the strong tradition of social policy, the government has sought agreements with employer organizations and unions in the different industries to address health problems at the workplace and has supported a variety of activities including research, information, pilot projects, and evaluation. The Working Conditions Act in 1990 promoted risk management at the source and called for initiatives through the Ministry of Social Affairs and Employment and the Ministry of Public Health, Welfare and Sports. As a result, several studies were performed in different settings: a hospital, a construction company, a metal products company, and in regional institutes for mental welfare. The four successful projects aimed at improving the health, safety, and welfare of workers, thus reducing absenteeism and work incapacity. These studies provided a breakthrough as they showed that workplace health promotion (WHP) can generate benefits in a variety of settings and produce positive financial outcomes. For example, the program estimated that for each Dutch guilder invested in the construction company intervention, 1.5 guilders were returned over a period of two years due to decreased levels of absenteeism (Pot & Gründemann, 1999). The hospital project showed similar results. Neither calculation took into account the benefits of increased productivity or improved working atmosphere.

Since its inception in 1995, the Dutch Center for Workplace Health Promotion has been an active force in the Netherlands and Europe to get health promotion recognized as a priority in social security laws, occupational health services, and health insurance packages. The Center perceives the need to market the concept to employers and employees more effectively by emphasizing the benefits and profits. As a result of these efforts, an increase from 9 to 13% in the number of companies offering WHP programs occurred between 1996 and early 1998 (Baart, 1998). In addition, 20% of companies indicated the intention to introduce WHP in the near future.

Finland

Finland is another European country at the forefront of new approaches to workplace health promotion. Finland has a strong tradition of occupational health services. These services have shifted from a traditional focus on safety to more comprehensive workplace health services, including the "maintenance of work ability program" (Pot & Gründemann, 1999). This program has the goal of helping aging employees to continue working as long as possible. The maintenance of work ability program has been implemented in response to the rising average age of the working population and the high figures of early retirement and disability. Under this program, numerous studies were conducted between 1990 and 1996 and showed positive results with regard to work ability and satisfaction. In order to take on the extended role of workplace health promotion, the occupational health services must train their professionals with the skills needed for a broader approach and cooperate with health promotion agencies. This has not been the case on a broad scale in Finland. In addition, the privatization of the occupational health services has not yet contributed to a broader perspective.

Sweden

Sweden has a long tradition of improving working conditions for employees. The Occupational Health Services, to which 70% of Swedish organizations belong, and the unions have played a significant role in workplace health promotion. Legislation is plentiful regarding the work environment; the responsibility for the employees' health is placed primarily on the employers. Recent legislation includes "internal control," which requires the employer to audit once a year and improve the work environment; a rehabilitation law that requires the employer to offer a rehabilitation plan and pay for rehabilitation; and a regula-

tion that the employer has to pay for the first two weeks of sick leave. Sweden has an extensive social insurance system; but, as in many European countries, costs are increasing rapidly and major cutbacks have been undertaken. This has resulted in an increase in the provision of private health insurance, and this in turn has evoked an interest in keeping healthy. In Sweden, all parties in the workplace are involved in decisions with regard to the work environment. Workplace health promotion programs address the psychosocial environment and the impact of management and organization on the health of employees, with a focus on stress reduction, which addresses both the organizational and the individual perspective.

Some of the companies that extensively integrated workplace health promotion and which are recognized as models of good practice are: ASTRA (pharmaceutical company), Länsförsäkringar Wasa (insurance company), and the Malmö Fire Brigade. They have all created a healthy work place, physically, psychologically, and socially, with different solutions. The workplace health promotion program at ASTRA includes developing and implementing policies (e.g., alcohol and drug policy, maternity policy); personnel care projects for groups at risk (holistic analysis of work situation, including hours, health profiles, attitude surveys, ergonomics); and a selection of health promotion activities including exercise facilities, culture room, education, massage, etc.

The workplace health promotion strategy at Länsförsäkringar Wasa is also based on a holistic view of health. Health and work profiles are compiled as a base for the program design. The management is committed to undertake necessary changes that are revealed in the profiles. All program components feature a yearly follow-up and evaluation. At the Malmö Fire Brigade, the Fire Chief is leading the development of a healthy organization, which was initiated by an alcohol and drug program nine years ago. The program has now expanded to include a work environment policy, rehabilitation policy, and a leadership policy with the slogan "We care." Suggestions for improvement of the work environment are often implemented; and, if not approved, employees always hear the reason. An open and straightforward dialogue between all parties is a trademark of the organization.

An increasing number of managers are recognizing the need for health promotion at the workplace in order for their business to succeed in the future. A Swedish survey undertaken in 1998 showed that Swedish middle-sized information technology companies invest in the health of their personnel. The emphasis is on leadership and organizational development and on extensive health promotion activities programs (e.g., 90% offer exercise activities) (Frisemo, 1998).

Germany

The German approach to health promotion differs from the U.S. approach. Lifestyle issues of health are part of a structural approach, which primarily aims at influencing health-related living and working conditions. Forms of work organization (e.g., issues of control) and working conditions are regarded as a high priority, and specific behavior-related interventions are only implemented within this context.

In order to understand health promotion at the workplace in Germany and its economics, one must take a look at the German social security system and the legal framework. Germany is a wealthy country with a heavily structured social security. The system represents a middle-of-the-road approach between a state welfare system, as in Britain, and a primarily market economy welfare system, like the U.S. German health care is based on a federally mandated insurance system in which each employee contributes a certain percentage of his or her wages to a nonprofit insurance company. Almost two thirds of all social benefits are covered by insurance systems, which are financed by premiums with the exception of accident insurance (which is half paid each by employees and employers). The employers' premiums are part of the wage costs and are included in their pricing. All other social benefits are financed by taxes, such as welfare, child, and housing benefits. The costs for health care and health insurance have grown steadily over the years. Reasons for this development are the increasing percentage of elderly people in the population, the growing number of chronic diseases, and medical and technical progress. Meanwhile, incomes have not grown as fast as costs, and a relatively high unemployment rate has also contributed to a financial crisis in the insurance system.

Workplace health promotion holds a special position in Germany. As a result of the change in the national occupational health and safety regulations necessitated by the European framework legislation, health promotion was included in the catalogue of tasks of the statutory accident insurance sector, which was previously responsible for regulating industrial accidents and occupational diseases. Economic incentives to introduce workplace health promotion programs in Germany are based on the costs for sick leave, which are absorbed by employers during the first six weeks of sickness absence. According to the Federal Institute for Occupational Safety and Health (Breucker, 1999), the costs due to absenteeism in 1994 were approximately DM 91 billion (about $45 billion) in Germany. The 1997 morbidity statistics surveyed annually by the company health insurance funds show that disease-related causes for absenteeism fell into six categories (Breucker, 1999):

1. musculo-skeletal injuries (29.2%)
2. respiratory tract illnesses (16.8%)
3. injuries and intoxication (14.1%)
4. disorders of the digestive system (7.7%)
5. cardiac and circulatory illnesses (7.3%)
6. mental disorders (5.3%)

After the recent changes, general health promotion services outside the workplace were largely privatized. However, this mainly applies to primary prevention. Secondary and tertiary preventive services can still be financed by the statutory health insurance funds. Direct economic incentives for prevention services are therefore very limited in Germany. The fee regulations within the medical care system with which incentives for health promotion services on the provider side could be created are, like everywhere else, aimed at medical and technical services.

Nevertheless, many private and public enterprises have invested in health promotion activities through encouragement and support by the statutory health insurance funds. In this context, a specific health promotion concept, known as the health circle approach, has gained widespread acceptance. The health circle approach should be viewed as a methodology similar to the quality circle concept and is part of corporate health and human resource management. The health circle approach consists of a series of group meetings during paid working time which focus on short- and medium-term improvements of working conditions and aspects of job design. The health circle members represent all involved stakeholders of a target area within an organization: human resource department, company physician, safety officer, employee representatives, etc.

An important precondition to help ensure the effective running of a health circle is the establishment of an overall steering group with representation from key members (including management, health and safety officers, personnel department, union representatives, and works council members). Furthermore, a health circle needs to be based on a sound needs analysis, including an analysis of absenteeism data, staff turnover, productivity, and health-relevant risks. The results of a health circle are presented to the steering committee which decides about the implementation of specific suggestions while monitoring the whole process.

Health circles have been implemented in many enterprises in different branches and business sectors. The general results indicate:

- a high acceptance by employees as well as employers
- a reduction in health complaints
- an improved working climate and satisfaction at work

The health circle concept has been further developed into several specific applications, one of which addresses communication and management style issues in particular. The enormous success of this approach is due to the fact that health circles are able to address the social factors of health within enterprises. They contribute to an improved mutual understanding of each others' perspective and facilitate the identification of practical solutions to highly ranked problems, which in most cases are related to the so-called soft factors such as cooperation, communication, settling of conflicts, and management style. In this way, employees are empowered, and their capacity to influence their own working environment is strengthened.

In those cases in which enterprises utilize the health circle concept more and more in a systematic way (i.e. on a regular basis and addressing all levels and areas of an organization), the contribution to building social capital, which is understood as the capacity of an organization to manage the needs and goals of all members in a coherent and sustainable way, is also supported (Breucker, 1999).

Japan

Health promotion at the workplace in Japan started in 1972 when the Industrial Safety and Health Law was passed. The law mandated that employers provide periodic physical checkups for all employees. The primary purpose of the checkups was to identify and screen employees with diseases. Primary prevention started in 1979 with the "Silver Health Plan," which addressed the promotion and maintenance of physical fitness programs among middle-aged and older employees in order to prevent chronic diseases and work-related injuries. An amendment to the law in 1988 resulted in the formation of the Total Health Promotion Plan. This more comprehensive health policy facilitated health promotion activities at the workplaces for employees of all ages. Target areas were expanded to other lifestyle issues such as nutrition, mental health, smoking, alcohol consumption, and sleeping patterns. To facilitate the implementation of this plan, the government provided incentives for employers by subsidizing associated costs, including for the training of qualified professionals. However, a number of companies ceased their programs when subsidies expired. This points towards a lack of recognition of the benefits of workplace health promotion and a need for more sound cost/benefit research and improved communication of the benefits to the employers. In addition, extended education and training of health promotion professionals is necessary for more effective implementation of worksite programs (Chikamoto, 1998).

Most Japanese companies face increasing health care costs, aging of employees, an increasingly demanding business environment, an increase in "lifestyle" diseases, and an increase in premature death from cancer among their employees. Osaka Gas Company has taken a progressive and noteworthy approach in tackling these health and business issues. A company of 10,000 employees in 65 cities and 39 towns, Osaka Gas has a history of health promotion programs dating back to the early 1970s. Early programs included the establishment of health fitness centers and counseling activities based on results of annual checkups. The comprehensive program now involves centralized management of employee health information, a physician referral system, qualified staffing at each individual office (including a public health nurse and fitness specialist), a mandatory annual medical checkup with follow-up system, and personalized health counseling. Stress management is an especially important component in the counseling sessions. In addition, employees taking sick leave or who are at high risk for disease are visited at home or in their office to obtain advice on health promotion and care utilization. Evaluation measures cover premature death, health care expenditures, absenteeism, and productivity. The most prominent factor of the Osaka Gas Company program is the personalized attention each employee, and to a lesser degree the employee's family members, receives with regard to their health status (personal interview with Toshio Yamazaki on 2/14/00).

Singapore

Major investments have been made in workplace health promotion in Singapore over the last decade with the government being a leading initiator. In many ways Singapore can be regarded as a model for the Southeast Asian region. In 1987, the Workplace Health Education Unit was set up by the Ministry of Health in response to the increased need for more comprehensive workplace programs. The Workplace Health Education Unit has provided assistance in the form of training, consultation, and resources to many organizations, both private and governmental. Several national campaigns were launched in the 1990s.

The National Lifestyle Campaign advanced the goal of "developing new ideas and programs which will excite and gather greater participation in healthy sports and lifestyles among all sectors of the public: schools, workplace, and the community at large" (Cashmore, 1999, p. 5).

A number of large corporations in Singapore have become major stakeholders in workplace health promotion. Hewlett Packard (HP) Singapore has been one of the frontrunners in creating healthy workers and workplaces. The wellness program is coordinated by a work life management team comprised of senior human resource managers. HP regards wellness as an extension of health by adding a positive dimension beyond the mere absence of disease. While emphasizing self-responsibility, HP offers an integrated and comprehensive program focusing on quality of life. An on-site 3 million Singapore dollar (S$) sport and recreation clubhouse was built in 1989 for the employees and their families. The staff pays affordable membership fees at S$5 per employee or S$9 for each family member per month. The wellness programs include sports programs, individual fitness assessments, healthy food service, and social programs. For example, to encourage employees to take short holidays to relax and recuperate, HP gives each a S$90 subsidy every year for trips. Also, other cruises and tours are organized at discounted rates. HP is considering introducing a medical copayment to encourage staff to take responsibility for their own health. In addition, in-house nurses organize health talks and thematic health fairs in different sites. The human resource management has also looked into flexible work options and the reduction of work stress. One of the key factors of the HP wellness program is the emphasis on marketing. Each department has a volunteer Wellness Facilitator who promotes and publicizes wellness activities and disseminates health information among his or her colleagues. In addition, HP has created a wellness website to provide relevant health information and a channel for feedback and communication between management and employees. Intranet technology (not accessible to the general public) enables the employees to order and customize their daily menus on-line.

The HP program is evaluated through regular informal feedback and process evaluation monitoring participation. Clubhouse membership has increased from 1,067 in 1989 to 2,512 in 1998. In addition, health costs and absenteeism are monitored. The average annual sick leave per staff member has been maintained at five days per employee since the implementation of the program. Also, HP's turnover is among the lowest in the industry. The resignation rate of 0.8% is below the 1997 national average monthly staff resignation rate of 2.7% (Cashmore, 1999, p. 4). The Work Life Management Team is convinced that the wellness program works because of the following factors: top management support and linking with company mission, comprehensive and integrated programming, regular evaluation with target performance indicators, and sustainability.

Another frontrunner in Singapore is Motorola, which is often regarded as the most innovative company with regard to health promotion. Workers at most plants are being financially compensated in benefits (up to S$200) for regular participation in fitness and healthy lifestyle programs. Senior wellness officer Ms. Yap Lai Ping summed up Motorola's health and human resource philosophy in the following words: "At first we wanted to raise awareness and teach skills, so we rewarded people for taking part in activities, but the program has been so successful we are ready to put some of the responsibility back to the individual. Good companies go beyond just paying their people, they work with employees to achieve balance in their lives" (Cashmore, 1999, p. 5).

The Ministry of Health's Workplace Health Education Unit has recently been focusing on the training of health promotion facilitators. In 1998, about 330 facilitators were trained to plan, implement, and evaluate their health promotion programs. Facilitators were mostly from workplaces and included human resource managers, occupational health and safety professionals, union leaders, company physicians, nurses, and Healthy Lifestyle Program committee members (Ministry of Health, of Singapore, 1998). The goal is to have trained facilitators in 25% of private workplaces by 2003. With the gathering and publication of best practices, the Ministry of Health has adopted a model for workplace health promotion and

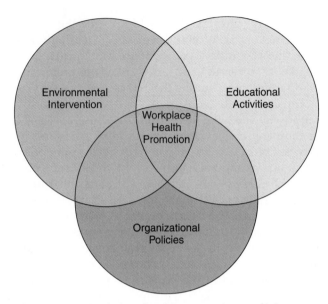

Figure 20-2 Workplace health promotion model.
Source: R. S. Parkinson. Managing health promotion in the workplace: Guidelines for implementation and evaluation (1999).

a "Health-at-Work" framework. The model combines environmental intervention, educational activities, and organizational policies (see Figure 20-2).

The framework comprises eight practical steps:

1. Obtain management support
2. Set up a working committee
3. Conduct a needs assessment
4. Define goals and objectives
5. Plan activities
6. Plan to evaluate
7. Implement program
8. Evaluate program

Taiwan

The country of Taiwan has only recently adopted the concept of health promotion at the worksite but is destined to catch up quickly with some of the more developed countries, parallel to the rapid development of their economy. The first formal workplace health promotion program in Taiwan was initiated in 1990 by Taiwan Power Company, Taiwan's largest national enterprise, in collaboration with the Departments of Physical Education and Health Education of

National Taiwan Normal University. The director and senior assistant of the occupational health department of Taiwan Power Company were very supportive of the ground-breaking project and convinced their highest authority, the CEO, of the benefits to be gained from an effective health promotion program. The support from the top ensured financial backing and available time for the employees to use work time to participate in the intervention (Jwo, 1999).

An initial experimental study of 250 employees at Taiwan Power Company headquarters included a 20-hour fitness workshop and 12-week long intervention activities. This was the first scientific study on workplace health promotion, including process and outcome evaluation, to have been conducted in Taiwan. The results showed improvements in cardiorespiratory endurance, muscular strength, flexibility, and self-image. Taiwan Power Company has continued the activity programs and expanded the workshops to other sites on the island. Based on the results at Taiwan Power Company, it was concluded that workplace health promotion programs can be successful within the Taiwanese culture and help employees improve their fitness and lead a more active lifestyle. The Taiwan Power Company physical activity intervention has served as a model for other companies. More companies are becoming aware of the importance of health promotion, especially because of the rise in "lifestyle" diseases in Taiwan.

South Africa

Workplace health promotion activities are still rare on the African continent. However, with the growing economic development, an increasing number of companies are being forced to deal with the same health and productivity issues as companies in more industrialized countries. South Africa is one of the fastest developing countries in Africa and has a number of functioning workplace health initiatives. One of these expanding initiatives is on the verge of having international application.

Since 1997 the South African Association for Biokinetics has been managing the "SANGALA" program for middle and senior management of South African companies. SANGALA stands for South African National Games and Leisure Activities. The program was originally started by former Minister of Sport, Mr. Steve Tshwete, and is aimed at the dissemination of knowledge on the value of physical activity, recreation, and sport for enhancing health, wellness, and quality of life. The "Corporate SANGALA" program is led by Prof. Gert Strydom of Potchefstroom University and is endorsed by the South African Heart Foundation. The aim is to supply all members of top and middle management of participating companies with the means to change their lifestyles for the better. It is envisioned that individual lifestyle changes will eventually lead to a better and more healthy company profile. The program contains the following elements:

- invitation to companies to participate in the Corporate SANGALA
- assessment questionnaire of individual lifestyle and physical activity profile to all middle and top-level managers of a company
- collection of data and analysis
- preparation of individualized feedback brochures and company profile
- feedback to a company on an individual and company basis
- handout of information and brochures.

International Organizations in Health Promotion

In most countries the concept of health promotion is relatively new. To date, few of the major international health-related organizations have addressed this issue as a key priority. As a result, international cooperation in this area is sparse. However, there are some promising signs within some organizations. The following section highlights some of these international initiatives.

World Health Organization (WHO)

Founded in 1948, the objective of the World Health Organization (WHO) is the attainment by all peoples of the highest possible level of health. Health, as defined in the WHO constitution (WHO website, 2000), is "a state of complete physical, mental, and social well-being and not merely the absence of disease or infirmity." Therefore, WHO has four main functions:

1. To give worldwide guidance in the field of health
2. To set global standards for health
3. To cooperate with governments in strengthening national health programs
4. To develop and transfer appropriate health technology, information, and standards

The WHO has not yet designated the workplace as a key setting to advance health promotion. A variety of setting approaches such as Healthy Cities, Health Promoting Schools, and Health Promoting Hospitals have been implemented incorporating health promotion strategies into health policies, programs, and projects in order to add value to the attainment of positive health outcomes. This is a result of the Sundsvall Statement in 1991, which focused on settings instead of individuals as a key issue to bring about change (WHO, 1991). However, the implementation of health promotion in work settings has not resulted in a similar comprehensive and unified approach.

In response to this shortcoming, the Healthy Work Approach was created in 1997 as a realization of the Global Strategy on Occupational Health for All (WHO, 1997). Based on the four fundamental principles of health promotion, occupational health and safety, human resource management, and sustainable development, the Healthy Work Approach is defined as: "A continuous process for the enhancement of the quality of working life, health and well being of all working populations through environmental (physical, psychosocial, organizational, economic) improvement, personal empowerment and personal growth" (WHO, 1997, p. 9). As stated in the strategy, it is assumed that the twenty-first century will bring a working population exceeding 2.7 billion people, of whom a great majority (around 80%) will be in developing countries. The goal of the Healthy Work Approach is to improve the quality of working life and to benefit the health and well-being of all sectors of the workforce, whether participating in working life in the formal or informal sector. However, due to the lack of strategies and the promotion of the health of the people working in the informal sector, this tar-

get group, specifically in developing countries, is of central concern.

As shown in Figure 20-3, eight guiding principles concern all phases of the application of the Healthy Work Approach from planning to implementation to evaluation.

Equity aims at the improvement of unfair and unjust living and working conditions. Practical tools toward attaining an equitable implementation require accountability and equal accessibility to resources. Leadership and commitment of all concerned parties are central for a Healthy Work project. The same can be said for an involvement based upon partnership and active participation of all people affected. These eight principles are directed towards intersectoral cooperation and the empowerment of individuals and communities to learn how to take responsibility and control over the determinants of their health and well-being.

Likewise, seven different action settings can be distinguished for the Healthy Work Approach. These are

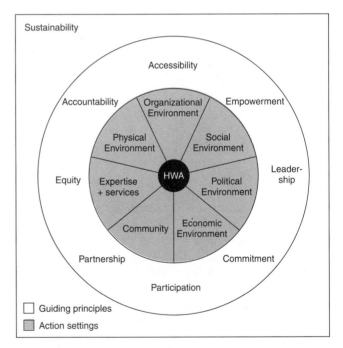

Figure 20-3 Guiding principles and action areas of the healthy work approach (HWA)

Source: World Health Organization (WHO), *WHO's Global Healthy Work Approach*, 1997.

physical environment, organizational environment, social environment, political environment, economic environment, community, and expertise and services. In most cases, one appropriate action area has to be chosen for the initiation of a project. However, other areas should be considered as soon as possible in the strategy development in order to establish a broad basis for support.

The Pan American Health Organization (PAHO) is a Regional Office of the WHO based in Washington, DC, working to improve health and living standards of the countries of the Americas, with a primary focus on Central and South America and the Caribbean Basin. PAHO's workplace health promotion activities are restricted to the improvement of the working environment and safety. The Program on Environmental Quality, within the division of Health and Environment, promotes the development and conservation of healthy environments. One of its actions is aimed at promoting comprehensive health care for workers with a preventive approach to guarantee workers a right to a healthy environment. Specifically, special attention is given to the preparation of public and social policies to protect workers' health, improvement of working conditions and environments, promotion of comprehensive health services provided to workers and their families, prevention of diseases and occupational accidents, and support of automated information systems to monitor and detect occupational risks.

The World Health Organization Europe is a Regional Office of WHO based in Copenhagen, Denmark. It consists of 51 Member States within an area stretching from Greenland to the North, the Mediterranean in the south, and the Pacific shores of the Russian Federation in the east. In 1998, in order to ensure a better quality of life for the citizens of these countries, WHO Europe introduced Health21: the "Health for All" policy framework for the WHO European Region. It was adopted (a) to promote and protect people's health throughout their lives and (b) to reduce the incidence of the main diseases (see Table 20-1) and injuries and alleviate the suffering they cause. Included is a call for stronger action to be taken to promote a healthier working environment through better legislation, standards, and enforcement mech-

anisms. The recommendation is for a "healthy company or enterprise" concept, which includes three elements: health promotion for staff, making company products as health-supportive as possible, and being socially responsible by supporting local community or countrywide health programs.

European Network for Workplace Health Promotion

The European Network for Workplace Health Promotion is an international organization that has been very active in the field over the past five years. Established in 1996 by the European Commission, the European Network includes organizations from all 15 member states (Austria, Belgium, Denmark, Finland, France, Germany, Great Britain, Greece, Ireland, Italy, Luxembourg, Netherlands, Portugal, Spain, and Sweden) and the countries of the European Economic Area (Iceland, Norway, and Switzerland). Before the European Network for Workplace Health Promotion was put in place, the European Foundation for the Improvement of Living and Working Conditions, based in Dublin, Ireland, played a major role in the development of workplace health promotion in Europe, including a large research program from 1989 to 1997. The objective of the European Network is to identify and disseminate examples of good practice of workplace health promotion by exchanging experience and knowledge. By so doing, the European Union encourages the Member States to place workplace health promotion high on their agenda and to incorporate workplace health issues in all respective policies.

This objective, outlined in the 1997 Luxembourg Declaration, created a political platform for the first time at the European level and laid down a common understanding of workplace health promotion. This common approach compares with the past when the promotion of health in the workplace differed among member states. In this context, the Network for Workplace Health Promotion is an important and sensible supplement to the activities of the European institutions responsible for statutory occupational safety and health. Therefore, in the few years of its activities, the Network has produced three important results: (a) the establishment of international cooperation structures, (b) the creation of a consulting concept for workplace health promotion, and (c) the collection of models of good practice in workplace health promotion (Conference of the European Network, 1999).

The Luxembourg Declaration (European Network for Workplace Health Promotion, 1997, p. 1) defines workplace health promotion as "the combined efforts of employers, employees, and society to improve health and well-being of people at work. This can be achieved through a combination of:

- improving the work organization and the working environment
- promoting active participation
- encouraging personal development."

While recognizing the value of traditional occupational health and safety legislation and practice, the Network regards workplace health promotion as a modern corporate strategy that aims at preventing ill health at work and enhancing health-promoting potentials and well-being in the workforce. Workplace health promotion contributes to the following work factors which improve health:

- management principles and methods that recognize employees are a necessary success factor for the organization instead of a mere cost factor
- a culture and corresponding leadership principles that include participation of the employees and encourage motivation and responsibility of all employees
- work organization principles that provide the employees with an appropriate balance between job demands, control over their own work, level of skills, and support
- a personnel policy that actively incorporates health promotion issues
- an integrated occupational health and safety service.

One of the recent projects undertaken by the Network is the development of success factors of workplace health promotion. Four principles need to be featured in any successful program: participation, integration, comprehensiveness, and effective management. A European Quality Frame for WHO has been developed that contains building blocks of corporate policy, health and human resources management, planning, social responsibility, implementation of comprehensive activities, and outcomes. The project paper "Success Factors of Workplace Health Promotion" (European Network for Workplace Health Promotion, 1998) explains this framework and points toward future priorities for joint work within the Network.

Although many good examples and success stories have been collected, the Network finds very few companies that are implementing health promotion programs due to a lack of resources, information, and know-how, as well as top management attitudes that view employees as a mere cost factor. Over the next two years, the Network will be focusing on workplace health promotion activities in small and medium-sized companies.

International Institute for Health Promotion (IIHP)

The International Institute for Health Promotion (IIHP) is another international organization active in workplace health promotion. The Institute was established as part of the National Center for Health Fitness of American University in 1994. This came about as a result of the Center's extensive health promotion efforts within the international community and as a response to requests from health promotion professionals throughout the world to assist them in their efforts to establish high quality and cost-effective health promotion programs. The IIHP has made it a priority to advocate the global advancement of health promotion. The overriding goal is to approach and convince governments, international organizations, academia, corporations, and decision makers worldwide to push forward health promotion policies and put more resources into promoting healthy lifestyles. The IIHP now consists of an interdisciplinary network of approximately 200 institutions involved in health promotion from 50 countries. More than 50 of them have signed cooperative agreements with American University. Successful initiatives include four strategic international meetings to build partnerships, discuss specific topics, and exchange information about the latest trends and best practices. As a result of the most recent meeting in Curitiba, Brazil (October 1999), the IIHP has published the "Curitiba Declaration," which calls for an increased focus on health promotion in the twenty-first century (see Appendix B). The IIHP has hosted or cohosted training seminars, scientific conferences, and international planning sessions, and its staff serves as the editors of the global newsletter "Health Promotion: Global Perspectives," which is published by the American Journal of Health Promotion, Inc.

One of the recently formed IIHP committees focuses on workplace health promotion. The committee is currently discussing such joint international research projects as combating hypertension at the workplace in the Americas and expanding a corporate fitness program originated in South Africa. The IIHP has also hosted numerous training seminars for human resource managers in several countries. The interest in sharing information on good practices and cost/benefit research has prompted the IIHP to expand this area with additional seminars, conferences, and collaborative projects. For example, the IIHP was one of the few organizations hosting a session on workplace health promotion at the 5th Global Conference on Health Promotion in Mexico City in June of 2000. The IIHP also hosted a seminar on April 10–11, 2000, for multinational corporations that are in the process of developing workplace health promotion programs for their global workforce.

DIFFERENCES BETWEEN PROGRAMS IN THE UNITED STATES

Judging by the amount of resources and research in this area, one could argue that the United States is the most advanced nation in the world when it comes to science and the profession of health promotion. Whether it is the National Institutes of Health, the Centers for Disease Control, or the many excellent university programs, information and expertise on specific health-related issues is abundant. Naturally, this does not mean that American health promotion professionals are right on target and cannot learn from their international colleagues. It is often said that one cannot learn from a program or approach of a different country because the distinct culture and

reality would not permit application in the home country. However, in spite of all the differences between countries, lessons are to be learned from other cultures and value systems. This is even more the case in today's world of globalization and the increasing exposure to other cultures. Not surprisingly, numerous multinational corporations are in the process of attempting to leverage resources and successful programs across borders.

One of the main factors accounting for international differences in programming is the regulatory environment and health care system. Decreasing health care claims, and thereby costs, is often cited in the U.S. as the main reason to implement health promotion programs. This comes as no surprise because employers have to bear most of the care-related costs. In many other countries (e.g., Canada, the United Kingdom, and Germany), health care is largely paid for by the government. The incentive is not as great to lower claims; therefore, other factors, such as decreasing absenteeism or increasing productivity, provide motivation to implement programs. Employers also list improved employee recruitment and retention as motivations, especially if they are competing in tight labor markets.

As mentioned above, numerous European countries have made it a priority to focus on improving work organization and the working environment. An optimal balance of productivity and health is the underlying goal. This approach targets organizational health and expands on the more traditional approach of behavior-related interventions geared toward the individual. This undoubtedly has its roots in the different mentality and societal norms of the U.S. and the countries of the European Union. Individuality is emphasized strongly in American society, whereas consensus and collective values find a greater resonance in western Europe. Therefore, a model like the "health circle" model, which emphasizes social factors and the involvement of all concerned parties at the workplace, is successful in Germany. The European tradition of social policies is reflected in the approach to workplace health promotion. The occupational health sector also still plays a major role in workplace health promotion in Europe due to its long tradition. Preventive measures, including safety and injury prevention, place high on the list of workplace health goals. However, this sector is expanding its services in many European countries as a result of a more proactive and health-oriented approach.

One can observe a gradual narrowing of differences between the U.S. and the western European approach to workplace health promotion. Three reasons stand out to explain this trend. The most obvious reason is the general dissolution of distinct cultural and ethnic differences between many countries due to the globalization trend and in spite of the many ethnic conflicts and splintering of nations worldwide. A second reason is the recognition among many U.S. health promotion professionals that programmatic and research efforts must focus more on social and organizational factors (as has been the case in western Europe and some other countries) than on physical risk factors. A third reason is the ongoing trend of privatization and dwindling state support in many European countries. No longer do programs have the luxury of receiving large amounts of public funds, rather they are now held accountable and asked to produce data that justify their existence. This more bottom-line-oriented approach in turn has been more prevalent in the U.S. Three recent studies on benchmarking best practices and success factors of workplace health promotion in different countries provided similar results. A U.S. study, conducted by Michael O'Donnell, Carol Bishop, and Karen Kaplan (1997), a study by the European Foundation for the Improvement of Living and Working Conditions (Wynne, 1998), and a Singaporean investigation by the Ministry of Health of Singapore (1999) found the following common success factors:

- management support
- program objectives linked to business objectives
- good communication policies and programs
- evaluation component
- supportive environment and presence of health policies
- involvement of nonhealth personnel (e.g., human resource management) in the process

Nevertheless, cultural differences remain clearly visible and leave their impact on health promotion programs (e.g., strong privacy concerns in Germany or the willingness to litigate in the U.S.). The statement issued in 1999 by Günther Goth, co-director of human resource management at Siemens, Germany, especially underlines the differences in the corporate perspective of workplace health promotion between the U.S. and western Europe: "It is totally nonsensible to compare the income and expense of a health management system in purely economic terms" (Goth, 1999). The key is to balance global economic and demographic trends with specific cultural nuances and to tailor programs to specific local conditions while basing them on a broader global framework.

CONCLUSION

The one resounding theme in statements by health promotion professionals from throughout the world is that the area of workplace health promotion will continue to grow and gain in significance. Trends affecting the workplace are evident: globalization, an aging population, increasing use of information technology, rising health care costs, changing employment patterns, increasing importance of the service sector, and increasing competition. These global trends are pushing companies more than ever to look for well-qualified, motivated, and healthy employees. Workplace health promotion can play a significant role in attracting employees, keeping them healthy, and assisting in facing the challenges posed by current trends.

The growing pressure to increase productivity and lower health care costs provides a unique opportunity for the field of workplace health promotion. According to the American Productivity and Quality Center, annual employee health and productivity losses to U.S. employers exceed $1 trillion, which is an all-time high (Landgreen, 1999). The ongoing challenge for the field is to demonstrate and document the benefits of health promotion programs and how they relate to increased productivity and cost savings in different settings and countries. Therefore, the need for objective data and evaluation measures will increase. In order to demonstrate the benefits, programs need to be tied to business objectives and accordingly justified to top level management. Mark Landgreen, Director of Health Management at the Coca-Cola Company, points toward the future by affirming the perspective of a progressive multinational corporation: "Understanding that good health is good business in all parts of the world produces a company with a competitive edge, led by a healthy, high-performing and productive workforce." (Landgreen, 1996b, p. 16) An increasing number of health professionals and human resource managers of global corporations follow this thinking and are making strides in developing global programs. The information technology boom has aided this development enormously as large numbers of employees worldwide can receive important health-related information very quickly and feel connected to headquarters.

The future also calls for the integration of health promotion with other health-related services. Work-life programs, fitness programs, occupational health services, medical services, disease management programs, etc., need to be incorporated into a multidisciplinary approach. This can be structured within a global strategy and leveraged as a best-practice as long as programs remain locally specific and tailored. The relationship between individual and organizational health will also be a hot topic for future investigation and will most likely leave an impact on program development. As mentioned above, working environment and organizational issues play a more prominent role in countries outside of the U.S. Building supportive environments and a healthy corporate culture is becoming a priority for companies worldwide. While companies in the U.S. may have to face the pressure of cost savings a while longer in the current health care system, organizations in other countries are looking to deepen their focus on the work environment and work organization, especially with the alarming increase of mental and stress-related health problems.

The future for workplace health promotion globally looks bright with the possible and logical linking of business and health strategies. The human being remains the most important factor within an organization and companies need to face a critical choice: whether to invest in their employees up-front to get and keep them healthy or to spend large amounts of capital to pay for the associated medical and lost-production costs. The overarching challenge for multinational corporations is to develop a global strategy with far-reaching policies and implement the most effective programs at the local setting. In order to be successful in this endeavor, it is necessary to increase international cooperation, maximize and improve existing local resources, and learn from success stories in different countries.

References

Adams, R. (September 1999). *Workplace Active Living Programs.* Paper presented at Health Economics seminar of CCN Consultores, Buenos Aires, Argentina.

Anderson, G. F. (1998). Multinational comparisons of health care: expenditures, coverage, and outcomes. The Commonwealth Fund. Available: *http://www.cmwf.org/programs/interntional/index.asp#cross.*

Applied Materials. (2000). *Wellness.* [On-line]. Available *http://www.appliedmaterials.com/careers/wellness.html.*

Associação Brasileira de Qualidade de Vida (ABQV). (2000). [on-line]. Available: *http://www.abqv.org.br.*

Baart, P. C. (1998). The implementation of WHP in the Netherlands. *WHP-Net-News 4* Newsletter. European Network for Workplace Health Promotion.

Brazilian Association of Quality of Life (ABQV). (2000). [On-line]. Available: *http://www.abqv.org.br.*

Breucker, G. (1999, May). *Experience of the European Network: Success factors and quality of workplace health promotion.* Paper presented at the conference of European Network for Workplace Health Promotion, Bonn, Germany.

Cashmore, M. (1999). Workplace health promotion in Singapore: Growth in times of economic crisis. *Global Perspectives of American Journal of Health Promotion,* 2 (1), 2.

Chikamoto, Y. (1998). Health policies affecting health promotion activities in the workplace in Japan. *Global Perspectives of American Journal of Health Promotion,* 1 (4), 4.

Department of Mass Exercise, Chinese Sports Committee. (1998). *Investigative report of Chinese workers' fitness in 1994.* Beijing: People's Sport Publishing House.

Dow Chemical Company (1995–2000). [on-line]. Available: *http://www.dow.com/about/aboutdow/vision.htm*. Accessed 3/11/2000.

European Network for Workplace Health Promotion. (1997). *Luxembourg Declaration on workplace health promotion*. Adopted in Luxembourg on November 27–28, 1997.

European Network for Workplace Health Promotion. (1998). Luxembourg Declaration. In G. Breucker et al. *Success factors of workplace health promotion* (pp. 9–13). Essen: Federal Association of Company Health Insurance Funds.

Frisemo, C. (1998). Workplace health promotion in Sweden: A tradition. *Global Perspectives of American Journal of Health Promotion, 2* (1), 2.

Ge Ke You. (1996). *The dietary and nutritional status of Chinese population. 1992 national nutrition survey.* Beijing: People's Medical Publishing House.

Goth, G. (1999, May). *A modern corporate health policy as an important factor in competition–Strategies and experiences on Siemens AG.* Paper presented at the conference of European Network for Workplace Health Promotion, Bonn, Germany.

Health Canada. (1998a). *Healthy settings: Canadian case studies.* Ottawa: Health Canada.

Health Canada. (1998b). *Workplace health system: Absenteeism.* Ottawa: Health Canada.

Health Canada. (1998c). *Workplace health system: Influencing employee health.* Ottawa: Health Canada.

Jwo, C. (1999). Health fitness promotion at Taiwan Power Company. *Global Perspectives of American Journal of Health Promotion, 2* (1), 2.

Karch, B. (1999). Workplace health promotion. *Global Perspectives of American Journal of Health Promotion, 2* (1), 1.

Landgreen, M. (1999a). Coca-Cola's global approach to associate employee management. *Global Perspectives of American Journal of Health Promotion, 2* (1), 6.

Landgreen, M. (1999b). Employee health management goes global. *AWHP's Worksite Health, 6* (4), 12–16.

Ministry of Health of Singapore. (1998). *State of health 1998.* Singapore: Ministry of Health.

Ministry of Health of Singapore. (1999). *Case studies on best practice in workplace health promotion.* Singapore: Cornfield Design Communication.

O'Donnell, M., Bishop, C., & Kaplan, C. (1997, March/April). Benchmarking best practices in workplace health promotion. *The Art of Health Promotion, 1*(1), 1–8.

Pan American Health Organization (PAHO). (2000). *About PAHO.* [On-line]. Available: *http://www.paho.org/english/aboutpaho.htm*.

Parkinson, R. S. (1982). Managing health promotion in the workplace: guidelines for implementation and evaluation. Reprinted from *Case studies on best practice in workplace health promotion*, p. 39, by Ministry of Health of Singapore, 1999, Singapore: Cornfield Design Communication.

Parkinson, R. S. (1999). Managing health promotion in the workplace: Guidelines for Implementation and Evaluation. In Ministry of Health of Singapore, *Case studies on best practice in workplace health promotion* (p. 39). Singapore: Cornfield Design Communication. (Reprinted from *Manual of Child Psychology*, pp. 703–705, by P. H. Mussen, Ed., 1970, New York: Wiley).

Pot, F., & Gründemann, R. (1999). *Workplace health promotion and modern occupational health and safety–Current state and perspectives.* Paper presented at the conference of European Network for Workplace Health Promotion, Bonn, Germany.

Schmitz, M. (2000). *The AIG global wellness initiative.* Unpublished manuscript.

United States Department of Agriculture (1999). World Cigarette Database. In Worldwatch Institute (1999). *Vital Signs 1999* (p. 109). New York: W.W. Norton Company.

World Health Organization (WHO). (1991). *Sundsvall statement on supportive environments for health.* Geneva: World Health Organization.

World Health Organization (WHO). (1997). *WHO's Global Healthy Work Approach.* Geneva: World Health Organization.

World Health Organization (WHO). (2000). *About WHO.* [On-line]. Available: *http://www.who.int/aboutwho/*

Wynne, R. (1998). European Foundation for the Improvement of Living and Working Conditions. What Makes Workplace Health Promotion work? In G. Breucker, et al., *Success Factors of Workplace Health Promotion* (pp. 15–25). Essen: Federal Association of Company Health Insurance Funds.

Zatonski, W. (1996). *Evolution of health in Poland since 1988.* Warsaw: Maria Sklodowska-Curie Cancer Centre.

A P P E N D I X

20-A

OTTAWA CHARTER FOR HEALTH PROMOTION

First International Conference on Health Promotion, Ottawa, Canada, 21 November 1986

The first International Conference on Health Promotion, meeting in Ottawa this 21st day of November 1986, hereby presents this CHARTER for action to achieve Health for All by the year 2000 and beyond.

This conference was primarily a response to growing expectations for a new public health movement around the world. Discussions focused on the needs in industrialized countries but took into account similar concerns in all other regions. It built on the progress made through the Declaration on Primary Health Care at Alma-Ata, the World Health Organization's Targets for Health for All document, and the recent debate at the World Health Assembly on intersectoral action for health.

HEALTH PROMOTION

Health promotion is the process of enabling people to increase control over, and to improve, their health. To reach a state of complete physical, mental, and social well-being, an individual or group must be able to identify and to realize aspirations, to satisfy needs, and to change or cope with the environment. Health is, therefore, seen as a resource for everyday life, not the objective of living. Health is a positive concept emphasizing social and personal resources, as well as physical capacities. Therefore, health promotion is

not just the responsibility of the health sector, but goes beyond healthy lifestyles to well-being.

Prerequisites for Health

The fundamental conditions and resources for health are:

* peace
* shelter
* education
* food
* income
* a stable ecosystem
* sustainable resources
* social justice and equity

Improvement in health requires a secure foundation in these basic prerequisites.

Advocate

Good health is a major resource for social, economic, and personal development and an important dimension of quality of life. Political, economic, social, cultural, environmental, behavioral, and biological factors can all favor health or be harmful to it. Health promotion action aims at making these conditions favorable through advocacy for health.

Enable

Health promotion focuses on achieving equity in health. Health promotion action aims at reducing differences in current health status and ensuring equal opportunities and resources to enable all people to achieve their fullest health potential. This includes a secure foundation in a supportive environment, access to information, life skills, and opportunities for making healthy choices. People cannot achieve their fullest health potential unless they are able to take control of those things that determine their health. This must apply equally to women and men.

Mediate

The prerequisites and prospects for health cannot be ensured by the health sector alone. More importantly, health promotion demands coordinated action by all concerned: by governments, by health and other social and economic sectors, by nongovernmental and voluntary organizations, by local authorities, by industry, and by the media. People in all walks of life are involved as individuals, families, and communities. Professional and social groups and health personnel have a major responsibility to mediate between differing interests in society for the pursuit of health.

Health promotion strategies and programs should be adapted to the local needs and possibilities of individual countries and regions to take into account differing social, cultural, and economic systems.

Health Promotion Action Means:

Build Healthy Public Policy

Health promotion goes beyond health care. It puts health on the agenda of policy makers in all sectors and at all levels, directing them to be aware of the health consequences of their decisions and to accept their responsibilities for health.

Health promotion policy combines diverse but complementary approaches, including legislation, fiscal measures, taxation, and organizational change. It is coordinated action that leads to health, income, and social policies that foster greater equity. Joint action contributes to ensuring safer and healthier goods and services, healthier public services, and cleaner, more enjoyable environments.

Health promotion policy requires the identification of obstacles to the adoption of healthy public policies in nonhealth sectors, and ways of removing those obstacles. The aim must be to make the healthier choice the easier choice for policy makers as well.

Create Supportive Environments

Our societies are complex and interrelated. Health cannot be separated from other goals. The inextricable links between people and their environment constitutes the basis for a socioecological approach to health. The overall guiding principle for the world, nations, regions, and communities alike is the need to encourage reciprocal maintenance—to take care of each other, our communities, and our natural environment. The conservation of natural resources throughout the world should be emphasized as a global responsibility. Changing patterns of life, work, and leisure have a significant impact on health. Work and leisure should be a source of health for people. The way society organizes work should help create a healthy society. Health promotion generates living and working conditions that are safe, stimulating, satisfying, and enjoyable.

Systematic assessment of the health impact of a rapidly changing environment—particularly in areas of technology, work, energy production, and urbanization—is essential and must be followed by action to ensure positive benefit to the health of the public. The protection of the natural and built environments and the conservation of natural resources must be addressed in any health promotion strategy.

Strengthen Community Actions

Health promotion works through concrete and effective community action in setting priorities, making decisions, planning strategies, and implementing them to achieve better health. At the heart of this process is the empowerment of communities—their ownership and control of their own endeavors and destinies.

Community development draws on existing human and material resources in the community to enhance self-help and social support and to develop flexible systems for strengthening public participation in and direction of health matters. This requires full and continuous access to information and learning opportunities for health, as well as funding support.

Develop Personal Skills

Health promotion supports personal and social development through providing information, education for health, and enhancing life skills. By so doing, it increases the options available to people to exercise more control over their own health and over their environments and to make choices conducive to health.

Enabling people to learn, throughout life, to prepare themselves for all of its stages and to cope with chronic illness and injuries is essential. This has to be facilitated in school, home, work, and community settings. Action is required through educational, professional, commercial and voluntary bodies, and within the institutions themselves.

Reorient Health Services

The responsibility for health promotion in health services is shared among individuals, community groups, health professionals, health service institutions, and governments. They must work together toward a health care system that contributes to the pursuit of health.

The role of the health sector must move increasingly in a health promotion direction, beyond its responsibility for providing clinical and curative services. Health services need to embrace an expanded mandate that is sensitive and respects cultural needs. This mandate should support the needs of individuals and communities for a healthier life and open channels between the health sector and broader social, political, economic, and physical environmental components.

Reorienting health services requires stronger attention to health research as well as changes in professional education and training. This must lead to a change of attitude and organization of health services refocuses on the total needs of the individual as a whole person.

Moving into the Future

Health is created and lived by people within the settings of their everyday lives—where they learn, work, play, and love. Health is created by caring for oneself and others, by being able to take decisions and have control over one's life circumstances, and by ensuring that the society one lives in creates conditions that allow the attainment of health by all its members.

Caring, holism, and ecology are essential issues in developing strategies for health promotion. Therefore, those involved should take as a guiding principle that, in each phase of planning, implementation, and evaluation of health promotion activities, women and men should become equal partners.

Commitment to Health Promotion

The participants in this Conference pledge:

- to move into the arena of healthy public policy and to advocate a clear political commitment to health and equity in all sectors;
- to counteract the pressures toward harmful products, resource depletion, unhealthy living conditions and environments, and bad nutrition, and to focus attention on public health issues such as pollution, occupational hazards, housing, and settlements;
- to respond to the health gap within and between societies and to tackle the inequities in health produced by the rules and practices of these societies;
- to acknowledge people as the main health resource, to support and enable them to keep themselves, their families, and friends healthy through financial and other means, and to accept the community as the essential voice in matters of its health, living conditions, and well-being;
- to reorient health services and their resources toward the promotion of health, and to share power with other sectors, other disciplines, and, most importantly, with people themselves;
- to recognize health and its maintenance as a major social investment and challenge; and
- to address the overall ecological issue of our ways of living.

The Conference urges all concerned to join them in their commitment to a strong public health alliance.

Call for International Action

The Conference calls on the World Health Organization and other international organizations to advocate the promotion of health in all appropriate forums and to support countries in setting up strategies and programs for health promotion.

The Conference is firmly convinced that if people in all walks of life, nongovernmental and voluntary organizations, governments, the World Health Organization, and all other bodies concerned join forces in introducing strategies for health promotion, in line with the moral and social values that form the basis of this CHARTER, Health For All by the year 2000 will become a reality.

CHARTER ADOPTED AT AN INTERNATIONAL CONFERENCE ON HEALTH PROMOTION—The move towards a new public health, November 17–21, 1986, Ottawa, Ontario, Canada

Co-sponsored by the Canadian Public Health Association, Health and Welfare Canada, and the World Health Organization

APPENDIX
20-B

Curitiba Declaration of the International Institute for Health Promotion, American University (2000)

CURITIBA DECLARATION

Background:
The International Institute for Health Promotion (IIHP) is an interdisciplinary network of health promotion institutions and individuals worldwide with the goal of exchanging information, building alliances, and developing strategies for the global advancement of health promotion. The IIHP, which is based at American University in Washington, DC, and consists of 200 institutions vested in health promotion in 50 countries, held its 4th Annual Meeting in Curitiba, Brazil, from October 10–13, 1999. One of the outcomes of the discussions in Curitiba is the following declaration which calls for an increased focus on health promotion in the 21st Century.

DECLARATION

The *Curitiba Declaration* calls for the global advancement of health promotion in the new millennium through sound policies supporting health promotion and enhanced resource allocation for the promotion of healthy lifestyles.

New Challenges In Global Health

The majority of chronic diseases, the number one killer in the world now, are related to unhealthy lifestyles and behaviors that are preventable. In line with economic growth, people in developing countries are acquiring the unhealthy behaviors of the industrialized countries (e.g., smoking, inactivity), resulting in a changing disease pattern. Most countries will face a tremendous economic burden in the next century as health care costs are on the rise. Improved medical technologies and more efficient care will not solve this global dilemma.

Health Promotion Is the Answer

Academic institutions, government authorities, international organizations, private corporations, insurance companies, schools, hospitals, medical groups, community groups, and individuals in health promotion have joined the universal effort to improve the quality of life. As a result, many multinational corporations are now taking a close look at the health status of their global workforce and are designing and implementing health promotion programs to respond to their needs. Numerous well-designed programs have shown an increase in productivity, reduction in health care costs, and improved morale among employees.

The IIHP believes that governments and decision makers around the world must make health promotion a high priority at the dawn of the new millennium. If they fail to do so, they will be regarded by future generations as having been grossly negligent because they had the knowledge and means to improve global health.

Call for Action

The IIHP calls on all government agencies (not just health ministries) to make health promotion a high priority on their agenda by developing and endorsing progressive health promotion policies, by allocating and providing more resources, and by creating supportive environments. The IIHP also calls on all health-related international organizations to advocate health promotion more aggressively in all available forums.

CHAPTER
21

Connecting the Workplace to the Community

Paul Terry and Michelle Nunn

INTRODUCTION

The definition of health as a state of complete physical, social, and mental well-being has long been accepted but seldom translated into practice in worksite health promotion. A preoccupation with somatic screenings, risk factor analysis, and fitness improvement has overshadowed the social and mental aspects of wellness. When cost containment was a primary goal of worksite health programs, focusing on fitness was an effective strategy. However, as employee recruitment and retention have become a business imperative in a thriving economy, corporations have come to recognize that the health needs of employees are broad and diverse.

Companies that realize the health of their workforce is closely aligned with the vigor of their surrounding communities will be more likely to build organizational commitment and employee job satisfaction. Employee health programs seeking to acknowledge a broad definition of health need to be extended to enrich the well-being of the community in which the company is located. The inherent interdependence between business and communities can be likened to the relationship of employee health to productivity—each affects the other, and both the profitability of the company and the resiliency of the workforce can improve when these relationships are effectively managed.

This chapter attempts to build a conceptual link in a chain that starts with social connections and ends with improved health. There is a persuasive body of literature demonstrating that improving social ties improves health. Evidence also points to the role of volunteerism in effectively connecting people to their communities. Indeed, several current studies show volunteerism produces direct health benefits. There is also data to illustrate the benefits companies derive from supporting social causes. Further, readers of this book can undoubtedly attest to the contribution worksite health programs make to improved employee health and productivity. What is missing in this chain of interrelated variables is the link that connects the worksite health promotion profession to the community.

If it is true that health benefits accrue from encouraging social connections, if companies benefit from healthy employees, and certainly if companies succeed best in healthy communities, then it should be apparent that worksite health promotion professionals have an active role to play in connecting employees to the community. This chapter offers scientific support for the above premise and advocates program options that can build the links needed to improve corporate and community health. Corporate volunteer programming is positioned as an effective strategy for improving employee health. After all, our understanding of the relationship between behavior and illness is derived from community epidemiology. Similarly, the theories that guide population health improvement interventions are grounded in empirical evidence from experimental community health trials. Given these roots, the worksite health promotion profession will achieve its greatest potential when it branches back into the community. This chapter describes how corporate community service policies and programs complement employee health programs. We offer evidence-based reasons for why health promotion practitioners need to provide leadership in community service. The reader will see that the goal of improving employee health through programming that addresses social and mental aspects of wellness is inexorably linked to the need to strengthen communities. This chapter is organized into three sections. In the first section, the benefits of connecting employees to the community are described, including the value to the organization, to the health promotion program, and to employees. The second section explains programming alternatives, particularly the role of volunteerism, and describes the role of the health promotion professional in advancing a social agenda. Finally, we offer information about resources available to the health promotion professional. Model community service policies will be described along with suggestions for the implementation of those policies through "City Care" organizations and "Hands On" groups.

THE VALUE OF CONNECTING THE WORKPLACE TO THE COMMUNITY

Burdened with the public distrust that follows an era of corporate downsizing, mergers, and acquisitions, companies are increasingly viewing community service as an important corporate strategy. Indeed, in a study conducted by the Points of Light Foundation, 92% of 454 U.S. corporations surveyed state they actively encourage employees to volunteer in their communities as a way to be the "neighbor of choice" (Miller, 1997). Companies have come to realize that the health of their future work force can be predicted by the vigor of their surrounding urban communities (Schlesinger et al., 1998). And urban community problems are rampant. Public policy debates make it clear that the urban sprawl that results from moving corporations from the cities to the suburbs has become untenable. Long-frustrating commutes, disparities in employment opportunity and incomes, and great variability in educational attainment between communities all threaten the vitality of the future work force. To complicate matters, as community landscapes are changing, so too is the American work force migrating from production to service professions. Competition to recruit and retain educated and motivated employees is more intense than ever, particularly in an era of very low unemployment.

Social Connections and Personal Health

Given the competitive demands that companies face, with access to a shrinking workforce and in the midst of urban problems, worksite health promotion could be elevated as an employee benefit that helps to differentiate an employer from other competitors. However, the trend toward targeting high-risk employees positions health promotion programs as a way to save money by focusing on the costs of certain individuals or health conditions rather than lending a hand to the majority of employees. Commonly accepted "demand-management" approaches are grounded in assumptions that individuals and their unhealthy choices are the reason health care expenditures have outpaced the rate of inflation (Breslow, 1999; Lynch & Vickery, 1993). In reality, individual health habits explain only a proportion of utilization, albeit lifestyle is one of the few known predictors of excess utilization (Hart, Smith, & Blane, 1998; Kingston & Smith, 1997; Terry, Fowler, & Fowles, 1998). The remaining variation in health services, as much as 75%, is largely unexplained.

For more than two decades, researchers have posited that the most significant precursor for health status relates to the social, economic, and environmental health of the community (Lannin, Mathews, Mitchell, et al, 1998; Salit, Kuhn, Hartz, Vu, & Mosso, 1998; Williams, 1998). Corporations with a broad perspective on employee health understand that health promotion and "demand management" programs can improve the health status of many employees. Nevertheless, community and social factors such as finding affordable housing, job advancement opportunities, income, and education are the most telling predictors of poor health for many employees (Lantz, House, Lepkowski, et al., 1998; Terry, Fowler, & Fowles, 1998). For example, Lantz found that after controlling for age, sex, race, urbanity, and education, the hazard rate ratio of mortality was 3.2 for low income groups as compared to 2.3 for middle income groups. When health risk behaviors were considered, the risk of dying was still significantly greater for the low income group.

In addition to the high cost of socioeconomic status, depression has been shown to be among the costliest health risk factors. In a recent study by the Health Education Research Organization, untreated depression was one of the most costly risk factors (Goetzel, et al., 1998). Even though the prevalence of depression is not as high as some other lifestyle risks, this finding is consistent with many other studies from community health research that demonstrate the insidious nature of depression. While it is often unclear whether depression results from social isolation or causes isolation, it is clear that the consequences of isolation are deleterious.

According to one large epidemiological trial, women have three times higher mortality rates when they lack social connections such as family, friends, clubs, or church groups (Winkleby, Kraemer, Ahn, & Varady, 1998). Similarly, a longitudinal study of adolescents showed parent-family connectedness and perceived school connectedness were protective against nearly every health risk behavior for young people (Lipman, Offord, & Boyle, 1994). Culture may also moderate depression. An analysis of the preterm birth rates of Latina and southeast Asian women showed that a strong sense of family and social support may be the most important buffer against the stresses of poverty (Guendelman, 1995). Companies cannot operate employee health programs in a vacuum. Addressing "nontraditional" risk factors such as isolation and depression will require action and collaboration at the community level.

Corporate volunteerism is an activity that mediates between the needs of the community and the individual. Table 21-1 highlights a number of recent studies that describe the relationship between variables such as volunteerism, community involvement, church affiliations, friendships, and other social connection factors in improving health. Such data suggest that facilitating employees in making connections to the community may be the disease management equivalent of building a fitness center.

Improving Health Program Effectiveness

While health promotion programming has matured considerably since its inception, the social dimension of programs is most often neglected. The past decade in employee health promotion has benefited from increasingly sophisticated lifestyle assessment and employee counseling. The era of clinical testing typical of the annual "physical exam" and the focus on executive health perks are long gone. Mature corporate health programs will use health risk assessment technologies to assess the prevention needs of their entire workforce, not just employees in need of special disease management services. Improving the health of the workforce has not only become a critical cost-containment imperative, it has become an expectation of employers managing self-insured risk pools. In the not-too-distant future, when company health benefits budgets are affected by larger segments of the population—including more Medicare- and Medicaid-funded enrollees—using traditional public health tools such as epidemiology, worksite health promotion, mass health screening, and mass communications will become commonplace (Reinertsen, 1995).

For the next generation of worksite programs to be effective, social issues will need to become paramount. When considering the resiliency of the work-

Table 21-1 The Health Benefit of Social Connections

Title/Author	Social Connection Factors	Type of Population	Study Results
Volunteering and mortality among older adults: findings from a national sample (Musick et al., 1999)	Civic involvement	Adults age 65 and older	Volunteering has a protective effect on mortality among those who volunteered for one organization or for 40 hours or less over the past year. The protective effects of volunteering are strongest for respondents who report low levels of informal social interaction and who do not live alone.
Older people—the reserve army of volunteers?: An analysis of volunteerism among older Australians (Warburton et al., 1998)	Self-efficacy among volunteers	Older Australians in immediate pre- or postretirement stages	Logistic regression analysis revealed that volunteers are significantly more likely to come from the higher occupational classes, are less likely to be self-employed, and are more likely to view their health positively.
Predictors of volunteer status in a retirement community (Okun, 1993)	Active church members, belong to several clubs and organizations	Retirement community	Actual volunteers attend church frequently, are free of activity limitations due to health, have volunteered previously, and belong to several clubs and organizations.
Psychosocial differences between elderly volunteers and non-volunteers (Hunter & Linn, 1981)	Civic involvement	Volunteer workers over age 65 compared to nonactive, retired elderly persons	Volunteers were found to have significantly higher degree of life satisfaction, stronger will to live, and fewer symptoms of depression, anxiety, and somatization.
Does public and private religiosity have a moderating effect on depression? A biracial study of elders in the American South (Husaini et al., 1999)	Perceived social support	955 African American and White elderly residents of Nashville	Levels of perceived social support were higher among the African American respondents than among others.
Lack of social participation or religious strength and comfort as risk factors for death after cardiac surgery in the elderly (Oxman et al., 1995)	Social/Community groups	232 patients who had open heart surgery	Lack of participation in groups was independently related to risk for death during the 6-month period after cardiac surgery.

(continued)

Title/Author	Social Connection Factors	Type of Population	Study Results
Are social supports in late midlife a cause or a result of successful physical aging? (Vaillant et al., 1998)	Social supports	223 men	Alcoholism, smoking, and premorbid psychopathology may mediate much of the association between poor social supports and mortality.
Social relations and mortality. An eleven year follow-up study of 70-year-old men and women in Denmark (Avlund et al., 1998)	Social network, education, income, and functional ability	734 70-year-old men and women in Glostrup (county of Copenhagen)	Men who did not help others with repairs and who lived alone, and women with no social support had increased risk of dying during the follow-up period.
Relation of social network characteristics to 5-year mortality among young-old versus old-old white women in an urban community (Yasuda et al., 1997)	Availability of network resources, contact with network resources, and integration into the neighborhood	806 65-year-old or older women who lived in Baltimore, MD	Both age and specific aspects of network structure were found to influence the association between social networks and mortality in elderly women.
Social networks, host resistance, and mortality: A nine-year follow-up study of Alameda County residents (Berkman & Syme, 1979)	Social and community ties	6,928 adults in Alameda County, California	The findings show that people who lacked social and community ties were more likely to die in the follow-up period than were those with more extensive contacts.
The association of social relationships and activities with mortality: Prospective evidence from the Tecumseh community health study (House et al., 1982)	Social relationships and activities	2,754 adult men and women in the Tecumseh Community Health Study	Men reporting a higher level of social relationships and activities in 1967–1969 were significantly less likely to die during the follow-up period. Trends for women were similar.
Facets of support related to well-being: quantitative social isolation and perceived family support in a sample of elderly women (Thompson & Heller, 1990)	Network embeddedness and perceived social support	271 community-dwelling women	Isolated participants had poorer psychological well-being and functional health than did nonisolated participants. Elderly women with low perceived family support had poorer psychological well-being, regardless of perceived support from friends or network embeddedness.
Social network and social support influence mortality in elderly men (Hanson et al., 1989)	Social network, social support, and social influence	621 male residents of Malmo, Sweden, who were born in 1914; 500 were examined and interviewed in 1982–83	A higher mortality risk was found among men with low adequacy of social participation and among men living alone.

(continued)

Table 21-1 The Health Benefit of Social Connections—*(continued)*

Title/Author	Social Connection Factors	Type of Population	Study Results
Social networks and mortality in an inner-city elderly population (Cohen et al., 1987)	Social network	155 residents of midtown Manhattan single-room-occupancy hotels	Discriminant function analysis indicated that 10 of 19 network variables were relatively strong discriminators between survivors and nonsurvivors.
Inequalities in mortality by social class measured at three stages of the life-course (Hart et al., 1998)	Social class for childhood, at labor-market entry, and at screening.	5,567 employed Scottish men	Mortality risk was similar at each stage of life, with men in the higher social classes having the lowest risk. Social class at screening produced the greatest relative indices of inequality.
The relation between religiosity, selected health behaviors, and blood pressure among adult females (Hixson et al., 1998)	Religious services	112 females at least 35 years of age and of Judeo-Christian faiths	Church affiliation may be associated with lower levels of blood pressure (BP) via direct pathway, such as improving the ability to cope with stress. In general, diastolic BP was more influenced by religiosity than systolic BP.
Population-based study of social and productive activities of survival among elderly Americans (Glass et al., 1999)	Social and productive activities	2,761 men and women from a random population sample of 2,812 people aged 65 or older	Social and productive activities that involve little or no enhancement of fitness lowered the risk of all-cause mortality as much as fitness activities. Activity may confer survival benefits through psychosocial pathways.

force, preventing urban decay can be likened to preventing back injuries in the workplace. The one is accomplished through corporate service and philanthropy, the other through education and fitness programs. Both strategies are critical to the productivity and health of the future workforce (Fries et al., 1993; Showstack, Lurie, Leatherman, Fisher, & Inui, 1996; Terry ,1998). Both strategies are represented at Honeywell, a multinational corporation with its headquarters in the city of Minneapolis. This large diversified manufacturing firm offers a prime example of a company intent on cultivating its work force through both employee and community health programs. Like other large corporations, Honeywell has

offered comprehensive employee health programs for over 10 years, including health screenings, disease management programs, fitness and nutrition programs, and much more (Terry, Fowles, Isham, & Wetzell, 1994). Unlike many other companies, Honeywell also recently invested over ten million dollars in housing redevelopment projects in the neighborhoods surrounding its headquarters. Working with city planners, Honeywell has led an effort to demolish a one-block area of houses that accounted for 13% of the crime in the surrounding neighborhood. It has been replaced with "Portland Place," 54 low-income housing units that have returned beauty and stability to the neighborhood. Also, in collaboration with

Habitat for Humanity, hundreds of Honeywell employees from around the country are volunteering to build new houses for low-income residents. Honeywell leaders simply state that they hope to keep their business located in the city and believe that the company's future is tied to the community's future.

Examining the relationship between corporate social responsibility and employee health promotion reveals conflicts or compatibility, depending on one's perspective. Some corporations have entered health care reform debates with strong convictions about the need for greater individual responsibility for health. Some benefits packages were designed to penalize employees with high health risks. ERISA (Employee Retirement Income Security Act)-exempt self-insured companies characterized such cost-shifting approaches as incentives that would motivate employees to improve their health (Terry, Fowles, Isham & Wetzell, 1994). In 1996, federal insurance laws changed to prohibit basing insurance premiums on individual risks. This legal challenge, along with the Americans with Disabilities Act, signaled a need for caution in designing demand reduction programs that could be deemed to blame the victim rather than offering support for employees with costly health conditions. Health promotion programs that target employees with certain conditions or lifestyles can diminish accusations of lifestyle discrimination when they have a concomitant social agenda. While the health care cost reduction motive in health promotion is legitimate, the prospect of success in engaging employee participation is considerably higher when the program is viewed as preventive rather than curative, as compassionate instead of castigatory.

Organizational Benefits of a Social Agenda

Aside from the health benefits to employees and communities, health promotion professionals advocating community involvement are also helping to advance company marketing objectives. Marketing messages from for-profit organizations show consistent attempts to demonstrate their concern for the health of the community. The American Express Corporation coined the phrase "cause-related marketing" in response to the realization that consumers are more likely to purchase products from organizations with a charitable mission (Stallings, 1998). According to a 1999 Roper survey, 67% of consumers say that if price and quality are equal, they are more likely to switch to a brand or retailer associated with a good cause (Society for the Advancement of Education, 1999). Similarly, nonprofit organizations, abetted by tax-exemption statutes, are keenly sensitive to public trust mandates that they demonstrate charitable work and community benefit. Peter Drucker, a renowned management consultant, characterizes this as "enlightened self-interest." Indeed, "City Care" organizations have volunteer ranks burgeoning with employees looking to find more meaning in their days. That an employee's contributions to the community will reflect favorably on their employer is a meritorious, albeit distant, motivation.

Worksite health promotion professionals advance many health improvement initiatives by showing the relationship between risks and costs (Abelson, Terry, & Sullivan, 1994). Mounting data show that the annual health care resource use for high-risk individuals can be more than double than that for low-risk people (Fries et al., 1993). Most corporate programs, then, focus on traditional risk factors such as smoking or obesity (U.S. Department of Health and Human Services & Public Health Service, 1993). Health promotion professionals, with their understanding of population health principles, are also well-equipped to help companies understand the health improvement opportunities that reside in the community. Too much focus on an individual's health behavior inordinately shifts the burden of health care cost containment to the poorest and least educated (Gazmararian et al., 1999; Sapolsky, 1998). One study, for example, used data from the National Longitudinal Mortality Study, a survey base of over a half million lives, to demonstrate that race, employment, income, and education are the strongest predictors of early mortality (Sorlie, Backlund, & Keller, 1995). Indeed, improvements in mortality have diverged sharply along racial lines. In the late 1980s, white men gained nearly a year in life expectancy while black men lost nearly a year in the same time period, mostly attributable to heart disease rates (Kochanek,

Maurer, & Rosenberg, 1994). Poverty has also been shown to be an independent variable for predicting psychosocial risk factors in children. A study using measures such as poor school performance, psychiatric disorders, and social impairment showed dramatically higher psychosocial morbidity rates for children of poor families (Salit et al., 1998). Such studies indicate that "targeting high risk" in the workplace should as often lead to low-paid single mothers as to heavy-set smokers. Moreover, effective corporate interventions are as likely to be community-based as worksite focused.

WORKSITE PROGRAM OPPORTUNITIES FOR CONNECTING TO THE COMMUNITY

Promoting community service programming in the workplace is strikingly similar to selling employers on employee health programming. In an educational session conducted at the International Conference of the Association for Worksite Health Promotion (1998), a role-playing game was enacted that simulated a corporate setting and its constellation of managers and decision leaders. The health promotion leader in the game was "convening a meeting" to advocate a policy allowing 40 hours of paid release time for community service. The "advocate" was armed with data concerning the health benefits of service to employees and the community.

Role players in the educational game about volunteerism advocacy acted out the positions of typical company supporters and detractors of such policies. There were those playing corporate curmudgeons, ever wary of activity that could detract from productivity or cost too much money. There were others who were mindful of company image in the community that could be both positively and negatively affected by community volunteers. Some roles in the game related to supporting the program for the wrong reasons, such as an easy excuse to get out of work. Others played roles of those genuinely interested in volunteering because it was the right thing to do for the company, its employees, and the community.

Game participants at the conference readily agreed that the discussions that ensued from this role playing were nearly identical to dialogue related to making the case for or against worksite health promotion. Just as there are those who believe employee health programs bolster morale, productivity, and reduce costs, there are also those who think such programs encroach on valuable work time and remain skeptical of the cost effectiveness of prevention. Philosophical positions concerning paternalism and the limits of the employee/employer relationships also emerged. This tension between private and corporate interests and individual versus social responsibility is familiar territory for health promotion professionals. The alliance between health promotion and community service is a natural and logical match.

Volunteerism and Service Programs Led by Employees

In spite of compelling evidence that community health and social support issues are strongly linked to employee health, some may view these as social services or medical issues outside of a company's sphere of influence (Peterson & Wilson, 1996). This concern is ratified, in part, by the fact that the greatest proportion of the variance in health between affluent and the poor remains unexplained. For example, only a small proportion of the relationship between socioeconomic status and health can be attributed to lack of access to health care (Olsen & Frank-Stromborg, 1993). Although some indigent populations use health services more often than affluent populations, they invariably have greater incidence of chronic health problems (Showstack, Lurie, Leatherman, Fisher, & Inui, 1996). These realities lead some to conclude that allocating additional resources to improving social factors, such as housing or underemployment would be more effective than investing in more health care (Barnett, 1997; J. Abdul-Mu'min, personal communication, September, 1998). Such intractable issues may discourage some companies from confronting community problems; however, for many other businesses, it is just such polarity that has led to mobilization of resources dedicated to meeting community needs.

"Business Shares," a model developed by the Greater DC Cares organization, is a working example of how a community service agency can provide support and direction to the community service strategies of industry. Progressive companies will look for ways to address community needs in the same strategic manner that they plan health care benefits. Indeed, with employee health benefits representing one of the most significant marginal costs of doing business, employers may increasingly view community service as a means of protecting their investment in the company's greatest assets, its human capital.

MANAGING PROGRAMS THAT INCREASE COMMUNITY CONNECTIONS

The above discussion leads to two conclusions. First, particularly for disadvantaged groups, many of the most significant preventable health problems can be traced to socioeconomic inequities and the health of the community. Second, social isolation, depression, and lack of meaningful connections to a community are significant determinants of individual health problems. Still, with health promotion professionals struggling to improve traditional risk factors, where is the incentive to take on community problems? When attracting participation in health programs is already difficult, why add another responsibility to the corporate health agenda? There is remarkable synergy and mutuality between community service programming and health education in the workplace. Mobilizing employees to volunteer in service of community needs improves community health, an imperative for the health of today's and tomorrow's workforces. What's more, connecting employees to the community addresses the isolation and depression that remains one of the most insidious and costly of risk factors. Much more than stress management or other self-management programs, involving people in meaningful ways in the lives of others is powerful therapy (Putnam, 1995). Often—and most important from a program administration standpoint—there is significant, and frequently free, support from community and nongovernment organizations to assist companies with community service programs.

The Role of the Health Promotion Professional

While corporate volunteerism is a time-honored tradition in many companies throughout the country, it is usually the employees rather than the employers who lead these efforts. Worksite health promotion professionals are uniquely positioned to advocate both employee and employer goals in community benefit programming. Just as worksite health promotion needs both top-down and bottom-up support to be successful, community benefits programming needs to be instigated by employees and supported by management. Moreover, similar to the most successful health screenings, such activities should be clearly voluntary for employees, but management can show it values such activities by allowing it to occur on company time. Additionally, managers must model their philosophy by becoming involved in community efforts in a demonstrable fashion. Table 21-2 illustrates the community service policies of several corporations committed to volunteerism. While release time is not necessary for successful volunteerism to occur, it is one of the most convincing ways to demonstrate that community service is a corporate value, a testament to the employer's interest in improving community health.

Community Agencies that Support Corporate Volunteerism

Companies are clearly not alone in their interest in sustaining healthy communities. Health care organizations, nonprofit organizations, public and private health agencies, and nongovernmental organizations have population health improvement missions. Collaboration and productive partnerships are watchwords of organizations that understand that population health improvement is a complex and prodigious task. One new organization, "The Coalition for Healthier Cities and Communities," is building a national network of partners working on community health improvement. The coalition is dedicated to creating partnerships, offering resources, and developing policy. Priority community health concerns are not determined by health care organizations; rather,

Table 21-2 Corporate Volunteer Policies

Corporate Volunteer Policy	Release Time	Community Service Examples	Policy Limitations	Application Process
Institute for Research and Education, Education Division, HealthSystem Minnesota	40 hours per year	Minnesota Food Share, nursing homes, free blood pressure screenings, Minneapolis Crisis Nursery	Paid time off to volunteer for not-for-profits	Management approval, two weeks notice expected
Reliastar (two plus two program)	Two percent of normal work time, 3–4 hours a month, up to 42 hours per year	Community Agencies Events during the workday; no "time off" but encouraged during workdays	Not-for-profit; no corporate time off for political, religious, fraternal organizations, social clubs, labor organizations	Application form describing activities; manager approval needed prior to volunteer commitment
American Express	Company supports volunteer center meetings and sponsors projects; time off to be made up by employees	Holidazzle Food Drive, Meals on Wheels, Junior Achievement, AIDS Walk, Habitat for Humanity	Employees and committees choose types of organizations and organizing committees	Employee networks organized around specific areas of interest; committees plan projects throughout the year
Northern States Power Company	Four hours per month, 48 hours per year maximum.	United Way agencies, speaker's bureau, and environmental protection programs	Nonprofits qualify; religious and political activities not included	Manager approval required
Home Depot	Store volunteer leaders—two paid hours per week; others are strictly volunteer.	Affordable housing, at-risk youth, environmental programs, national partnerships with Christmas in April, Youthbuild USA	Generally done with nonprofit organizations that have received donations; excluding labor organizations and social and veterans' groups	Team leaders are encouraged to get store manager buy-in
Coca Cola	Teambuilding activities occurring during regular work hours are given with permission of manager/supervisor	Hands On Atlanta Day Serve-a-thon, United Way Campaign, Toys for Tots, Genesis Shelter	Nonprofits qualify; religious and political activities are excluded	Manager approval required; employees are organized through specific interests and employee volunteer programs

they emerge from dialogue with public and private sector partners. This collaborative process has been well-documented in materials published by several health care organization stakeholder associations, including the Hospital Research and Education Trust (HRET) division of the American Hospital Association (AHA), the HealthCare Forum, and the Catholic Health Association of the United States. The coalition's agenda includes improving health systems' accountability and responsiveness to community needs and promoting the value of diversity and inclusion in community coalitions. Company leaders and their volunteer workforces have played a critical role in advancing the coalition's initiatives. The coalition can be contacted through their website: http://www.healthycommunities.org/.

City Cares Groups

In most cities, worksite health professionals are well-positioned in their organizations to mobilize employees for developing and organizing community service activities. Just as employee health program staff routinely call on hospitals, clinics, and HMO's for support in offering traditional health programs, there are numerous community agencies dedicated to enlisting citizens into community action. A national model in the service community is an Atlanta-based network of more than 24 volunteer service organizations called "City Cares of America." Table 21-3 lists Care Groups currently active in cities throughout America. City Cares recruits, identifies, and nurtures city volunteer groups. An example of these affiliates is "Hands On Atlanta, Inc."

(www.handsonatlanta.org/home/), a nonprofit volunteer service organization that promotes volunteerism and directs community involvement among concerned people in Atlanta. Founded in 1989, Hands On Atlanta has grown from a few dozen volunteers to a volunteer corps of more than 20,000 and partners with community-based agencies and public schools to address Atlanta's most critical needs. Every day of the year, volunteers are placed in service projects, including house-building and renovation for low-income and homeless individuals, tutoring and mentoring activities, providing assistance to seniors, working at soup kitchens and homeless shelters, addressing the needs of HIV-positive individuals, and coordinating outings for children. Hands on Atlanta currently offers more than 250 monthly projects serving the community and its citizens.

While humanitarian services and connecting employees to the community in meaningful ways are a primary objective, cultivating employee leadership and organization skills is an additional benefit. For example, volunteers play a large role in Hands On Atlanta structure and organizational direction. Each project is coordinated by a project coordinator, a Hands On Atlanta volunteer, who assumes responsibility for recruiting volunteers and ensuring the success of the project. Volunteers serve on committees that develop and coordinate Hands On Atlanta's special events and assist with public relations and fundraising efforts. In conjunction with its volunteer projects, Hands on Atlanta sponsors regular educational events and volunteer gatherings, which provide members with an opportunity to share experiences and learn more about problems facing the

Table 21-3 "City Cares" Groups

Hands On Atlanta, Atlanta, GA	Boston Cares, Boston, MA
Hands On Charlotte, Charlotte, NC	Greater DC Cares, Washington, DC
Volunteer Impact, Southfield, MI	Hands On Greenville, Greenville, SC
Kansas City Cares, Kansas City, MO	Hands On Nashville, Nashville, TN
New York Cares, New York, NY	Philadelphia Cares, Philadelphia, PA
Pittsburgh Cares, Pittsburgh, PA	San Diego Cares, San Diego, CA
Hands On San Francisco, San Francisco, CA	Community Impact, Palo Alto, CA
Seattle Works, Seattle, WA	

Atlanta community. It recruits and trains its volunteers and then leads them in community service projects. After participating in an orientation, each Hands On Atlanta volunteer receives *The Citizen,* a monthly magazine that lists volunteer opportunities and news. Volunteers sign up for projects according to their interest and availability.

The list of accomplishments by "Hands On" groups and their systematic documentation of activities afford employee health program planners the credibility they need to make volunteerism a supported and sustainable corporate activity. For example, in 1999, Hands On Atlanta engaged a corps of 19,500 metro Atlantans in community service, resulting in 34,676 opportunities for citizens to volunteer; this was 307,546 volunteer service hours spanning 2,184 community service projects. These activities cultivated 1,700 service leaders and partnered with 24 Atlanta Public Schools, delivering 156,999 hours of service to over 5,060 Atlanta Public School students. These efforts decreased disciplinary actions by 25% at schools with Hands On Atlanta AmeriCorps members and increased parental participation at PTSA meetings by 25%. Hands On Atlanta directly assists companies in organizing their employees into community volunteer teams or directly recruits corporate volunteers for service projects. For example, serve-a-thons offer companies an efficient way to involve a large number of employees for hands-on service for a high-profile event that makes a visible difference for the community. Hands On Atlanta engaged 11,000 volunteers and generated 63,000 service hours to the community during Hands On Atlanta Day.

Hands On Atlanta is one example in this growing network of local "City Cares" organizations known as "Cares," or "Hands On," groups (see www.citycares.com). These "Care" (CCA's) groups engage over 100,000 individuals in direct, hands-on service within their communities each year. Local Cares organizations were formed in response to the challenges groups and individuals have finding time to contribute to the community when work and family commitments can be so demanding. With the goal to make volunteering possible for even the busiest individuals, the Cares model of service is an ideal one for companies that seek to engage their employees in meaningful volunteer service in areas which they support, both geographically and philanthropically. For companies seeking to fulfill The President's Summit commitments or other community commitments, CCA's Corporate Partners Program (in partnership with CCA affiliates) offers a wealth of resources, including knowledgeable staff sensitive to corporate cultures, a wide range of hands-on projects that address different community needs, and team volunteer opportunities for large or small groups. The President's Summit commitments from corporations range from building low-income housing or cleaning up parks to reading to kids or coaching sports teams. City Cares' groups also provide unique team-building and leadership opportunities, access to a network of affiliates across the country, and flexible scheduling and commitment levels that need not interfere with the workday. Working with an entity such as CCA's corporate partners program will likely reduce the time-consuming and often costly efforts of forming a new corporate volunteer structure or developing new volunteer opportunities so that employees can participate in volunteering with ease and achieve maximum impact in the community.

CONCLUSION

Health Promotion professionals use self-care and disease management programs to reduce unnecessary utilization in the short-term. Although such consumer-focused education strategies are vital components of an employee health improvement program, such efforts are "downstream" of the major causes of premature disease, disability, and death. Common risk factors such as smoking, poor diet, lack of exercise, and excess alcohol use are commonly attributed to unnecessary suffering, and such risk factors have social, behavioral, and environmental antecedents. It is the community that is the keeper of these antecedents. It is in our neighborhoods and schools where healthful or deleterious life choices are cultivated. Progressive program planners will connect their worksites with the community to get "upstream" of employee health problems and, in so doing, will be challenged to explore the balance between individual and social responsibility for health.

The term "demand reduction" has come to represent contemporary intervention strategies targeted at individuals (Fries et al., 1993). The concept is limited as it relates to health improvement for large populations. If employee health improvement programs are to be cost effective, increasing the employee's role in disease management will be imperative. "Demand management" programs are reportedly achieving 7–17% lower rates of utilization associated with patient disease management instruction, self-care education, or nurse-based phone counseling interventions. Demand management proponents argue that lowering demand for service holds more promise than containing the costs of service delivery. By implication, cost-containment strategies that focus on reducing the cost of patient care services will never compensate for the presumed bottomless pit of patient demand for service.

Interpersonal health behavior theories, such as the "health belief" model, are operational in the demand management-oriented programs. Such theories assert that if people are educated about their personal susceptibility to health problems, they will be motivated to become more involved in self-management of their conditions. Companies that focus on individual patient behavior maintain that teaching employees to make safe, appropriate, and informed health care choices will yield a short-term cost benefit. This belief counters the argument that long-term economic benefit can result from programs designed to optimize personal health and well-being. Since health promotion is positioned as a strategy for managing demand for health services, emphasis must be placed on teaching consumers skills related to appropriate utilization. This orientation, however, comes at the risk of diverting scarce resources away from primary prevention education, which has been the mainstay of health promotion (Friedman, 1993). When consumers are expected to pay a greater share of costs in the future, they will, in turn, expect greater value from each visit.

In some cases the advantage accrues to the conservative, those who save time and money by learning from the tribulations of others. However, the monumental challenge of improving population health will not be met if the worksite health promotion agenda does not move at a more exponential pace. It will be the most judicious organizations—those that can balance the pressure of a competitive market-sensitive corporate culture with tenets of corporate social responsibility—who will serve as role models for the next millennium in worksite health promotion and community service.

References

Abdul-Mu'min, J. (1998, September). Personal communications with the Executive Director. A. Wooten Jr. Heritage Center.

Abelson, D., Terry, P. E., and Sullivan, S. (1994). Preventive screening: Guidelines for primus non nocere (first do no harm). *The Bulletin, 38*(2):70–79.

Avlund, K., Damsgaard, M. T., & Holstein, B. E. (1998). Social relations and mortality: An eleven-year follow-up study of 70-year-old men and women in Denmark. *Social Science and Medicine, 47*(5), 635–643.

Barnett, K. (1997). *The future of community benefit programming.* Berkeley, CA: The Public Health Institute.

Berkanovic, E., & Telesky, C. (1985). Mexican-American, Black-American, and White-American differences in reporting illnesses, disability and physician visits for illnesses. *Social Science and Medicine, 20*(6), 567–577.

Berkman, L. F., & Syme, S. L. (1979). Social networks, host resistance, and mortality: A nine-year follow-up study of Alameda County residents. *American Journal of Epidemiology, 109*(2), 186–204.

Breslow, L. (1999). From disease prevention to health promotion. *Journal of the American Medical Association, 281*(11), 1030–1033.

Cohen, C. I., Teresi, J., & Holmes, D. (1986–87). Social networks and mortality in an inner-city elderly population. *International Journal of Aging and Human Development, 24*(4), 257–269.

Community accountability: Meeting the challenge. (1996, November). Irving, TX: VHA Inc.

Friedman, E. (1993). An ounce of compassion. *Healthcare Forum Journal, 36*(6), 11–13, 15, 17.

Fries, J. F., Koop, C. E., Beadle, C. E., Cooper, P. P., England, M. J., Greaves, R. F., Sokolov, J. J., & Wright, D. (1993). Reducing health care services by reducing the need and demand for medical services. The Health Project Consortium. *New England Journal of Medicine, 29,329*(5), 321–325.

Gazmararian, J. A., Baker, D. W., Williams, M. V., Parker, R. M., Scott, T. L., Green, D. C., Fehrenbach, S. N., Ren, J., & Koplan, J. P. (1999).

Health literacy among Medicare enrollees in a managed care organization. *Journal of the American Medical Association, 281*(6), 545–551.

Glass, T. A., de Leon, C. M., Marottoli, R. A., & Berkman, L. F. (1999). Population-based study of social and productive activities as predictors of survival among elderly Americans. *BMJ, 319*(7208), 478–483.

Goetzel, R. Z., Anderson, D. R., Whitmer, R. W., Ozminkowski, R. J., Dunn, R. L., & Wasserman, J. (1998). The relationship between modifiable health risks and health care expenditures: An analysis of the multi-employer HERO health risk and cost database. The Health Enhancement Research Organization (HERO) Research Committee. *Journal of Occupational and Environmental Medicine, 40*(10), 843–854.

Guendelman, S. (1995, October). *Immigrants may hold clues to protecting health during pregnancy.* Los Angeles, CA: The California Wellness.

Hanson, B. S., Isacsson, S. O., Janzon, L., & Lindell, S. E. (1989). Social network and social support influence mortality in elderly men. The prospective population study of "Men born in 1914," Malmo, Sweden. *American Journal of Epidemiology.* 1989 Jul, 130(1), 100–111.

Hart, C. L., Smith, G. D., & Blane, D. (1998). Inequities in mortality by social class measured at three stages of the lifecourse. *American Journal of Public Health, 88*(3), 471–474.

Hixson, K. A., Gruchow, H. W., & Morgan, D. W. (1998). The relation between religiosity, selected health behaviors, and blood pressure among adult females. *Preventive Medicine, 27*(4), 545–552.

House, J. S., Robbins, C., & Metzner, H. L. (1982). The association of social relationships and activities with mortality: prospective evidence from the Tecumseh Community Health Study. *American Journal of Epidemiology, 116*(1), 123–140.

Hunter, K. I., & Linn, M. W. (1980–1981). Psychosocial differences between elderly volunteers and non-volunteers. *International Journal of Aging and Human Development, 12*(3), 205–213.

Husaini, B. A., Blasi, A. J., & Miller, O. (1999). Does public and private religiosity have a moderating effect on depression? A bi-racial study of elders in the American South. *International Journal of Aging and Human Development, 48*(1), 63–72.

Kingston, R. S., & Smith, J. P. (1997). Socioeconomic status and racial and ethnic differences in functional status associated with chronic diseases. *American Journal of Public Health, 87*(5), 805–810.

Kochanek, K. D., Maurer, J. D., & Rosenberg, H. M. (1994). Why did black life expectancy decline from 1984 through 1989 in the United States? *American Journal of Public Health, 84*(6), 938–944.

Lannin, D. R., Mathews, H. F., Mitchell, J., Swanson, M. S., Swanson, F. H., & Edwards, M. S. (1998). Influence of socioeconomic and cultural factors on racial differences in late-stage presentation of breast cancer. *Journal of the American Medical Association, 279*(22), 1801–1807.

Lantz, P. M., House, J. S., Lepkowski, J. M., Williams, D. R., Mero, R. P., & Chen, J. (1998). Socioeconomic factors, health behaviors and mortality: Results from a nationally representative prospective study of U.S. adults. *Journal of the American Medical Association, 279*(21), 1703–1708.

Lipman, E. L., Offord, D. R., & Boyle, M. H. (1994). Relation between economic disadvantage and psychosocial morbidity in children. *Canadian Medical Association Journal, 151*(4), 431–437.

Lynch, J. W., Everson, S. A., Kaplan, G. A., Salonen, R., & Salonen, J. T. (1998). Does low socioeconomic status potentiate the effects of heightened cardiovascular responses to stress on the progression of carotid atherosclerosis? *American Journal of Public Health, 88*(3), 389–394.

Lynch, W. D., & Vickery, D. M. (1993). The potential impact of health promotion on health care utilization: An introduction to demand management. *The American Journal of Health Promotion, 8*(2), 87–92.

Miller, W. (1997). Volunteerism: a new strategic tool. *Industry Week, 246,* 13–14.

Musick, M. A., Herzog, A. R., & House, J. S. (1999). Volunteering and mortality among older adults: Findings from a national sample. *Journals of Gerontology. Series B, Psychological Sciences and Social Sciences, 54*(3), S173–80.

Okun, M. A. (1993). Predictors of volunteer status in a retirement community. *International Journal of Aging and Human Development, 36*(1), 57–74.

Olsen, S. J., & Frank-Stromborg, M. (1993). Cancer prevention and early detection in ethnically diverse populations. *Seminars in Oncology Nursing, 9*(3), 198–209.

Oxman, T. E., Freeman, D. H. Jr., & Manheimer, E. D. (1995). Lack of social participation or religious strength and comfort as risk factors for death after cardiac surgery in the elderly. *Psychosomatic Medicine, 57*(1), 5–15.

Peterson, M., & Wilson, J. (1996). Job satisfaction and perceptions of health. *Journal of Occupational and Environmental Medicine, 38*(9), 891–898.

Putnam, R. D. (1995, June). Bowling alone: America's declining social capital. *Current, 373,* 3–9.

Reinertsen, J. L. (1995). Collaborating outside the box: When employers and providers take on environmental barriers to guideline implementation. *Joint Commission Journal of Quality Improvement, 21*(11), 612–618.

Salit, S. A., Kuhn, E. M., Hartz, A. J., Vu, J. M., & Mosso, A. L. (1998). Hospitalization costs associated with homelessness in New York City. *New England Journal of Medicine, 338*(24), 1734–1740.

Sapolsky, R. (1998). How the other half heals: one secret of health is more straightforward than you think: money, (impact of wealth and poverty on health and well-being). *Discover, 19*(4), 46–52.

Schlesinger, M., & Gray, B. (1998). A broader vision for managed care, Part 1: Measuring the benefit to communities. *Health Affairs* (Millwood), *17*(3), 152–168.

Schlesinger, M., Gray, B., Carrino, G., Duncan, M., Gusmano, M., Antonelli, V., & Stuber, J. (1998). A broader vision for managed care, Part 2: A typology of community benefits. *Health Affairs* (Millwood), *17*(5), 26–49.

Showstack, J., Lurie, N., Leatherman, S., Fisher, E., & Inui, T. (1996). Health of the public: The private sector challenge. *Journal of the American Medical Association, 276*(13), 1071–1074.

Society for the Advancement of Education (1999, August). Good Deeds Attract Customers and Workers. *USA Today* (Magazine), 28 (2651), 15.

Sorlie, P. D., Backlund, E., & Keller, J. B. (1995). U.S. mortality by economic, demographic, and social characteristics: The National Longitudinal Mortality Study. *American Journal of Public Health, 85*(7), 949–956.

Stallings, B. B. (1998, September). Volunteerism and Corporate America. *U.S. Society and Values,* 23–26.

Terry, P. E. (1994). A case for no-fault health insurance: from the "worried well" to the "guilty ill." *American Journal of Health Promotion, 8*(3), 165–168.

Terry, P. E. (1998). Four stages of maturation in managed care health promotion. *The HealthCare Forum Journal, 21*(5), 12–21.

Terry, P. E., Fowler, E. J., & Fowles, J. B. (1998). Are health risks related to medical care charges in the short-term? Challenging traditional assumptions. *American Journal of Health Promotion, 12*(5), 340–347.

Terry, P. E., Fowles, J., Isham, G., & Wetzell, S. (1994). Beyond report cards: A health profile for Health-Partners Health Plan and the Business Health Care Action Group. *HMO Practice, 8*(4), 171–175.

Thompson, M. G., & Heller, K. (1990). Facets of support related to well-being: Quantitative social isolation and perceived family support in a sample of elderly women. *Psychological Aging, 5*(4), 535–544.

U.S. Department of Health and Human Services Public Health Service and Public Health Service. (1993). 1992 National Survey of Worksite Health Promotion Activities: Summary. *American Journal of Health Promotion, 7*(6), 452–464.

Vaillant, G. E., Meyer, S. E., Mukamal, K., & Soldz, S. (1998). Are social supports in late midlife a cause or a result of successful physical aging? *Psychological Medicine, 28*(5), 1159–1168.

Warburton, J., Le Brocque, R., & Rosenman, L. (1998). Older people—the reserve army of volunteers?: An analysis of volunteerism among older Australians. *International Journal of Aging and Human Development, 46*(3), 229–245.

Williams, M. V., Parker, R. M., Baker, D. W., Parikh, N. S., Pitkin, K., Coates, W. C., & Nurss, J. R. (1995). Inadequate functional health literacy among patients at two public hospitals. *Journal of the American Medical Association, 274*(21), 1677–1682.

Winkleby, M. A., Kraemer, H. C., Ahn, D. K., & Varady, A. N. (1998). Ethnic and socioeconomic differences in cardiovascular disease risk factors: findings for women from the Third National Health and Nutrition Examination Survey, 1988–1994. *Journal of the American Medical Association, 280*(4), 356–362.

Yasuda, N., Zimmerman, S. I., Hawkes, W., Fredman, L., Hebel, J. R., & Magaziner, J. (1997). Relation of social network characteristics to 5-year mortality among young-old versus old-old white women in an urban community. *American Journal of Epidemiology, 145*(6), 516–523.

CHAPTER

22

The Future of Workplace Health Promotion

Don R. Powell and Elaine Frank

INTRODUCTION

Yogi Berra once said, "The future ain't what it used to be." Having been involved in the field of health promotion and wellness for over 25 years, we are amazed at the evolution that has taken place. Twenty-five years ago, we used to argue over how "health promotion" differed from "wellness." Twenty-five years ago, we were without data to justify the cost benefits of health promotion programs. Twenty-five years ago, hospitals were satisfied to simply treat illness rather than prevent it, and corporations just expected to pay ever-increasing health insurance premiums. In the early years, wellness was belittled and was called a fad.

Today, it is different. We have corporate fitness centers, smoking bans both in communities and at worksites, employee assistance programs, managed-care options, and warning labels on cigarettes and alcohol.

There are also some very positive signs for the next 25 years. The Environmental Protection Agency has documented the dangers of sidestream smoke and, together with the Occupational Safety and Health Administration (OSHA), will probably be developing more stringent guidelines for smoking at the work-

place. Forty-nine states (all except New Hampshire) and the District of Columbia have passed mandatory seatbelt laws (Insurance Institute for Highway Safety). In 1990, the Year 2000 Health Objectives, (*http://www.health.gov/healthypeople*) guidelines for all communities and corporations to strive for, were launched in Washington, DC, and we are now planning for the launch of the Year 2010 Health Objectives (*http://www.health.gov/healthypeople*). In 1994, health care reform was debated; and although not passed, the reasons for it remain. Today, we see that wellness is not a fad. It is a movement that took us away from a lopsided focus on treatment and the resultant lack of focus on prevention. Health promotion in the workplace is here to stay.

Unfortunately, there are some negative signs. The adult U.S. population is becoming more overweight, while at the same time consuming more diet food and fewer calories (Heini & Weinsier, 1997). Lung cancer has replaced breast cancer as the most common cause of cancer deaths in women (American Cancer Society, 1998). The Centers for Disease Control and Prevention (1999) estimate that between 650,000 and 900,000 people are living with HIV, and that 1 in every 400 people has AIDS. Alcohol and drug abuse continue to be major problems for individuals in particular and society as a whole. Currently, nearly 14 million Americans, 1 in every 13 adults, abuse alcohol or are alcoholic (National Institute on Alcohol Abuse and Alcoholism, 1996), and 6.1% of Americans 12 years of age and older report illicit drug use in the past 30 days (U.S. Department of Health and Human Services, 1996). Just as the fields of fashion, economics, and business follow trends, so does health promotion.

What future can we expect for health promotion? Some of the future trends are already starting to occur today and will accelerate as we move into the future. Others have yet to occur, but we can expect to see them in the coming years. What follows is a glimpse into our crystal ball on health promotion.

CHANGING OF THE GUARD: WHO PROVIDES WELLNESS?

In the twenty-first century, we will see a continuation of the changing of the guard in terms of who provides wellness programs. The organizations that benefit the most from keeping people healthy will have the greatest growth in wellness programming. Continuing a trend that has already begun, corporations will expand their wellness offerings more than any of the other providers of wellness programming. Insurance providers will continue to expand the number of wellness programs that they offer as well, but to a lesser extent. Hospitals will increase their programming only slightly, while community agencies will offer fewer wellness programs. Figure 22-1 shows our prediction for the change in who will be providing wellness programming in the twenty-first century. This prediction is based on a survey done during the summer of 1999 at a major conference of health education professionals (Frank, 1999). Sixty-three health educators completed the one page survey that asked for their "best guess" on several aspects of what health promotion would be like in the twenty-first century. Thirty-eight percent of those surveyed were corporate health educators, 32% worked for hospitals or other health care providers, 11% worked for community health organizations, 10% were educators, 6% worked for insurance providers, and 3% were in the military.

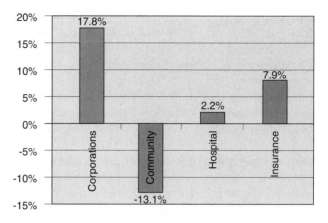

Figure 22-1 Change in who provides wellness in the twenty-first century.
Source: E. Frank, Predict the Future Survey, 1999.

NEW ROLES EMERGE FOR WELLNESS PROVIDERS

Community Wellness Programs Continue to Be Important, But in a New Way

The focus of community programs will be on those not in the active workforce: stay-at-home parents, retirees, and children. Corporations will be offering so much health promotion programming onsite that employed people will not be as likely to participate as much in the community programs. Corporate health educators may be contracted by community agencies to offer wellness programs for them as these agencies reduce their own staff of health educators. Some of the larger corporations will invite the community to participate in some aspects of their health promotion programs as a community service. These corporations will take some of their programming out into the community to reach retirees, spouses, and dependents. Especially in the case of medical self-care, the corporation will want to reach the family to be able to save the greatest amount of money.

Case Study: United Auto Workers and General Motors Communities Program

General Motors decided that in order to cut their health care costs, they needed to look at how health care is provided and utilized in the communities that cost them the most and compare that to the communities that cost them the least (Larkin, 1998). They started their review in Anderson, Indiana, where the company spends 83% more on health care per employee than in Rochester, New York, their lowest cost market. What they found was that the better-performing plans had strong ties to well-organized, high-quality medical groups and hospitals. It appeared that lower cost care could be synonymous with higher quality care. From there they enlisted the support of the United Auto Workers (UAW) in what both organizations believe will become a win-win situation for the company and the employees.

The UAW and GM worked together with the city government of Anderson to form the Citizens' Action Group. The goal of the committee was to work with the providers to improve health care for everyone in the community. They hired health care consultant Lewin-VHI to assess resources and needs. The study found 10 areas of concern, including a shortage of primary care doctors, excessively high rates for some procedures, a prevalence of risky behaviors like smoking and overeating, and poor results for cardiac and cancer care. As a result, they established a clinic that uses disease management techniques to improve the treatment of asthma and an education program for doctors and patients aimed at increasing use of generic drugs.

The asthma clinic cut hospital admissions dramatically and is going to be offered communitywide. The program to cut the use of high-cost drugs has reduced prescription costs by 30%. Educational programs for the medical staffs at the three hospital systems serving the county are a great success; St. John's has cut its inpatient costs and length of stay about 10% annually over the last three years. However, the big challenge of consolidating duplicated clinical services remains to be resolved.

GM and the UAW are pleased with the results and plan to continue working with their communities and providers to ensure high quality care at a competitive price. The communities and providers are joining them in what seems so far to be a winner all the way around.

Insurance Companies Will Offer Wellness Incentives

People will earn incentives for cost-saving/healthy behaviors from their insurance provider. Nonsmokers, exercisers, healthy eaters, and citation-free drivers will receive incentives to encourage continued healthy behavior. People will be "risk rated," as they are for auto insurance, based on their health behaviors. People will complete a behavior profile, which asks questions about their health behaviors, similar to a health risk appraisal questionnaire. This profile will be used to determine the level of incentive that the person qualifies for based on their responses to the profile questions. Most companies will ask for a doctor's signature to certify the behavior profile. Other companies will spot check the behavior profiles for accuracy.

Insurance incentives will include reduced or waived co-pays, increased benefits, and lower rates. Some companies will partially or fully pay for health club memberships, healthy cooking classes, massage therapy, and other "healthy" incentives. These incentives act not only as a reward, but also help people learn and practice healthy behaviors.

Participants will feel the pressure to participate and perform in the area of health promotion as close to half of the insurers implement incentives such as lower co-pays and deductibles (Frank, 1999). Not participating and not improving one's wellness behaviors will start to be very expensive as these savings are withheld. Currently, some providers are uncertain about what they can and can't offer and still be in compliance with the Health Insurance Portability & Accountability Act of 1996 (HIPAA, *http://hcfa.gov/reg/hipaac.htm*). Disincentives are not allowed under HIPPA, rather this law requires that incentives must be positive, not punitive. The law prohibits any provider from applying a surcharge or additional premium charge to specific individuals based on a health status-related factor.

Will court rulings on this law disallow incentives for healthy behavior because they are not available to everyone and could thus be interpreted as a disincentive? We think not. It is our prediction that the legal pendulum will swing in favor of wellness. Incentives clearly designed to encourage a measurable improvement in any health behavior will be important in the future of successful health promotion programming.

Providers Will Partner to Offer Programs

Health care providers, insurance providers, and employers will partner to offer programs that provide win/win/win/win opportunities. Medical self-care is one such program. Health care providers win because their resources are used more appropriately. Insurance providers win because they can offer better insurance at a lower cost if it is not being abused. Employers win because the cost of health insurance for their employees does not continue to climb. Employees win because they get the treatment they need, when they need it, and save time and discomfort when they can treat problems on their own. Other future win/win/win/win programs might include programs to reduce antibiotic overuse, prenatal education, seatbelt use, breastfeeding in the workplace, and marriage strengthening programs.

Participants will benefit from the increase in quality and amount of health promotion programming. As the providers see that everyone wins, more funds will be allocated to health promotion.

CHANGE IN THE COMPOSITION OF WELLNESS PROGRAMS

Wellness programs in the twentieth century have been limited in the amount of technology involved and, for the most part, have been poorly marketed and underresearched. There have been a few standard topics covered, such as stress management, smoking cessation, weight control, and fitness. Their format has been mostly lecture and group discussion. The twenty-first century is going to bring radical changes in the composition of wellness programs. We are going to see a dramatic increase in the use of technology and significant growth in the areas of format, topics, marketing, and research as indicated in Figure 22-2 (Frank, 1999).

Technology Is King

Technology will permeate every corner of health promotion. The materials we use will no longer be predominantly printed. The methods of marketing, presentation, and research will all change to include the computer, e-mail, and the Internet. The health educator will have to know these technologies and be able to communicate well using them. Health care has become the sixth largest content area on the Internet.

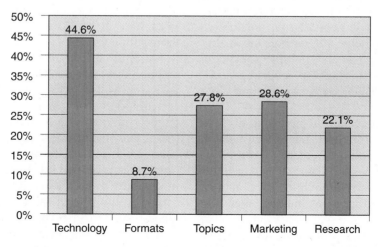

Figure 22-2 Predicted change in composition of wellness programs in the twenty-first century.
Source: E. Frank, Predict the Future Survey, 1999.

Two-thirds of all those going online seek out health information at least once, while one-third do so regularly (Menduno, 1999). The Internet has become an extremely important avenue for health information. Unfortunately, it can also be a source of misinformation. This has led to the development of a type of "Good Housekeeping Seal of Approval" on portals and their content called Health on the Net, or HON for short (Health on the Net Foundation, 1995). The HON code of conduct requires, amongst many other things, that any medical/health advice provided will only be given by trained and qualified professionals unless a clear statement is made that a piece of advice offered is from a nonmedically/health qualified individual or organization.

Participants will expect programs and materials to be available in high-technology formats. Information that is presented only in print will be viewed as being less valuable and attention worthy. Reports and materials will be customized at the participant's educational level, with tailored messages geared to the kinds of food the participant likes and the activities in which they are most likely to participate. They will be offered multiple alternatives from which to choose. Getting people to participate will be dependent on having all of these technologies incorporated into a company's program.

People will increasingly turn to the web for a sense of community, not just information. They will participate in programs via the Internet in a chat room type format. Some sessions will have a group facilitator, and others will be self-help-style with group members facilitating the chat. In self-help-type groups, individuals will be responsible for reporting their progress to the group leader via e-mail or other electronic communication.

Participants will record their own version of their medical history on the Internet. This history will be referenced during office and emergency room visits and will supplement the verbal history typically given at such visits. It will contain information about family history, past illnesses and surgeries, allergies, wellness activities, personal goals, and self-evaluation.

Patients will get health promotion information from their health care provider from the provider's home page. After a visit to the doctor, a patient may stop in the waiting room or go online at home to pull up and print diet, exercise, medication, or presurgery information. Test results will be e-mailed or made available in a password-protected format on the provider's home page. Treatment instructions based on test results will be provided in this way as well.

People will communicate their progress on health improvement goals with their medical providers and their worksite health promotion program via e-mail or by updating their progress record via the Internet. Both medical and worksite providers will check these records periodically and provide feedback.

Program materials will include more interactive CD-ROMs. The same interactive programs will be available on their employer's home page and through links to the home pages of other providers. This content will be more highly trusted than the content of the Internet-at-large because the employer will have checked the sources before selecting the content to provide. Health risk appraisal and other interactive programs will be provided on the employer's home page for the employee to use from their workstation, break room, or home.

Drug and equipment companies will provide more educational material on the Internet. This material will not be sales-oriented and thus may be hard to identify as coming from a drug or equipment company. If the material is completely generic, employers may agree to use such material on their home page and in their programs. But beware, the sales message will probably still be there, just in a more subtle form.

Each individual's biochemical uniqueness will be mapped out in detail. This information will be used to design wellness programs that are customized to accommodate not just diverse cultural, racial, and ethnic differences, but diversity at the individual level. This biochemical uniqueness could also be used in health risk appraisals (HRAs), where presently an epidemiological model is used. Currently individuals are given results that come from a comparison of their health behaviors, histories, and blood results to others in the population with similar characteristics. We believe that with new tools and measurements, such as genetic mapping, enhanced biochemical testing, and better methods of evaluating the data, we may be able to accurately predict what a person will die of and when. This prediction would also include a list of healthy changes that the person could make and exactly what impact they would have on his or her health. If individuals knew definitely what the future held for them regarding their health and longevity, rather than just the probabilities, they would be much more likely to participate in health promotion programs and change their unhealthy behaviors. These predictions, of course, only would hold true if the person were not killed prematurely in some form of accident.

Technology will bring us a variety of other interesting advances, including some of the following:

- at-home testing for everything from AIDS, arteriosclerosis, cancer, and diabetes, to heart disease, multiple sclerosis, and stroke
- 3-D virtual reality sound machines for stress management
- virtual reality to allow people to experience how they would feel during and after various types of medical procedures
- virtual reality to help people overcome phobias
- improved electronic displays and technology for exercise equipment
- smart shoes to take the stress out of walking, running, and jumping (Sensors measure the pressure produced by the wearer. Collected data is sent to a microchip embedded in the sole. The data is analyzed and an adjustment made in the support the shoe provides as a result of the opening and closing of valves inserted beneath the sensors.)
- computers and wireless technology to help patients remember to take their medications
- transcranial stimulation to treat addictive behaviors (such as smoking, alcohol, and drug abuse) and for pain management
- smart cards to show what an individual recently ate and what should be eaten for proper nutrition at the next meal
- exercise machines that automatically adjust the seat height; change the weight and/or resistance; display a suggested workout regimen; and automatically adjust weight, speed, incline, or tension to keep the user in the target heart range
- genetic screening and gene mapping to eliminate certain disorders

- new types of surgeries
- more organ and body part transplants
- the ability to identify predisposition toward more diseases and the resultant ability to begin intervention much earlier
- more genetic and recombinant DNA interventions to repair weaknesses in the individual's genome
- insulin spray rather than shots
- a vaccine for cocaine addiction
- a new generation of break-through drugs to transform the treatment of pain, offering unprecedented relief to people with arthritis, cancer, migraines, and back pain
- a parasite-containing pill to aid in weight control by helping consume the food eaten

Technology will also give us more and different nutritional supplements and engineered foods. These products will be better researched and contain more real food. "Organically grown" will be replaced by "chemically enhanced production." These products will offer more real benefit to the consumer. Because of the increased research and the proven benefit, doctors, dietitians, and health educators will endorse this new breed of wellness products that will help aging Baby Boomers look and feel younger by helping them maintain good health as they make their trek "over the hill."

Case Study: Celebration Health

In Celebration, Florida—Walt Disney Companies' "community of tomorrow"—neighbors tell each other jokes via e-mail, view calendars of events electronically, send notes to their children's teachers, and view their health records over a city-wide intranet.

Celebration Health (Cross, 1997), a 60-acre health campus, is one of the cornerstones of Celebration, Disney's planned city in central Florida. Residents have unprecedented communication with health professionals. For example, after an appointment with a physician, a patient can use their home computer to view billing and other information about their visit. They are able to type in notes on their reaction to a treatment and renew a prescription. They can send messages to their physician and request health information from an electronic library. The Celebration

Health clinic also has computers in every exam room, a full-scale computer-based patient records system, and the ability to move X-rays and other large health data files over a local area network that uses asynchronous transfer mode technology.

"Celebration Health is a living laboratory, so it has forced us to have some foresight and provide technologies that can be utilized today as well as position us for the future," says Frederick L. Balusha, Vice President of Management Information Systems at Florida Hospital, which operates Celebration Health.

Florida Hospital is working with several information technology vendors, including Columbia, SC, -based HealthMagic, which developed a program called HealthCompass to enable consumers to read and report personal medical information over intranets and the Internet. Some day hospitals and emergency rooms around the world may be able to access this information, with the patient's permission, to secure lifesaving information. On a less dramatic note, the corporate health promotion director may send a progress report to the employee's physician using the same program.

Program Formats Expand

Blended programs will increase in popularity. One or two group meetings interspersed with periods of self-help activities that are supported by periodic health educator contact will be more popular. A program with more than four class sessions will be unheard of. The savvy health educator will plan more, shorter programs so that people can work participation into their schedule.

Health education programs will be made into computer games for children and adults. Learning is more likely with repetition, and repetition is more likely to occur if the learner is having fun. Computer games will be designed specifically to teach concepts important to health and wellness, without being as obvious as the current educational games. The bullets will be donuts, the car will spin out and crash after hitting a patch of saturated fat, and the dying player will be brought back to life with energizer veggies. The action will be fast paced, and the graphics and sound effects equal to the most popular computer games on the market.

Health education lending libraries for books, videos, games, etc. will be available in more workplaces and provider offices. Use of these materials will be encouraged through a wellness "bucks" incentive program. Each book, video, or game will come with a quiz for the employee to complete and return for incentive credits. These wellness "bucks," which are especially important in programs that require independent action on the part of the employee, will be used to purchase incentives.

The team approach will be used to motivate people to participate and succeed. Employees will earn wellness "bucks" for bringing more members on to the team. Departments and department managers with the best participation rates will win valuable incentives.

Topic Explosion Occurs

Health promotion topics of the past 30 years focused on the major risk factors of smoking, obesity, hypertension, high cholesterol, stress, and lack of exercise. Other topics were covered but to a much lesser degree. The topic balance within most health promotion programs was like a pyramid, with the base being frequently offered topics like smoking cessation, weight control, and stress management. The tip of the pyramid was occupied by the infrequently offered topics often grouped under the title "alternative health." The levels in between were occupied by topics such as nutrition, humor, self-esteem, mental health, and self-care (see Figure 22-3).

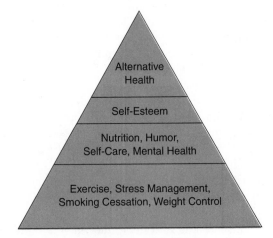

Figure 22-3 Twentieth century wellness topics.

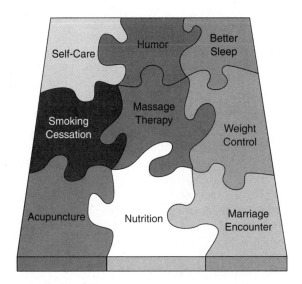

Figure 22-4 Twenty-first century wellness topics.

The twenty-first century is going to witness a topic explosion. It will be just as commonplace to see a program on nurturing a healthy marriage as it will be to see a smoking cessation program. Breastfeeding stations will be as common as blood pressure monitoring stations. Virtual reality centers will be as well equipped as the fitness center. The topics of the twenty-first century will be like the pieces of a puzzle, none more important than the other in the construction of an employee wellness program (see Figure 22-4).

Studies such as the one conducted at Johns Hopkins University School of Medicine (Thomas, Krush, Brown, Shaffer, & Duszynski, 1982) are fueling this topic explosion. The Johns Hopkins study indicates that healthy adults appear to possess the following:

- Positive relationships with their parents during childhood
- Strong self-esteem
- An optimistic outlook
- Relative lack of depression
- A marked ability to cope with stress

All five are psychological characteristics, and all but the first can be addressed in worksite health promotion programs. Many corporations are already offering stress management programs. The future promises continued emphasis on stress management and an increased emphasis on programs addressing self-esteem, depression, attitude, and optimistic outlook.

Mental health issues are increasingly being treated in a seminar/training atmosphere rather than in a one-on-one psychotherapy setting. Currently assertiveness training, stress management, and self-esteem enhancement are being successfully taught in this manner. In the future you will see other mental health issues (such as depression, relationship disorders, obsessive/compulsive behaviors, fears and phobias, and anorexia nervosa) being treated in a seminar/training approach. Health care expenditures were 46% higher for employees reporting high stress levels and 70% higher for employees with depression or anxiety (Goetzel, Anderson, Whitmer, Ozminkowski, Dunn, Wasserman, et al., 1998). Because of the high cost to business of these mental health issues, corporate health promotion is going to receive the mandate to address them at the worksite.

Two studies (Wickrama, Conger, & Lorenz, 1995; Wickrama, Lorenz, Conger, Matthews, & Elder, 1997) at Iowa State University demonstrated how important a happy marriage is to employee health, and conversely, how important job satisfaction is to a happy marriage. Among their findings:

- The connection between marriage and well-being holds only when the marriage is happy.
- Couples whose marriages got better over the course of the study also reported improvements in their health.
- The spouses whose relationships lost their luster got sick more often, more severely, or both.
- The happily married employees are more involved in better physical health behaviors and have better mental health.
- If individuals have better marriages, they are involved in better mental health behaviors.

In another study (Bergmann, Grahn, Hannaford, & Wenner, 1993), it was found that better working conditions (e.g., a shorter commute, lower work demands, work flexibility, less intensive hours, work autonomy), overflow to the family and contribute to a happy marriage. The worksite health promotion team will be involved in recommending and supporting policies that improve working conditions because of their role in marital and mental health.

Corporate health educators will address the importance of a healthy sex life. Employees without sex partners will be given referrals to clinics that offer safe sex via virtual reality. Employees who travel in their work will be provided electronic connections with their distant partners. Social issues are sure to occur as a result of robotic sexual partners, or sexbots. There will be concern that they will replace real people rather than act as a temporary substitute. Some people will become addicts. While you probably won't see these technologies in the break rooms of corporate America, you will find corporate health educators making referrals to such services.

More focus will be placed on topics giving short-term results. These are often programs that work to change less complex (easier to change) behaviors. Companies will continue to be interested in offering lifestyle-change programs, but a smaller proportion of the wellness dollar will be spent on those programs. With employee turnover on the rise, companies are not as interested in long-term results. Health promotion managers will be expected to show results at the end of one or two years. Some areas currently showing good short-term results include hand washing, seatbelt usage, self-care, wise health consumerism, prenatal care, and disability management. A future program likely to offer good short-term results would be an ergonomic program to prevent carpal tunnel syndrome that teaches voice control of the computer. A future technology that should offer quick results is a smart chair that will give you feedback on proper posture to reduce back pain. These programs will also be popular because most people are more motivated by quicker, easier results.

Topics will be dictated by high cost ICD9 (International Classification of Disease, 9th revision) codes. Health promotion managers will receive mandates of which diseases should be the focus of their major efforts and funds. Employee preference will carry less weight than it has in the past, as companies find it easier to track actual savings.

Marketing Intensifies

We have learned from Madison Avenue that traditional marketing approaches are limited in who they reach. This has led to the use of micro- or guerilla marketing, which can reach narrowly targeted groups of people. This form of marketing makes use of special events to promote programs and activities such as health fairs, fitness events, and stop-by-educational displays. You may already be familiar with focused advertising on home videos or in movie theaters. In supermarkets, focused advertising takes the form of a computerized shopping cart. This shopping cart can provide brand advertising at the moment the shopper is in front of the appropriate shelf. A coupon dispenser on the shelf spits out a discount coupon as the cart describes the benefits of the product. The more novel and targeted the approach is in reaching employees, the greater the participation in wellness programs will be.

Advertising will be more focused. It will be designed to appeal to people with specific individual characteristics. Manufacturers of automobiles with large trunks will design ads to appeal to golfers, large families, and car pool parents. They will show us their product doing what we need done, whether it be carrying four sets of golf clubs, a dozen bags of groceries, or sports equipment for five soccer players. Readiness to change is one of the individual characteristics that will be targeted in marketing for health promotion. The ads geared toward precontemplaters will be different than the ads geared toward those who are in the action stage. Targeted marketing will help the health educator get the participants that the program is most likely to help.

Most employers have sophisticated marketing departments. Those resources will be made available to the health promotion department to advance the marketing of wellness to employees. Businesses have learned that the marketing department pays for itself by increasing the sales of whatever the business sells. In the twenty-first century, businesses are going to realize that if they want to sell the wellness lifestyle to their employees, they are going to have to dedicate resources to the marketing effort.

Proving Cost Savings Increases in Importance

Evaluation of programs will continue to increase in importance, as proving the savings resulting from health promotion programming becomes more important. All of the feel-good reasons for offering health promotion programs will continue to be seen as benefits by companies, but only cost savings will cause companies to continue to offer such programming.

How many people participate will still be important, but what long-term changes they make and the savings that are incurred will increase in importance. Employee change will be monitored through self-report as well as through monitoring in the workplace. Where possible, claims data will be used to measure change and progress towards goals.

Outcome measures will broaden in scope to supplement research that proves cost savings. Health promotion departments will measure positive healthy behavior changes. Sales of healthy food from the cafeteria, generic drug selection by employees, and seatbelt utilization upon entering and exiting the employee parking area will be measured, and improvements over time will be used to demonstrate the positive impact of the corporate health promotion activities.

Cost savings will be measured by reductions in costs related to targeted ICD9 codes. It will become standard practice for health insurance companies to assist employers in gathering data on claims. Employees will be more involved in understanding the impact their health behaviors have on costs.

TOPICS OF SPECIAL INTEREST

Medical Self-Care

Medical self-care exploded as a health promotion program in the last decade of the twentieth century. Suddenly we had a program with very good short-term results. Now the health promotion department could show that it had a measurable impact on the bottom line. Medical self-care brought life back to health promotion in corporate America.

Medical self-care consists of many elements, some much more important than others. The backbone of every good medical self-care program is a book or booklet that guides a person through a process of assessing their problem and directs them to an appropriate level of care, including self-care instructions for those problems that do not require professional intervention. Medical self-care may also include a nurse call service, a computer and/or Internet component, and group sessions for instruction and practice.

Medical self-care will continue to increase in popularity as the research continues to show significant financial savings. While it may seem to many that it must have reached its peak by now, it has not. Many more companies will offer medical self-care programs, and the current programs will broaden their scope.

Self-care information will be given out by an increasing number of employers and insurance providers. Self-care information will be available at virtually every work place, in every conceivable format. Employee newsletters will provide self-care tips that are pertinent to the season and/or activities currently occurring at work. Supervisors will be instructed to bring up self-care at staff meetings and in their communications with their subordinates. Self-care information will literally permeate most organizations.

Self-care information will be available in every home as well. Every home will have a self-care book or two. If technology is king, the printed word is still queen. Nothing will replace a book. Written information has withstood the test of time. It will still be important in twenty-first century wellness.

It is our prediction that the nurse call line aspect of medical self-care will peak in the first few years of the twenty-first century and then decline in popularity. All homes will have at least one, in many cases more than one, medical self-care guide publication. These publications will offer Internet resources for additional information. The Internet resources will provide video and audio clips that show and describe signs and symptoms. At the same time that the information available to the consumer grows, the consumers' concern over being a primary care provider to themselves and their families will shrink. With increasing education and resources available at work and a self-care publication in every home, the need to call for additional clarification will be almost eliminated for problems that can be self-treated. The reduced role of answering phone questions will revert back to the medical provider and his or her staff.

Alternative Health

Alternative therapies will no longer be alternative, but instead will be offered alongside allopathic remedies. Integrative therapy is the combination of traditional and alternative methods. Wellness professionals will increasingly be required to work with concepts such as energy medicine, metaphysical concepts, intuitive healing, and changes in consciousness. The things that really make most people sick are a result of how we have chosen to view life and the human experience. Things that get labeled as quackery are often the very future of our work. Research suggests that as many as 83 million Americans already use alternative medicine (Eisenberg, Davis, Ettner, Appel, Wilkey, Van Rompay, & Kessler, 1998). With this many Americans looking to alternative medicine, we are sure to see more of it in our worksite health promotion programs.

Non-conventional medical treatments including acupuncture, chiropractic, homeopathy, massage body work, and dietary therapies will be included in the educational materials that health educator's use. Employees will be encouraged to explore these options with their providers. In most cases, medical coverage will pay for what we currently classify as nonconventional treatments.

Guided Self-Help Wellness Programs Grow

Phone, fax, and e-mail contact with participants will overtake personal contact with a health educator. The corporate health educator will be available in the chat room rather than in the conference room. Participants will have more contact with their health educator but less of it will be face-to-face. Many factors will lead to the increase in popularity of the guided self-help program.

The American workforce is becoming more dispersed. This happens as a result of mergers and acquisitions. It also has occurred as a result of the technologies that make working at home or in the car not only possible but practical. We need self-help programs so that employees who work in remote sites can access high-quality health promotion programs.

We feel like we live in a time-deprived society. We have so many leisure time options that it seems like work gets in the way of what we want to do. Americans are working roughly the same number of hours per week now as they were 50 years ago, but they feel like they are working more (Kacapyr, 1998). People study time management, hoping that if they are more efficient in doing what they must do, that they will have more time to do what they want to do. We try to eat, drink, sleep, and work fast in order to accomplish all we wish to do during the course of a day. This limits the amount of time people are willing to spend on activities designed to maintaining good health. Thus, it becomes advantageous for us to educate people in shorter periods of time and/or at the times that are most convenient.

Employees will sign up at work, or from their remote worksite, to participate in self-help health promotion programs. They will receive their materials at the health educator's office at the worksite, by mail, or download them from the corporate intranet or Internet site. They will be contacted by the health educator on a predetermined schedule to review program concepts, application of the program in the employee's life, and behavior change progress. Likewise, the employees will contact the health educator with periodic questions, concerns, and updates on their progress in using techniques and changing behaviors.

Companies will provide self-help health promotion information at employee workstations and in community areas such as the fitness center, break rooms, and cafeterias. This information will be in the form of educational pieces that can be printed out, interactive programs, and prescreened websites that can be accessed.

Participating in self-help programs will be rewarded with incentives. As discussed earlier in the Program Formats Expand section, employees will receive wellness "bucks" for program completion. Most programs will also offer "bucks" for incremental behavior changes and reporting in with the health educator. Wellness "bucks" will be cashed in for incentive items from the company store or for paying the employee portion of health insurance.

Case Study: United Auto Workers and Ford Motor Company

In the mid 1980s UAW/Ford offered smoking cessation, weight reduction, stress management, and other traditional wellness programs (Powell, 1993). Each plant was responsible for selecting a vendor from a list of approved vendors to provide the programs. For several years participation in group sessions was excellent, but toward the end of the 1980s it started to decline. Hoping to find a way to continue to reach employees with these programs, they decided to offer the same topics in self-help versions.

The company and union together selected a self-help smoking cessation program. It contained the same materials as a group program and an additional cassette tape of the instructor explaining the use of the materials. Employees could request the kit by faxing or mailing a request form or by calling a toll-free number. Since its implementation in 1989, over 9,000 UAW/Ford employees have participated in the self-help smoking cessation program, and 22% of those contacted 12 months afterward have quit smoking.

In 1995 UAW/Ford began offering a self-help program for employees who wanted to lose weight. Along with the self-help kit, the employees received phone calls over a six-month period to encourage them and answer any questions they may have had. Nearly 2000 employees have participated in that program, and 13% of those who could be contacted have lost weight.

Targeting High-Cost Diseases and High-Cost Drugs

Education will be targeted toward high-cost diseases as tracked by the ICD9 codes that doctor's record when providing services. Insurance companies will provide health educators with information on the claims costs associated with particular ICD9 codes. Programs will be planned and offered that specifically address the costliest diseases of the particular employee population.

Insurance companies will also provide health educators with information on the drug costs of their employee population. Programs encouraging generic drug substitution will be offered and incentives given to employees who request generic substitutions. Employees will not have to pay copayments if they request a generic substitution.

Programs targeting the high-cost diseases and drugs will be increasingly common as health educators start to receive performance incentives based on how well they lower the health care costs of the corporation. Health educators who ignore the significance of the bottom line may find themselves out of a job. Normally only executives have performance clauses in their contracts. It is our prediction these clauses will become commonplace for health educators as well.

Comprehensive Corporate Wellness Programs Grow

Comprehensive corporate wellness programs contain many of the elements that have already been reviewed in earlier sections. They will be mentioned again briefly as elements of a comprehensive program. In addition, this section will cover some characteristics that are unique to the most comprehensive corporate health education programs.

Health education will be available around the clock at these workplaces. It will include many of the technologies discussed earlier, such as videotaped programs, interactive CD programs, intranet and Internet programs, and some stop-by and short group programs. What is unique is that this programming will be offered at all hours of the day and night.

High-risk follow-up will become more important. High-risk employees will be invited back for continued screening and education related to their risks. Health educators will work proactively with these employees to help them set realistic goals and monitor their progress toward these goals. Participation will be tracked for all employees, and those who lower their risk will receive substantial incentives.

Improvements in risk levels will be tracked. At companies that offer adequate financial and organizational support to run a comprehensive wellness program, health educator performance will be evaluated by how well they help employees lower their risks. Innovation and motivation will be required to be a successful health educator.

Management support will increase as cost savings are more frequently demonstrated. The companies that have been saying "prove it to me before I budget the money" will see that it has been proven so many times that they can't afford *not* to offer a comprehensive program. This increase in management support, and the budget money that comes with it, will expand the role of the health educator in corporations. Health promotion will be a staffed department, with a mission, a budget, and the bottom line to answer to.

Case Study: UAW and DaimlerChrysler Corporation

From 1986 to 1998 DaimlerChrysler Corporation worked in conjunction with the UAW to implement a comprehensive on-site health promotion program at all 34 of their sites in North America that employ 500 or more workers (Duff, 1999). The company, Chrysler Corporation at that time, was looking for ways to save money; and, acting on the belief that keeping employees healthy would save money, they started the wheels rolling. The program is also offered remotely to employees at the smaller sites. Sites that can accommodate it also have a fitness center.

The UAW/DaimlerChrysler National Wellness Program is confidential and voluntary. Outside vendors provide the staff and programming elements. DaimlerChrysler, in cooperation with the UAW, provide the guidelines, corporate atmosphere, and oversight that ensure the program will be successful. Employees are offered a yearly health risk appraisal and blood screening, with confidential report. High-risk employees are invited back to be rescreened every six months. Risk reduction programs are offered year-round by highly trained staff who know the employees and can customize the topics and the approach to meet their needs.

Employees earn incentive "bucks" for participation and can save them up to purchase incentives ranging in value from less than a dollar up to just under $25. The employees find the incentive aspect of the program to be fun and rewarding. T-shirts and other wellness program apparel are worn proudly by employee participants.

Chrysler Corporation made a very large commitment to health promotion at a time when the research to support such a comprehensive program didn't exist. Now that research is showing the benefit, the comprehensive corporate wellness program is sure to spread.

CONCLUSION

The future of health promotion is seen today in some of the premier programs around the country. We won't be reinventing health promotion in the twenty-first century, just refining what we already have. To expect and receive corporate support in the twenty-first century, health promotion programs must be:

- well-promoted
- interesting
- educational
- motivating
- fun
- supported by those important to the participant
- providing long-term follow-up

In short, they must work! And, they must be researched to prove that they work. It isn't enough to be high-tech, new, and different. While these traits may help to catch the participant's attention, they do not define a successful program. Look for substance. Look for a good track record. Remember the past. It is your best guide to a successful future.

References

American Cancer Society. (1998). Cancer facts & figures. [On-line]. Available: http://www.lungusa.org

Bergmann, T., Grahn, J., Hannaford, W., & Wenner, J. (1993). Relationship of family satisfaction to employee job satisfaction. *Journal of Nursing Administration, 23,* 34.

Centers for Disease Control & Prevention. (1999). *National center for HIV, STD, and TB prevention web site.* [On-line]. Available: http://www.cdc.gov/nchstp/hiv_aids/pubs/faq/faq13.html

Cross, M. A. (1997). *Disney's city of the future.* [On-line]. Available: http://www.health-compass.com/press3.html

Duff, S. (1999). Winning hunch: DaimlerChrysler's award-winning wellness program started on instinct. *Employee Benefit News, 13,* 1, 46.

Eisenberg, D., Davis, R., Ettner, S., Appell, S., Wilkey, S., Van Rompay, M., & Kessler, R. (1998). Trends in alternative medicine use in the United States, 1990–1997: Results of a follow-up national survey. *Journal of the American Medical Association, 280,* 1569–1575.

Frank, E. (1999, July). *Predict the future survey.* Unpublished research survey conducted at the National Wellness Institute Conference, Stevens Point, WI.

Goetzel, R. Z., Anderson, D., Whitmer, W., Ozminkowski, R., Dunn, R., Wasserman, J., & the Health Enhancement Research Organization (HERO) Research Committee (1998). The relationship between modifiable health risks and health care expenditures: An analysis of the multi-employer HERO health risk and cost database. *Journal of Occupational and Environmental Medicine, 40,* 843–854.

Health on the Net Foundation (HON). [On-line]. Established 9/7/95. Available: http://www.hon.ch/HONcode/conduct.html

Heini, A. F., & Weinsier, R. L. (1997). Divergent trends in obesity and fat intake patterns: The American paradox. *American Journal of Medicine, 102,* 259–264.

Insurance Institute for Highway Safety. (1999, August). *Child restraint/belt laws as of August 1999.* [On-Line]. Available: http://www.highwaysafety.org

Kacapyr, E. (1998). Hours at work—the long view. [On-line]. Available: http://www.demographics.com

Larkin, H. (1998). *Count on quality.* [On-line]. Available: http://www.hhnmag.com

Menduno, M. (1999, March). Net profits. *Hospitals & Health Networks.* [Magazine] 44–50.

National Institute on Alcohol Abuse and Alcoholism. (1996). *Alcoholism: Getting the facts Booklet No. 96.* [On-line]. Available: http://www.nih.gov

Powell, D. R. (1993). A guided self-help smoking cessation intervention with white-collar and blue-collar employees. *American Journal of Health Promotion, 13,* 1, 46.

Thomas, C., Krush, A., Brown, C., Shaffer, J., & Duszynski, K. (1982). Cancer in families of former medical students followed to mid-life: Prevalence in relatives of subjects with and without major cancer. *John Hopkins Medicine, 151,* 193–202.

U.S. Department of Health and Human Services. (1996). *National household survey on drug abuse.* [On-line]. Available: http://www.whitehousedrugpolicy.gov/drugfact/drugtrends/table1.html

Wickrama, D. A., Lorenz, F. O., Conger, R. D., Matthews, L., & Elder, G. H., Jr. (1997). Linking occupational conditions to physical health through marital, social, and intrapersonal processes. *Journal of Health and Social Behavior, 38,* 363–375.

Wickrama, K. A. F., Conger, R. D., & Lorenz, F. O. (1995). Work, marriage, lifestyle, and changes in men's physical health. *Journal of Behavioral Medicine, 18*(2), 97–111.

INDEX